Manual of
Pathology of the Human Placenta

Rebecca N. Baergen, MD

New York Presbyterian Hospital—Weill Medical College of
Cornell University, New York, NY, USA

Manual of
Pathology of the
Human Placenta

Second Edition

Foreword by Kurt Benirschke, MD

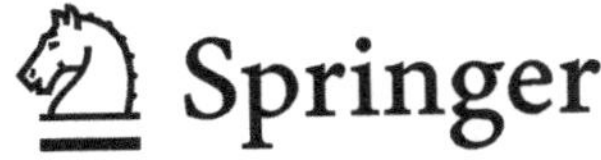 Springer

Rebecca N. Baergen, MD
New York Presbyterian Hospital—Weill
Medical College of Cornell University
New York, NY 10021
USA

ISBN 978-1-4419-7493-8   e-ISBN 978-1-4419-7494-5
DOI 10.1007/978-1-4419-7494-5
Springer New York Dordrecht Heidelberg London

© Springer Science+Business Media, LLC 2011
All rights reserved. This work may not be translated or copied in whole or in part without
the written permission of the publisher (Springer Science+Business Media, LLC, 233
Spring Street, New York, NY 10013, USA), except for brief excerpts in connection with
reviews or scholarly analysis. Use in connection with any form of information storage and
retrieval, electronic adaptation, computer software, or by similar or dissimilar methodology
now known or hereafter developed is forbidden.
The use in this publication of trade names, trademarks, service marks, and similar terms,
even if they are not identified as such, is not to be taken as an expression of opinion as to
whether or not they are subject to proprietary rights.
While the advice and information in this book are believed to be true and accurate at the
date of going to press, neither the authors nor the editors nor the publisher can accept any
legal responsibility for any errors or omissions that may be made. The publisher makes
no warranty, express or implied, with respect to the material contained herein.

Printed on acid-free paper

Springer is part of Springer Science+Business Media (www.springer.com)

To Steve

Foreword

Over the past 50 years, the human placenta has gradually become better understood so far as its function is concerned, and, simultaneously, pathologic features have been more clearly delineated. Some features are characteristic of certain maternal diseases, and others specify fetal conditions. But for some other features, while they are well described and their consequences are well characterized, their etiology has remained a mystery. Aspects of placental pathology leading to an understanding of perinatal problems have also been widely used in medicolegal disputes in recent years. When they adequately studied, these pathologic findings have often been useful in settling many difficult cases of perinatal mortality and of neonatal diseases, such as the cause of cerebral palsy. All of this has led to a more frequent demand for placental examination, even of "routine" deliveries, but certainly of all those leading to premature birth and of neonates that experience perinatal problems.

As the perinatal mortality has decreased substantially over the past decades, largely because of better prenatal care, modern sonographic studies, and the elimination of the common "hyaline membrane syndrome" of premature infants, attention has now been focused on understanding preeclampsia and the causes of prematurity, the major obstetric challenges remaining. But as some diseases have now become aspects of the historical past, new challenges are being created, in part through the advent of assisted reproductive technology (ART) and intracytoplasmic sperm injection (ICSI). The multiple gestations created by this technology have produced new challenges in our understanding placentation of multiples, especially the relatively common production of additional multiple offspring from the division of one or more of the transferred blastocysts. All of these features continue to make it mandatory that the detailed study of the placenta after delivery be continued.

The book before us is designed to assist the general pathologist, whose interests have usually been with neoplasms and other diseases, to get a handle on an organ that all too often is described as "mature placenta" when it reaches the pathologist's desk. Dr. Baergen endeavors and succeeds in presenting the essential features of placental pathology to the uninitiated pathologist; she carefully lays out what is a "must-observe" aspect of each of the placental structures, and how to assess the findings in the context of normal findings. The book is easily followed, directions and diagnostic features are clearly spelled out, and suggestions for their description in diagnostic terms are provided. The book does not endeavor to be encyclopedic, but it is well illustrated – an essential aspect for the morphologist – and the essential references are provided. No doubt, this book will be a welcomed addition to the shelves of the practicing pathologist in which to find answers to the major questions sought for care by the neonatologist, to provide answers to the obstetricians and the parents, and to serve as the basis for possible medicolegal questions of the future.

San Diego, CA   Kurt Benirschke

Preface to the First Edition

The primary objective of this book is to be a concise, practical manual of placental pathology. When I began studying placental pathology I was intimidated by its complex anatomy and pathology. Although Benirschke and Kaufmann's *Pathology of the Human Placenta* was, and is, a comprehensive text, I often wished for a more basic book that would be appropriate for the neophyte in placental pathology but based on this respected volume. I hope that this book will fulfill this goal. In an effort to be true to this ideal, Kurt Benirschke graciously agreed to review and comment on every chapter – a task for which I am profoundly grateful. Furthermore, in each chapter, there are references to the Fourth Edition of *Pathology of the Human Placenta* (PHP4), which direct the reader to the corresponding discussion and references in that book.

The book is designed to be a user-friendly, practical guide, and bench manual that can be used in the grossing room as well as at the microscope. The first section discusses the approach to the placental specimen. These chapters provide suggestions on what to do, as well as when and how to do it. In Chaps. 3 and 4, there are tables of gross and microscopic lesions, respectively, which give specific figure numbers where the lesions and associated disease processes are discussed and illustrated. Inclusion of figure numbers, I believe, make the text quite usable and give quick access to the remainder of the book. As it turned out, listing figure numbers rather than chapter or subject headings, was a labor-intensive process for me as well as for the editorial and production staff at Springer. Although every attempt has been made to ensure the accuracy of the figure numbers, errors may occur. If any are noted by the reader, it would be greatly appreciated if they were communicated to us.

The second section covers detailed development and normal histology of all parts of the placenta for those wanting to learn about specific areas of the placenta. Subsequent sections discuss placental lesions, disease processes related to the placenta, neoplasms, and trophoblastic lesions. The subjects discussed in these chapters are all referenced in the tables in Chaps. 3 and 4. The last section gives an overview of the legal implications of placental examination and discusses future directions. The last chapter has been kindly written by Kurt Benirschke. Finally, since the study of placental pathology is intimately associated with clinical history and has significant implications for neonatal and maternal health, an appendix is included which provides definitions and explanations of pertinent clinical and pathologic terms.

Specific features have been included throughout the book to enhance readability and usability. Bold type has been used to highlight important lesions, diseases, or concepts, while italic type has been used for features and definitions of bolded items. After discussion of each diagnostic entity, a subheading entitled "Suggestions for Examination and Report" includes key points in gross examination, sectioning, and diagnosis. Suggestions for comments that may be included in the surgical pathology report are included for problematic situations or when the diagnosis or diagnostic implications are unclear. Tables are included in many chapters to summarize pertinent information and to provide easy access to the differential diagnoses of various lesions. Attempts were made to create images of the highest quality, many of them in color. Original art was also created for line drawings to provide a uniform feel to the book.

It is my hope that this book will make examination of the placenta as enjoyable and rewarding for the reader as it has been for me.

New York, NY   Rebecca N. Baergen

Preface to the Second Edition

The primary objective of the first edition was to create a concise, practical manual of placental pathology; a basic book, appropriate for the neophyte in placental pathology based on the more comprehensive *Pathology of the Human Placenta*. I have been gratified to hear positive feedback from readers, and so I hope this goal has been fulfilled. I have attempted to stay true to that goal. As in the first edition, there are references to the *Pathology of the Human Placenta*, fifth edition (PHP5), that direct the reader to the corresponding discussion and references in that book. The use of bold and italic type and the inclusion of multiple summary tables have been retained, as has the "Suggestions for Examination and Report" for each diagnostic entity. This edition has been updated with more recent information from the literature, but a number of other changes have also been made. The first eight chapters have been reorganized and rewritten and follow, what I feel is, a more logical progression. The discussion of normal histology has been streamlined, as have the tables in Chaps. 3 and 4. The use of tables throughout the book continues to provide important summary information, but in this edition the tables have been duplicated in one convenient place in Appendix B for easy access. Finally, many new, high-quality color images have been added or have replaced previous black and white images, and color has been added to many of the line drawings.

New York, NY   Rebecca N. Baergen

Contents

Section IV   Abnormalities of the Placenta

Section V   Disease Processes and the Placenta

Section VI   Neoplasms and Gestational Trophoblast Disease

Section VII   Legal Considerations and New Directions

Section I

Approach to the Specimen

This section is concerned with the approach to gross and microscopic placental examination. The chapters provide a systematic "bench" approach to examination of first-, second-, and third-trimester specimens, which includes initial handling of the specimen, specific steps of the gross examination, sections to submit, special studies, fixation, and storage. The first chapter covers gross and microscopic evaluation of first-trimester abortion specimens. The second chapter covers second-trimester specimens and briefly discusses handling of dilatation and evacuation specimens in the setting of fetal anomalies. The third and fourth chapters cover the macroscopic and microscopic examination of the placenta, respectively. Both these chapters feature a series of tables that list pathologic features for each part of the placenta, that is, fetal membranes, umbilical cord, fetal surface, and so on. When the reader is confronted with a particular gross or microscopic finding, the tables at the end of each chapter provide possible diagnoses, instructions on special handling, and special studies and references to where in the text the lesions are discussed and illustrated. This arrangement enables the reader to diagnose even complex lesions quickly and efficiently.

Chapter 1

Evaluation of the First-Trimester Products of Conception

General Considerations

Early abortion specimens are one of the most common specimens submitted to pathology. They are quite varied in their composition, as they may consist of blood clot, decidua, fragmented villous tissue, and fetal parts in various combinations. There may be minimal tissue, a completely intact gestational sac, or anything in between. Evaluation of these specimens is enhanced by an understanding of the purpose of pathologic examination, and how it may be helpful to both the patient and the clinician. Goals of examination include:

- Documentation of **pregnancy**
- Documentation of an **intrauterine** pregnancy
- Documentation of suspected or unsuspected **anomalies**
- Confirmation of **gestational age**
- **Interval of retention** after embryonic or fetal death
- **Etiology** of pregnancy loss
- Exclusion of **gestational trophoblastic disease**

R.N. Baergen, *Manual of Pathology of the Human Placenta,*
DOI 10.1007/978-1-4419-7494-5_1, © Springer Science+Business Media, LLC 2011

Macroscopic Examination

Macroscopic examination of first-trimester products of conception is primarily concerned with the identification of **decidual tissue**, **villous tissue**, and **embryonic** or **fetal tissue**. Often the components are disrupted and intermixed, but each component should be identified and examined individually, if possible. It is convenient to examine the fetal tissues first, and, in this endeavor, several general questions should be addressed:

- Is there embryonic or fetal tissue present
- If present
  - Is the embryo or fetus intact and complete
  - Is the embryo or fetus macerated and if so, to what extent (Fig. 1.1)
  - Is the embryo or fetus the appropriate size for the stated gestational age? This is best accomplished by comparison of crown-rump length, foot length, or weight with standard tables (see Table 3.7 Chap. 3)
  - Does the embryo or fetus have grossly normal features, major growth disorganization, or focal defects such as cleft lip or spina bifida (Figs. 1.2 and 1.3)

Each of these points should be addressed in examination and then included in the gross description of the report. Detailed examination of fetal anomalies is beyond the scope of this text, and the reader is referred to the Selected References (see end of chapter) for several excellent monographs on the subject.

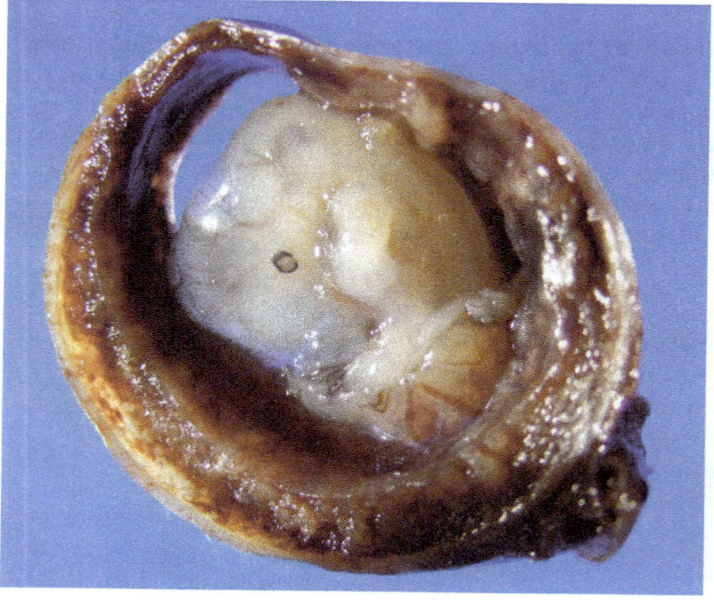

Figure 1.1. Intact gestational sac with embryo in an early spontaneous abortion. Note placental/villous tissue is present circumferentially around the embryo. Maceration is not present in this specimen.

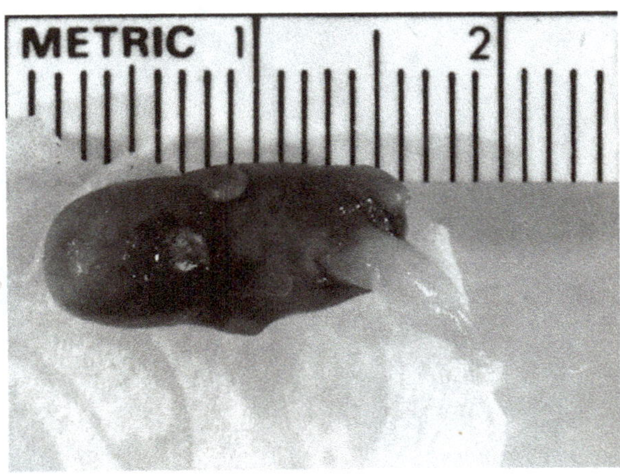

Figure 1.2. Spontaneous abortus at 9 weeks showing major growth disorganization and a cylindrical embryo. It was also small for the gestational age (expected crown rump length 2.5 cm).

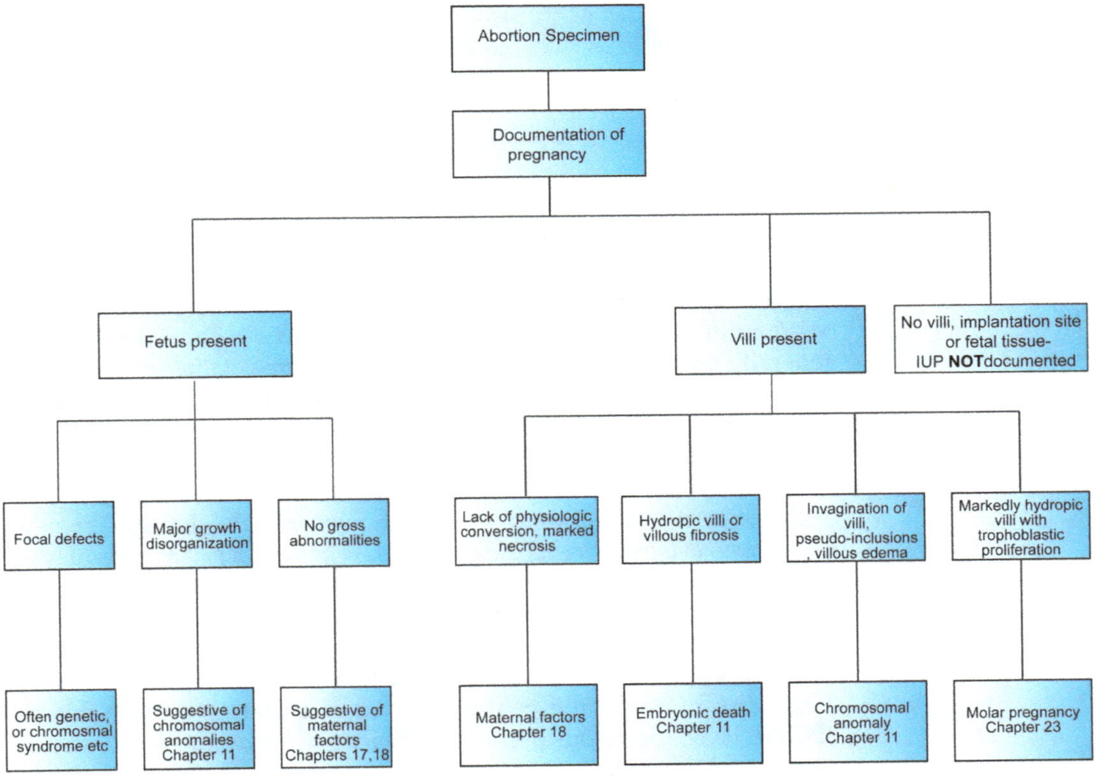

Figure 1.3. Etiologic significance of gross and microscopic findings in abortion specimens. IUP, intrauterine pregnancy.

The nonembryonic tissues are usually more abundant than the embryonic tissue in early pregnancies. **Decidual tissue** usually appears as *small, flattened sheets of tissue that are relatively smooth on one surface*

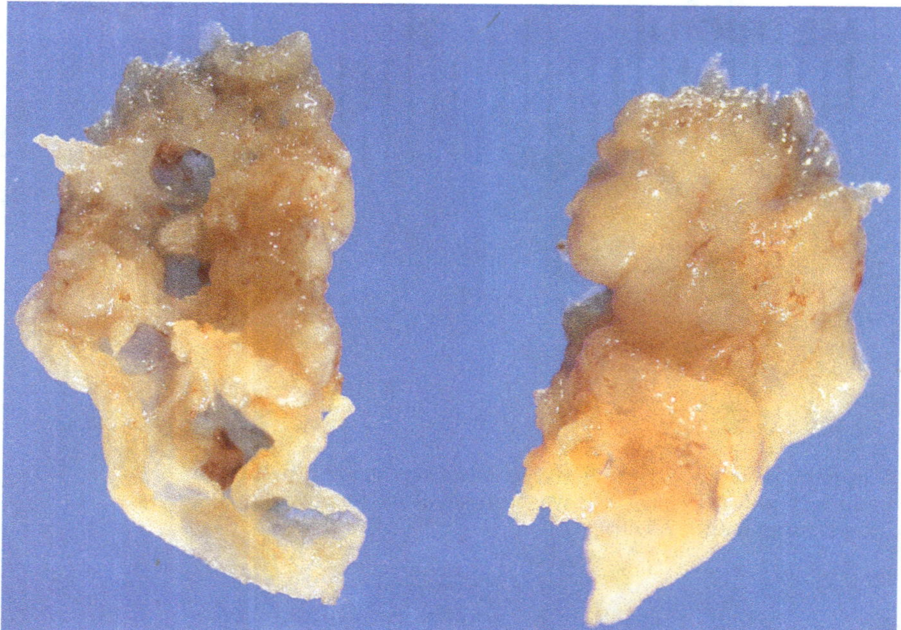

Figure 1.4. Fragment of decidual tissue. Note the membranous character with one smooth (*right*) and one granular (*left*) surface.

and granular or nodular on the opposite surface (Fig. 1.4). Grossly identifiable decidual tissue often contains the implantation site and may show important pathology. Therefore, contrary to the widely held belief that one should submit only villous tissue, some decidual should always be submitted for microscopic examination. Grossly, **chorionic villi** are generally *fine, soft and white, papillary fronds representative of their villous structure* (Fig. 1.5). Villous tissue is often attached to fragments of *shiny, delicate, and translucent* **fetal membranes** (Fig. 1.6). Both should be submitted for microscopic examination along with a fragment of umbilical cord if it can be identified. The blood clot that is often present usually does not contain diagnostic material; however, *if the clot is granular or firm, it may contain fragments of degenerated chorionic villi within.* This may be helpful when villous tissue is not easily identified on gross examination. In this case, several fragments of blood clot can be submitted in the hopes of identifying chorionic villi. In general, macroscopic examination of nonfetal tissue in early products of conception provides little diagnostic information except in the case of **gestational trophoblastic disease.** Here, the villous tissue shows *enlarged, hydropic vesicles* (see next section and Chap. 23).

Cytogenetics, Flow Cytometry, and Other Special Studies

In up to 50% of spontaneous abortions, chromosomal anomalies are present. Therefore, in spontaneous abortions, it is advantageous to send material for *cytogenetic analysis.* This may not be possible on every spontaneous abortion for financial or practical reasons. However, in

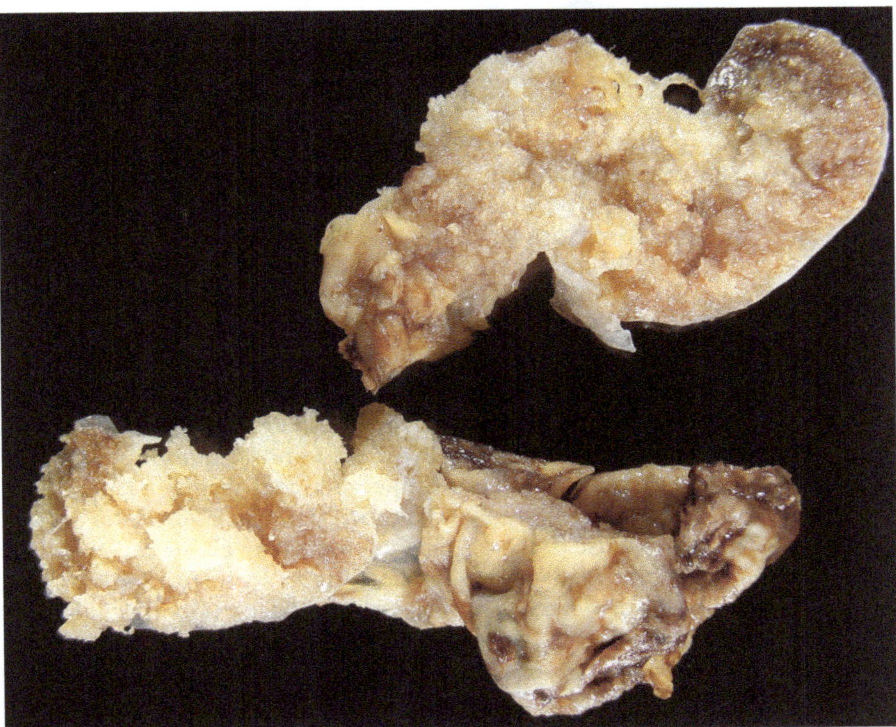

Figure 1.5. Fragment of villous tissue in early abortus. Note the fine, delicate papillary structures characteristic of early pregnancies. Some decidual tissue is also present on the *lower right*.

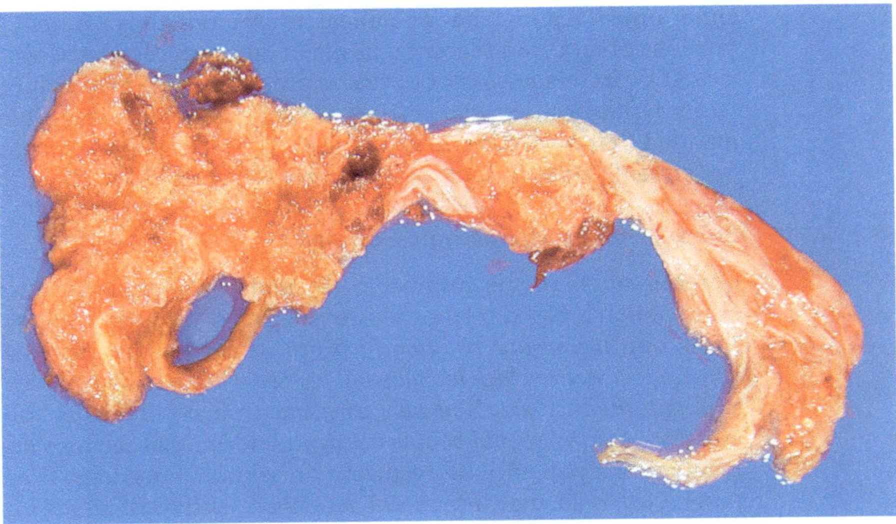

Figure 1.6. Translucent fetal membranes (at *right*) cover a portion of villous tissue.

the case of *recurrent or habitual abortion, cytogenetics should always be sent* as the incidence is much higher in these specimens. Some advocate sending only fetal tissue due to the presence of possible confined placental mosaicism (see Chap. 11) while others point out that fetal tissue may be macerated and so does not grow in culture. For these reasons, it is recommended that *fetal tissue be sent if it appears viable, otherwise villous tissue should be sent.* Although skin or connective tissue is often taken, skeletal muscle tends to grow better in culture. If resources allow, both tissues may be submitted separately for optimal results. Then, if the fetal tissue does not grow, the placental tissue may be used for analysis.

Grossly hydropic villi are usually not present except in the case of a partial or complete hydatidiform mole. Hydropic abortuses generally do not show the grossly cystic villi seen in molar pregnancies (see Fig. 23.1). If these are identified, the specimen may be *sent for flow cytometry* or prepared in such a way that flow cytometry can be done if necessary, as differentiation between a molar pregnancy and a hydropic abortus may be difficult on histology alone. Flow cytometry and immunohistochemical stains can often be done on paraffin-embedded fixed tissue (see Chap. 23 for discussion on differential diagnosis of moles). The testing available and the ease of use of the various methods to evaluate moles and abnormal conceptuses will vary from institution to institution, and familiarity with available resources can help direct the pathologist on how to prepare tissue in these circumstances.

Rarely, requests for molecular testing of fetal tissue are made to rule out specific diseases or conditions. In this situation, it is best to communicate directly with the laboratory that will be handling the test **prior** to receiving the specimen, if at all possible, since there may be specific handling requirements. Unfortunately, advance notice is not always given. Therefore, if one suspects a special test may be requested, due to either unusual anomalies or clinical information, it is prudent to freeze portions of fetal and placental tissue in liquid nitrogen and store at −70 to −80°C. In this way, tissue will be preserved and may be utilized for many types of molecular testing. If tissue is to be frozen, it is recommended that *connective tissue and tissue from a fetal organ such as liver be frozen, along with chorionic villi and a portion of chorionic plate.*

Submission of Microscopic Sections

Determination of the number of sections to submit for microscopic examination is based on the index of suspicion for underlying pathology. Thus, *in a therapeutic abortion in which no macroscopic abnormalities are noted, one cassette, which includes villous tissue and a small portion of decidua with implantation site, is usually adequate.* In a spontaneous abortion, *at least two cassettes should be submitted,* and additional sections are recommended in a patient with recurrent or habitual abortions. If an ectopic pregnancy is in the differential diagnosis, sufficient tissue should be submitted to ensure the diagnosis of an intrauterine pregnancy. If no chorionic villi are grossly identified, or when there is a small amount of tissue, the entire specimen should be submitted. If on initial microscopic examination, an intrauterine pregnancy cannot be documented, the remaining tissue, if any, should be submitted. Finally, if fetal anomalies are noted, sections should also be taken to optimize diagnosis of those lesions. In cases in which the embryo is small, submission of the entire embryo in a single cassette may be accomplished.

Microscopic Examination

Therapeutic or Induced Abortion

Therapeutic abortions are performed by dilatation and curettage, dilatation and evacuation, suction curettage, the use of prostaglandins (with or without the use of cervical laminaria), intraamniotic injection of hypertonic saline or urea solutions, and other means. The pathological findings in the aborted specimen differ to some degree for each procedure. For the pathologist, examination generally entails one or more of the goals stated in the beginning of this chapter. First and foremost is confirmation of an intrauterine pregnancy, which can be accomplished by identification of **chorionic villi, trophoblastic cells,** *or* **portions of implantation site**. The latter consists of *decidual tissue and vessels infiltrated by trophoblast and abundant fibrinoid* (Fig. 1.7). The presence of decidualized endometrium alone does **not** confirm **an intrauterine pregnancy** as this change is hormonally dependent and can be seen outside of pregnancy.

Rarely, a few chorionic villi or trophoblastic cells may be transported to the endometrial cavity from an ectopic pregnancy. Therefore, if only a few chorionic villi are present in the entire specimen and there is no implantation site, communication with the submitting physician is essential in determining if an ectopic pregnancy is likely. If it is, a comment in the report should indicate that rare trophoblastic elements or chorionic villi do not confirm an intrauterine pregnancy. On the contrary, *presence of an implantation site* is *confirmation of an intrauterine pregnancy.* The normal *physiologic conversion of decidual vessels* into uteroplacental vessels should be identified in every specimen (Fig. 1.7). Converted

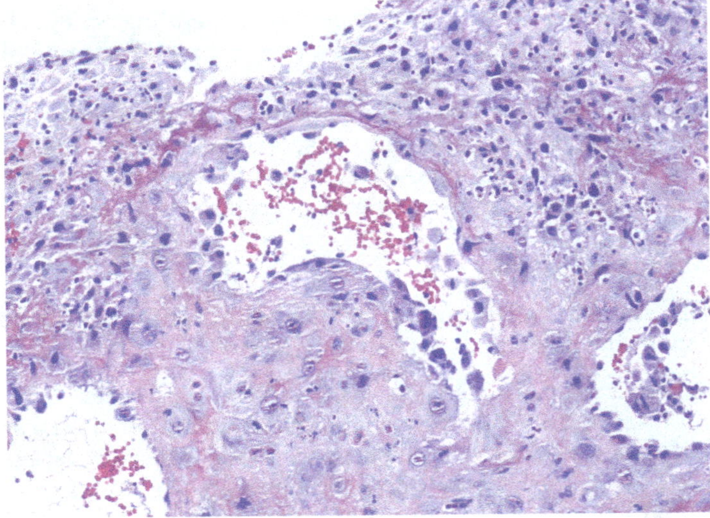

Figure 1.7. Curettings from a spontaneous abortion. Note the fibrinoid material admixed with large extravillous trophoblast. There is normal physiologic conversion of decidual vessels seen with infiltration by trophoblast, a large, irregular lumen, and thin vascular wall with fibrinoid. Despite the absence of chorionic villi and syncytiotrophoblast, this histologic picture suffices for the diagnosis of placental site and thus an intrauterine pregnancy. H&E ×260.

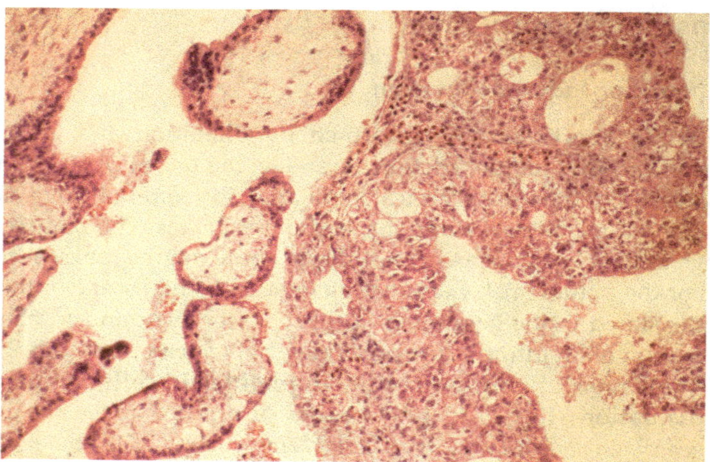

Figure 1.8. Yolk sac at 6 weeks gestation. Note the large sinusoids filled with erythropoietic cells. The tissue is rich in glycogen and occasionally endodermal epithelium may be seen within. H&E ×240.

vessels should have *large, irregular lumens and a thin wall composed primarily of fibrinoid and scattered extravillous trophoblast.* These findings are diagnostic of a normal implantation site. If an ectopic pregnancy is suspected, and microscopic sections do not show villi, implantation site, or trophoblastic cells, the entire specimen should be submitted for microscopic examination. Rarely, in early abortions, curettage is not successful in removing all products of conception, and, again, only a few villi may be present in the specimen. There have been unusual cases in which this occurred, the pregnancy continued undiscovered until abortion was no longer possible and there was subsequent legal action on the part of the patient. Therefore, depending on the clinical circumstances, it is prudent to suggest in a comment that retained or remaining products of conception may be present.

Occasionally the remnant of the **yolk sac** may be present in early abortion specimens (Fig. 1.8) and cause confusion with other structures. The yolk sac remnant has a lacy, reticular appearance with many glandular-like spaces and the presence of erythropoietic cells.

Spontaneous Abortions

The spontaneous abortion often arrives with various designations, which have clinical definitions:

- **Threatened** – uterine bleeding without cervical dilatation
- **Inevitable** – uterine bleeding with cervical dilatation or effacement
- **Incomplete** – all tissue (products of conception) has not yet passed
- **Missed** – intrauterine retention after embryonic or fetal death
- **Habitual** – three or more consecutive spontaneous abortions

The goals in examination of these specimens include the goals stated for an induced abortion, with the increased likelihood of pathologic findings. Special studies are more commonly requested. Unfortunately, pathologic changes that are present *are often more related to the timing of embryonic or fetal death rather than the etiology of the demise.* In previous embryonic death, the **chorionic villi** often show hydropic change and sclerosis, and because many villi are degenerating, there is often much *finely granular mineralization (calcification) along the trophoblastic basement membrane* (see Chap. 20 and Fig. 20.13). Hydropic change is more likely to be present with early embryonic death when the villi are not well vascularized, i.e., less than 6 weeks embryonic age, whereas sclerosis occurs more often when death occurs after this period.

The early abortion specimen may show abnormalities that suggest possible etiologies of the pregnancy failure, and this is illustrated in Fig. 1.3. Abnormalities of the implantation site associated with spontaneous abortions are most suggestive of maternal factors such as preeclampsia and other conditions of decreased uteroplacental perfusion (see Chap. 18). For example, small spiral arterioles with persistent muscle and small lumens in an area in which trophoblast is present are diagnostic of **lack of physiologic conversion**. In addition, *marked inflammation and necrosis* in the implantation are also abnormal findings. Caution must be used, however, as normally there is a mild chronic inflammatory infiltrate in the decidua and implantation site. Fetal anomalies are most suggestive of a genetic or chromosomal disorder as is irregularity of the villous contour, with or without trophoblastic pseudoinclusions or invaginations (see Chap. 11). Mild hydropic change in the villi will usually be seen with embryonic death, while markedly hydropic villi suggest a molar pregnancy (see Chap. 23). Massive chronic intervillositis is occasionally present in first-trimester specimens. This lesion is characterized by the presence of massive numbers of mononuclear cells, primarily histiocytes, in the intervillous space, and has been associated with pregnancy loss in all three trimesters (see Chap. 16). Other abnormalities that may occasionally be seen are subinvolution of the placental site (see Chap. 12), trophoblastic disease other than hydatidiform moles (see Chaps. 26 and 27), and infections (see Chap. 16). These pathologic processes are discussed in more detail in the respective chapters. It is important to remember that although examination of early pregnancy specimens may not give a definitive answer, it may direct additional testing of the mother, fetus, or placental tissue, thus enabling identification of the underlying etiology of the pregnancy loss.

Suggestions for Examination and Report

Diagnosis: If normal appearing chorionic villi are present along with gestational endometrium (decidua), implantation site and fetal tissue, a descriptive diagnosis including all components present is sufficient. An example is "immature chorionic villi, gestational endometrium and implantation site." Use of the term "products of conception" is NOT recommended because this is really a clinical term and does not have the specificity of a descriptive diagnosis. If villi and/or implantation site show pathologic changes, those specific lesions should be specified (see above).

(continued)

Suggestions for Examination and Report (continued)

Comment: Certain circumstances deserve an additional comment. If villi and implantation site are not identified, then a comment such as "No chorionic villi, trophoblastic cells or implantation site are identified, and therefore an intrauterine pregnancy cannot be confirmed. Clinical correlation is suggested." is warranted. If only a few villi are present and there is no implantation site, this information should be included in the diagnosis and a comment made such as "As only rare villi are present, the possibility of retained products of conception should be considered." Depending on the clinical history, a comment about ectopic pregnancy not being entirely excluded can also be made. It is prudent to call the clinician in these cases as significant and important clinical history that may explain the findings may be lacking on the pathology requisition. Finally, if the clinical history specifically indicates that an ectopic pregnancy was in the differential diagnosis, a comment should be made as to whether this can or cannot be ruled out.

Selected References

PHP5, pages 762–796 (Abortions).

Baldwin VJ, Kalousek DK, Dimmick JE, Applegarth DA, Hardwic DF. Diagnostic pathologic investigation of the malformed conceptus. Perspect Pediatr Pathol 1982;7:65–108.

Dimmick JE, Kalousek DK (eds). Developmental pathology of the embryo and fetus. Philadelphia: JB Lippincott, 1992.

Fox H. Histological classification of tissue from spontaneous abortions: a valueless exercise? Histopathology 1993;22:599–600.

Kalousek DK. Pathology of the abortion. Chromosomal and genetic correlations. Monogr Pathol 1991;33:228–256.

Kalousek DK, Pantzar T, Tsai M, Paradice B. Early spontaneous abortion: morphologic and karyotypic findings in 3912 cases. Birth Defects 1993;29:53–61.

Kaplan CK. Embryonic pathology of the placenta. In: Lewis SH, Perrin E, eds. Pathology of the placenta. New York: Churchill Livingstone, 1999:89–106.

Keeling JW. Fetal pathology. Edinburgh: Churchill Livingstone, 1994.

Szulman AE. Examination of the early conceptus. Arch Pathol Lab Med 1991;115:696–700.

Chapter 2

Evaluation of the Second-Trimester Products of Conception

General Considerations

Second-trimester products of conception with no history of fetal demise, anomalies, or other problems can be handled in much the same way as first trimester specimens, with *documentation of intrauterine pregnancy and identification of any unexpected abnormalities*. When there are fetal anomalies, additional attention is required to document the specific anomalies present and in some cases, to submit tissue for special testing. Like first trimester specimens, there is marked variability in the type of tissue received and the extent of disruption. If the specimen is delivered spontaneously or after induction of labor, the fetus may be relatively intact, although the placenta often does not survive undamaged. When surgical procedures are performed to terminate the pregnancy or remove uterine contents, both the placenta and fetus can be quite disrupted, making examination problematic. In addition, in cases of fetal demise, autolysis may further hamper evaluation. For these reasons, examination of these specimens creates unique challenges to the pathologist. Although detailed examination for fetal anomalies is beyond the scope of this text, it is the author's hope that this chapter, covering the *general approach and overview* to the handling these types of specimens, will assist in initial evaluation of these specimens. The reader is referred to the Selected References at the end of the chapter for several excellent texts detailing fetal examination in the setting of congenital anomalies.

R.N. Baergen, *Manual of Pathology of the Human Placenta,*
DOI 10.1007/978-1-4419-7494-5_2, © Springer Science+Business Media, LLC 2011

Macroscopic Examination and Description

The first step in gross examination is separation of *fetal tissue from the nonfetal tissue*. With practice, the fine papillary villi can be identified and separated from the remaining tissue along with membranes and fragments of umbilical cord (see Figs. 1.4–1.6). This is a relatively simple procedure in the second trimester, as the components are better defined compared to the first trimester specimen. Once the placental tissue is separated, *the placental tissue should be measured and weighed in aggregate, and the cord length and cord diameter should be ascertained if possible.* Abnormalities of the cord, such as excessive twisting, knots, constrictions, discolorations, or abnormal length, should be noted at this time, as these are important causes of demise even in the second trimester (see Chap. 15). If a cord abnormality is noted, a photograph is recommended before further examination and sectioning. The fetal membranes should be evaluated for opacity or discoloration as well as identification of the rare amnionic band (see Chap. 14). The villous tissue should be examined for blood clots, infarcts or other lesions (see Fig. 3.8).

After the fetal tissue has been separated, an attempt to "reconstruct" the fetus should be made, placing the fetal parts in anatomic position (Fig. 2.1). This will provide an opportunity to make an inventory of the fetal organs and fetal parts and possibly gain some insight into their relationships. *If any major skeletal structures are missing, it may be prudent to contact the clinician, as this could indicate that tissue is retained in the uterus.* It is important to try and identify each major organ, but disruption and maceration may prohibit identification of all organs even if they are present. If identification of each organ is not possible, it is suggested that sections be taken of "unidentifiable" tissue or "possible" organs in the hopes that additional organs will be recognized microscopically. Photographs should be taken if any abnormality is noted. In cases of fetal anomalies and in particular, fetuses with complex or unusual anomalies, photographs are invaluable for later study or consultation. Radiographs should also be taken at this time, if necessary (see below).

Many specimens show marked disruption, and it is notable that different portions of the fetus are more or less prone to disruption. Usually, the extremities are the most likely to remain intact, while the abdomen is usually the most disrupted. The pelvis, chest, and head are variably disrupted. Adequate clinical history is extremely helpful in directing examination for anomalies, but is not always forthcoming. Therefore, *a systematic approach is suggested in which each portion of the fetus is examined* in order to maximize the information gained.

The following is an example of a systematic approach to these specimens:

- External examination
  - Measurements
    - Crown-rump
    - Crown-heel
    - Head, abdominal, and chest circumferences

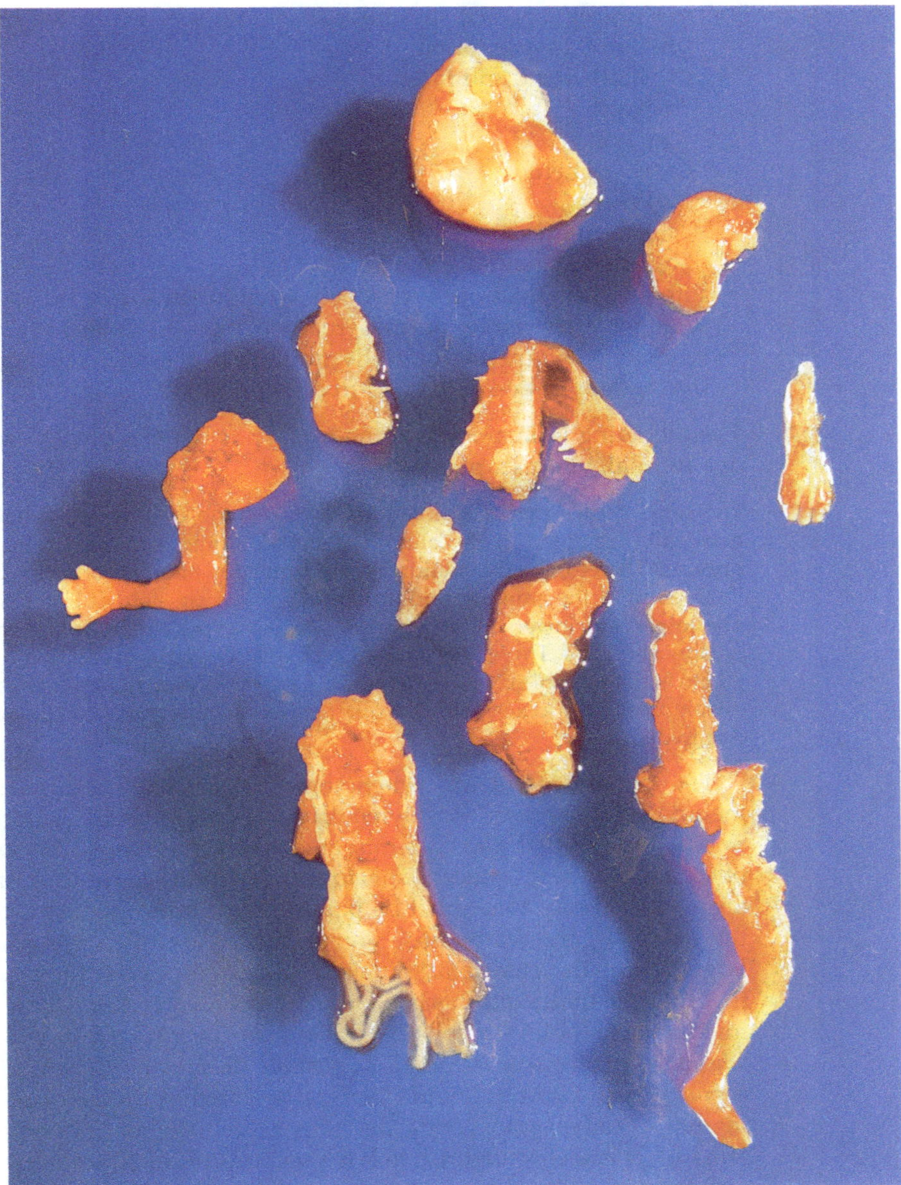

Figure 2.1. Fetus after pregnancy termination procedure with typical disruption. The fetal parts have been arranged such that the normal anatomical position has been approximated. The skull became collapsed during the procedure. This is a common artifact.

- • Foot length – may be the only measurement possible in severe disruption but it has a good correlation with gestational age (Table 3.7)
- ■ External appearance – initially give an overall evaluation of the extent of disruption. Then for each region below, describe each structure that can be identified indicating whether is anomalous

> or normal and list structures that cannot be evaluated or identified due to disruption
> - Skull, head, and face
> - Neck
> - Chest
> - Abdomen
> - Pelvis
> - Extremities
> - External genitalia

- Internal examination – describe what organs can be identified, whether they have normal relationships to other organs and whether they are anatomically normal, if possible. Then list those that cannot be evaluated due to disruption

The following is an *example* of the initial portion of a gross description of a normal, but disrupted fetus:

The fetus shows marked disruption and is quite fragmented. The head is markedly disrupted, with collapse of the skull and minimal brain tissue is present. Therefore, examination of the brain for anomalies is not possible. Evaluation of the cranium and upper face is not possible due to disruption. The lower jaw, lower lip, and portions of the upper lip are intact and show no abnormalities. There is no evidence of a cleft lip, but evaluation for a cleft palate is not possible due to disruption. One ear is present and shows normal development and placement. No other craniofacial features can be evaluated due to disruption.

It is recommended that when some portions are not present, one include what **is** present and what **cannot** be identified. It is not recommended to say that parts are missing, as this may imply that portions of the fetus were misplaced. This format is continued for the remaining areas of the body. One must be particularly careful in examination of the external genitalia because young fetuses are often missexed. The large size of the clitoris in female fetuses often gives the impression that they are male, and this is a common mistake made by novices. One must not just look at the phallus but *examine the genital folds and identify whether they are fused (scrotum) or separate (labia) and if there is a patent vagina.* These findings should be clearly stated in the gross section of the report rather than saying the fetus is "female" or "phenotypically female." It is always helpful to have sections of the gonads to confirm sex. The sex is often important information both medically and personally for the family. If the external genitalia are entirely consistent with male or female sex, but the gonads could not be identified to confirm, then it is suggested that the diagnosis read "phenotypically male (or female) fetus" rather than "male (or female) fetus," the latter being used when gonads are able to be examined microscopically.

The same systematic approach is used for the internal organs. Each visceral organ should be identified, and the organ relationships should be evaluated, if possible. This is particularly important in the setting of congenital heart defects where relationships with the lungs and great vessels are essential to diagnosis. Finally, anatomic defects in each organ are evaluated. Although each organ and portion of the fetus is examined individually, attempts should be made to integrate the findings and provide as much information about each organ systems as possible. Organ weights should be included for intact organs only. The following is an example of a description of disrupted organs.

The abdomen and pelvis are markedly disrupted. Organs that can be identified are liver, bowel, stomach, kidneys, bladder, and gonads, all of which are grossly unremarkable and show no anatomic defects. Normal entrance of both ureters into the bladder is present, but the kidneys are partially disrupted and their relationship to the ureters cannot be ascertained. Other organ relationships cannot be evaluated due to disruption. Organ weights of intact organs are as follows…

When there is marked disruption, it is recommended that a comment be made indicating that "interpretation is limited due to disruption." In addition, the report should indicate whether or not the specific anomalies indicated in the clinical history may or may not be ruled out, and if the latter, why not. When specimens are macerated and autolyzed, additional artifacts are introduced. Specifically, the joints may be lax such that abnormalities of positioning of the extremities, such as arthrogryposis, cannot be evaluated. Dehydration also occurs and may make the diagnosis of hydrops or nuchal edema difficult if not impossible. The brain may not be able to be examined due to liquefaction. With fetal death, there is often hemorrhage, discoloration, and softening in many of the fetal tissues. These artifacts may also limit meaningful interpretation. In these circumstances, a "disclaimer" should also be included indicating that examination is limited due to marked autolysis.

Special Procedures

In certain situations, special procedures may be required. **Cytogenetic analysis** *is essential in cases of fetuses with multiple malformations.* Sometimes this is done prenatally via amniocentesis or chorionic villus sampling. If one is aware that these procedures have been done and has knowledge of these results, cytogenetic testing need not be repeated. In some states, it is required that these results be confirmed by sending a sample from the abortion specimen. Pathologists should be conversant with the health statutes in their area in order to be compliant. If a specimen is to be submitted for cytogenetic analysis, *it is prudent to send samples of both placenta and fetus.* The rationale for this is the following. The fetal tissue is optimal as it will be representative of the fetal genetic makeup. Placental tissue may or may not be reflective of the fetal genotype due to **confined placental mosaicism** (see Chap. 11), in which there is a variation of the placental genetic makeup disparate from the fetus. However, if the fetal tissue is macerated, fetal tissue will often not grow in culture. Therefore, it is best if both are submitted separately so that placental tissue may be used if the fetal cells do not grow. For the fetal sample, connective tissue such as tendon is often used, but skeletal muscle often grows better in culture. Chorionic villi or chorionic plate tissue is suggested for the placental sample, as this will avoid the maternal tissue that is present in the basal plate.

The specimen should be submitted in a sterile fashion in the appropriate medium as required by the specific laboratory. In cases without a significant clinical history suggesting a chromosomal anomaly and lack of fetal anomalies, the yield of karyotypic analysis is usually low, depending on the patient population.

If the constellation of malformations does not fit into one of the various chromosomal syndromes, e.g., trisomies, and the diagnosis is not apparent from prenatal testing or gross examination, it *may be sensible to freeze a portion of fetal tissue.* This requires minimal labor but the rewards are great if tissue is needed for molecular studies to make the diagnosis. If the tissue is found to be unnecessary, it may easily be discarded. Usual recommendations are to snap freeze organ tissue, such as the liver, and connective tissue in liquid nitrogen and then store at −70 to −80°C. Placental tissue may be frozen as well.

If the fetus has obvious limb or bony abnormalities, radiographs should be taken. These are necessary for the diagnosis of **skeletal dysplasias** as well as many malformation syndromes with bony anomalies. Bony abnormalities include *shortened, missing or abnormally formed limbs or digits and abnormalities of the spine, ribs, or skull.* On occasion, severe growth restriction of the fetus has been confused with skeletal dysplasias, and radiographs will help differentiate these cases. The fetal parts should be positioned anatomically with an attempt to straighten them into an anterior–posterior position. The exposure of the radiograph should be adequate for evaluation of bony structures (Fig. 2.2). In cases of suspected skeletal dysplasia, *longitudinal sections of a long bone should also be submitted for routine histology* and a portion of bone should be snap frozen and stored at −70 to −80°C, in addition to organ tissue and connective tissue.

Uncommonly, fetuses may suffer from metabolic disorders. If these are suspected, a small amount of fetal tissue should be fixed for later **electron microscopy** as well as snap-frozen. Finally, in some cases, **bacterial cultures** of the fetus or placenta may be indicated. This is particularly true when the fetal surface of the placenta is opaque, which is suggestive of an ascending infection. To take the culture, the amnionic membrane is lifted from the chorionic plate and the surface of the plate should be swabbed. This will usually avoid bacterial contamination. Unless the clinical history or gross examination suggests an ascending infection or acute chorioamnionitis, bacterial cultures are usually not recommended.

Submission of Microscopic Sections

Sections of each organ identified should be submitted for microscopic examination. At times, marked disruption may make identification of solid organs difficult, particularly the liver, spleen, and adrenals. In this situation, there are often additional fragments of tissue that cannot grossly be identified as a particular organ but are clearly of fetal origin. It is suggested that these fragments also be submitted for microscopic examination. Depending on the type of anomaly identified, special sections of the anomalous part are submitted. For example, in anencephaly

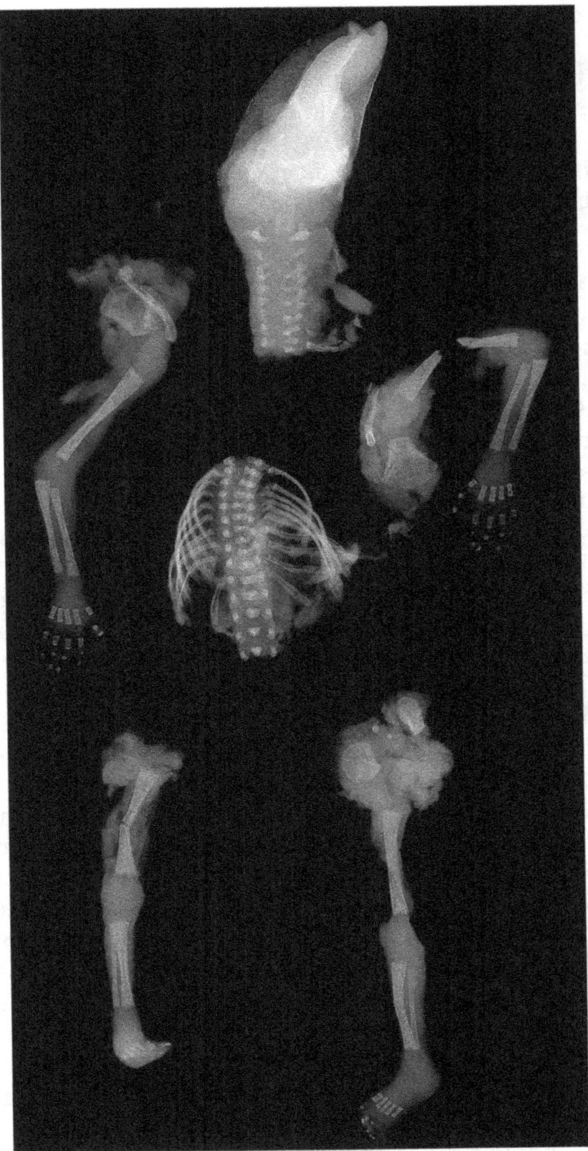

Figure 2.2.   Radiograph of the fetus depicted in Fig. 2.1. The X-ray has been taken with the fetal parts placed in an approximation of the normal anatomical position. An attempt should be made to ensure that there is minimal twisting so that a typical anterior–posterior (A–P) position is achieved. This fetus showed no gross, radiographic, or microscopic abnormalities.

sections through the base of the skull are particularly illustrative of the lack of brain tissue and the presence of the cerebrovasculosa. Thus, sectioning must be tailored to the anomalies that are present as well as those that are suspected. The reader is referred to the many excellent texts on the subject of fetal anomalies and the best techniques for the dissection of those anomalies. Sections of the placenta should also be submitted similar to that for third trimester placentas (see Chap. 3), including two sections of the membranes, two sections of umbilical cord, and several sections of villous tissue. The latter should include both fetal and maternal surfaces if possible. If grossly identifiable decidual tissue is present, a small fragment should also be submitted for microscopic examination.

Microscopic Description, Diagnosis, and Report

Microscopic sections of each organ should be examined for appropriateness for stated gestational age as well as the presence of abnormalities. In some cases, this is confirmation of a grossly identified abnormality, while in others it may be primarily a microscopic finding. The gross and microscopic findings should be integrated with the goal of making a specific diagnosis. This is important in that different syndromes have markedly different recurrence risks and so have significance to the family in making decisions about future pregnancies.

A statement about whether or not the fetus is the appropriate size for the gestational age is obligatory. Tables of normative values with crown-rump, crown-heel, and foot length can be used for this purpose (see Table 3.7). The sex of the fetus should also be stated if this is known. If the determination of sex is based solely on external genitalia, it is wise to indicate that the fetus is "phenotypically" male or female. Thus, one can state "Phenotypically male fetus, size consistent with 17 weeks' gestation." If a diagnosis of a particular syndrome can be made, this should follow in the next statement. If a particular syndrome is suspected clinically, but cannot be confirmed, a statement such as "Clinical history of ..." may be used instead. This should be followed by the specific anomalies noted on gross and microscopic examination. Each abnormality indicated in the clinical history should be addressed as *present, absent, or unable to be evaluated due to disruption or maceration*. This is important because lack of specific anomalies may rule out certain syndromes that are in the differential diagnosis. Unfortunately, with disrupted fetuses, limitations in examination often make meaningful diagnosis impossible. In that case, it should be clearly stated that a diagnosis cannot be made and why. A general comment may also be added indicating that pathologic evaluation is limited due to marked disruption.

Selected References

PHP5, pages 1–11 (Examination of the Placenta).

Baldwin VJ, Kalousek DK, Dimmick JE, Applegarth DA, Hardwic DF. Diagnostic pathologic investigation of the malformed conceptus. Perspect Pediatr Pathol 1982;7:65–108.

Dimmick JE, Kalousek DK. Developmental pathology of the fetus and infant. Philadelphia: Lippincott, 1992.

Gilbert-Barnass E (ed). Potter's pathology of the fetus and infant. St. Louis: Mosby, 1997.

Gilbert-Barnass E, Debich-Spicer DE. Handbook of pediatric autopsy pathology. Totowa, NJ: Humana Press, 2005.

Gilbert-Barnass, Debich-Spicer DE, Williams M. Embryo and fetal pathology: color atlas with ultrasound correlation. Cambridge, UK: Cambridge University Press, 2004.

Jones KL. Smith's recognizable patterns of human malformation, 5th ed. Philadelphia: WB Saunders, 1997.

Kalousek DK, Fitch N, Paradice BA. Pathology of the human embryo and previable fetus. An atlas. New York: Springer-Verlag, 1990.

Keeling JW. Fetal pathology. Edinburgh: Churchill Livingstone, 1994.

Keeling JW, Khong TY. Fetal and neonatal pathology, 3rd ed. London: Springer, 2007.

Wigglesworth JS, Singer DB. Textbook of fetal and perinatal pathology, 2nd ed. Malden, MA: Blackwell Science, 1998.

Chapter 3

Macroscopic Evaluation of the Second- and Third-Trimester Placenta

Selection of Placentas for Pathologic Examination

In general, tissue removed or spontaneously passed from the body must be sent for pathologic examination. Placentas are the notable exception in that they are the only specimens for which routine examination is not required. The Joint Commission on the Accreditation of Hospitals states that "normal placentas" from "normal deliveries" are not required to be examined or submitted to pathology. However, a definition of what is normal is not forthcoming. Although there are a number of options for placental selection, this task is frequently left to obstetricians or other health care workers involved in the delivery, and thus selection is seldom based on specific criteria. This is the least desirable of the possible options discussed below.

R.N. Baergen, *Manual of Pathology of the Human Placenta,*
DOI 10.1007/978-1-4419-7494-5_3, © Springer Science+Business Media, LLC 2011

Examination of All Placentas

Most placentas are normal, as are most babies; therefore, examination of all placentas may not be warranted, and from a practical standpoint, may not be possible due to time constraints and other practical and financial considerations, particularly in hospitals with large numbers of deliveries. Nonetheless, a case can be made for this option. First, sporadic examination does not allow the general surgical pathologist or pathology resident *to obtain sufficient background knowledge as to what constitutes a truly normal placenta.* Gross and microscopic examination of many placentas is necessary to have a good base of knowledge of what is and what is not normal. Another reason examination of all placentas may be desirable is today's litigious climate, which makes *the study of placentas highly valuable, particularly in the defense of obstetricians* (see Chap. 26).

Selection Based on Consensus Indications

Another option is selection of placentas based on *relevant indications for submission,* which is a reasonable compromise. The College of American Pathologists coordinated a multidisciplinary working group on placental pathology, which developed indications for submission of placentas for pathologic examination that included **placental, fetal, and maternal indications.** An adapted version is shown in Table 3.1. When delivery personnel are responsible for the selection of placentas, it is recommended that these indications be provided to them and adopted for routine use. If these indications are followed, the likelihood that a placenta with any significant pathology will not be examined is very small.

Initial Selection with Storage of Remaining Placentas

In this approach, *placentas are initially selected for examination* by consensus criteria as above and the remaining placentas are stored in a refrigerator at 4°C. This method is particularly desirable as *a number of neonatal problems are not apparent until several days of life.* Furthermore, it provides a way to "catch" those placentas that should have been submitted but for some reason or another, were not. One week is usually sufficient time for storage, and placentas are almost perfectly preserved for meaningful examination when stored for this time period. If this approach is to be implemented, a refrigerator with seven shelves labeled with the days of the week is recommended. The placentas are placed on the shelf corresponding to the day of delivery, and each day the placentas not selected from 1 week prior are discarded. During that week of storage, neonatologists, obstetricians, or other personnel may request placental examination based on development of neonatal or postpartum problems. This is method used in our institution.

Gross Examination of All Placentas with Microscopic Examination on Selected Placentas

In this scheme, *all placentas are initially examined macroscopically.* Based on gross examination and clinical information, a *portion of them is submitted for microscopic examination.* Those with no significant gross abnormalities and normal pregnancy and delivery history would only be examined macroscopically. The success of this approach is partially dependent on the skill and experience of the examiner as well as the availability of clinical history. A variation of this technique is macroscopic examination along with *submission of tissue for processing into blocks on all placentas*. Histologic sections are then cut only on selected cases based on gross examination and history as above. If problems occur in the future, the blocks may then be cut. This approach has not commonly been used, and at some institutions regulations may prohibit such a system from being implemented. However, in recent years some malpractice insurance companies have shown interest in this approach as a type of "insurance" against future litigation.

Storage

Placentas should ideally be examined *in the fresh state or at least prior to fixation*. Placentas should **never be frozen** prior to examination, as it makes macroscopic examination difficult and obliterates the most useful histologic characteristics. Specimens that have been *previously frozen will show reddish discoloration of the fetal surface, cord, and membranes due to hemolysis*. Formalin fixation prior to examination is not optimal, as it obscures many macroscopic features, makes examination more difficult, and causes difficulties in the submission of specimens for tissue culture, cytogenetics, and bacteriologic examination. Although some lesions are better visualized after fixation, examination of unfixed placentas affords the opportunity to view lesions in both fresh and fixed states. If storage is needed, placentas should be stored in tightly sealed containers at 4°C.

During storage, the placenta loses some weight to a small extent by evaporation but predominantly by leakage of blood and serum. The freshly examined placenta is thus softer, bloodier, and thicker than one that has been stored. Weight loss is most significant in hydropic or edematous placentas. *After formalin fixation, the placenta will gain approximately 5% in weight.*

Macroscopic Examination

As with examination of any specimen, it is wise to *follow a routine protocol*. This will not only enhance subsequent interpretation, but also provide a systematic approach so that nothing will be omitted. The following is an example of such a procedure for placental examination. Readers are encouraged to tailor this to their personal style and needs. Specific gross lesions are listed by location in tables at the end of the chapter (Tables 3.2–3.6), and Fig. 3.1 gives an example of a gross reporting form useful for macroscopic evaluation.

Instruments

The instruments needed are basic, and consist of a *ruler or tape measure; a long, sharp knife; forceps with teeth; scissors; and a scale.* Mounting the ruler directly over and perpendicular to the cutting board is advantageous, as the cord length, placental diameter, and other measurements can be easily made. The knife should be long, relatively thin, and very sharp. Often

SYNOPTIC REPORT OF MACROSCOPIC PLACENTAL EXAMINATION

Name :________________________   Path. #____________   Medical Record #________________

History:____

____

____

____

GENERAL:

Weight (disk only)__________g

   ☐ Formalin-fixed

   ☐ Unfixed

Size______ x ______ x ______ cm

CORD:

Insertion: ☐ Central

      ☐ Eccentric

      ☐ Marginal

      ☐ Furcate

      ☐ Interpositional

      ☐ Velamentous

         ________cm from margin

Velamentous vessels:

      ☐ Intact

      ☐ Disrupted

      ☐ Thrombosis

MEMBRANES:

Insertion: ☐ Marginal

      ☐ Circumvallate

      ☐ Circummarginate

Color: ☐ Green

      ☐ Opaque

      ☐ Brown

      ☐ Normal

      ☐ Other__________________

Point of rupture from margin: ________cm

☐   Amnion nodosum

☐   Squamous metaplasia

Other________________________________

SURFACE VESSELS ABNORMALITIES:__________________

TWINS: ☐ Yes

      ☐ No

HIGHER MULTIPLES:__________________

Fused: ☐ Yes

      ☐ No

      ☐ DiDi

      ☐ DiMo

      ☐ MoMo

Anastomoses____________________________

Cord Vessels: ☐   3

            ☐   2

            ☐   4

Thrombosis: ☐ Yes

      ☐ No

Knots: ☐ Yes

      ☐ No

Length: ________ cm   Diameter______ cm

Coiling: ☐ Left

      ☐ Right

      ☐ None or minimal

      ☐ Marked

Discoloration: ☐ Green

      ☐ Yellow

      ☐ Brown

      ☐ Other________________

Other lesions________________________

MATERNAL SURFACE:

Intact: ☐ Yes

      ☐ No

Color: ☐ Normal

      ☐ Pale

      ☐ Congested

Retroplacental hematoma: Size ________cm,

          ________% of surface

      ☐ Old

      ☐ Recent

CUT SURFACE/VILLOUS TISSUE:

Infarct(s):   ☐ Yes

      ☐ No

   Multiple (no.)____________

   Largest size(cm)__________

   % of total placenta________

      ☐ Old

      ☐ Recent

Intervillous thrombi__________

Increased Fibrin______________

Other Lesions:__________________

Pictures taken?

      ☐ Yes

      ☐ No

Special Studies ____________________

Figure 3.1.   Suggested macroscopic worksheet.

the best knife for this use is obtained from a butcher supply house or cutlery store rather than conventional sources. The forceps, scissors, and scale are all standard items and easily obtained. In addition, an adjacent sink is optimal, as this facilitates rinsing of the placenta for easy, gentle removal of blood and other fluids. This will assist in accurate identification of lesions and discolorations of the membranes, cord, or surfaces of the placenta and makes for a cleaner work area. The placenta should never be wiped off, as this will damage the surfaces.

Procedure for Examination

After removing the placenta from the container and rinsing briefly in water, perform the following steps:

- **General characteristics:**
  - **Check for odors** – may indicate bacterial growth.
  - **Ascertain shape** – irregular, discoid, etc. Immersion of the placenta in water will return the placenta to its shape in utero and thus demonstrate the shape of the uterine cavity. This is particularly useful with abnormally shaped placentas (see Chap. 13) and in cases of uterine anomalies.
- **Membranes (Table 3.2):**
  - **Check for completeness** – sufficient membranes should be present to enclose the fetus.
  - **Measure membrane rupture site** – this is the distance from the placental edge to the nearest rupture site (Fig. 3.2). If it is greater than zero in a vaginally delivered specimen, a placenta previa is ruled out.

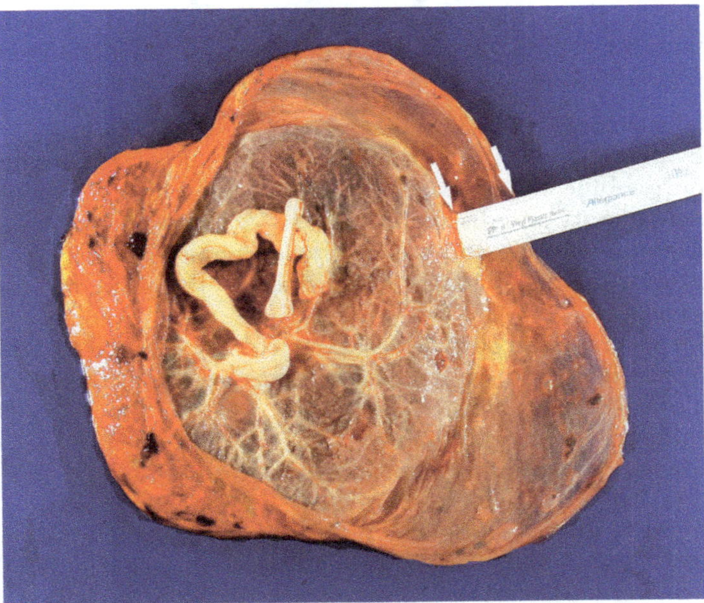

Figure 3.2. Demonstration of the measurement of the shortest distance between the membrane rupture site and the margin of the placenta. The two *arrows* along the *ruler* indicate this measurement.

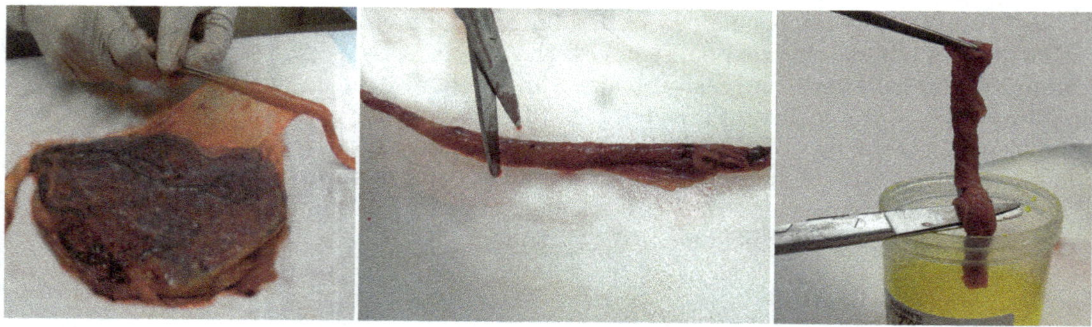

Figure 3.3. Rolling of membranes for fixation and later sectioning. It is best to use a standardized protocol, rolling the membranes with the amnion inside, starting at the site of rupture and proceeding toward the edge of the placenta as shown at *left*. A segment is taken from the rolled portion (*center*) and fixed (*right*) before sectioning.

- **Evaluate color and appearance** – the membranes are normally translucent and shiny, but may be opaque or discolored yellow, green, brown or red-brown.
- **Identify membrane insertion** – the normal insertion is at the margin; insertion other than at the edge indicates circumvallation or circummargination (Figs. 13.4–13.6 in Chap. 13).
- **Remove fetal membranes** – use sharp scissors and keep the orientation to rupture site.
- **Make a "membrane roll"** – take a strip approximately 10 cm wide, and with forceps grasp the portion representing the rupture site (furthest from the placental margin). Roll the membranes with the rupture site in the center and with the amnion inward (Fig. 3.3).

- Fetal surface (Table 3.3):
  - **Evaluate color and appearance** – the fetal surface is normally purple-blue and translucent (Fig. 3.4). As with the membranes, note opacity and discoloration.
  - **Examine surface and subchorionic region** – identify nodules, plaques, amnionic bands, hemorrhage, cysts, fibrin, masses and, so on.
  - **Inspect the fetal surface vessels** – look for vascular thrombosis, hemorrhage or disruption; *arteries cross over veins* (Fig. 3.5).
- Umbilical cord (Table 3.4):
  - **Measure length and diameter.**
  - **Identify spiraling of the umbilical cord** – right or left twist (Fig. 3.6); excessive or minimal twisting or constriction.
  - **Identify insertion of the umbilical cord** – marginal, eccentric, central, paracentral, or velamentous (see Fig. 15.17); if velamentous, measure the distance from the insertion to the placental edge, and note hemorrhage, disruption, or thrombosis of vessels.

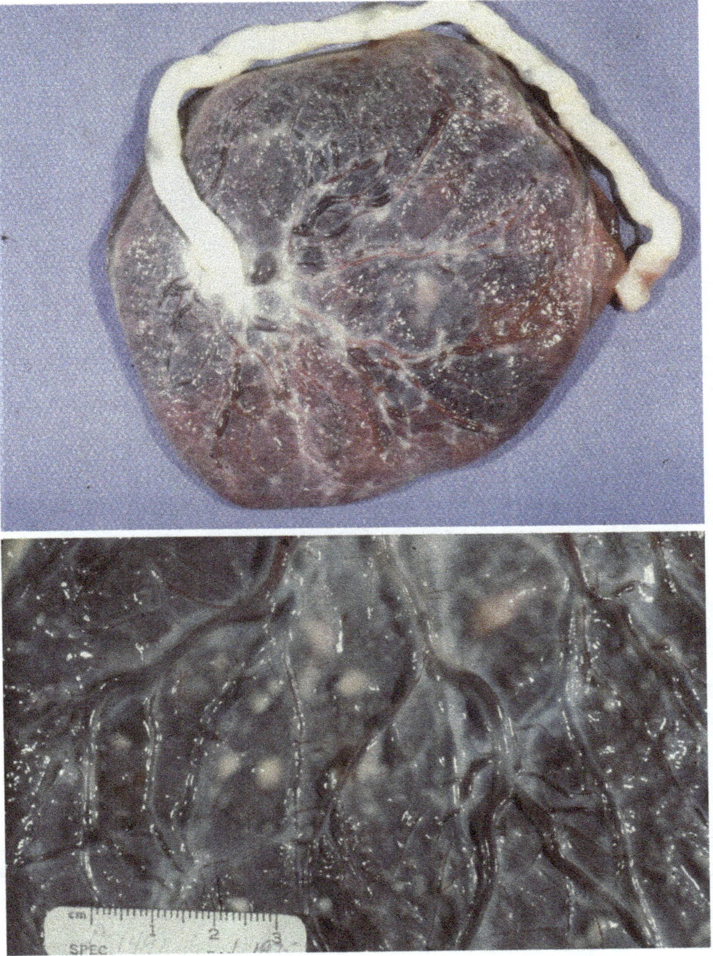

Figure 3.4. Normal fetal surface of the placenta. The surface is blue to purple and translucent with a pearly white, eccentrically inserted umbilical cord (*top*). Normally, subchorionic fibrin/fibrinoid deposits are present which appear as irregular white patches on the fetal surface (*bottom*).

- **Knots** – identify true knots; note whether tight or loose and if congestion is present.
  - **Umbilical vessels** – normally three, but two or four vessels may occur.
  - **Other** – discoloration, thrombosis, hemorrhage, cysts, surface nodules, masses, etc.
  - **Remove the cord from the placenta at the insertion site**.
- **Placental disk (Tables 3.5–3.7):**
  - **Measure the placenta in three dimensions.**
  - **Weigh the placenta** – without cord or membranes.
  - **Evaluate shape of placental disk** – discoid, irregular, bilobed, succenturiate, etc. Evaluate membranous vessels if present.

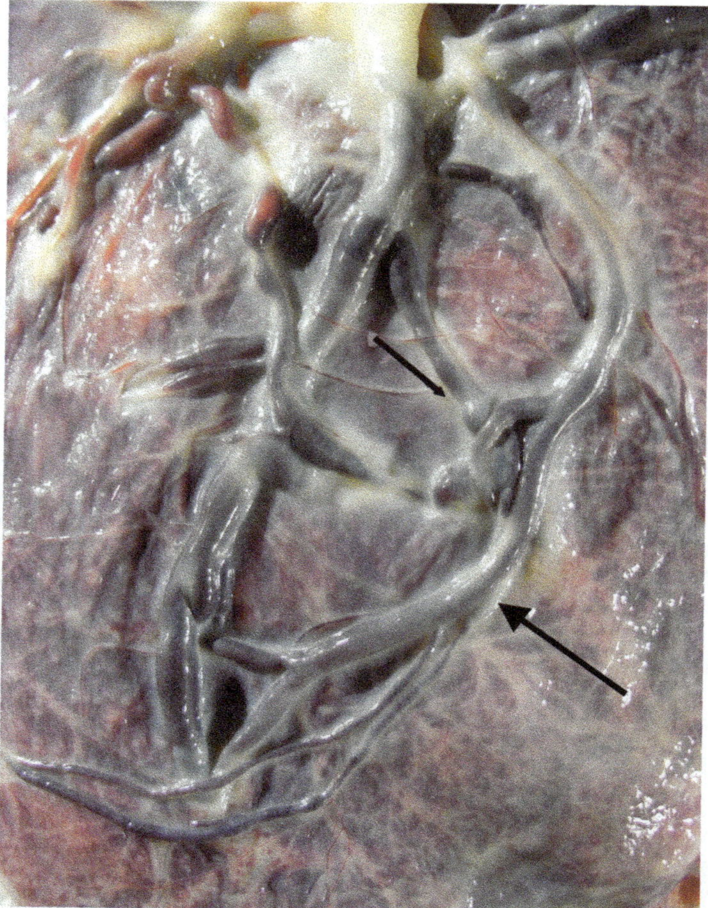

Figure 3.5. Entrance of the vessels on the chorionic plate into the cotyledon. One artery (*large arrow*) brings in the fetal blood and the vein (*small arrow*) returns it to the fetus. Note that the arteries cross over the veins.

- **Maternal surface** – check for completeness, cotyledonary development, blood clots, calcifications (Fig. 3.7).
- **Retroplacental hematoma (abruptio placentae)** – look for adherent blood clot, compression of villous tissue, underlying infarct (Fig. 3.8).
- **Serially section the placental tissue at 5-mm intervals.**
- **Evaluate the color of villous tissue – pale, congested or normal.**
- **Identify and describe villous lesions – measure, note location (fetal versus maternal surface; peripheral versus central), single or multiple and percentage of placenta involved (Fig. 3.8).**

Normal Macroscopic Appearance

In 90% of the cases, the placenta is disk-like, flat, and round to oval. Abnormalities of shape occur in about 10% of cases and include **bilobed placenta**, **succenturiate lobes**, and **placenta membranacea**

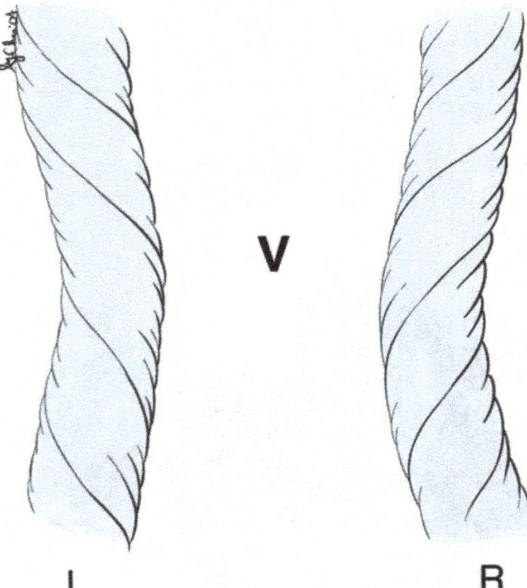

Figure 3.6. Diagram of cord twisting. When cord is placed vertically, the direction of the spiral is compared to the arms of the letter "V." If the spiral is in the direction of the left arm, the cord is left twisted, and if it is in the direction of the right arm, it is a right twist. This method ensures the same results no matter which way the cord is oriented.

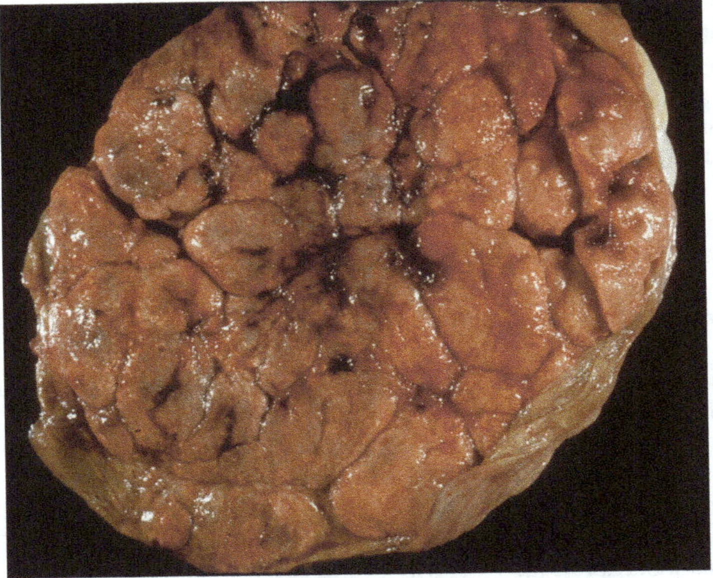

Figure 3.7. Normal maternal surface of the term placenta. Note the divisions into lobules or cotyledons and the small white speckled areas representing calcifications.

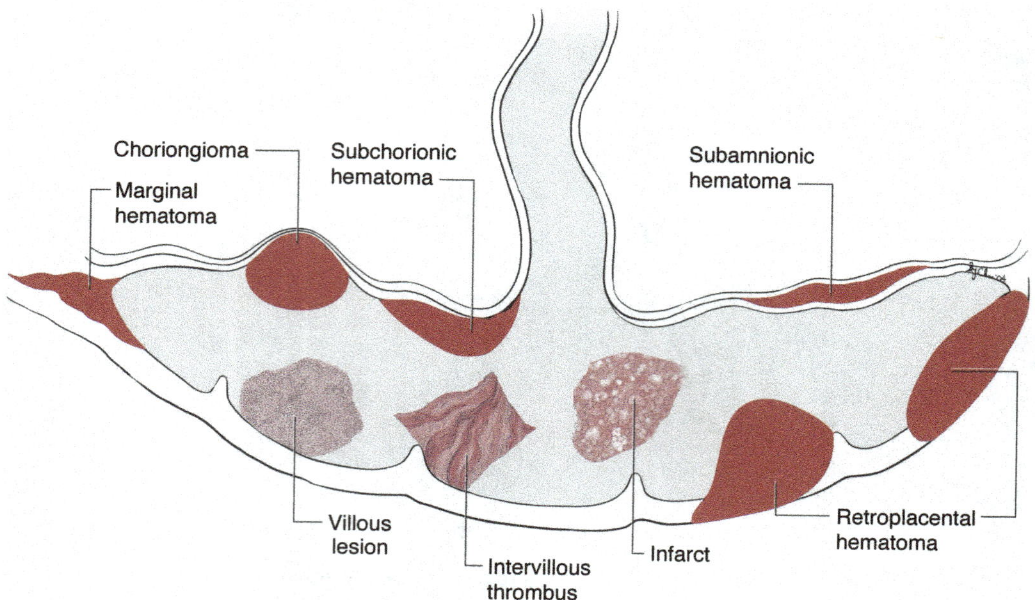

Figure 3.8. Diagram of selected, grossly visible lesions of the placenta. Miscellaneous lesions include acute or chronic villitis, fibrinoid deposition, intervillous abscesses and various tumors.

(see Chap. 13). At term, the average diameter is 22 cm, thickness is 2.5 cm, and weight is 470 g (Table 3.7). The umbilical cord is normally pearly white and measures an average of 55 cm in length and 1.0–1.5 cm in diameter at term (Table 3.4). It most commonly inserts **eccentrically** and usually contains three vessels, two arteries, and one vein. It may have a **marginal, velamentous,** or **furcate insertion.** Occasionally a single artery or a persistent second vein occurs (see Chap. 15). Care must be taken when evaluating the cord for the presence of a single umbilical artery, as the arteries commonly anastomose close to their insertion on the placental surface. The cord is left twisted in about 70% of cases (Fig. 3.6). The coiling index is sometimes used to evaluate the amount of twisting, although this may vary throughout the length of the cord. A normal coiling index is 0.2 ± 0.1 coils/cm, i.e., one coil for every 5 cm.

The **fetal membranes** are generally translucent and shiny but in pathologic conditions may be **opaque** or **discolored** (Table 3.2). The **fetal surface,** facing the amnionic cavity, is usually blue to purple with a **glossy** or **shiny** appearance. Pathologic conditions may lead to discoloration or opacity (see Chap. 14). The **chorionic vessels** run underneath the amnion and branch is a star-like pattern, centrifugally from the cord insertion (Fig. 3.4). *Arteries cross over veins* (Fig. 3.5, Table 3.3). Around the larger vessels, the **chorionic plate** is more opaque due to increased numbers of collagen fibers. White plaques or nodules are due to **subchorionic fibrinoid** and in moderate amounts are not significant. Occasionally, the remnant of the **yolk sac** can be identified underneath the amnion, consisting of a chalky white, flattened ovoid of tissue (see Fig. 14.7a).

After delivery of the placenta, some **decidua basalis** is left in utero and some remains as part of the **basal** plate. The plate is composed of a heterogeneous population of trophoblastic and decidual elements embedded in **extracellular debris, fibrinoid,** and **blood clot.** An incomplete system of "grooves" subdivides the basal surface into 10–40 lobes or **cotyledons** (Fig. 3.7), which correspond to the **septa** seen histologically.

On cut section, the villous tissue is **red** to **red-brown,** and **spongy** on cut section. Its color is almost wholly determined by its content of *fetal blood and thus the fetal hemoglobin/hematocrit* (Tables 3.5 and 3.6). If the fetal hemoglobin is high, the villous tissue is dark and congested; if the hemoglobin is low, the villous tissue is pale. In the center of many delivered placentas are holes or so-called lakes, which were filled with blood in utero, they are of no consequence. At the periphery of many term placentas, the villous tissue may show areas of tan-white and firmer tissue and thus may appear "infarcted." These are not true infarcts but rather villous atrophy due to poor circulation at the periphery.

Suggested Gross Description

The following is a suggested gross description with options in parentheses. It can be used as a template for dictation and transcription.

Received **(fresh/unfixed/in formalin),** labeled with the patient's name and ID, is a **(discoid/bilobed/irregularly shaped)** placenta measuring ______×______×_____cm in greatest dimensions with a trimmed weight of _________ g. The **(three/two)** vessel umbilical cord has a **(right/left/minimal/ marked)** twist. It measures __________cm in diameter by __________cm in length and has **(an eccentric/a marginal/a velamentous/a central)** insertion. There **(is/is no)** evidence of hemorrhage, thrombosis, discoloration or true knots. The membranes are **(complete/incomplete)** and are ruptured ______cm from the placental margin. The fetal surface is **(purple, translucent/discolored yellow/opaque, etc).** The maternal surface is **(intact/disrupted/incomplete)** with **(no/a recent/an old)** retroplacental hematomas. Cut section reveals spongy, **(pale/congested/friable/unremarkable)** soft spongy tissue with **(no/a single/numerous)** infarct **(s). (The infarcts comprise** _________**% of the placental tissue.)** No other gross lesions are identified. Representative sections are submitted. Summary of sections: A1 – umbilical cord (×2) and membrane roll (×2), A2–A4 – villous tissue, A4 – lesion, A6 – maternal surface.

Submission of Microscopic Sections

Routine sections that should be taken on every placenta are listed below. Additional sections should be taken when abnormalities are present, and the reader is directed to Tables 3.2–3.6 for descriptions of specific lesions. The routine sections should include:

- **Two sections of membrane roll, one from the rupture site and one from the placental margin**
- **Two sections of umbilical cord from each of two areas**

- **Two full-thickness sections of villous tissue including fetal and maternal surfaces**
- **Sections of the maternal surface**

Several small sections of the maternal surface in one cassette may enhance one's examination of decidual vessels. The sections of the villous tissue should be *taken away from the margin of the placenta*, as the perfusion is not consistent throughout the placenta and abnormalities exist in peripheral areas of poor perfusion that *may not be reflective of the remainder of the specimen*. Sections of the **fetal surface with chorionic vessels** should be included in those sections of villous tissue. This requires taking at least one section near the insertion of the umbilical cord to obtain vessels of sufficient caliber.

Fixation

Pathologists commonly fix tissue for histological study in **10% buffered formalin** solution (a 1:10 dilution of the commercial 40% formaldehyde). However, brief fixation in formalin is usually insufficient for placental tissue, which tends to be quite bloody. Inadequate fixation makes trimming of the tissue and sectioning on the microtome more difficult, giving poor results in final sections. This is particularly true of the sections of the membrane roll. One option is to *fix the initial sections of placental tissue for a longer period*, at least overnight before trimming and processing. Another option is to *briefly fix the tissue in* Bouin's solution prior to trimming and processing. Bouin's solution makes tissue considerably harder and allows one to trim the tissue more readily before embedding. Bouin's solution is made by preparing a saturated solution (1.2%) of picric acid in water and adding 40% formaldehyde solution and glacial acetic acid in proportions of 15:5:1. After 1–3 h fixation, the tissue is ready to be trimmed. Ideally, the Bouin's-fixed sections are immersed in a *saturated lithium carbonate solution* before embedding. This step is not required, but it helps to remove extraneous pigments. Moreover, some intervillous blood is lysed, and pigments derived from blood ("formalin pigment," acid hematin) are more frequently present when lithium carbonate is omitted. This is also important when one wishes to do immunohistochemistry.

Special Procedures

The placenta is a good source of tissue for **chromosome analysis**, particularly when the fetus is macerated, as tissue from that source will often not grow in culture. The procedure is to disinfect the amnion with alcohol and then strip the amnion off a portion of placental surface. With sterile instruments, a piece of chorion is taken, placed in culture medium, and then transferred to the cytogenetics laboratory. Multiple areas of the placenta may need to be sampled if one needs to rule out confined placental mosaicism (see Chap. 11). **For bacterial culture**, tissue swabs or tissue samples from the undersurface of the amnion should be taken as contamination of the amnion is likely.

Photography should be an integral part of any gross examination. The old adage that "a picture is worth a thousand words" is most applicable in this instance, and particularly true when the placenta is the subject of future litigation. Any unusual or clinically significant lesion should be photographed, as dissection will usually destroy the macroscopic lesion. Photography is particularly important when the macroscopic appearance, and not the microscopic appearance, demonstrates the lesion best.

Table 3.1. Indications for placental examination.

Maternal indications

History of reproductive failure – ≥1 spontaneous abortions (Abs), stillbirths, neonatal deaths,
or premature births

Maternal diseases

Coagulopathy
Hypertension (preeclampsia, pregnancy induced or chronic)
Diabetes mellitus
Prematurity (<2 weeks)
Postmaturity (>42 weeks)
Oligohydramnios
Polyhydramnios
Fever or infection
Repetitive bleeding
Abruptio placentae

Fetal and neonatal indications

Stillbirth or perinatal death
Fetal growth restriction (intrauterine growth retardation, IUGR)
Hydrops
Severe neonatal central nervous system (CNS) restriction or neurologic
problems such as seizures
Apgar score of 3 or less at 5 min
Suspected infection
Congenital anomalies
Thick meconium

Placental indications

Any gross abnormality of the placenta, membranes or umbilical cord, such as masses, thrombi, excessively long, short or twisted umbilical cord, etc.

Optional recommendations

Prematurity between 32 and 36 weeks
Low 1-min Apgar score
Fetal distress or non-reassuring fetal status
Multiple birth

Adapted from the College of American Pathologists (Altshuler and Deppisch 1991).

Table 3.2. Macroscopic lesions of the fetal membranes (see Chap. 14).

Type of lesion	Diagnosis		Comment	Figure number
Discoloration				
Green, green-yellow	Meconium		Check for staining of umbilical cord (see Table 3.4)	14.15a
Opaque, white to yellow	Acute inflammation (chorioamnionitis)		Check for odor. Consider culture	16.2
Brown to yellow	Hemosiderin		Old bleeding – retromembranous or retroplacental hematoma	14.19a
Red-brown, red-pink	Hemolysis		Most often due to fetal demise or freezing	–
Focal lesions	*Description*	*Diagnosis*		
Plaques	Red to brown, shaggy	Retro-membranous hematoma	May be secondary to ruptured membranes, decidual bleeding or iatrogenic due to amniocentesis	14.12
	Yellow to white, ragged	Decidual necrosis	May be due to decidual vascular lesions but most commonly nonspecific	–
	Tan, roundish, plaque-like	Fetus papyraceous	Ascertain placentation if possible	10.1–10.3
	Pasty, hydrophobic material	Vernix caseosa	Usually secondary to membrane rupture and is of little consequence	14.8
Strings or bands of membrane	Usually tethered to base of umbilical cord	Amnionic bands	Chorionic plate will be devoid of amnion. May be associated with isolated amputations, various fetal anomalies or cord entanglement. Take photograph	14.24–14.29

Table 3.3. Macroscopic lesions of the fetal surface and chorionic plate (see Chaps. 14, 21, and 22).

Description	Diagnosis	Comment	Figure number
Plaques or nodules			
White, hydrophobic plaques	Squamous metaplasia	Adherent to surface. DDx: amnion nodosum	14.21a
Translucent, white or yellow nodules	Amnion nodosum	Can be scraped off. Due to oligohydramnios. DDx: squamous metaplasia	14.22
Oval, chalky disk, under amnion	Yolk sac remnant	Normal embryonic remnant	14.7a
Firm, white subchorionic nodules or plaques	Subchorionic fibrin/fibrinoid	Usually of no consequence	3.4, 3.8
Well-circumscribed, hemor-rhagic, fibrous or myxoid nodule	Chorangioma	Note size, consistency. Villous tissue may be pale due to associated hemorrhage	3.8, 22.1–22.4
Cyst	Subchorionic cyst	Usually of no consequence	14.4, 14.5

(continued)

Table 3.3. (continued)

Description	Diagnosis	Comment	Figure number
Plaques or nodules			
Hemorrhage or hematoma	Amnionic cyst	Usually of no consequence	14.2
	Subchorionic hematoma	Note size and % surface	3.8, 14.13
		If large, may be associated with demise	14.14
	Subamnionic hematoma	Usually iatrogenic	3.8, 14.11
		Look for source of bleeding – disrupted fetal vessels in chorionic plate (rare)	
Chorionic vessels			
White streak or firmness in vessel	Thrombosis	Extra sections of fetal surface vessels	21.1–21.3
		May be associated umbilical cord problems	
Dilated and tortuous vessels	Acute cord compression	May be associated with cord problems, e.g., hypercoiling, long cords, knots, entanglements, etc.	–
	Mesenchymal dysplasia	May be associated with cystically dilated villi	19.18a

DDx differential diagnosis.

Table 3.4. Macroscopic lesions of the umbilical cord (see Chap. 15).

Description	Diagnosis	Gross examination	Figure number
Insertion			
Insertion at placental margin	Marginal	Usually of no consequence unless there are associated velamentous vessels (velamentous insertion)	15.17
Insertion into/ within membranes	Velamentous	Measure from insertion to placental margin	15.17, 15.18, 15.21, 15.22
		Note disruption, hemorrhage or thrombosis of vessels	
		Submit separate membrane roll of velamentous vessels	
Cord divides before insertion	Furcate	Check that all vessels are intact	15.17, 15.19
Cord inserts and runs in membranes without branching	Interpositional	Usually of no consequence	15.17, 15.20
Length: **Normal 55 cm**			
<40 cm	Short cord	Difficult to diagnose without measurement of total cord length at delivery	–
>70–80 cm	Long cord	Check for associated chorionic plate vascular thrombosis	15.9
Diameter: **Normal 1–1.5 cm**			
Increased	Thick cord	If focal, may represent a cyst	15.10
		May be associated with diabetes, macrosomia or hydrops	

(continued)

Table 3.4. (continued)

Description	Diagnosis	Gross examination	Figure number
Diameter: **Normal 1-1.5cm**			
Decreased	Thin cord	May be associated with growth restriction	15.8
Focal constriction	Stricture	Measure diameter and take sections through stricture Check for associated chorionic plate vascular thrombosis	15.8
Knot	True knot	Document Loose or tight Congestion on one side of the knot If, after untying, cord stays coiled Take sections through untied knot	15.12, 15.13, 15.16
	False knot	Redundant vessels of no consequence	15.15
Twisting or coiling			
Excessive twist		Check for associated thrombosis or stricture May be associated with adverse outcome	15.6, 15.7
Minimal or no twist		May be associated with adverse outcome	15.6
Vessels: **Normally three**			
Two vessels	Single umbilical artery	Avoid sections near insertion site due to arterial anastomosis	15.23
Four vessels	Persistent vein	Avoid sections with false knots	–
Thrombosis	Thrombosis	Ensure it is not in an area of cord clamping or due to false knots Serially section and submit Take photograph	15.24
Discoloration: **Normal – white**			
Pink, red, or red-brown	Hemolysis	Usually due to fetal demise or freezing of the placenta	–
Brown, yellow-brown	Hemosiderin	Due to old bleeding	14.19a
Green or yellow-green	Meconium	Note if focal or diffuse Take extra sections of stained cord	14.15a
Yellow	Bile	Note in report May be due to maternal hyperbilirubinemia	14.18
Chalky deposits	Calcification	Usually due to infection – necrotizing funisitis	16.21
Mass			
Cyst	Embryonic remnants	Measure and take extra sections	15.2
White, tan, or yellow surface nodules	*Candida* infection	Take additional sections of lesions	16.16
Hemorrhage	Hemorrhage, hematoma, or hemangioma	Ensure it is not in an area of cord clamping	15.26, 15.27
Miscellaneous			
Edema	Edema	If localized, may represent a cyst May be associated with macrosomia or hydrops	15.10
Rupture	Rupture	Look for associated lesions that could explain rupture, such as hematoma, meconium, masses, etc.	15.26

Table 3.5. Macroscopic lesions of the maternal surface (see Chaps. 16, 18, and 19).

Description	Diagnosis	Comment	Figure number
White, chalky, stippled, gritty lesions	Calcifications	Normal finding	3.7
Shaggy, tan loosely adherent plaques	Decidual necrosis	Usually a nonspecific finding but may be associated with decidual vascular disease	–
Adherent blood clot	Retroplacental hematoma (abruptio placentae)	Note size and % of maternal surface involved Note compression of villous tissue Note if old or recent Note if there is an underlying infarct	3.8, 18.13, 18.14, 19.5, 19.6
	Marginal hematoma	Often due to ascending infection (acute chorioamnionitis) Note size and % of maternal surface involved Note compression of villous tissue	3.8 16.3
Yellow discoloration; firm, corrugated surface	Maternal floor infarction (massive perivillous fibrinoid)	Note % involvement of placental parenchyma Note if diffuse or multifocal	19.13 19.14
Firm, white or reddish lesions	Infarct, intervillous thrombus or fibrin deposition	Note size and % involvement Take extra sections of lesions	3.8, 18.7–18.9, 19.6

Table 3.6. Abnormalities of placental shape and macroscopic lesions of the villous tissue (see Chaps. 13, 18–23).

Description	Diagnosis	Comment	Figure number
Shape alterations			
Two equal lobes	Bilobed	Check membranous vessels to ensure they are intact and without thrombosis	13.1, 13.2
Two or more unequal lobes	Succenturiate lobe	Check membranous vessels to ensure they are intact and without thrombosis	13.1, 13.3
Extremely large, thin placenta	Membranacea	May be associated with bleeding and/or placenta accreta	13.1, 13.12
Membranes do not insert into placental margin	Circumvallate or circummarginate	Note if partial or complete Measure distance from insertion to placental margin	13.4–13.6, 13.8
	Extrachorial or extramembranous pregnancy	Measure distance from insertion to placental margin	13.9, 13.10
Full thickness defect in placenta	Fenestra	Usually of no consequence	13.1, 13.13
Ring shaped placenta	Zonary placenta	Usually of no consequence	13.1, 13.14

(continued)

Table 3.6. (continued)

Description	Diagnosis	Comment	Figure number
Diffuse lesions of villous tissue			
Firm, net-like, white deposits throughout villous tissue	Maternal floor infarction/massive perivillous fibrin deposition	Note extent – % of villous tissue involved Note if multifocal or diffuse Note involvement of maternal floor	19.15–19.17
Mottling of villous tissue	Chronic villitis	Usually very subtle Note the extent – % of villous tissue involved	3.8, 16.29
Focal lesions			
Well-circumscribed, round lesion with granular surface	Recent infarct (pink to red discoloration)	Note if single or multiple Note % of placenta involved	3.8, 18.8
	Old infarct (white discoloration)	Note if single or multiple Note % of placenta involved	3.8, 18.7–18.9, 19.6
Well-circumscribed, angular lesion with shiny surface	Intervillous thrombus	Usually of no consequence If large or multiple may be associated with fetomaternal hemorrhage	3.8 19.1 19.2
Well-circumscribed nodular lesion with consistency of blood clot, myxoid or "fibrous" tissue	Chorangioma	Benign hemangioma Usually of no consequence unless large	3.8, 22.1–22.4
Poorly demarcated white, granular lesion	Intervillous abscess	Associated with bacterial infection, most commonly *Listeria*	16.12
Cystically dilated villi	Mesenchymal dysplasia	Dilated, tortuous vessels on fetal surface may also be present	19.18a
	Hydatidiform moles	Additional sections should be taken Consider cytogenetics, flow cytometry, etc.	23.2, 23.3, 23.6
Nodular lesion with consistency of blood clot, myxoid or "fibrous" tissue	Chorangioma	Benign hemangioma	3.8, 22.1–22.4
	Chorangiomatosis	Multiple lesions – various clinical associations	19.10
Color of villous tissue – reflective of fetal hematocrit			
Pale	Fetal anemia	May be associated intervillous thrombi May be associated with fetomaternal hemorrhage or hydrops	20.1
	Twin-to-twin transfusion	Note type and size of vascular anastomoses	9.7, 10.13
Congestion	Villous congestion	May be associated with maternal diabetes or obstruction of venous return (possible umbilical cord problems)	17.3

Table 3.7. Normative values.

Pregnancy week postmenstrual	Crown–rump length (mm)	Foot length (cm)	Embryonic/ fetal weight (g)	Placental weight (g)	Fetal/ placental weight ratio	Placental thickness (cm)	Placental diameter (cm)	Umbilical cord length (cm)
3								
4								0.2
5	2.5							0.4
6	5							0.7
7	9							1.2
8	14		1.1	6	0.18			2.0
9	20		2	8	0.25			3.3
10	26		5	13	0.38			5.5
11	33		11	19	0.58			9.2
12	40		17	26	0.65			12.6
13	48	1.2	23	32	0.72		5.0	15.8
14	56	1.7	30	41	0.73	1.0	5.6	18.8
15	65	1.9	40	50	0.80	1.1	6.2	21.5
16	75	2.2	60	60	1.00	1.2	6.9	24.0
17	88	2.5	90	70	1.29	1.2	7.5	26.4
18	99	2.8	130	80	1.63	1.3	8.1	28.7
19	112	2.9	180	101	1.78	1.4	8.7	30.9
20	125	3.3	250	112	2.23	1.5	9.4	33.0
21	137	3.6	320	126	2.54	1.5	10.0	35.0
22	150	3.9	400	144	2.78	1.6	10.6	36.9
23	163	4.2	480	162	2.96	1.7	11.2	38.7
24	176	4.5	560	180	3.11	1.8	11.9	40.4
25	188	4.7	650	198	3.28	1.8	12.5	42.0
26	200	5.0	750	216	3.47	1.9	13.1	43.5
27	213	5.3	870	234	3.72	1.9	13.7	45.0
28	226	5.5	1,000	252	3.97	2.0	14.4	46.4
29	236	5.8	1,130	270	4.19	2.0	15.0	47.7
30	250	6.0	1,260	288	4.38	2.1	15.6	49.0
31	263	6.2	1,400	306	4.58	2.1	16.2	50.2
32	276	6.5	1,550	324	4.78	2.2	16.9	52.0
33	289	6.7	1,700	342	4.97	2.2	17.5	53.0
34	302	6.9	1,900	360	5.28	2.3	18.1	54.0
35	315	7.1	2,100	378	5.56	2.3	18.7	54.9
36	328	7.4	2,300	396	5.81	2.4	19.4	55.7
37	341	7.6	2,500	414	6.04	2.4	20.0	56.5
38	354	7.8	2,750	432	6.37	2.4	20.6	57.2
39	367	8.0	3,000	451	6.65	2.5	21.3	57.9
40	380	8.1	3,400	470	7.23	2.5	22.0	58.5

Portions of this table were modified from Kalousek et al. (1992)

Selected References

PHP5, pages 1–12 (Examination of the Placenta), pages 13–15 (Macroscopic Features of the Delivered Placenta).

Altshuler G, Deppisch LM. College of American Pathologists Conference XIX on the examination of the placenta: report of the working group on indications for placental examination. Arch Pathol Lab Med 1991;115;701–703.

Altshuler G, Hyde S. Clinicopathologic implications of placental pathology. Clin Obstet Gynecol 1996;39:549–570.

Baergen RN. Macroscopic examination of the placenta immediately following birth. J Nurse Midwif 1997;42:393–402.

Benirschke K. Examination of the placenta. Obstet Gynecol 1991;18:309–333.

Booth VJ, Nelson KB, Dambrosia JM, et al. What factors influence whether placentas are submitted for pathologic examination? Am J Obstet Gynecol 1997;176:567–571.

Gruenwald P. Examination of the placenta by the pathologist. Arch Pathol 1964;77:41–46.

Kalousek, DK, Baldwin VJ, Dimmick JE, et al. Embryofetal-perinatal autopsy and placental examination. In: Dimmick JE, Kalousek DK, eds. Developmental Pathology of the Embryo and Fetus. JB Lippincott, Philadelphia, 1992:55–82.

Kaplan CG. Color Atlas of Gross Placental Pathology, 2nd ed. Springer, New York, 2007.

Kaplan CG. Gross pathology of the placenta: weight, shape, size, colour. J Clin Pathol 2008;61:1285–1295.

Langston C, Kaplan C, MacPherson T, et al. Practice guidelines for examination of the placenta. Developed by the placental pathology practice guideline development task force of the College of American Pathologists. Arch Pathol Lab Med 1997;121:449–476.

Naeye RL. Functionally important disorders of the placenta, umbilical cord, and fetal membranes. Hum Pathol 1987;18:680–691.

Chapter 4

Microscopic Evaluation of the Second- and Third-Trimester Placenta

Approach to the Specimen

A systematic and straightforward approach to microscopic examination of the placenta is to review each part of the placenta separately and in a specific order, which will ensure that no area or structure is omitted. It is thus convenient to review the extraplacental fetal membranes, umbilical cord, and placental disk separately. To this end, each component of the placenta is listed below with specific features that should be evaluated and possible abnormalities that may be present. Tables at the end of the chapter list lesions along with a microscopic description, possible diagnoses, and the location in the text where figures depicted the abnormality or feature can be found.

Fetal membranes (Table 4.1):

- **General:**
  - macrophages, which may contain pigment such as hemosiderin or meconium
  - acute or chronic inflammatory cells
  - bacteria
  - hematoma or other masses
- **Amnionic epithelium** (Fig. 4.1):
  - "metaplastic" change to keratinized stratified squamous epithelium
  - degenerative changes, piling up of cells, sloughing, or cytoplasmic vacuolization
  - deposition of amniotic fluid debris

R.N. Baergen, *Manual of Pathology of the Human Placenta,*
DOI 10.1007/978-1-4419-7494-5_4, © Springer Science+Business Media, LLC 2011

Epithelial Abnormalities

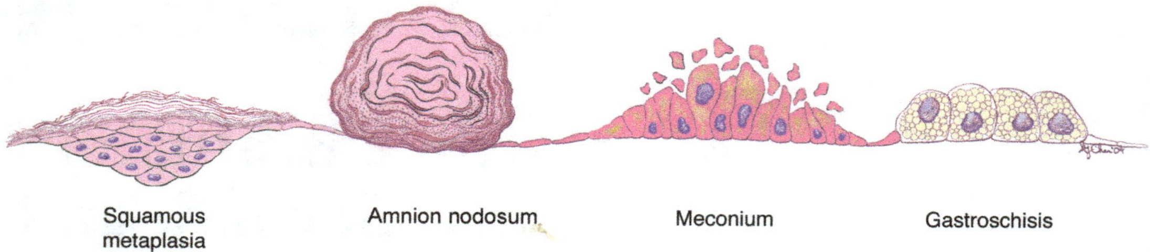

Figure 4.1.   Various epithelial abnormalities of the amnionic epithelium are depicted. These lesions are referenced and described in Table 4.1.

- **Decidua capsularis:**
  - necrosis, inflammation
  - abnormalities of vessels such as thickening, necrosis, inflammation, or thrombosis

Umbilical cord (Table 4.2):
- **General:**
  - edema
  - ulceration
  - inflammation
  - calcification
  - hemorrhage
  - masses including hematoma, tumors, cysts, or epithelial remnants

- **Umbilical vessels:**
  - single umbilical artery or second umbilical vein
  - disruption
  - thinning of the wall
  - degeneration of smooth muscle
  - thrombosis

Placental disk:

- **Chorionic plate** (Table 4.3):
  - masses, cysts, hematomas
  - excessive fibrinoid
  - fetal membranes of chorionic plate (see above)
- **Chorionic and stem vessels** (Table 4.3):
  - inflammation
  - thrombosis or other vascular lesions
- **Intervillous space** (Table 4.4):
  - intervillous thrombosis
  - excessive fibrinoid
  - cellular infiltrate including:
    - (a) inflammatory cells
    - (b) abnormal or atypical cells

- **Chorionic villi** (Table 4.5):
  - size and morphology:
    - (a) appropriate for gestational age
    - (b) enlarged (delayed maturation) or small (hypermature)
    - (c) increased or decreased syncytial knots
  - simplified outlines, invaginations or irregularities of the surface
  - hydropic change
  - ischemic change or infarction
- **Villous stroma** (Table 4.5):
  - inflammatory cell infiltrate
  - microcalcification
  - edema
  - hyalinization
  - hemorrhage
- **Villous capillaries** (Table 4.5):
  - increased or decreased
  - thrombosis
  - disruption or extravasation of red blood cells into the stroma
- **Basal plate including decidua basalis** (Table 4.6):
  - excessive fibrinoid
  - necrosis
  - chronic inflammation with plasma cells
  - hematoma

- **Decidual vessels** (Table 4.6):
  - thrombosis
  - other vasculopathy

Abnormalities in each area of the placenta should be noted and the findings correlated with all other findings and with the clinical history if possible. See Tables 4.1–4.6 for more specific information on each lesion and corresponding figures for more specific information. Certain clinical conditions are associated with specific placental lesions and the most common are listed in Table 4.7.

Routine and Special Stains

For histological examination, the standard **hematoxylin and eosin (H&E)** stain is usually adequate. Special stains such as trichrome or mucin rarely have use in diagnostic placental pathology. On some occasions, however, it is useful to employ special stains for microorganisms. These include tissue **Gram stains**, silver stains such as **Warthin-Starry, Steiner,** or **Gomori methenamine silver stains**, or **periodic acid–Schiff** (PAS), **Giemsa,** and **acid-fast stains**. However, generally speaking, bacterial organisms causing acute chorioamnionitis are difficult to identify in tissue sections even if special stains are performed. Specific immunohistochemical stains that disclose the presence of viruses, e.g., cytomegalovirus and herpes antigens, are sometimes helpful if a specific organism is suspected. Thus, immunohistochemistry may be helpful in identification of specific organisms causing chronic villitis and congenital infections. See Chap. 16 for more information on specific infections.

Immunohistochemical Markers

Immunohistochemical stains may be used for reasons other than identification of infectious organisms. First, certain stains are used to differentiate trophoblastic cells from other cells, particularly in the setting of trophoblastic disease (see Chapts. 24 and 25). Since *all trophoblastic cells are epithelial*, they will stain strongly positive for all **cytokeratins**. There are many different antibodies on the market, most of which work well in paraffin sections. These include **AE1/AE3, CAM 5.2,** and others. The *amnionic epithelium* will also stain for these antibodies. *Syncytiotrophoblasts* stain strongly for **human chorionic gonadotropin (hCG),** while *extravillous trophoblastic cells* are either negative or weakly positive. Extravillous trophoblast stain for **human placental lactogen (hPL), placental alkaline phosphatase (PLAP), α-inhibin, Mel-CAM,** and **placental protein 19 (PP19).** Some of these markers are able to differentiate different types of extravillous trophoblast (see Chap. 25 for more specific information). **Anti-vimentin** antibodies stain all mesenchymal-derived cells such as *connective tissue cells, macrophages, decidual cells, smooth muscle cells, and endothelial cells.* Generally, most cells in the placenta will be positive for either cytokeratin or vimentin. **Vimentin** will also stain decidual cells as they are stromal in origin, and so *vimentin and cytokeratin are useful markers in distinguishing extravillous trophoblast, particularly intraarterial trophoblast, from decidual cells in the implantation site.* Therefore, they may often be used together and are particularly helpful in possible ectopic pregnancies to document or rule out intrauterine pregnancy.

The antibodies **Ki-67, MIB-1,** and **anti-PCNA** (clones PC10, 19A2, 19F4) bind to nuclear proteins and are expressed in proliferating cells. Ki-67 is only applicable on frozen sections, but MIB-1 is its analogue and works wells in both formalin-fixed paraffin sections as well as frozen sections. Anti-PCNA can be used only for paraffin material. These antibodies are useful markers *to distinguish proliferating stem cell populations from differentiated ones and identifying growth zones.* They are also useful in the differential diagnosis of trophoblastic lesions, particularly lesions of extravillous trophoblast (see Chap. 25).

Other immunohistochemical stains may be helpful when abnormal or atypical cells are present in the intervillous space. The differential diagnosis of these lesions is generally between a metastatic malignancy to the placenta from the mother (see Chap. 17) and choriocarcinoma (see Chap. 22). In this case, characterization of these cells with immunohistochemistry is usually necessary.

Table 4.1. Lesions of the fetal membranes (see Chap. 14).

Description	Diagnosis	Comment	Figure number
Pigment in macrophages			
Yellow-brown	Meconium	Often associated with degenerative change of the amnion	4.1, 14.15b 14.16
Brown, particulate, refringent	Hemosiderin	Look for source of bleeding – often from decidua Iron stain may be needed to confirm	14.19b
Inflammation – see also Table 16.1			
	Acute inflammatory cells	Acute chorioamnionitis Gram stain done rarely – usually negative	16.4, 16.5
	Chronic inflammatory cells	Chronic chorioamnionitis May be associated with chronic villitis Often only present in decidua	16.20, 16.32
	Acute inflammatory cells with necrosis	Subacute chorioamnionitis – acute chorioamnionitis of longer duration	16.10
Hemorrhage	Retromembranous hematoma	May be associated with rupture of membranes, but usually nonspecific finding	14.12
Cyst			
Epithelial	Amnionic cyst	No clinical significance	14.1
Squamous	Epidermoid cyst	No clinical significance	14.2
Extravillous trophoblast	Subchorionic cyst	No clinical significance	14.3
Epithelial change			
Squamous change	Squamous metaplasia	Normal finding near term	4.1, 14.21b
Anucleate squames and debris forming nodules	Amnion nodosum	Usually secondary to severe oligohydramnios and associated with fetal renal anomalies	4.1, 14.23
Vacuolization	Gastroschisis	Specific finding associated with gastroschisis	4.1, 14.20
Degenerative change of epithelium	Meconium	Degenerative change may indicate that meconium discharge is more remote	4.1, 14.16

(continued)

Table 4.1. (continued)

Description	Diagnosis	Comment	Figure number
Miscellaneous			
Cartilage, bone, skin	Teratoma	May represent acardiac twin	–
	Embryonic remnants	No clinical significance	–
	Fetus papyraceous	Document and identify membranes relationships if possible	10.4
Anucleate squames and debris	Vernix caseosa	No clinical significance Often occurs with membrane rupture	14.9, 14.10
Necrotic tissue	Decidual necrosis	May be associated with decidual vasculopathy or hemorrhage but often non-specific	–
Inflammation in decidua	Acute deciduitis	May be associated with acute chorioamnionitis, otherwise is non-specific	16.6
	Chronic deciduitis	May be associated with chronic villitis Diagnosis usually made only with intense infiltrate and/or presence of plasma cells	16.20
Abnormal vessels	Decidual vasculopathy	May be associated with other changes of placental malperfusion	18.1–18.5

Table 4.2. Umbilical cord (see Chap. 15).

Description	Diagnosis	Comment	Figure number
Skin, cartilage, bone	Teratoma	May represent an acardiac twin	–
Vessels	Hemangioma	May be associated with hematoma or rupture	15.25
Epithelial elements	Embryonic remnants	Allantoic duct remnant Omphalomesenteric duct remnant Vitelline vessel remnant	15.1 15.3–15.5

(continued)

Table 4.2. (continued)

Description	Diagnosis	Comment	Figure number
Edema	Focal – embryonic cyst	Usually develops from embryonic remnants	15.2
	Diffuse – edema	May be associated with fetal hydrops	15.10
Acute inflammation	Acute funisitis	Fetal inflammatory response	16.7
See also Table 16.1	*Candida* infection	Focal lesions of umbilical cord surface	16.17
		Usually not associated with acute chorioamnionitis	
		PAS or Gomori methenamine silver (GMS) to confirm	
	Necrotizing funisitis	May be associated with calcification	16.8 16.22
		Classically seen in syphilis but may be seen in other infections	
Pigmented macrophages	Meconium	Meconium filled macrophages rarely identified in cord despite gross staining	–
		May be associated with myonecrosis of umbilical vascular smooth muscle	
Single umbilical artery	Single umbilical artery	May be associated with other fetal anomalies	15.23
Four umbilical vessels	Super- numerary vessel	Rare, may be associated with fetal anomalies	–
Thrombosis	Thrombosis	Often associated with thrombosis in chorionic or stem vessels	15.24b
Hemorrhage	Hematoma	May be associated with other cord lesions	15.27
		May compress umbilical vessels (particularly the umbilical vein) leading to vascular embarrassment	
Thinned vessels	Varix or aneurysm	May lead to hemorrhage or rupture	15.30
Vascular necrosis	Meconium induced ascular necrosis	Usually due to prolonged meconium exposure in utero	14.17

Table 4.3. Chorionic plate (see Chaps. 14, 21, and 22).

Description	Diagnosis	Comment	Figure number
Focal lesions			
Oval, lacy structure	Yolk sac remnant	Embryonic remnant of no clinical significance	1.8, 14.7b
Fetal skeleton	Fetus papyraceous	Note membrane relationship if possible	10.4
Fibrinoid	Subchorionic fibrinoid	If excessive, may be ssociated with placental malperfusion or maternal floor infarction	3.4
Cyst	Subchorionic cyst	Usually of no clinical significance	14.6
Hematoma	Subchorionic hematoma	If large, may be associated with stillbirth	–
	Subamnionic hematoma	Fresh blood under amnion, most commonly an artifact secondary to excessive traction on cord during delivery Rarely due to disruption of fetal chorionic vessels	–
Vascular mass	Chorangioma	Benign vascular neoplasm – similar to hemangioma	22.5–22.7
Chorionic vessels			
Thrombosis	Thrombosis	Look for other associated thrombotic lesions in villous tissue: avascular villi, villous stromal karyorrhexis	21.4–21.7 21.10
Inflammation See also Table 16.1	Acute chorioam-nionitis	Ascending infection May be associated with thrombosis	16.4 16.5 16.9
	Chronic chori-oamnionitis	Often associated with chronic villitis	16.32
	Subacute chorioam-nionitis	Due to long standing ascending infection	16.10
Degeneration of muscle	Meconium induced damage	Usually due to long standing meconium	14.17

Table 4.4. Intervillous space.

Description	Diagnosis	Comment	Figure number
Blood clot	Intervillous thrombus	If large or multiple, may be associated with fetomaternal hemorrhage	3.8 19.3
Fibrin/fibrinoid	Increased perivillous fibrin	If excessive, may represent maternal floor infarction	19.12 19.15 19.16 19.17
Inflammation – see also Tables 16.1 and 16.2	Intervillous abscess	Most commonly due to *Listeria* infection. Rarely due to maternal sepsis	3.8 16.13
	Chronic intervillositis	Idiopathic disorder with infiltrate of histiocytes and lymphocytes	16.33
Abnormal or atypical cells	Malignancy – fetal or maternal metastatic	Cells may present as clusters in intervillous space or invade villi. Immunohistochemistry may be necessary for specific diagnosis	3.8 22.8–22.10
	Intraplacental choriocarcinoma	Markedly atypical syncytiotrophoblast and cytotrophoblast	24.10–24.12
Collapse of intervillous space	Early villous ischemic change	Often associated with infarction	18.10
Expansion of intervillous space	Villous hypoplasia – terminal villus deficiency	Often associated with other changes of placental malperfusion	18.16

Table 4.5. Chorionic villi.

Description	Diagnosis	Comment	Figure number
Villous morphology			
Increased syncytial knots	Increased syncytial knots	Associated with placental malperfusion	18.15 18.17
Delayed maturation	Villous immaturity	Associated with maternal diabetes. May be associated with IUGR, IUFD	17.4

(continued)

Table 4.5. (continued)

Description	Diagnosis	Comment	Figure number
Villous morphology			
Straight, unbranched villi	Villous hypoplasia/ terminal villus deficiency	Indicative of profound decrease in perfusion Usually associated with abnormal Doppler (absent or reversed end diastolic flow)	18.15 18.16
Invagination, irregular contour	Trophoblastic inclusions	Suggestive of chromosomal defect Also seen in hydatidiform moles	11.7 23.9
Clear space inside villi	Cisterns	Hydatidiform moles Beckwith–Wiedemann syndrome Mesenchymal dysplasia	23.4 20.6 19.19
Degeneration, smudging of nuclei	Ischemia	Evidence of early infarction Associated with placental malperfusion	18.11
Ghost villi	Infarction	Old infarction	18.12
Vacuolization of trophoblast or other cells	Storage disorder	Various cells may show vacuolization See Table 20.1	20.9
Trophoblastic proliferation	Hydatidiform mole	Associated with hydropic villous change See Tables 23.2 and 23.3	23.4 23.5 23.8 23.9 23.10 23.12
Edema	Villous edema	Focal villous edema (if diffuse, may be seen in hydrops – see below)	19.21 20.5
Villous stroma			
Inflammation See also Tables 16.1 and 16.2	Acute villitis	Generally due to *Listeria* infection May be due to maternal sepsis	16.13
	Chronic villitis	Differential diagnosis is chronic villitis of unknown etiology versus infectious etiology	16.18 16.19 16.23 16.25 16.30 16.31
Fine stippled calcification of stroma or basement membrane	Microcalcification	Seen in fetal death, twin–twin transfusion and hydrops	20.13
Hyalinization of stroma	Avascular villi	Associated with thrombosis in fetal circulation	21.8

(continued)

Table 4.5. (continued)

Description	Diagnosis	Comment	Figure number
Villous stroma			
Hemorrhage	Intravillous hemorrhage	May be secondary to acute injury, ischemia, abruption	19.4
Red blood cells in stroma	Villous stromal karyorrhexis/ hemorrhagic endovasculopathy	Generally associated with other thrombotic lesions	19.4 21.12 21.13
Edema or hydropic change	Mesenchymal dysplasia	Developmental abnormality of villous tissue Also associated with tortuous chorionic vessels	19.19
	Molar pregnancy	Marked hydropic change Trophoblastic hyperplasia is necessary for the diagnosis – see Tables 23.2 and 23.3	23.4 23.5 23.8 23.9 23.10 23.12
	Villous edema	May be secondary to acute injury or ischemia	19.21 20.5
	Villous immaturity	Diffuse villous immaturity for gestational age	19.20
	Hydropic abortus	Seen in early pregnancy and may be confused with a hydatidiform mole	11.8 11.9 23.11
	Hydrops	Placental and/or fetal hydrops (diffuse edema) May be secondary to etomaternal hemorrhage	20.2 20.3
	Immature intermediate villi	Residual immature villi in term placenta may be confused with villous edema	7.4
Villous capillaries			
Increased vessels	Diffuse – chorangiosis	Placental response to hypoxia	19.8
	Multifocal – chorangiomatosis	Focal, segmental, or multinodular diffuse	19.11
	Single lesion– chorangioma	Localized lesion – increased capillaries representing a benign neoplasm	22.5–22.7
	Diffuse – congestion	Not true increase in vessels but may be confused with chorangiosis Associated with decreased venous return and maternal diabetes	19.9
Disruption of vessels	Villous stromal karyorrhexis/ hemorrhagic endovasculopathy	Associated with disruption of vessels and extravasated red blood cells and thrombosis	21.11– 21.13
Thrombosis	Thrombosis	May be associated with other thrombotic lesions	21.12 21.13
Nucleated red blood cells	Nucleated red blood cells	Fetal response to hypoxia or anemia	20.7

Table 4.6. Basal plate.

Description	Diagnosis	Comment	Figure number
Increased fibrinoid	Maternal floor infarction – massive perivillous fibrin deposition	Some fibrinoid is normal. If excessive may represent a "maternal floor infarction". May be associated with proliferation of extravillous trophoblast	19.12 19.15 19.16 19.17
Necrosis	Decidual necrosis	Look for associated lesions such as hemorrhage or decidual vasculopathy	–
Inflammation	Acute deciduitis	May be associated with acute chorioamnionitis	16.6
	Chronic deciduitis	May be associated with chronic villitis	16.20
Hemorrhage	Retroplacental hematoma	Underlying tissue may be ischemic or infarcted. May be associated with other changes of placental malperfusion	3.8 18.14 19.7
Abnormal vessels	Decidual vasculopathy	Usually associated with other changes of placental malperfusion	18.1–18.5
Adherent myometrium	Placenta accreta	Diagnosis based on lack of decidua between chorionic villi and myometrium	12.6

Table 4.7. Placental lesions in specific clinical situations.

Clinical situation	Placental conditions	Maternal conditions	Fetal conditions
Preterm delivery	Placental malperfusion Infarction Decreased weight Retroplacental hematoma Circumvallate membrane insertion Maternal floor infarction Acute chorioamnionitis	Poor nutrition Uterine anomalies	Fetal anomalies

(continued)

Table 4.7. (continued)

Clinical situation	Placental conditions	Maternal conditions	Fetal conditions
Intrauterine growth restriction	Maternal floor infarction Villitis of unknown etiology Fetal thrombotic vasculopathy Shape abnormalities Umbilical cord Excessively long cord Velamentous insertion	Drug use Tobacco Alcohol Poor nutrition Uterine anomalies Systemic disease Diabetes mellitus with vascular disease Preeclampsia Gestational hypertension Renovascular disease Autoimmune disease Thrombophilias	Genetic conditions Confined placental mosaicism Chromosomal disorders Genetic disorders
Intrauterine fetal demise	Maternal floor infarction Villitis of unknown etiology Fetal thrombotic vasculopathy Abruptio placentae Umbilical cord Entanglement True knots Torsion Constriction Rupture Excessive length or twisting Velamentous insertion and rupture	Systemic disease Diabetes mellitus with vascular disease Preeclampsia Gestational hypertension Renovascular disease Autoimmune disease Thrombophilias	Infection TORCH Ascending infection Fetomaternal hemorrhage

TORCH toxoplasmosis, other agents, rubella, cytomegalovirus, and herpes simplex titer

Selected References

PHP5, pages 16–29 (Microscopic Survey).

Benirschke K. Examination of the placenta. Obstet Gynecol 1961;18:309–333.

Khong TY, Lane EB, Robertson WB. An immunocytochemical study of fetal cells at the maternal-placental interface using monoclonal antibodies to keratins, vimentin and desmin. Cell Tissue Res 1986;246:189–195.

Naeye RL. Functionally important disorders of the placenta, umbilical cord and fetal membranes. Hum Pathol 1987;18:680–691.

Section II

Development and Normal Histology

This section presents the development and histology of the normal placenta. Chapter 5 discusses the early development of the placenta. Normal histology of chorionic villi is covered in Chap. 6, along with a discussion of the development of different villous types, including mesenchymal villi, immature intermediate villi, mature intermediate villi, stem villi, and terminal villi. Chapter 7 provides an overview and microscopic survey of both the first-trimester placenta and placentas of the second or third trimester. Histology of the fetal membranes, umbilical cord, the placentone (placental lobule), and the intervillous space are also presented here. Finally, Chap. 8, covers histology and development of the extravillous trophoblast and components of the implantation site such as decidua, fibrinoid, and uteroplacental vessels.

Chapter 5
Early Placental Development

General Considerations

For many years, it was thought that the understanding of placental pathology required only a limited knowledge of implantation and early placental development, as disturbances of these early steps of placentation seemed to cause abortion, rather than affecting placental structure and function. Increasing experience with assisted reproductive technology (ART), as well as clinicopathologic correlation of placental pathology with fetal well-being, however, has taught us that improper conditions during implantation can handicap early development and result in inappropriate functioning of the fetoplacental unit and impaired outcome. For this reason, basic understanding of early placental development has become increasingly important.

Prelacunar Stage: Day 1–8 Postconception

The **prelacunar stage** is defined as the period from conception to day 8 PC (postconception). After fertilization, the zygote develops into a **blastocyst,** a flattened vesicle composed of between 107 and 256 cells.

R.N. Baergen, *Manual of Pathology of the Human Placenta,*
DOI 10.1007/978-1-4419-7494-5_5, © Springer Science+Business Media, LLC 2011

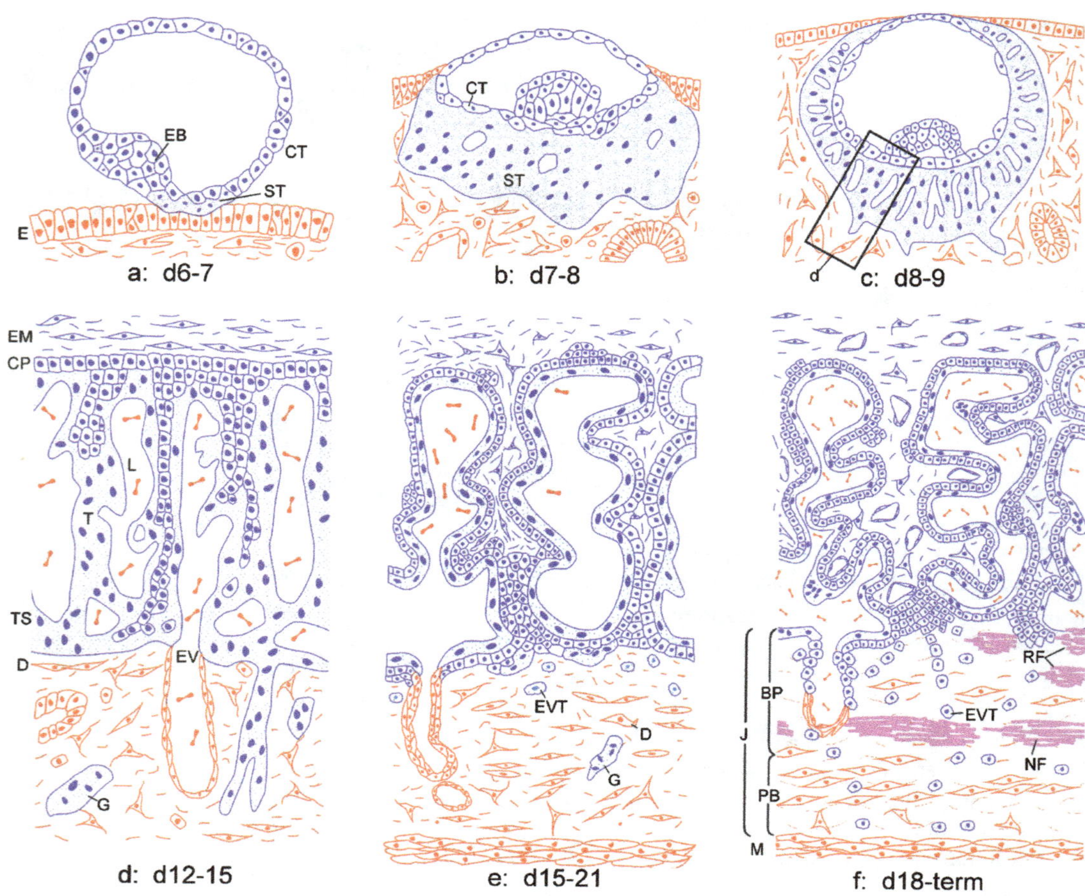

Figure 5.1. Simplified drawings of the stages of early placental development. (**a, b**) Prelacunar stages. (**c**) Lacunar stage. (**d**) Transition from lacunar to primary villous stage. (**e**) Secondary villous stage. (**f**) Tertiary villous stage. Note that the basal segments of the anchoring villi (**e, f**) consist only of trophoblast and form cell columns. All maternal tissues are in *red*, and all fetal tissues are in *blue*. *E* endometrial epithelium, *EB* embryoblast, *CT* cytotrophoblast, *ST* syncytiotrophoblast, *EM* extraembryonic mesoderm, *CP* primary chorionic plate, *T* trabeculae and primary villi, *L* maternal blood lacunae, *TS* trophoblastic shell, *EV* endometrial vessel, *D* decidua, *RF* Rohr's fibrinoid, *NF* Nitabuch's or uteroplacental fibrinoid, *G* trophoblastic giant cell, *x* X-cells or extravillous cytotrophoblast, *BP* basal plate, *PB* placental bed, *J* junctional zone, *M* myometrium (modified from Kaufmann and Scheffen 1992, with permission).

The cells of the outer wall are the **trophoblast**, which surround the **blastocystic cavity** (Fig. 5.1a). The **inner cell mass** is a small group of larger cells on the inner surface. The trophoblast is the forerunner of the placenta, while the inner cell mass forms the **embryoblast**, from which the embryo, umbilical cord, and amnion are derived. Both embryoblast-derived mesenchyme and embryoblast-derived blood vessels contribute to the formation of the connective tissue and blood vessels of the chorionic villi.

The first step in implantation of the **blastocyst** is called apposition and takes place around day 6–7 PC. In most cases, the blastocyst is oriented so that the **embryonic pole** attaches to the endometrium, thus forming the **implantation pole**. If, during implantation, the blastocyst rotates so that the embryonic pole and the implantation pole are not identical, abnormal cord insertions will occur (see Chap. 15). The **implantation window** is a short, specific phase during which attachment of the blastocyst occurs. To find or to generate this window is the most important prerequisite for successful implantation in in vitro fertilization and other forms of ART.

In the following days, the trophoblastic cells proliferate to form a double layer as they progressively invade the endometrial epithelium. *The inner layer, which does not initially contact the maternal tissues, is composed of* **cytotrophoblast**. *The outer layer, facing the maternal tissue, becomes the* **syncytiotrophoblast** by fusion of neighboring cytotrophoblastic cells (Fig. 5.1b). The syncytiotrophoblast is a continuous system, not interrupted by intercellular spaces and is thus not composed of individual cells or units (see Chap. 6). At the implantation pole, the syncytial mass forms branching, finger-like extensions that deeply invade, and interdigitate with, the endometrium. This is the **trophoblastic shell**.

Lacunar Stage: Day 8–13 Postconception

On day 8 PC, *small vacuoles appear in the syncytiotrophoblastic mass*. The vacuoles grow and become confluent, forming a system of **lacunae** (Fig. 5.1b, c). The lacunae are separated from each other by bands of syncytiotrophoblast, called **trabeculae**. The syncytiotrophoblastic mass and the lacunar system expand circumferentially over the entire blastocystic surface. By day 12 PC, the blastocyst is deeply implanted and the uterine epithelium closes over the implantation site. The cytotrophoblastic cells extend into the trabeculae and, by day 13 PC, reach the trophoblastic shell, eventually coming into contact with the endometrium (Fig. 5.1d–f).

Trophoblastic proliferation and syncytial fusion start at the implantation pole, making the trophoblast thicker here. This area of preferential growth is *later transformed into the placental disk*. The opposing thinner trophoblastic circumference eventually *atrophies and becomes the smooth chorion*, or the **chorion laeve**. At this point, the trophoblastic covering of the blastocyst is divided into three layers (Fig. 5.1c, d):

- The **primary chorionic plate**, facing the blastocystic cavity
- The **lacunar system** including the trabeculae
- The **trophoblastic shell**, facing the endometrium

Primary Chorionic Plate

The **primary chorionic plate** is composed of cytotrophoblast covered by syncytiotrophoblast on the "maternal" side (Fig. 5.1d). On day 14 PC, **embryonic mesenchyme** spreads around the inner surface of the blastocyst cavity and cytotrophoblast layer. This forms a *triple-layered chorionic plate composed of mesenchyme, cytotrophoblast, and syncytiotrophoblast*. At the same time, the first villous outgrowths form from the trabeculae (Fig. 5.1d, e). The trabeculae are henceforth called the **villous stems, which** later become the stem villi. The lacunar system is transformed into the **intervillous space**. The chorionic plate creates a "lid" over the intervillous space and serves as the base from which the villous trees are suspended.

Lacunar System

Below the primary chorionic plate is the **lacunar system** (Fig. 5.1c). Around day 12 PC the trabeculae are invaded by cytotrophoblastic cells (Fig. 5.1d) from the primary chorionic plate. At the maternal surface, *the trabeculae join together to form the* **trophoblastic shell**. The syncytiotrophoblast is present at the "luminal" surface of the lacunae; below that is a zone of cytotrophoblast. Below the latter and facing the endometrial connective tissue is an additional discontinuous layer of syncytiotrophoblastic elements.

During the early stages of implantation, erosion of the maternal tissues occurs under the lytic influence of the syncytial trophoblast. Subsequently, there is proliferation and migration of trophoblast, resulting in deep invasion of the endometrium and superficial myometrium. This is accomplished by *multinucleated and mononucleated trophoblastic elements far removed from the trophoblastic shell* – the **extravillous trophoblast**. The extravillous trophoblast are intimately involved in development of the implantation site including invasion and remodeling of the decidual vessels (see Chap. 8). Meanwhile, the endometrial stromal cells transform into the **decidual cells**. On day 12 PC, invading trophoblast cause disintegration of the endometrial vessel walls and the expanding extravillous trophoblast replaces the capillary walls in a stepwise fashion, from beginning to end.

Trophoblastic Shell

Around day 12 PC, as the cytotrophoblast expands into the trabeculae, the distal ends of the trabeculae join together and form the outermost layer of the trophoblast, the **trophoblastic shell**. Initially, this is a syncytiotrophoblastic structure, but when the cytotrophoblast reaches the shell at about day 15 PC, the shell becomes more heterogeneous (Fig. 5.1e). The syncytiotrophoblast face the lacunae, followed by cytotrophoblast and then a discontinuous layer of syncytiotrophoblastic elements facing the endometrial connective tissue. From day 22 PC onward, the term **trophoblastic shell** is usually replaced by **basal plate**, a term that includes the base of the intervillous space together with all placental and maternal tissues that adhere to it after parturition.

Early Villous Stage: Day 13–28 Postconception

In the early villous stage, cytotrophoblast invades the trabeculae, and **trophoblastic sprouts** grow into the lacunae to form the **primary villi** (Fig. 5.1d, e). *Primary villi are composed only of an outer layer of syncytiotrophoblast and a core of cytotrophoblast.* Their presence marks the beginning of the villous stages of placentation. Further proliferation and subsequent branching initiate the development of primitive **villous trees**, the stems of which are derived from the former trabeculae (Fig. 5.1e). The villi that keep their contact to the trophoblastic shell are called **anchoring villi**. Subsequently, cells derived from the mesenchymal layer of the primary chorionic plate invade the villi, transforming them into **secondary villi** (Fig. 5.1e). *Secondary villi consist of an outer layer of syncytiotrophoblast, an inner layer of cytotrophoblast, and a core of connective tissue.* Within a few days, the mesenchyme expands peripherally to the villous tips. The expanding villous mesenchyme does not completely reach the trophoblastic shell. Clusters of cytotrophoblast surrounded by an incomplete layer of syncytiotrophoblast persist as **cell columns** (Fig. 5.1e, f). They are places of *longitudinal growth of the anchoring villi as well as sources of extravillous trophoblast.* Focally, the villous tips of free-floating villi may not be invaded by villous mesenchyme, and these become the **trophoblastic cell islands** (see Chap. 8).

The first **fetal capillaries** appear in the villi on day 18–20 PC. They are derived from hemangioblastic progenitor cells, which locally differentiate from the mesenchyme. *The appearance of capillaries in the villous stroma marks the development of the first* **tertiary villi**. When enough capillary segments are fused with each other to form a capillary bed, a complete fetoplacental circulation is established. This occurs at the beginning of the fifth week.

The early villous trees expand in the following way: At the surfaces of the larger villi, cytotrophoblastic cells proliferate and subsequent syncytial fusion produces **syncytial (trophoblastic) sprouts**. These *sprouts are comparable to the early primary villi* as they consist of only cytotrophoblast and syncytiotrophoblast. Most degenerate, but a few are invaded by villous mesenchyme and transformed into **villous sprouts**, which *are comparable to the secondary villi.* Fetal vessels then form within the stroma, *similar to the development of tertiary villi.* Fetal and maternal blood comes into close contact with each other as soon as a fetoplacental circulation is established. The two bloodstreams are always separated by the **placental barrier** (see Fig. 6.1), which is composed of **syncytiotrophoblast, cytotrophoblast, basal lamina, connective tissue**, and **fetal endothelium**. In the last trimester, the cytotrophoblast is discontinuous and the fetal endothelium is surrounded by endothelial basal lamina.

Second Month and Beyond

Starting with the second month PC (Fig. 5.2), the connective tissue layer of the chorionic plate becomes more densely fibrotic and fibrous tissue extends into the villous stems. Subsequently, the tertiary villi undergo a complex process of differentiation that results in various villous types, which differ from each other in structure and function (see Chap. 7). With maturation, the *syncytiotrophoblast is reduced in thickness and the cytotrophoblast becomes rarefied.* The *mean villous diameter decreases, and the fetal capillaries are more numerous and closer to the villous surfaces.* This results in considerable reduction of the thickness of the placental barrier and thus a reduction in the mean maternofetal diffusion distance.

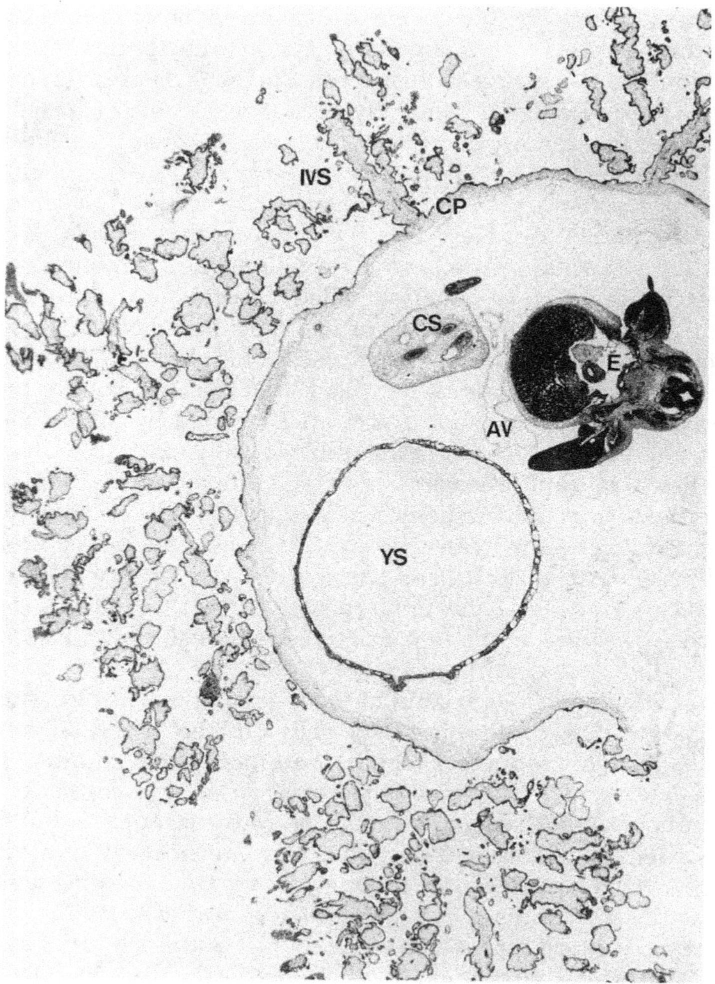

Figure 5.2. Semithin section across embryo and placenta of the fourth week after conception. Underneath the embryo (E), one can identify the connective stalk (C) as precursor of the cord, the yolk sac (YS), and a small amnionic vesicle (AV). The chorionic cavity is surrounded by the chorionic plate (CP); from the latter, numerous placental villi protrude into the surrounding intervillous space (IVS). The basal plate is missing in this specimen (×9.5) (from Kaufmann 1990, with permission).

Development of the Fetal Membranes

Depending on its spatial relation to the implanting chorionic sac, the decidua is subdivided into several segments (Fig. 5.3). The decidua at the implantation site, below the blastocyst and later the placenta, is the **basal decidua** or **decidua basalis**. When the embryo becomes completely embedded in the endometrial wall, the decidua closes over the blastocyst. Growth of the embryo and placenta causes the decidua to *protrude* into the uterine cavity. This protruding portion of the decidua, which has lost a direct connection with the uterine wall, is the

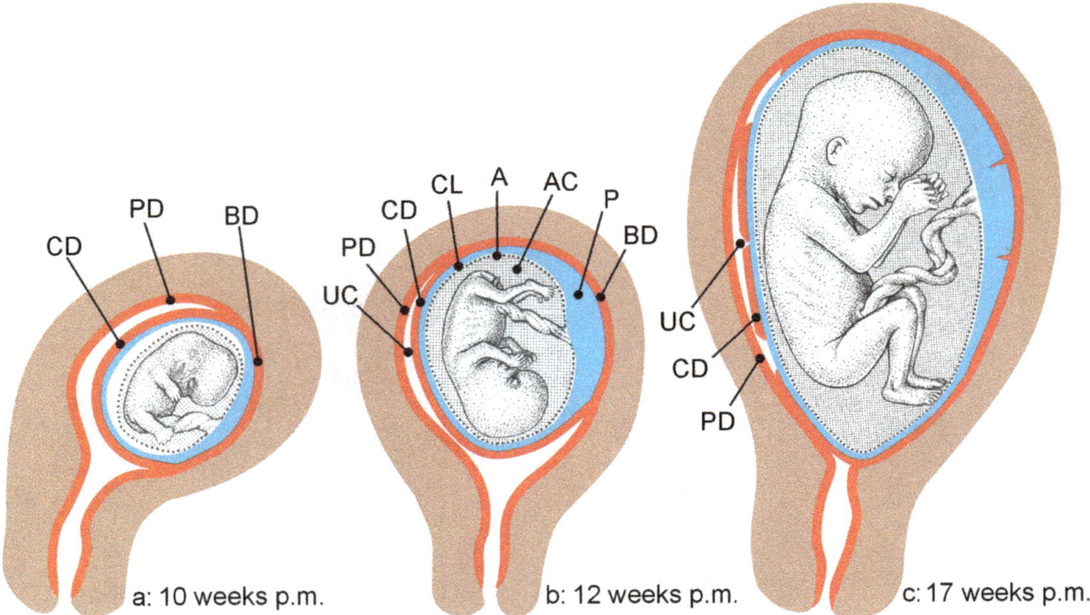

Figure 5.3. Development of the fetal membranes. The fetus and amnion are *black,* trophoblast is *blue,* decidua is *red,* and myometrium is *brown.* (**a**) Up to 10 weeks postmenstruation, the embryo is surrounded by the chorion frondosum (*blue*); later, it develops into the chorion laeve and the placenta or chorion frondosum, indicated on the diagram by only a slight thickening. The capsular part of the chorion frondosum is covered by the capsular decidua (CD), which is continuous with basal decidua (BD) at the placental site, and with the parietal decidua (PD), which lines the uterine cavity (UC). The amnion (*black dotted line*) is not fused in most places with the chorion frondosum. (**b**) Two weeks later (12th week postmenstruation), the original chorion frondosum has differentiated into the placenta (P) and the thinner fetal membranes that surround the inner amniotic cavity (AC). At this stage, the membranes are composed of the amnion (A), chorion laeve (CL), and capsular decidua (CD). Because of the embryo's small size, the uterine cavity (UC) still is quite large. (C) From 17 weeks on, the membranes come into close contact with the uterine wall. The remainder of the capsular decidua (CD) fuses with the parietal decidua (PD) and obliterate the uterine cavity (UC). From then on, the chorion laeve contacts the parietal decidua (modified from Kaufmann 1981).

capsular decidua or **decidua capsularis**. The remaining decidua, that which is without contact with the blastocyst (i.e., on the opposite uterine wall), is the **parietal decidua** or **decidua vera**. With growth of the chorionic sac, the capsular decidua focally degenerates, and eventually touches the parietal decidua (Fig. 5.3c). Between the 15th and 20th weeks PC, *the smooth chorion, together with its attached residual capsular decidua, locally fuses with the parietal decidua, thereby largely obliterating the uterine cavity* (Fig. 5.3c). From this date onward, the smooth chorion has contact with the decidual surface of the uterine wall over nearly its entire surface. However, there is no true fusion between the decidua capsularis and the decidua vera.

Small cells lining the inner surface of the trophoblast, the *amniogenic cells,* are the forerunners of the **amnionic epithelium**. A cleft separates these cells from the embryoblast, which ultimately becomes the **amniotic cavity** (Fig. 5.4, day 13). Before the 12th week PC, the amniotic cavity is separated from the chorion by chorionic fluid, the **magma**

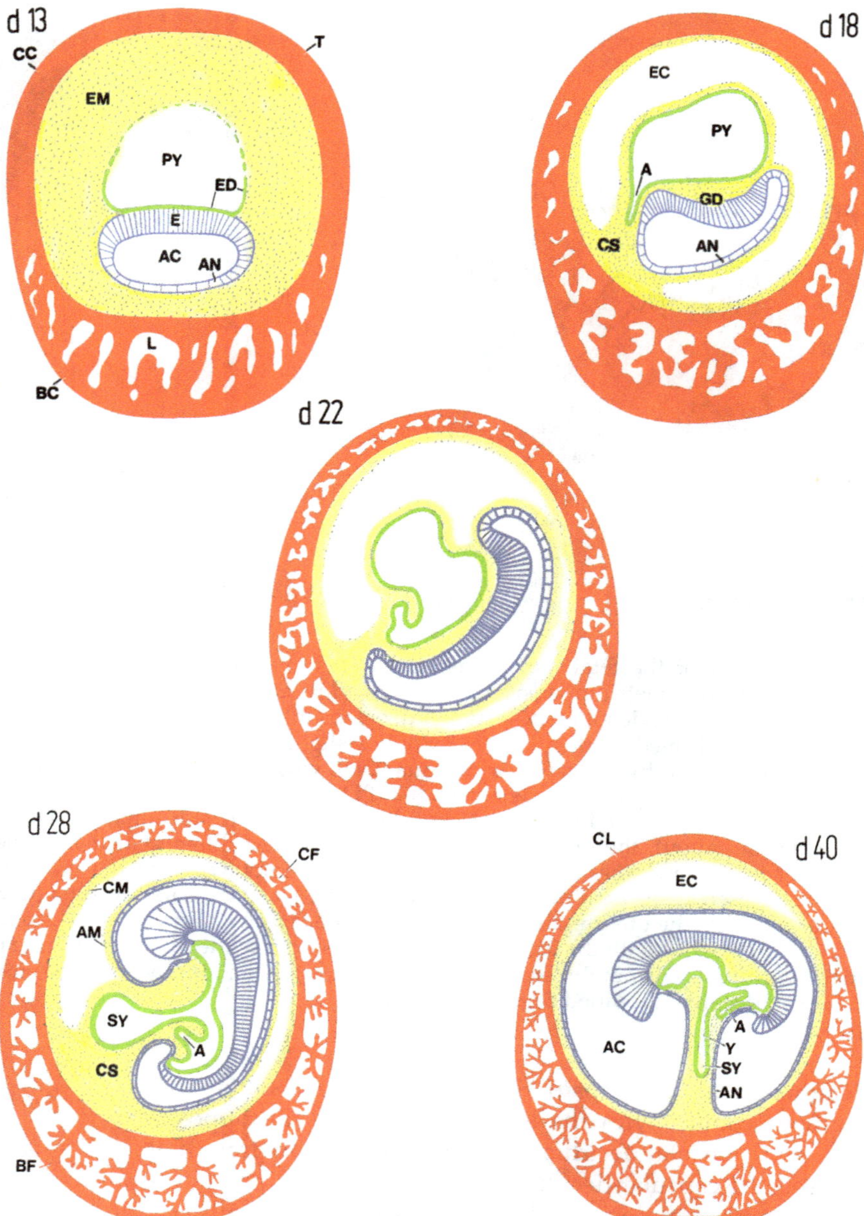

Figure 5.4. Simplified representation of the development of the umbilical cord and amnion. (**a**) Day 13 postconception. The embryonic disk consists of two epithelial layers: the ectoderm (E), which is contiguous with the amnionic epithelium (AN), and the endoderm (ED), which partially surrounds the primary yolk sac cavity (PY). Both vesicles are surrounded by the extraembryonic mesoderm (EM). (**b**) Day 18 postconception. At this stage, the entoderm has become closely applied to the periphery of the yolk sac; and at the presumptive caudal end of the germinal disk, the allantoic invagination (a) has occurred. In the extraembryonic mesoderm, the exocoelom (EC) has cavitated. A mesenchymal bridge, the connecting stalk (CS) has developed that will ultimately form the umbilical cord. (**c**) Day 28 postconception. The embryo has begun to rotate and fold. The primary yolk sac is being subdivided into the intraembryonic intestinal tract and the secondary (extraembryonic) yolk sac (SY). Secondary yolk sac and allantois extrude from the future embryonic intestinal tract into the connecting stalk. The amnionic sac largely surrounds the embryo because of its folding and rotation. Villous formation has occurred

reticulare. Extraembryonic mesenchyme expands to cover the surface of the amnionic epithelium and becomes the **amnionic mesoderm**. During the sixth to seventh week PC, the amnionic mesoderm fuses with the chorionic mesoderm, near the cord insertion site at the chorionic plate (Fig. 5.4, day 28 and 40). This process is completed in the 12th week PC. However, *fusion of the amnion and chorion is never complete*, and thus the two membranes can always easily slide against each other. This is different from the situation in the umbilical cord, where the *expanding amnion becomes closely attached to the surface of the cord and firmly fuses with it.*

Development of the Umbilical Cord

The development of the umbilical cord is closely related to that of the amnion. At the end the second week PC, the embryoblast within the blastocystic cavity is surrounded by a loose meshwork of mesodermal cells (Fig. 5.4, day 13). The double-layered embryonic disk is between the **amnionic vesicle** and the **primary yolk sac**. Basal to the amnionic vesicle, the mesodermal cells condense and form the **connecting stalk** (Fig. 5.4, day 18), which is the *early forerunner of the umbilical cord*. During the same period, a duct-like extension of the yolk sac, originating from the future caudal region of the embryo, grows into the connecting stalk. This structure is the transitory **allantois**, the *primitive extraembryonic urinary bladder*. Remnants of allantoic elements may be found in sections of the umbilical cord at term (see Chap. 15).

The subsequent weeks are characterized by three developmental processes. First, the **embryo rotates** so that the yolk sac is turned toward the implantation pole rather than away from it. Second, the **amniotic cavity** enlarges and extends around the embryo. Lastly, the originally **flat embryonic disk is bent in both the anteroposterior and lateral directions** and thus "herniates" into the amniotic cavity. As the embryo bends, it subdivides the yolk sac into an intraembryonic duct (the gut) and an extraembryonic part (the omphalomesenteric duct), which is dilated peripherally to form the extraembryonic yolk sac vesicle.

Both the allantois and the extraembryonic yolk sac extend into the mesenchyme of the connecting stalk (Fig. 5.4, day 22). Between days 28 and 40 PC, the expanding amniotic cavity surrounds the embryo and *the connecting stalk, allantois, and yolk sac become compressed to a slender cord covered by amnionic epithelium* (Figs. 5.2 and 5.4, day 28 and 40), the **umbilical cord**. The cord lengthens as the embryo "prolapses" backward into the amniotic sac. During the same process of expansion,

---

Figure 5.4. (continued) at the entire periphery of the chorionic vesicle, forming the chorion frondosum (CF). **(d)** Day 40 postconception. The embryo has now fully rotated and folded. It is completely surrounded by the amniotic cavity and is attached to the umbilical cord. The latter has developed from the connecting stalk as it has become covered by amnionic membrane. The exocoelom has become largely compressed by the expansion of the amniotic cavity. At the anembryonic pole of the chorionic vesicle, the recently formed placental villi gradually atrophy, thus forming the chorion laeve (CL). Only that portion that retains villous tissue, that which has the insertion of the umbilical cord, develops into the placental disk.

the amnionic mesenchyme locally touches and finally fuses with the chorionic mesoderm, thus obliterating the exocoelomic cavity. This is completed at 12 weeks.

During the third week PC, the **extraembryonic yolk sac**, the **omphalomesenteric duct**, which connects with the embryonic gut, and the **allantois** become supplied with fetal vessels. Two allantoic arteries originate from the internal iliac arteries, and one allantoic vein enters the hepatic vein. These allantoic vessels invade the placenta and become connected to the villous vessels. The allantoic participation in placental vascularization is the reason that the human placenta is a "chorioallantoic" placenta.

Selected References

PHP5, pages 42–49 (Early Development of the Human Placenta).

Boyd JD, Hamilton WJ. The human placenta. Cambridge: Heffer & Sons, 1970.

Castellucci M, Scheper M, Scheffen I, et al. The development of the human placental villous tree. Anat Embryol (Berl) 1990;181:117–128.

Enders AC, King BF. Formation and differentiation of extraembryonic mesoderm in the rhesus monkey. Am J Anat 1988;181:327–340.

Hertig AT, Rock J. Two human ova of the previllous stage having an ovulation age of about eleven and twelve days respectively. Contrib Embryol 1941;29:127–156.

Heuser CH, Streeter GL. Development of the macaque embryo. Contrib Embryol 1941;29:15–55.

Kaufmann P, Scheffen I Placental development. In, Neonatal and Fetal Medicine-Physiology and Pathohysiology. R Polin and W Fox eds, pp 47-56, Saunders, Orlando, 1992.

Kaufamnn P, Placentation and Placenta. In, Humanembryologie. K.V. Hinrichsen, ed pp 159-204, Springer-Verlage, Heidelberg, 1990.

Kaufmann P. Entwicklung der Pazenta. In, Die Plazenta des Menschen. V. Becker, T.H. Schiebler and F. Kubli, eds. Thieme, Stuttgart, 1981.

Leiser R, Beier HM. Morphological studies of lacunar formation in the early rabbit placenta. Trophoblast Res 1988;3:97–110.

Luckett WP. Origin and differentiation of the yolk sac and extraembryonic mesoderm in presomite human and rhesus monkey embryos. Am J Anat 1978;152:59–97.

Pijnenborg R, Robertson WB, Brosens I, Dixon G. Trophoblast invasion and the establishment of haemochorial placentation in man and laboratory animals. Placenta 1981;2:71–92.

Chapter 6

Chorionic Villi: Histology and Villous Development

Histology

The **chorionic villi** are the site where virtually all *maternofetal and fetomaternal exchange* takes place. Most *metabolic and endocrine activities* of the placenta are localized there as well. The villi have a dual blood supply from both the fetal and maternal circulations. Despite the diversification of villous types, *all chorionic villi exhibit the same basic structure* (Fig. 6.1). They are covered by **syncytiotrophoblast**, an epithelial surface layer (Fig. 6.1a) that is in direct contact with the maternal blood and *functions as an endothelium*. Between syncytiotrophoblast and the basement membrane are the **villous cytotrophoblast, or Langhans' cells.** These are the villous stem cells of the syncytium, supporting its growth and regeneration. The trophoblastic basement membrane separates the trophoblast from the villous stroma. The stroma is composed of *connective tissue cells, connective tissue fibers, ground substance, and fetal vessels.* In the larger stem villi, the vessels are mainly arteries and veins, while in the peripheral branches most fetal vessels are capillaries or

R.N. Baergen, *Manual of Pathology of the Human Placenta,*
DOI 10.1007/978-1-4419-7494-5_6, © Springer Science+Business Media, LLC 2011

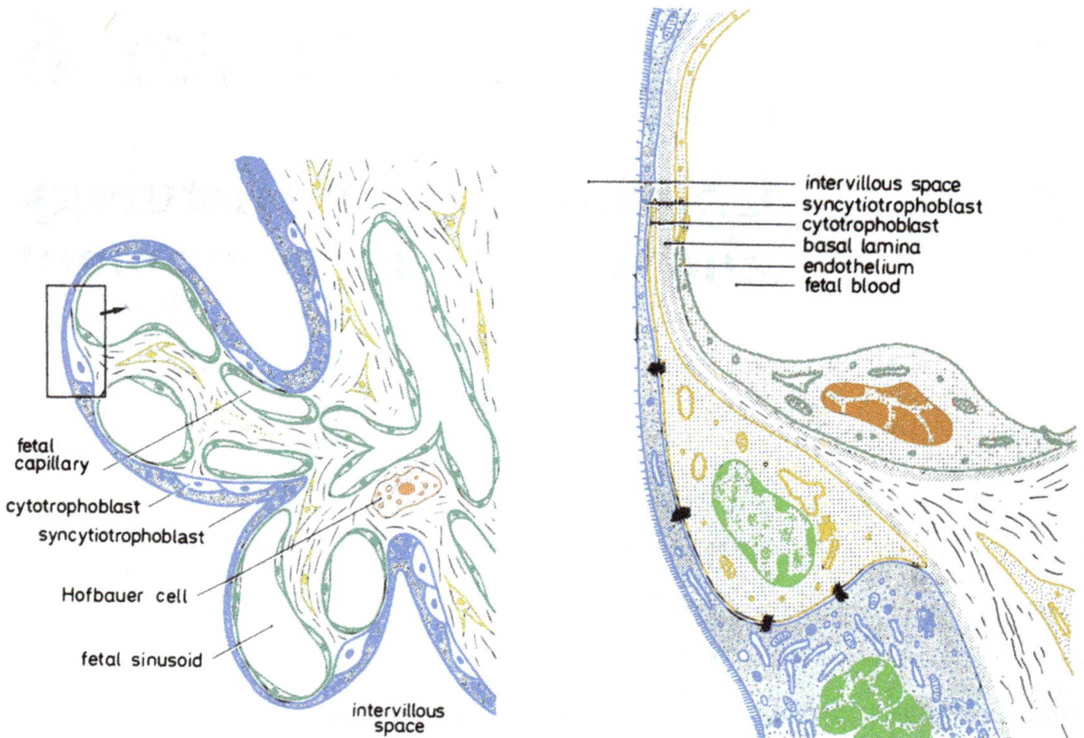

Figure 6.1. Morphology of human placental villi. On the *left* is a simplified light microscopic section of two terminal villi, branching off a mature intermediate villus. This is shown in greater detail on the *right*, with a schematic electron-microscopic section of the placental barrier, demonstrating typical layers (modified from Kaufmann P. Vergleichend-anatomische und funktionelle Aspekte des Placenta-Baues. Funkt Biol Med 1983;2:71–79, with permission).

"sinusoids." The human placenta is hemochorial in that the maternal blood has direct contact with trophoblast. The layers separating maternal from fetal blood are as follows (Fig. 6.1b):

- **Syncytiotrophoblast**
- **An incomplete layer of cytotrophoblast**
- **Trophoblastic basement membrane**
- **Connective tissue**
- **Endothelial basement membrane**
- **Fetal capillary endothelium**

These layers form the vasculosyncytial or placental "membrane."

Syncytiotrophoblast

The **syncytiotrophoblast** is a *continuous, normally uninterrupted layer* that extends over the surfaces of all villous trees and chorionic villi as well as over parts of the inner surfaces of chorionic and basal plates. It thus *lines the entire intervillous space* and is a single continuous structure for every placenta. Therefore, plural terms such as *syncytiotrophoblast*s and *syncytial cell*s, which are often used, are inappropriate and should be avoided. Their use indicates a misunderstanding of the true nature of the syncytiotrophoblast. The syncytium is involved in *complex, active maternofetal transfer mechanisms*, including:

- **Catabolism and resynthesis of proteins and lipids**
- **Synthesis of various hormones**
- **Diffusional transfer of gases and water**
- **The facilitated transfer of glucose**
- **Active transfer of amino acids and electrolytes**

The **syncytium** varies in thickness from 2 to about 10 mm (Fig. 6.2). On tissue sections of first-trimester placentas (Fig. 6.3), the syncytiotrophoblast appears as a single layer surrounding the cytotrophoblast with no cell border. The *nuclei are small, with moderately dense chromatin. The cytoplasm is homogeneous to finely granular, somewhat basophilic, and*

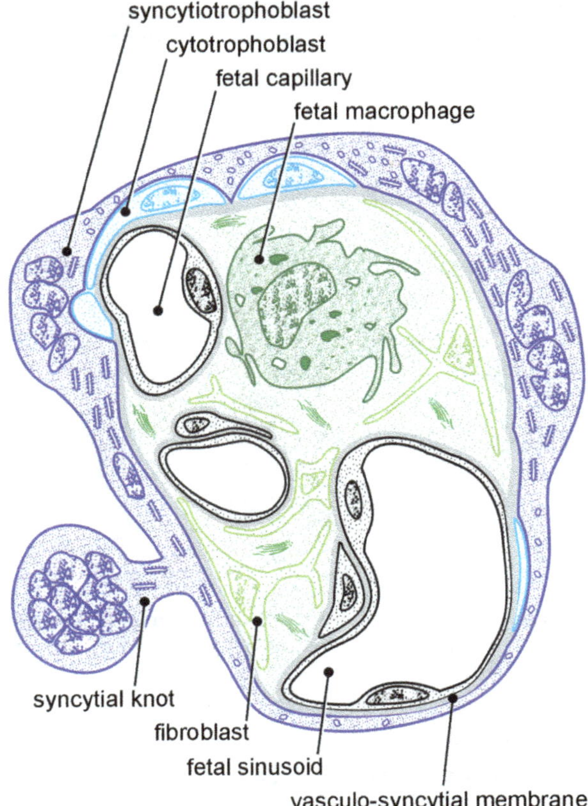

Figure 6.2. Simplified drawing of a cross section of a terminal villus demonstrating the structural variability of the syncytiotrophoblast. Depicted are vasculosyncytial membrane, syncytiotrophoblast with well-developed smooth and rough endoplasmic reticulum, cytotrophoblast, fetal sinusoid, fetal capillary, syncytial knot, and additional cells within the villus including macrophage and fibroblast (from Kaufmann P, Schiebler ThH, Biobotaru C, Stark J. Enzymhistochemische Untersuchungen an reifen menschlichen Placentazotten. II. Zur Gliederung des Syncytiotrophoblasten. Histochem 1974;40:191–207, with permission).

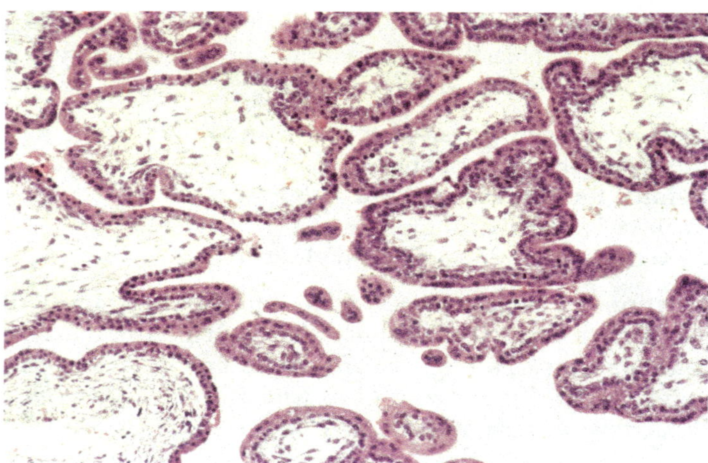

Figure 6.3. Light microscopic appearance of a first-trimester chorionic villus with relatively thick syncytiotrophoblast and well-defined cytotrophoblastic layer. H&E ×100.

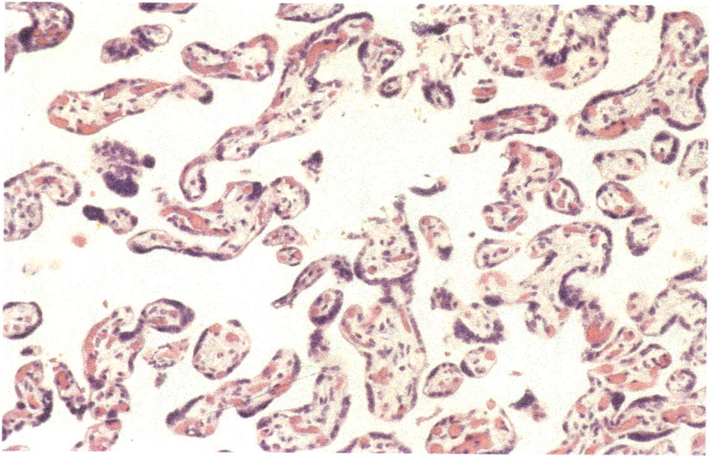

Figure 6.4. Light microscopic appearance of third-trimester chorionic villi with irregularly thinned syncytiotrophoblast and focally incomplete cytotrophoblastic layer. H&E ×100.

is often vacuolated. Later in pregnancy (Fig. 6.4), the syncytiotrophoblast varies markedly in thickness and focally may be thinned to almost invisibility, forming the **vasculosyncytial membrane** (Fig. 6.2a). In some areas it appears as a single layer of cells, while in other areas the nuclei are piled up forming **syncytial knots** (Fig. 6.2e). Nuclei may focally show degenerative change, but under normal circumstances mitotic figures are not identified in syncytiotrophoblast.

Syncytial Knots, Sprouts, and Bridges

Syncytial knots, sprouts, and bridges are a heterogeneous group of syncytiotrophoblastic specializations characterized by *aggregates of trophoblastic nuclei at the trophoblastic surface.* The term syncytial knots

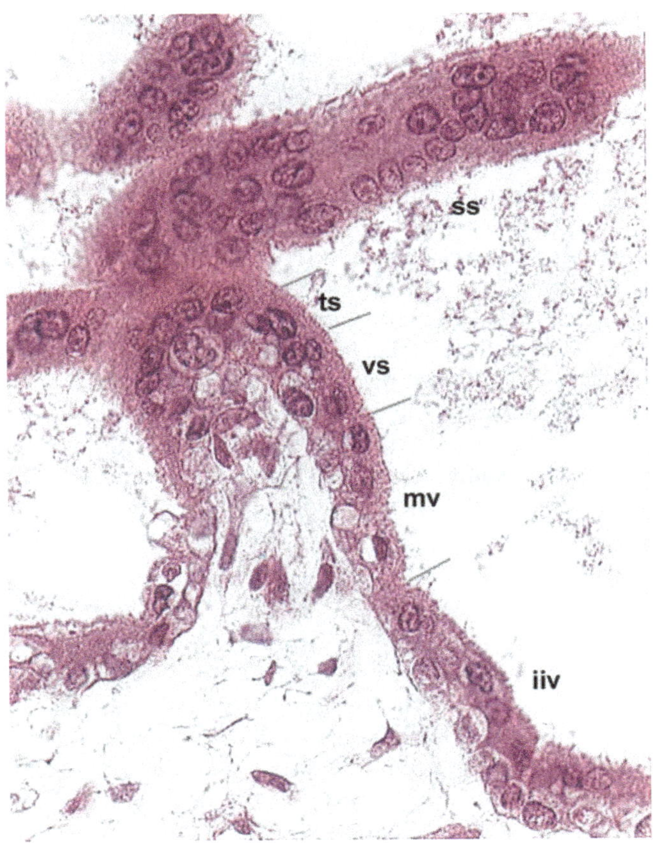

Figure 6.5. Longitudinal section of a newly sprouting villus demonstrates the stages of the sprouting process. In the upper third a group of syncytial sprouts (ss) is formed; they become invaded by cytotrophoblast to form a trophoblastic sprout (ts), followed by invasion of cellular stroma to form a villous sprout (vs). Development of fetal capillaries marks the transition to a mesenchymal villus (mv). The latter branches to form an immature intermediate villus (iiv), the starting point of the sprouting process. Paraffin section. H&E ×560.

is often used to refer to this entire group as they are generally indistinguishable on light microscopy. In the first half of pregnancy, most knots visible on histologic section are **syncytial sprouts** or **trophoblastic sprouts** (Fig. 6.5). These are characterized by *vermiform extensions from the villous surface with loosely arranged, large ovoid syncytial nuclei at the tip*. These are true proliferative outgrowths of the chorionic villi (vide infra). A minority of syncytial knots show apoptotic changes and are the sites of shedding of apoptotic nuclei into the maternal circulation. These **apoptotic knots** are characterized by *densely packed nuclei with condensed chromatin and occasional degenerative change*. **Syncytial bridges** are true bridges and they develop from *fusion of adjacent villi*. They are quite rare. In the third trimester of pregnancy, knots visible by light microscopy are most commonly the result of *tangential sectioning across syncytiotrophoblastic surfaces* (Fig. 6.4). The contour of the chorionic villi changes as the placenta matures, and as it does so, there is a corresponding increase in syncytial knots due to tangential sectioning. Thus, despite the fact that this is an artifact, it is a consistent one, and therefore is helpful in determining the age of placentas as well as evaluating uteroplacental perfusion (see Chap. 17).

Villous Cytotrophoblast (Langhans' Cells)

The **Langhans' cells** or **villous cytotrophoblastic cells** form a *second trophoblastic layer beneath the syncytiotrophoblast.* During early pregnancy, this layer is nearly complete (Fig. 6.3), but later in gestation it becomes discontinuous (Fig. 6.4). As the villous surface expands, the cytotrophoblastic cells become widely separated, and thus are less numerous in sectioned material. They have the characteristic features of undifferentiated, proliferating stem cells (Figs. 6.3 and 6.4). Typically they are *cuboidal, polyhedral, or ovoid cells with well-demarcated cell borders, and large, lightly staining nuclei containing finely dispersed chromatin.* The cytoplasm is usually clear to slightly granular and somewhat basophilic. In contrast to syncytiotrophoblast, mitotic figures are occasionally found.

Villous Stroma

The trophoblastic basement membrane separates the trophoblastic epithelium from the villous stroma. The stroma consists of fixed connective tissue cells, connective tissue fibers, free connective tissue cells (Hofbauer cells), and fetal vessels. **Undifferentiated stromal cells** or **mesenchymal cells** are the prevailing cell type until the end of the second month. In later pregnancy, they are generally found only in stem villi and in the few remaining villous precursors (vide infra). These cells are *small spindled cells* with little cytoplasm (Fig. 6.6). At the end of the second month, the mesenchymal cells differentiate into **fibroblasts**, which

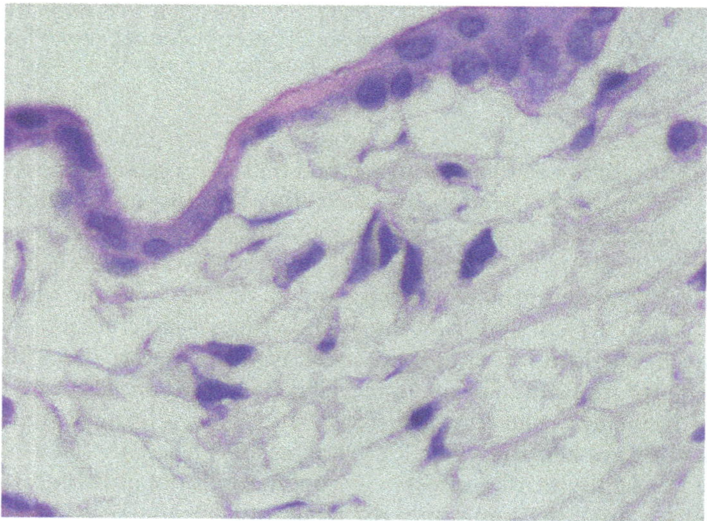

Figure 6.6. Immature chorionic villus with several typical undifferentiated mesenchymal cells present underneath the trophoblastic cover. H&E ×400.

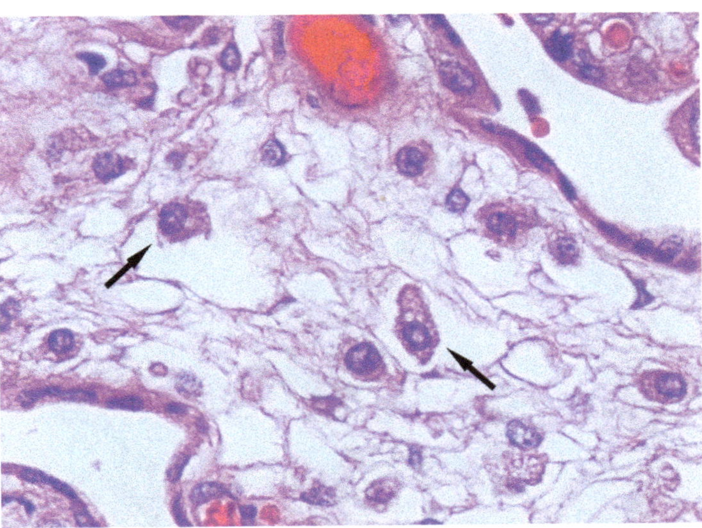

Figure 6.7. H&E-stained section of an immature chorionic villus with prominent Hofbauer cells (*arrows*) ×400.

have *elongated, bizarre-shaped cell bodies* from which several *long, thin, branching cytoplasmic processes* extend forming flat sails of cytoplasm. These form the stromal channels of the immature intermediate villi (vide infra). Later in pregnancy the mesenchymal cells differentiate into **myofibroblasts**, which have *abundant cytoplasm*, with only a *few short, filiform, or thick processes*.

Most free connective tissue cells of placental villi are tissue macrophages, the **Hofbauer cells**. However, there are a few mast cells and plasma cells. *Hofbauer cells are numerous in both the villous stroma and the chorionic plate throughout pregnancy.* Initially, they are derived from chorionic mesenchymal cells, but once fetal circulation is established, they likely derive, as other macrophages do, from fetal bone marrow-derived cells. Hofbauer cells are *large, isolated cells that are round, ovoid, reniform, or stellate in shape and have an eccentric nucleus* (Fig. 6.7). At term, Hofbauer cells are difficult to identify and difficult to differentiate from other cells. In the case of villous edema, the Hofbauer cells are said to be "unmasked" and are easier to appreciate.

General Considerations of Villous Development and Villous Types

The ramifications of the villous trees can be subdivided into five villous types based on caliber, stroma, vasculature, position within the villous tree, function and development (Fig. 6.8a–e). The five types are:

- **Mesenchymal villi**
- **Immature intermediate villi**
- **Mature intermediate villi**
- **Stem villi**
- **Terminal villi**

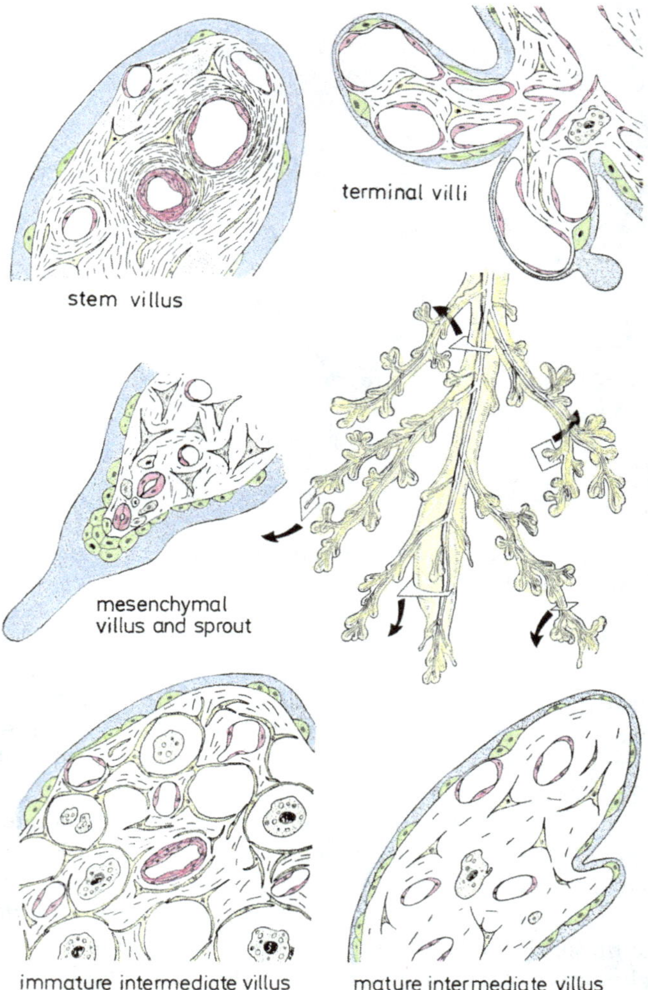

Figure 6.8. Simplified representation of the mature placental villous tree (**a**) and cross sections of the various villous types (**b–f**). For further details see text (from Kaufmann P, Scheffen I. Placental development In: Polin RA, Fox WW (eds) Neonatal and fetal medicine – physiology and pathophysiology, Vol 1. Saunders, Orlando, 1992:47–55, with permission).

Each of these types is present to a varying degree in most placentas. Therefore, identification and differentiation of these villous types is important so that they are not mistaken for pathologic changes. **Immature intermediate villi** develop from maturation of **mesenchymal villi** during the first two trimesters and are ultimately transformed into **stem villi** (Fig. 6.9a). In the third trimester, **mature intermediate villi** develop from mesenchymal villi and are later transformed into **terminal villi** (Fig. 6.9b). Thus, *"intermediate" villi are transitions from mesenchymal to mature villi*. Intermediate villi are typically found between the centrally located stem villi and the most peripheral terminal villi.

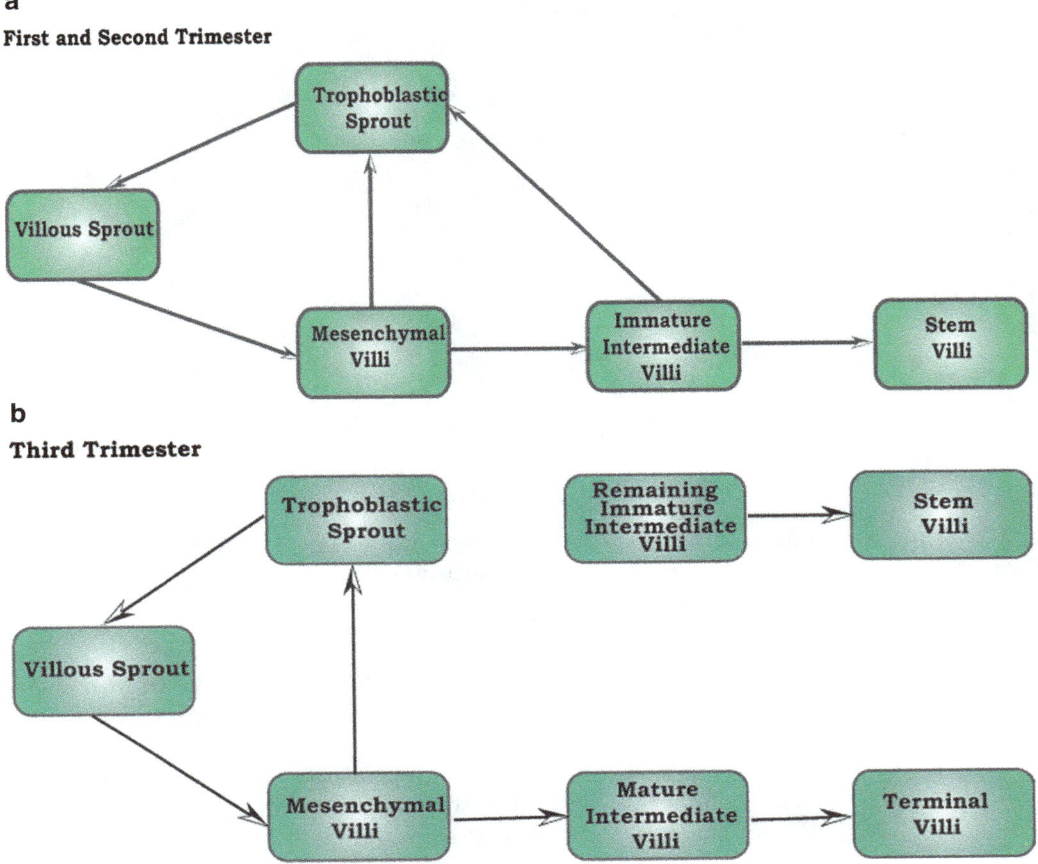

Figure 6.9. Routes of villous development during the first and second trimester (**a**) and third trimester (**b**). (**a**) Trophoblastic sprouts are produced along the surfaces of mesenchymal and immature intermediate villi. Via villous sprouts, they are transformed into mesenchymal villi. The latter differentiate into immature intermediate villi, which produce new sprouts before they are transformed into stem villi. (**b**) Throughout the third trimester, the mesenchymal villi differentiate into mature intermediate villi, which then may produce terminal villi. Mesenchymal villi no longer produce immature intermediate villi, but those still remaining continue to differentiate into stem villi. Thus, their number decreases with increasing gestational age. The source of new sprouts is also then reduced and therefore the growth capacity of the villous tress gradually slows.

Mesenchymal Villi

Mesenchymal villi are the first generation of the tertiary villi and *are the precursors from which all other villous types arise.* Mesenchymal villi develop beginning in the fifth week (from last menstrual period) at the onset of villous vascularization. From the fifth to the sixth week they develop from the tertiary villi via primary and secondary villi. After the sixth week, the villi develop syncytial outgrowths or **syncytial sprouts.** In growth of cytotrophoblast forms **trophoblastic sprouts,** and growth of connective tissue forms **villous sprouts.** Finally, fetal capillaries form in the connective tissue core to create new mesenchymal villi. From early gestation through the second trimester, mesenchymal villi

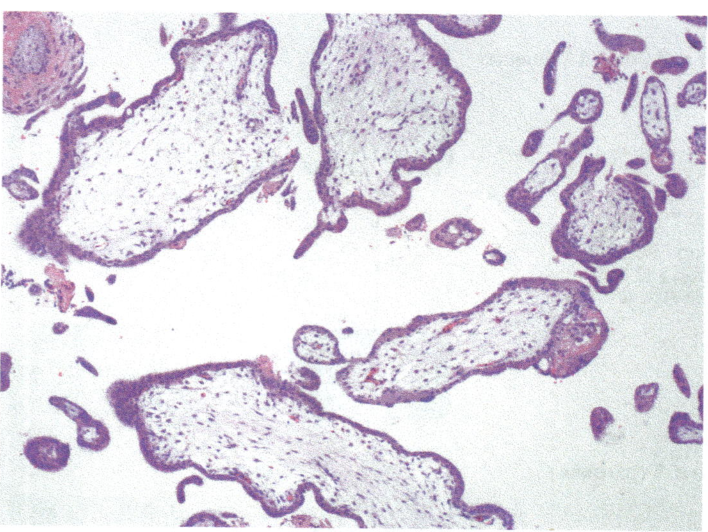

Figure 6.10. Mesenchymal villi; eighth week postmenstruation. As can be seen from the diffuse stromal structure, the villi still belong to the mesenchymal type ×100.

differentiate into **immature intermediate villi**. In the third trimester, mesenchymal villi primarily differentiate into **mature intermediate villi** (Figs. 6.8 and 6.9 and Table 6.1).

Mesenchymal villi have a *thick trophoblastic cover* with prominent cytotrophoblast. They have the highest mitotic index of all villous types. There is a *primitive stromal core with loosely arranged collagen, fibroblasts and a few Hofbauer cells* (Figs. 6.8b and 6.10). *Fetal capillaries are poorly developed.* Early on, mesenchymal villi are not only the source of *villous proliferation* but also the site of *maternofetal exchange* and *endocrine activity.* With advancing pregnancy their functional importance is reduced to villous growth. At term, they are only found in small numbers on the surfaces of immature intermediate villi in the center of the villous trees and comprise less than 1% of the placental volume.

Immature Intermediate Villi

The **immature intermediate villi** appear around the eighth week and comprise the majority of villi from the 14th to the 20th week. At term, only rare clusters are present in the center of the villous trees, where they comprise less than 5% of the placental volume. These villi mature into stem villi, a transformation that is a gradual process resulting in many intermediate forms. Morphologically, immature intermediate villi are *bulbous* in shape with a *thick trophoblastic cover, prominent cytotrophoblast,* and a distinctive *reticular stroma containing fluid-filled stromal channels* (Figs. 6.8c and 6.11). The stroma contains easily identifiable Hofbauer *cells.* The fetal capillaries are poorly developed. The reticular stroma may cause diagnostic problems, as it simulates villous edema. Starting at about the eighth week,

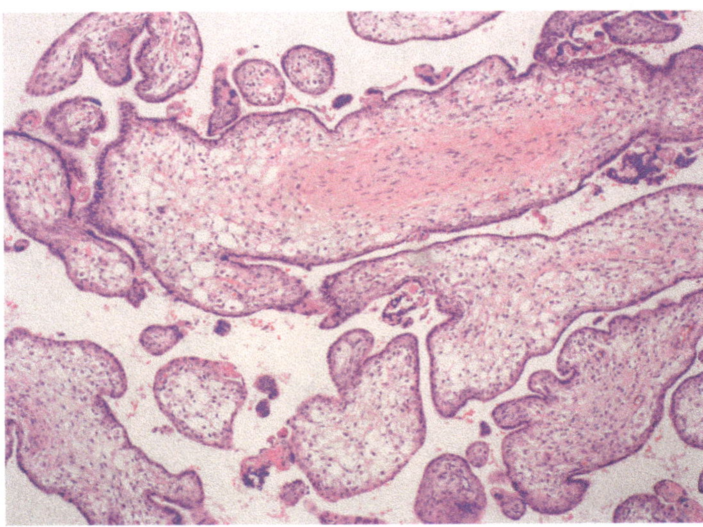

Figure 6.11. Immature intermediate villi and stem villi; 15th week. The larger immature intermediate villi exhibit the first signs of central stromal fibrosis, originating from the larger fetal vessels, thus establishing the first stem villi (SV). Several typical immature intermediate villi (IV) and mesenchymal villi (MV) can be seen. As is typical for mesenchymal villi of the second and third trimester, they are associated with degenerating villi and are becoming transformed into intravillous fibrinoid ×125.

the immature intermediate villi act as growth centers of the villous trees by forming new mesenchymal villi. Thus, new mesenchymal villi are formed from both old mesenchymal villi and immature intermediate villi.

Stem Villi

Stem villi are derived from immature intermediate villi and begin to appear at about the eighth week (Figs. 6.11 and 6.12). The large "trunks" and "branches" of the villous trees and the anchoring villi are all stem villi and differ only in caliber and position. At term, they make up to 20–25% of the placental volume because many are so large. Because of their branching pattern, their "volumetric" share is highest in the central subchorionic area of the placenta, particularly beneath the cord insertion site. *Functionally, stem villi serve to mechanically support the structure of the villous trees.* Their share in the function of maternofetal exchange is negligible.

Histologically, stem villi have a *thick trophoblastic cover with identifiable cytotrophoblast* on about 20% of the villous surfaces. In the mature placenta, the surfaces of these villi are often degenerative and partially replaced by fibrinoid, particularly in the large caliber stem villi. The stroma consists of *condensed bundles of collagen fibers with occasional fibroblasts and rare macrophages or occasional mast cells* (Figs. 6.11 and 6.12). In the larger stem villi, there is a central artery and corresponding

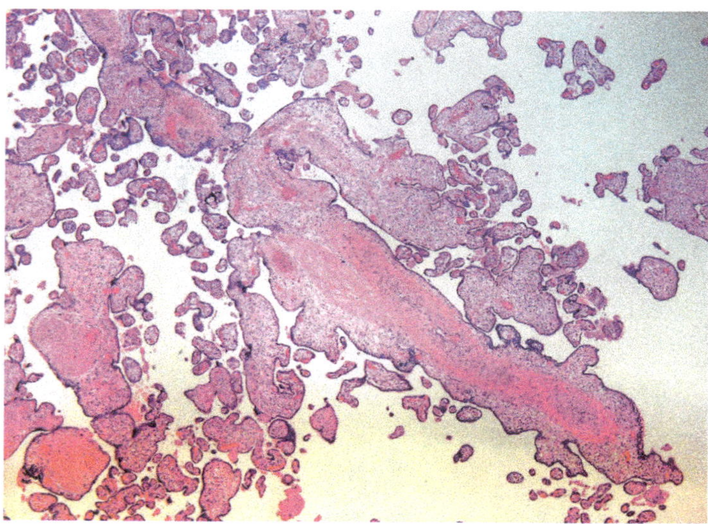

Figure 6.12. Stem villus. Cross section of a large stem villus. Note that the adventitias of the right and vein directly continue into the surrounding dense fibrous stroma of the villus. Superficially, numerous smaller vessels of the paravascular capillary net are seen. The trophoblastic covering has been replaced by fibrinoid in many places ×115 (from Leiser et al. 1985, with permission).

vein along with smaller arterioles, venules, and superficial paravascular capillaries (Fig. 6.12). The adventitia of the vessels continues without sharp demarcation into the surrounding fibrous stroma.

The transition from immature intermediate villi to stem villi is gradual. Initially, the vessels acquire a distinct media and adventitia, which expand to include the entire villus. Concurrently, an increase in the connective tissue leads to compression and finally disappearance of the stromal channels. In "immature" stem villi, there is a *superficial rim of reticular stroma surrounding the fibrous stroma*, which represents a differentiation gradient, the most central layer showing the highest degree of differentiation. Stem villi are established when the superficial reticular stroma beneath the trophoblast is thinner than the fibrous tissue surrounding the stem vessels.

Mature Intermediate Villi

In the third trimester, the mesenchymal villi switch from forming immature intermediate villi to forming **mature intermediate villi**. These are the precursors of the terminal villi. Mature intermediate villi are usually *long and slender*, but when their surfaces bear developing terminal villi they form a *zigzag configuration* as the terminal villi branch off (Fig. 6.13). The stroma consists of *unoriented, loose bundles of connective tissue fibers and connective tissue cells*. There are *numerous capillaries, small terminal arterioles, and collecting venules*. Cross sections contain less than 50% vascular lumens and therefore they participate

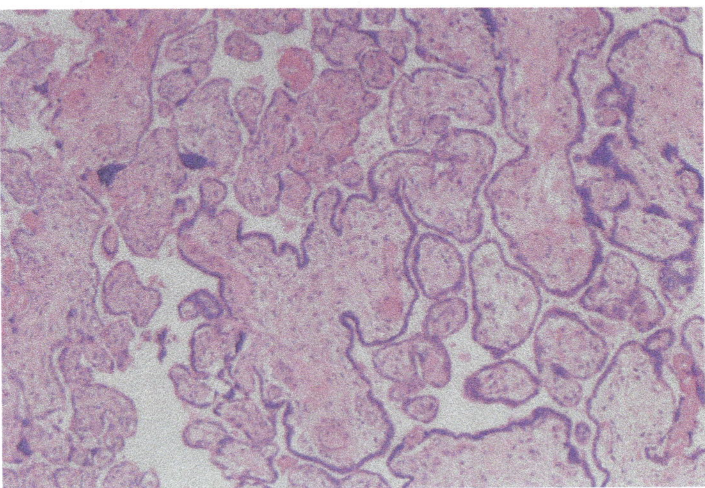

Figure 6.13. Mature intermediate villi; 29th week PM. During this period, the mature intermediate villi and the stem villi (*lower left*) are the prevailing villous types. Immature intermediate villi with typical reticular stroma (*lower right*) are less common ×125.

significantly in fetomaternal exchange. Approximately 25% of the placental volume at term consists of this villous type.

Terminal Villi

Terminal villi are the final ramifications of the villous tree. They are *grape-like outgrowths of the mature intermediate villi* and appear as single villi or as side branches (Fig. 6.13). The peripheral end of the mature intermediate villus normally branches into an aggregate of terminal villi and is connected to them by a narrow neck region. There are *scant connective tissue fibers and rare macrophages with a thin trophoblastic cover in intimate contact with sinusoidally dilated capillaries* (Figs. 6.13 and 6.14). The capillaries *possess a continuous endothelium and complete basal lamina*. Strictly speaking, terminal villi are those villi in which *the vascular lumens comprise at least 50% of the stromal volume and which contain no vessels other than capillaries and sinusoids*.

Contrary to the development of other villous types, the terminal villi are not formed by cellular outgrowths but rather are *formed passively by capillary growth and coiling*. This results in stretching of trophoblast and thinning of the vasculosyncytial membranes. Accordingly, maldevelopment of the terminal villi is a consequence of abnormal fetoplacental angiogenesis (see Chap. 17). These villi are the primary site of fetomaternal exchange. In the term placenta, they comprise 45% of the placental volume and approximately 60% of the cross sections.

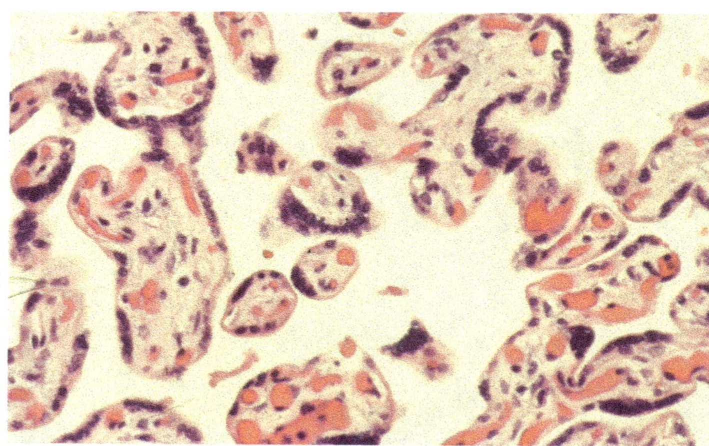

Figure 6.14. Terminal villi; 38th week PM. Dominating villous types are mature intermediate villi and terminal villi, both of small caliber. Several stem villi of varying caliber can also be seen in between. As is typical for term placentas, the trophoblastic cover of the stem villi is partly replaced by fibrinoid and the stroma in completely fibrosed. Reticular stroma or cellular connective tissue (a typical sign of immaturity, which is usually visible below the trophoblast in earlier stages) throughout the last few weeks is absent ×125.

Table 6.1 Villous characteristics.

Villous type	When present	When maximum	% Volume at term	Size	Characteristic features
Mesenchymal villi	5 weeks–term	0–8 weeks	<1%	120–250 µm (<8 weeks) 60–100 µm (>8 weeks)	Primitive stroma, thick trophoblastic cover, few vessels
Immature intermediate villi	8 weeks–term	14–20 weeks	5–10%	100–200 µm May be up to 400 µm	Reticular stroma with fluid-filled stromal channels
Stem villi	12 weeks–term	Term	20–25%	150–300 µm	Fibrotic stroma, myofibroblastic perivascular sheath, large vessels
Mature intermediate villi	Third trimester	Third trimester	25%	80–150 µm	Cellular stroma with <50% capillaries
Terminal villi	Third trimester	Term	40–50%	60 µm	>50% capillaries

Selected References

PHP5, pages 50–120 (Basic Structure of the Villous Trees), pages 121–173 (Architecture of Normal Villous Trees).

Boyd JD, Hamilton WJ. Electron microscopic observations on the cytotrophoblast contribution to the syncytium in the human placenta. J Anat 1966;100:535–548.

Cantle SJ, Kaufmann P, Luckhardt M, et al. Interpretation of syncytial sprouts and bridges in the human placenta. Placenta 1987;8:221–234.

Castellucci M, Scheper M, Scheffen I, et al. The development of the human placental villous tree. Anat Embryol (Berl) 1990;181:117–128.

Castellucci M, Zaccheo D. The Hofbauer cells of the human placenta: morphological and immunological aspects. Prog Clin Biol Res 1989;269:443–451.

Demir R, Kaufmann P, Castellucci M, et al. Fetal vasculogenesis and angiogenesis in human placental villi. Acta Anat 1989;136:190–203.

Demir R, Kosanke G, Kohnen G, et al. Classification of human placental stem villi: review of structural and functional aspects. Microsc Res Tech 1997;38:29–41.

Enders AC, King BF. The cytology of Hofbauer cells. Anat Rec 1970;167:231–252.

Graf R, Schoenfelder G, Muehlberger M, et al. The perivascular contractile sheath of human placental stem villi: its isolation and characterization. Placenta 1995;16:57–66.

Kaufmann P. Basic morphology of the fetal and maternal circuits in the human placenta. Contrib Gynecol Obstet 1985;13:5–17.

Kaufmann P, Scheffen I. Placental development In: Polin RA, Fox WW (eds) Neonatal and fetal medicine – physiology and pathophysiology, Vol 1. Orlando: Saunders, 1992:47–55.

Kaufmann P, Sen DK, Schweikhart G. Classification of human placental villi. I. Histology and scanning electron microscopy. Cell Tissue Res 1979;200:409–423.

Leiser R, Luckhardt M, Kaufmann P, Winterhager E, Bruns U The fetal vascularisation of term human placental villi. I. Peripheral stem villi., Anat Embryol 173:71-80, 1985.

Loukeris K, Sela R, Baergen RN. Frequency of syncytial knots in the placenta as different gestational ages. Mod Pathol 2007;20:289.

Wigglesworth JS. Vascular organization of the human placenta. Nature 1967;216:1120–1121.

Chapter 7
Overview and Microscopic Survey of the Placenta

Introduction

For the novice in placental pathology, histologic sections of the organ may look confusing since they contain not only a broad variety of differently structured villi but also many nonvillous structures as well. This chapter introduces those basic histologic features and architecture that leap out when inspecting a section of the placenta. Histology of the nonvillous portions of the villi is discussed in Chap. 8.

R.N. Baergen, *Manual of Pathology of the Human Placenta,*
DOI 10.1007/978-1-4419-7494-5_7, © Springer Science+Business Media, LLC 2011

Overview and Microscopic Survey of First-Trimester Placenta

Ideally, routine histologic examination of the human placenta starts with vertically oriented sections, which cover all placental structures from the chorionic plate, through the intervillous space, down to the basal plate (Fig. 7.1). Such sections are easily obtained from most second- and third-trimester placentas, but rarely from first-trimester specimens. In tissue from early abortions and curettages, the basal plate together with neighboring tissues such as septa, anchoring villi, and cell columns are often absent or at least difficult to identify since they are often destroyed or admixed with each other. However, knowledge of the ideal specimen will enhance recognition of structures in the disrupted specimen. Complete and well-oriented sections of the first-trimester placenta (Fig. 7.1a) include the following structures:

- **Chorionic plate** (Fig. 7.1b)
- **Intervillous space** (Fig. 7.1a), surrounding the
- **Chorionic villi** (Fig. 7.1c–f)
- **Cell islands** (Fig. 7.1g)
- **Basal plate** (Fig. 7.1j–m), from which
- **Septa** (Fig. 7.1h) protrude into the intervillous space
- **Anchoring villi** are connected via
- **Cell columns** to the septum (Fig. 7.1h) or to the basal plate (Fig. 7.1i)

The **intervillous space** (Fig. 7.1a) is the space between the chorionic plate and the basal plate. From the 13th week on, it *contains maternal blood*, which flows around the villi and other structures. The **chorionic plate** (Fig. 7.1b) in the first trimester is *usually devoid of amnion* as the amnion is only superficially attached to the chorionic plate and is commonly removed during preparation. The fetal surface, then, is usually covered by an inconspicuous, incomplete layer of mesothelium, and then a thick layer of chorionic mesoderm in which the chorionic vessels (branches of the umbilical vessels) are embedded. Towards the intervillous space, the surface is covered early on by a layer of syncytiotrophoblast, which, with progressing pregnancy, is replaced by acellular, eosinophilic fibrinoid (see Chap. 8).

The **placental villi** arise from the chorionic plate in a *progressive, branching, tree-like arrangement* and protrude into the intervillous space. The outer surfaces of the villi are bathed directly by maternal blood. The trophoblastic surface of the villi is composed of an outer continuous layer of **villous syncytiotrophoblast** beneath which is a discontinuous layer of **villous cytotrophoblast**. The villous **stroma** is *composed of fetal vessels, which are embedded in a mixture of fixed connective tissue cells, macrophages, and connective tissue fibers.* In the first 2 months of pregnancy, nucleated red blood cells are usually found in the villous vessels (Fig. 7.1c).

Before the eighth week PM (after the last menstrual period), the villi show a *homogeneous, rather dense cellular stroma* in which arteries and veins are absent. These are the **mesenchymal villi** (Fig. 7.1f). After the eighth week PM and through the second trimester, the majority of

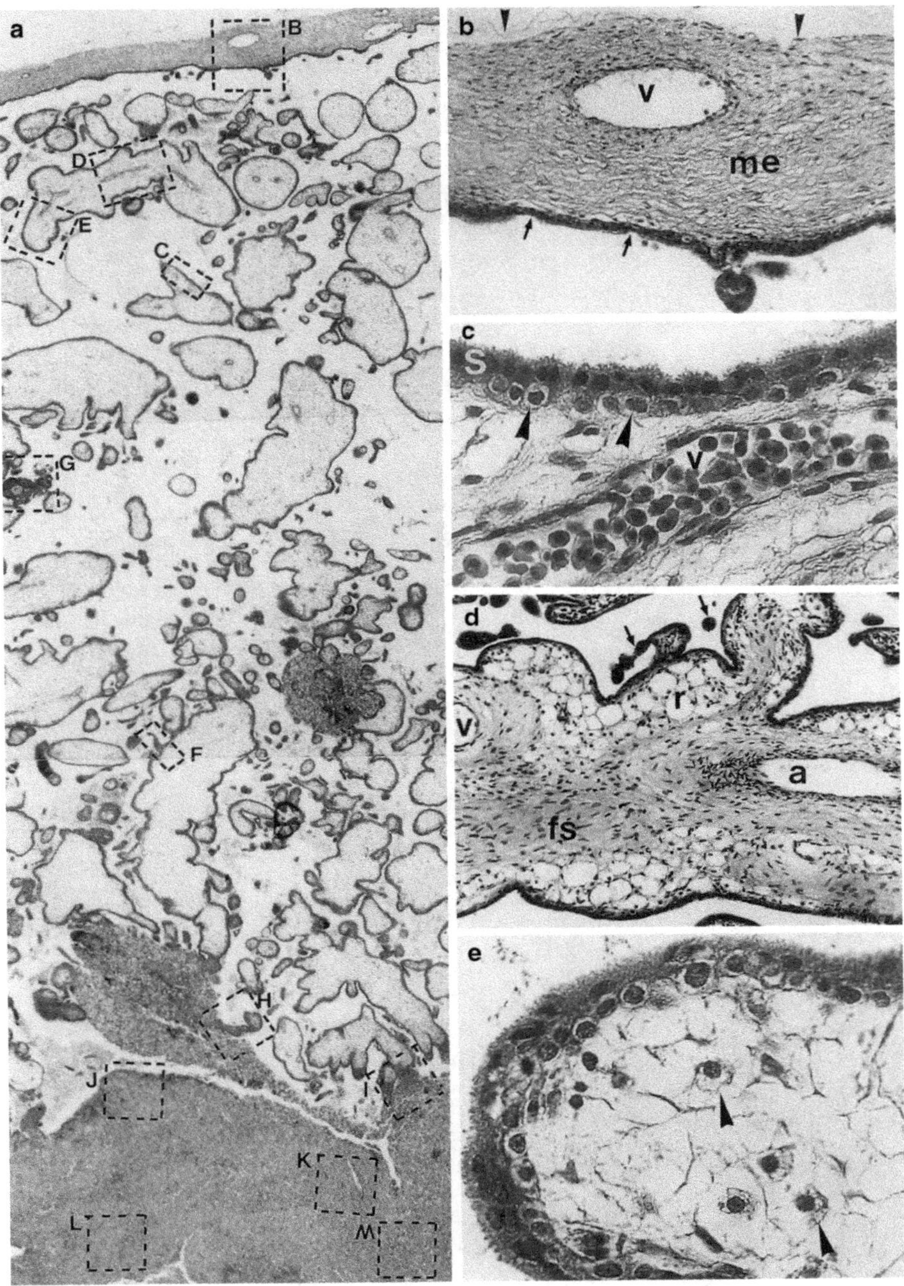

Figure 7.1. Typical features of the first-trimester placenta as seen in H&E-stained paraffin sections. All specimens are from the sixth week PM, except when otherwise stated. For details and explanation of the labeling, see text. (**a**) Vertical survey section of an in situ specimen. The marked frames refer to the following detailed pictures ×20. (**b**) Chorionic plate ×100. (**c**) Immature intermediate villus with a fetal vessel containing nucleated red blood cells ×400. (**d**) Transitional form of an immature intermediate villus becoming a stem villus (18th week PM) ×100. (**e**) Immature intermediate villus showing characteristic reticular stroma with macrophages (*arrowheads*) ×400. (**f**) Mesenchymal villus (m) arising from an immature intermediate villus (i) and extending into syncytial sprouts (ss) ×400. (**g**) Cell island attached to chorionic villi ×100. (**h**) Placental septum connected to a villus by a cell column (cc) ×200.

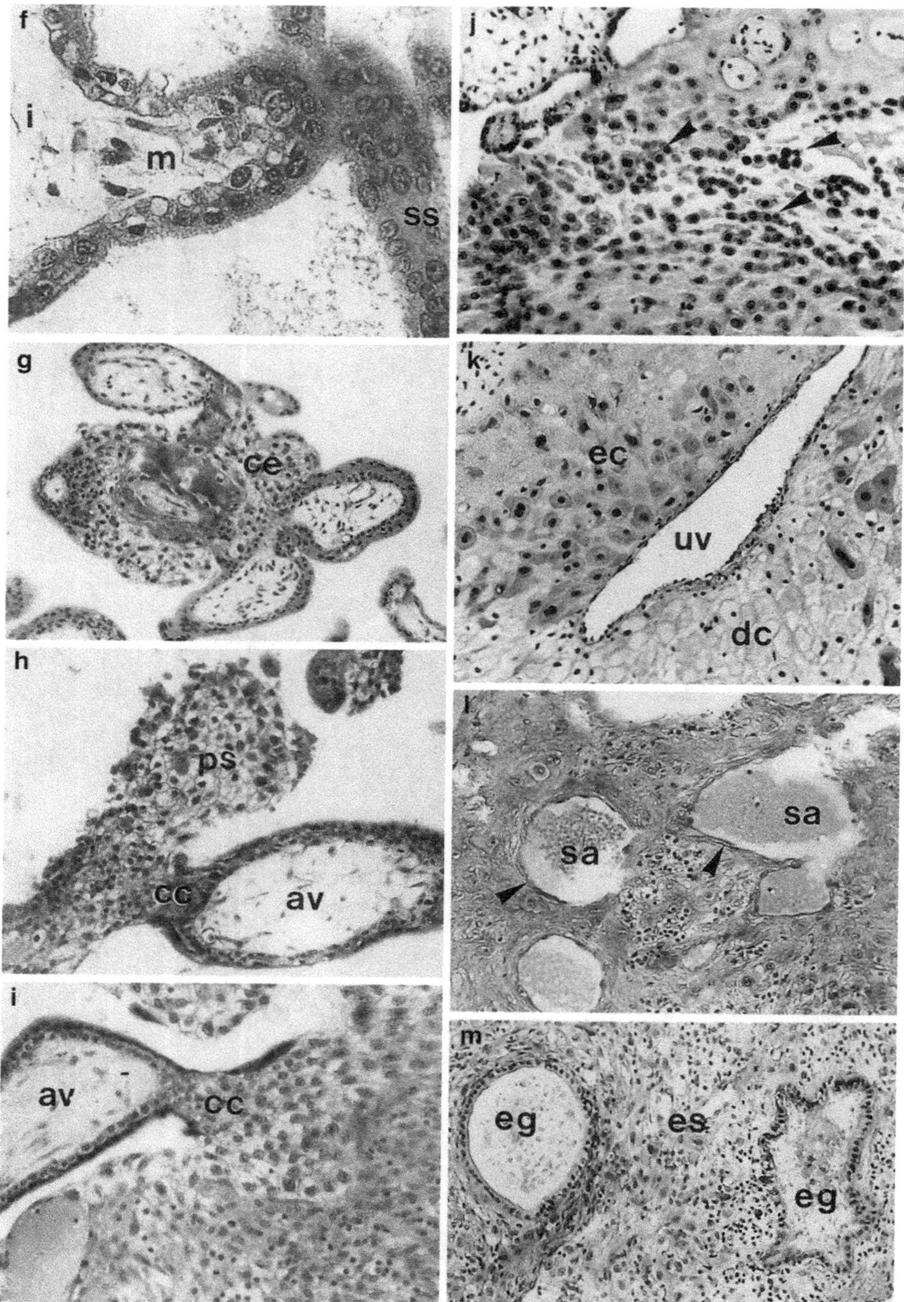

Figure 7.1. (continued) (**i**) Anchoring villus connected to the basal plate by a cell column ×200. (**j**) Superficial basal plate showing extravillous trophoblastic cells (*arrowheads*) embedded in fibrinoid (tenth week PM) ×100. (**k**) Deep part of the basal plate showing a uteroplacental vein (uv) surrounded by extravillous cytotrophoblast (ec) and decidua (dc) (37th week PM, similar to the first-trimester situation) ×140. (**l**) Multiple cross sections across a spiral artery the wall of which is replaced by fibrinoid (*arrowheads*) ×100. (**m**) Endometrial glands (eg) of the junctional zone embedded in endometrial stroma ×200.

villi are the **immature intermediate villi** (Fig. 7.1d, e), which are *large and bulbous with reticular stroma* and stromal macrophages. The central stems of the villous trees show fibrotic stroma around larger vessels and form the **stem villi** (see Chap. 6).

Cell islands (Fig. 7.1g) are accumulations of **extravillous trophoblastic cells**, usually embedded in fibrinoid and are *the still-proliferating remnants of the primary villi from early pregnancy.* **Placental septa** (Fig. 7.1h) are roughly *pillar-shaped extensions of the basal plate* that protrude into the intervillous space. They are rudimentary and do not completely subdivide the intervillous space. Structurally they have the *same composition as the basal plate, containing mostly extravillous trophoblastic cells admixed with fibrinoid and occasional decidual cells.* Cross sections of tips of septa may look like cell islands, the difference being that cell islands do not have decidual cells. Very often, **anchoring villi** can be seen attached to the septa of basal plate (Fig. 7.1h, i). *They stabilize the villous trees in the intervillous space.* **Cell columns** are the *trophoblastic feet of the anchoring villi.* Early in pregnancy they consist of several layers of proliferating extravillous trophoblast and serve as a source of proliferation of villous and basal plate cytotrophoblast.

The **basal plate** (Fig. 7.1j) is the bottom of the intervillous space and represents that part of the maternofetal junctional zone that adheres to the placenta after delivery. The deeper portion, the **placental bed**, remains in utero after delivery. The basal plate is composed of an admixture of *extravillous trophoblast, decidual cells, uteroplacental vessels, and endometrial glands embedded in abundant fibrinoid* (Fig. 7.1k). **Uteroplacental veins** are embedded in decidua and extravillous trophoblast, but are rarely invaded by extravillous trophoblast. **Uteroplacental arteries** (Fig. 7.1l) connect the maternal uterine arteries to the intervillous space. The *endothelial lining of the arteries, the arterial media, and the adventitia are largely replaced by extravillous trophoblast and fibrinoid.* These cells may form plugs that narrow or even occlude the arterial lumen early in gestation. In the depth of the basal plate, remainders of **endometrial glands** (Fig. 7.1m) may sometimes be found.

Overview and Microscopic Survey of Second- and Third-Trimester Placenta

The second- and third-trimester placenta has a similar structure to that of the early placenta, with the general exception that the layers are often better defined. The following is a list of those structures, roughly in order from the fetal to the maternal surface:

- **Chorionic plate** (Fig. 7.2c), including
- **Chorionic villi** of various types (Fig. 7.2d–g)
- **Intervillous space** (Fig. 7.2a)
- **Fibrinoid deposits** in various locations (Fig. 7.2c, f, h–l)
- **Cell islands** (Fig. 7.2j)
- **Septa** (Fig. 7.2k)

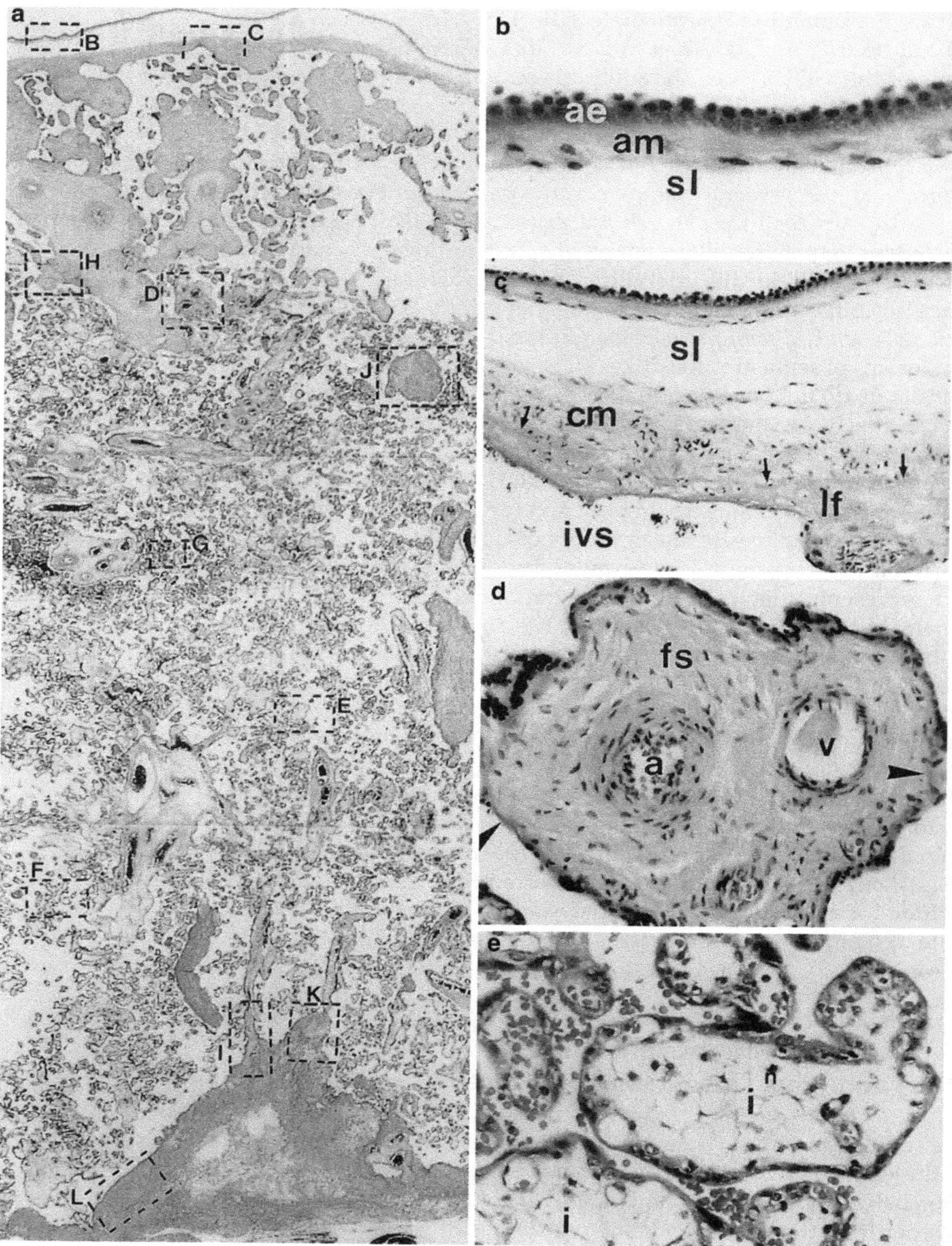

Figure 7.2. Typical features of the third-trimester placenta as seen in paraffin sections following H&E staining. All specimens are from the 40th week PM. For details and for explanation of labeling see text. (**a**) Vertical survey section. The marked frames refer to the following detailed pictures ×10. (**b**) Amnion ×120. (**c**) Chorionic plate, covered by the amnion ×60. (**d**) Peripheral stem villus ×180. (**e**) Two immature intermediate villi (i) surrounded by some mature intermediate (mv) and terminal villi (t) ×180. (**f**) A longitudinally sectioned mature intermediate villus (mv) together with some terminal villi and a villous fibrinoid necrosis (if) ×180. (**g**) A group of terminal villi showing considerable syncytial knotting

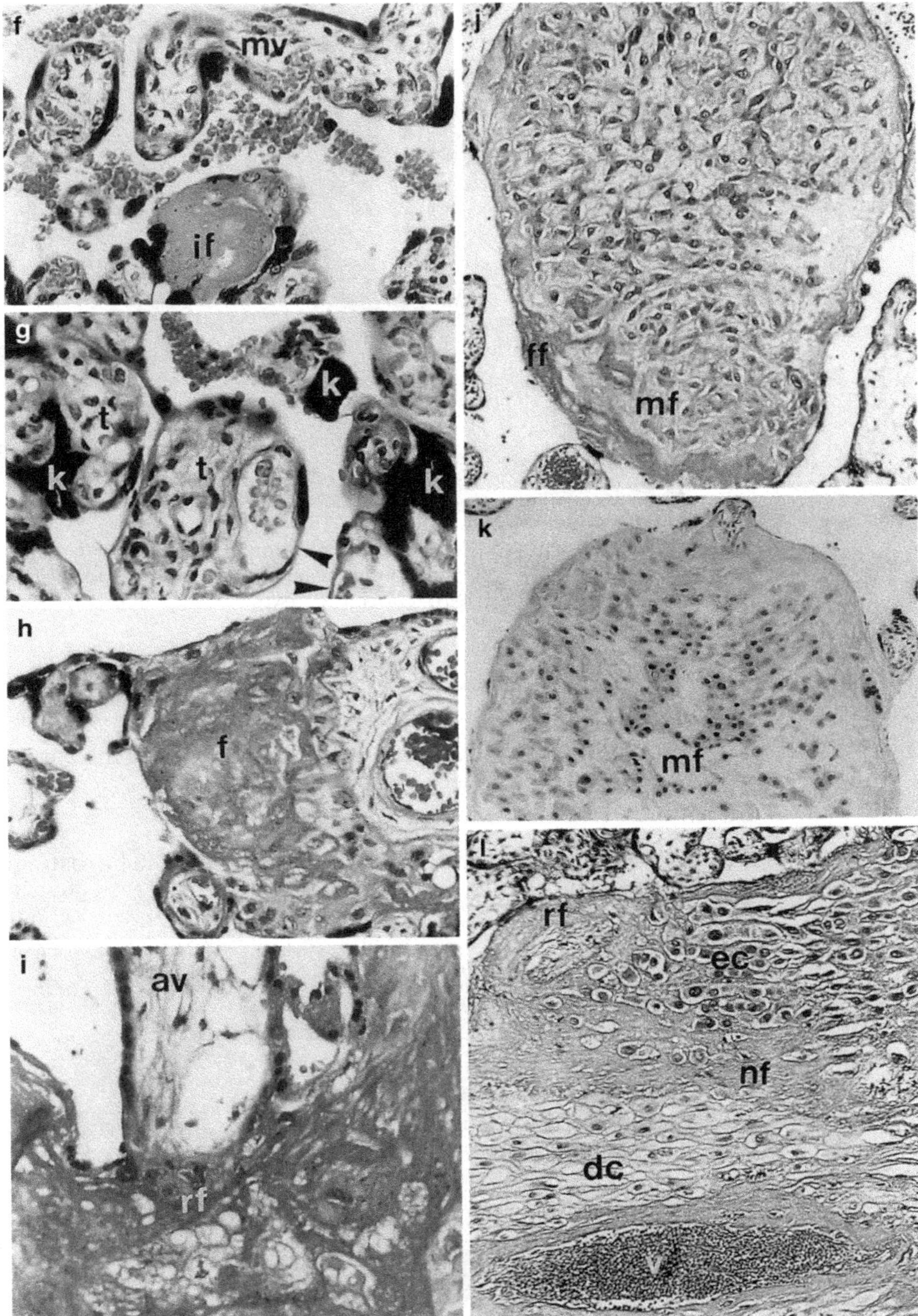

Figure 7.2. (continued) (k) ×360. (**h**) A small stem villus (sv), the trophoblastic cover of which is partly replaced by a thick plug of perivillous fibrinoid (f) ×180. (**i**) An anchoring villus (av), connected to the basal plate by fibrinoid (rf) as the originally connecting cell column has vanished ×180. (**j**) Cell island ×90. (**k**) Tip of a placental septum ×90. (**l**) Basal plate with obvious layering ×90.

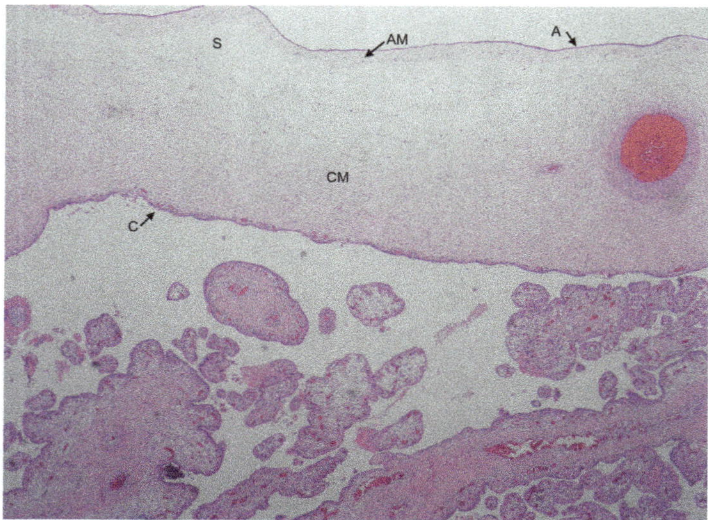

Figure 7.3. H&E-stained section of the chorionic plate at the 21st week PM. Amnionic epithelium (A), amnionic mesenchyme (AM), spongy layer (S), chorionic mesenchyme (CM), chorionic (extravillous) cytotrophoblast (C), Langhans' fibrinoid (L) ×100.

- **Basal plate** including
  - **Anchoring villi** connected via
  - **Cell columns** (Fig. 7.2i) to the septa (Fig. 7.2h) or the basal plate

Chorionic Plate

At term, the following layers of the chorionic plate can be distinguished (Figs. 7.3 and 7.4):

- **Amnion**
  - **Amnionic epithelium**
  - **Amnionic mesoderm**
- **Spongy layer, separating amnion and chorion**
- **Chorion**
  - **Chorionic mesoderm**
- **Extravillous trophoblast**
- **Langhans' fibrinoid layer encasing the extravillous cytotrophoblast**

The **chorionic plate** (Fig. 7.2c) is the cover of the **intervillous space** (Fig. 7.2a) directly below. The **amnion** (Fig. 7.2b) covers the chorionic plate toward the amniotic cavity. It consists of a single layer of cuboidal to columnar cells, beneath which is a thin layer of **amnionic mesoderm**. The chorion consists of the *spongy layer with clefts, then a compact layer of chorionic mesoderm, a rudimentary basement membrane, and finally fibrinoid* (Fig. 7.2c). On the lower side of this basement membrane, highly variable amounts of **extravillous trophoblast** can be found. Due to the instability of the spongy layer, and the fact that the amnion never really "fuses" with the chorion, the amnion may "detach" from the chorion or even become lost during preparation. The structure of the amnion and chorion are similar to that of the extraplacental fetal membranes

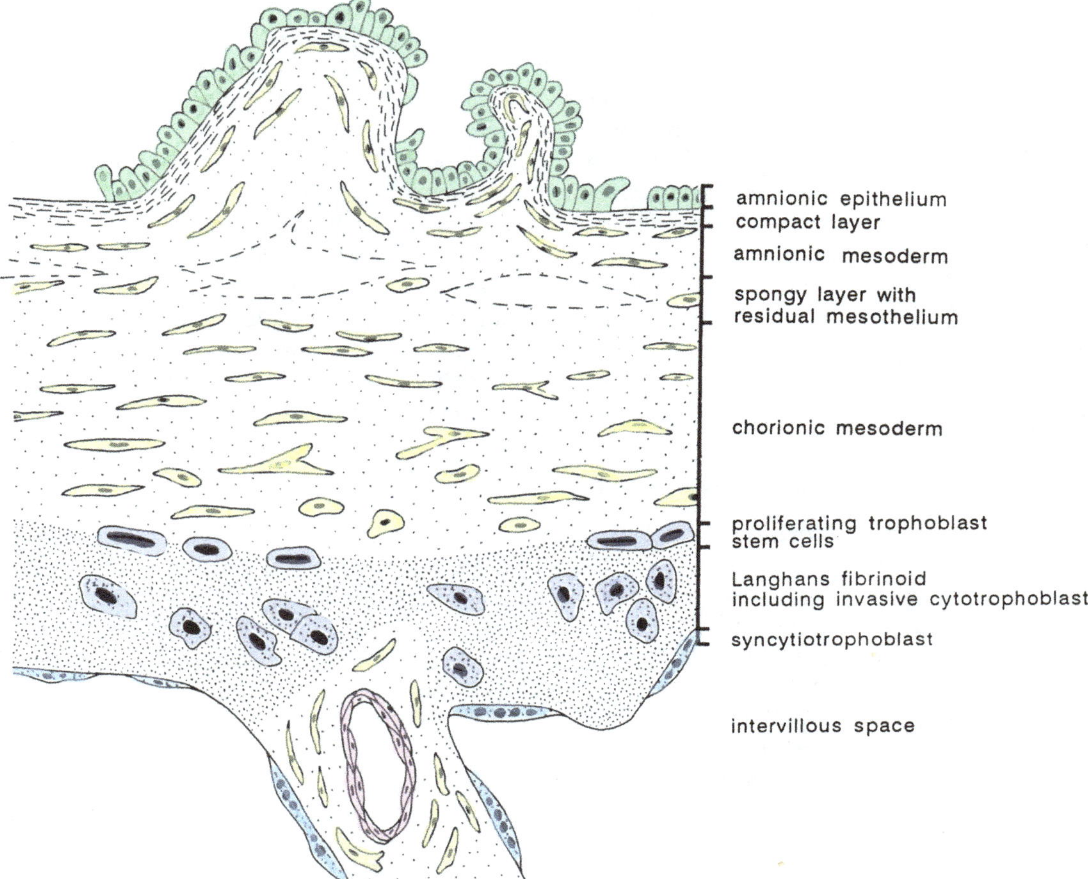

Figure 7.4. The layering and cellular composition of the chorionic plate.

except that the chorionic vessels, branching from the umbilical vessels, run in the mesoderm.

In its early stages, the intervillous surface of **Langhans' layer** is still mostly covered by syncytiotrophoblast, but this becomes completely replaced by fibrinoid during later pregnancy. Abundant scattered or aggregated extravillous trophoblast cells can be seen in the fibrinoid (Fig. 7.4). In some places, the chorionic mesoderm is directly in contact with the Langhans' fibrinoid without interposed trophoblast. *Subchorionic fibrinoid forms the "bosselations" and the laminated subchorionic plaques seen on the fetal surface of placentas.* These deposits vary markedly and result from eddying in the places where the intervillous blood is turned back toward the basal plate.

Villous Structures

Attached to or extending from the fibrinoid one finds numerous large **stem villi**, *representing the first branches of villous trunks (or villous trees) branching off from the chorionic plate* (see upper third of Fig. 7.2a). Different from the first trimester situation, the width of the **intervillous space** (Fig. 7.2a) is highly variable with large **subchorionic lakes** of maternal blood and narrow intervillous clefts between the terminal villi. In the term placenta, the width of the clefts is somewhat dependent on the mode of delivery and how much maternal blood is expelled during the process. The **villous trees** (Fig. 7.2d) branch into **stem villi**, which are the largest caliber villi and are found in highest concentration near the chorionic plate, particularly near the insertion of the umbilical cord. Histologically, they are characterized by *one or several arteries and veins, or arterioles and venules surrounded by a fibrous stroma.* Focally the trophoblastic cover of the stem villi may be replaced by fibrinoid near term. Although **immature intermediate villi** (Fig. 7.2e) and **mature intermediate villi** (Fig. 7.2f) are present in the term placenta, the predominant villous type is **terminal villi** (Fig. 7.2g). These are the grape-like terminal side branches of the mature intermediate villi and contain *loose stroma* and *sinusoidally dilated fetal capillaries* (see Chap. 6 for discussion of villous types).

Nonvillous Structures

Fibrinoid (Fig. 7.2h) is an *acellular, eosinophilic material* present in the intervillous space (Fig. 7.2c, d, f, h). Areas of prominent fibrinoid deposition are the chorionic and basal plates, the cell islands, and septa (Fig. 7.2c, i–l). Fibrinoid has two different compositions, fibrin and fibrinoid, which cannot be distinguished histologically and may be deposited close together or separately (see Chap. 8).

Cell islands (Fig. 7.2j) are round or irregularly shaped structures *connected to either the villous tree or the chorionic plate.* They vary in size from several hundred micrometers to 3 mm and are *composed primarily of extravillous trophoblastic cells encased in fibrinoid* (Fig. 7.5). They increase in

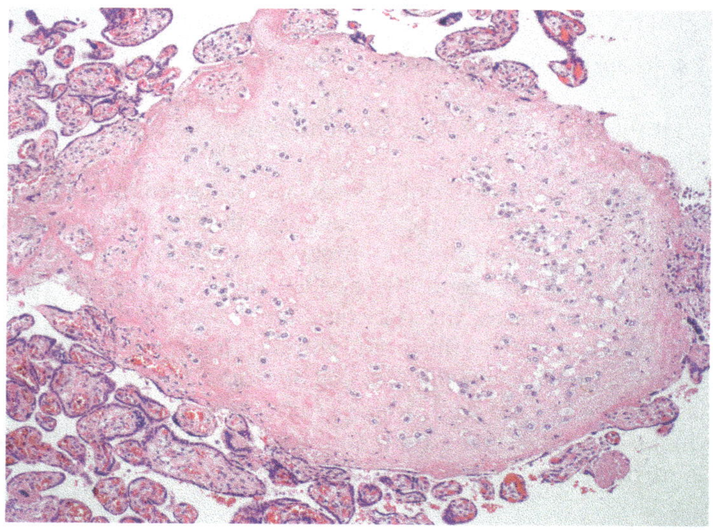

Figure 7.5. Cell island at 20 weeks' gestation. The mononuclear cells with dark cytoplasm in the center are the extravillous trophoblastic cells. They are surrounded by "fibrinoid." Note that there is no differentiation to syncytium among the extravillous trophoblast cells. Incorporated decidual cells are rare findings. The surrounding placental villi may be attached to the surface; sometimes they are incorporated into the fibrinoid. H&E ×160.

size throughout pregnancy due to continuous trophoblastic proliferation and increased fibrinoid. Large cell islands may contain central cavities or "cysts," which result from degeneration of trophoblast cells and subsequent liquefaction. They resemble septa in structure and composition except that they lack decidua. Cell islands are comparable to the basal ends of the anchoring villi, the **cell columns** (see below). *The major difference between a cell island and a cell column is the topographic relation: cell islands are freely floating cell columns; cell columns are anchored to the basal plate or to septa.*

Placental septa (Fig. 7.2k) are the result of folding of the basal plate, probably supported by tension of anchoring villi (see Chap. 8). They are found in nearly every mature placenta, and their absence is rare and is usually linked to pathologic conditions such as maternal floor infarction (see Chap. 19). They are *rudimentary pillar-shaped structures*, which are not true septa and are actually *irregular protrusions of the basal plate* into the placenta, partially subdividing the intervillous space. Because they develop from the basal plate, their composition generally resembles that of the basal plate (Fig. 7.2a), being composed of *extravillous trophoblast and decidual cells embedded in fibrinoid with occasional endometrial glands* (Fig. 7.6). Precursors

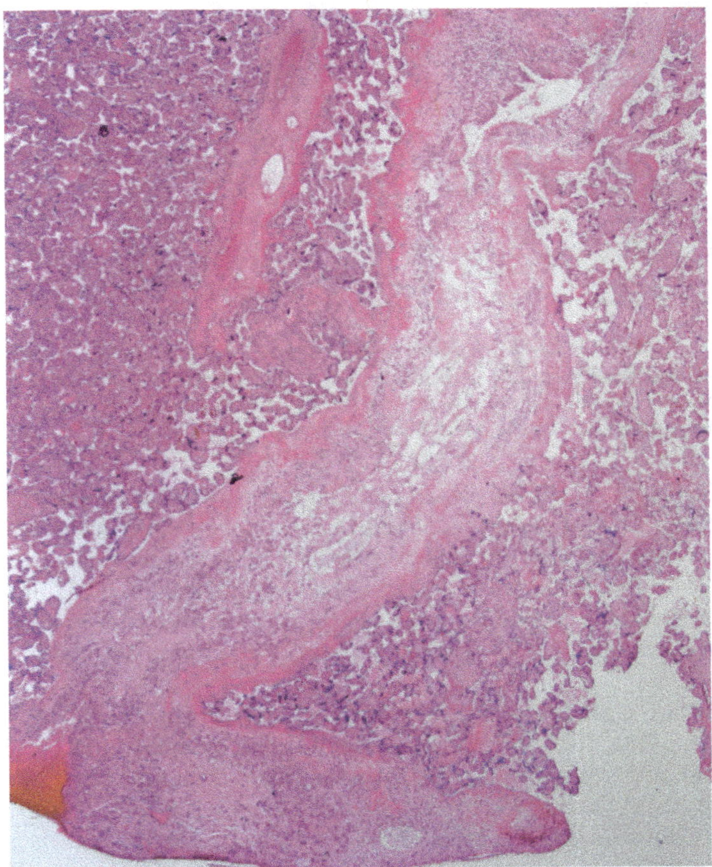

Figure 7.6. Paraffin section of a placental septum, 37th week PM. Note the numerous anchoring villi inserting at the septum. In its base several vessel cross sections (V) represent uteroplacental veins ×65.

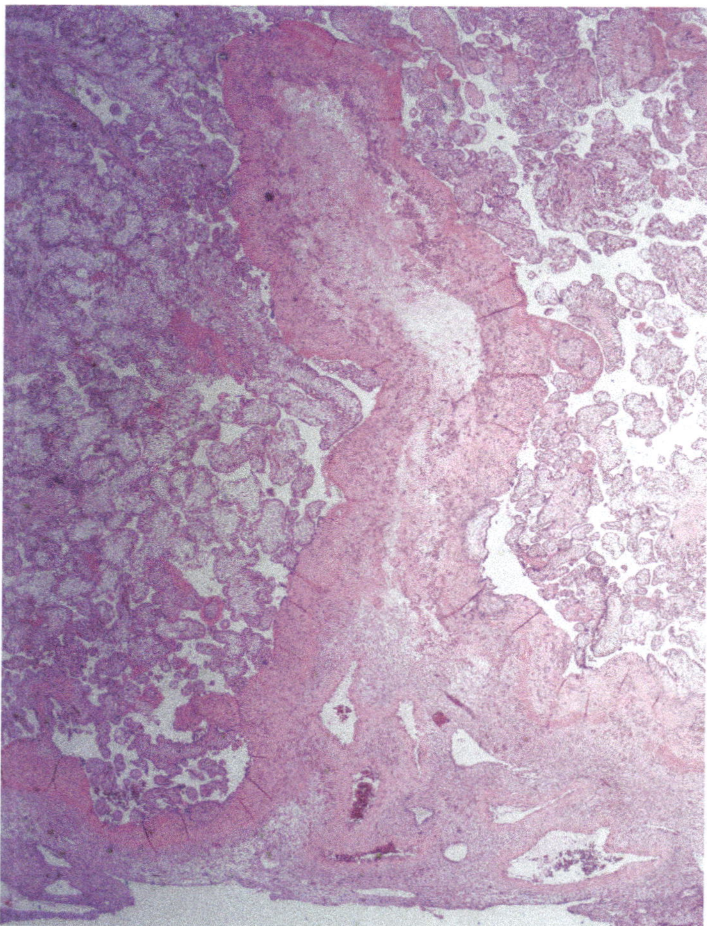

Figure 7.7. Paraffin section of an early placental septum (*middle*) during the early second trimester. The cellular composition is similar to that of the early basal plate. They are largely devoid of fibrinoid and can be interpreted as being extensions and folds of the early basal plate ×90.

of future septa are visible as early as in the sixth week postmenstruation (PM) (Fig. 7.7). These early septa consist of *cytotrophoblast with anchoring villi near their tips.* They develop further by traction on the anchoring villi combined with proliferation of their cytotrophoblastic feet. Ultimately, there is buckling or folding of the basal decidua induced by the pressure of expanding villous lobules without distention of the uterine wall (Fig. 7.6).

Septa are a frequent site of **placental cysts**, formerly called **X-cell cysts** (Fig. 7.8). They may occasionally be grossly visible and consist of fibrinoid and trophoblastic cells surrounding a cystic space. They often show necrosis, and thus it seems they are degenerative in nature.

Cell columns are the *trophoblastic connections between the anchoring villi and basal plate or placental septa.* The development of cell columns starts around day 15 postconception (PC) when the primary villi become invaded by extraembryonic mesenchyme and form tertiary villi. *The basal parts of the villous stems that are connected to the basal plate*

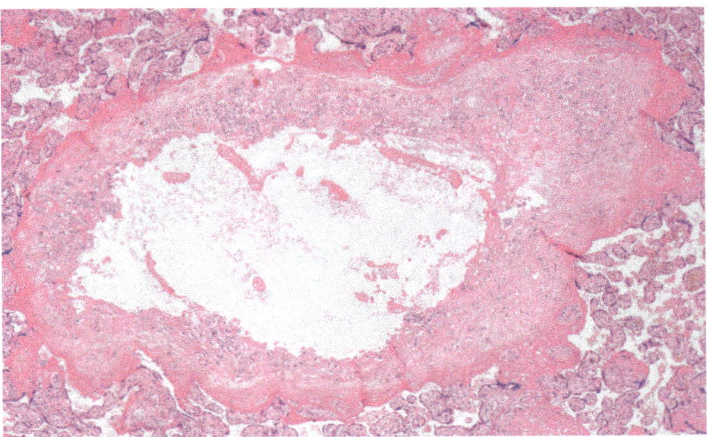

Figure 7.8. Cross section of a placental septum with cyst. It is similar in appearance to the typical "X-cell" cysts being composed of extravillous trophoblast and extracellular matrix ×100.

persist as primary villi and are called the **cell columns**. These developmental events are identical to those at some free-floating villous tips, leading to the formation of cell islands. Cell columns are composed of a *multilayered core of cytotrophoblast surrounded by an incomplete sleeve of syncytiotrophoblast*. As soon as cell columns are surrounded by fibrinoid and buried in the basal plate, their syncytiotrophoblastic cover becomes replaced by fibrin (Fig. 7.9). The cytotrophoblastic core continues without sharp demarcation into the anchoring villus. The cell columns represent the proliferative zones of extravillous trophoblast, and the various steps from trophoblastic proliferation via differentiation to invasion are present in these columns (see Chap. 6). All extravillous trophoblastic cells invading the basal plate and the placental bed derive from this stem cell population. These cells migrate laterally into the villi as well as basally into the basal plate. With advancing gestation, the number of proliferating cells is reduced; however, even at term, one can still can find intact cell columns.

Basal Plate

The **basal plate** (Fig. 7.2l) is a highly variable structure, ranging in thickness from 100 µm to 1.5 mm. At term, the basal plate has often lost it typical layering in most places, and only in a few exceptional places is it as clearly layered as depicted here (Fig. 7.10). In most places, there is no clearly defined fetomaternal border, and extravillous trophoblast, decidual cells, uteroplacental vessels, and endometrial glandular residues are intermingled with fibrinoid in a somewhat haphazard manner. Generally speaking, the following layers make up the mature basal plate (from the superficial surface to the deep maternal surface):

- **Inner surface**
- **Rohr's fibrinoid**
- **Principal layer**
- **Nitabuch's fibrinoid**
- **Separation zone**

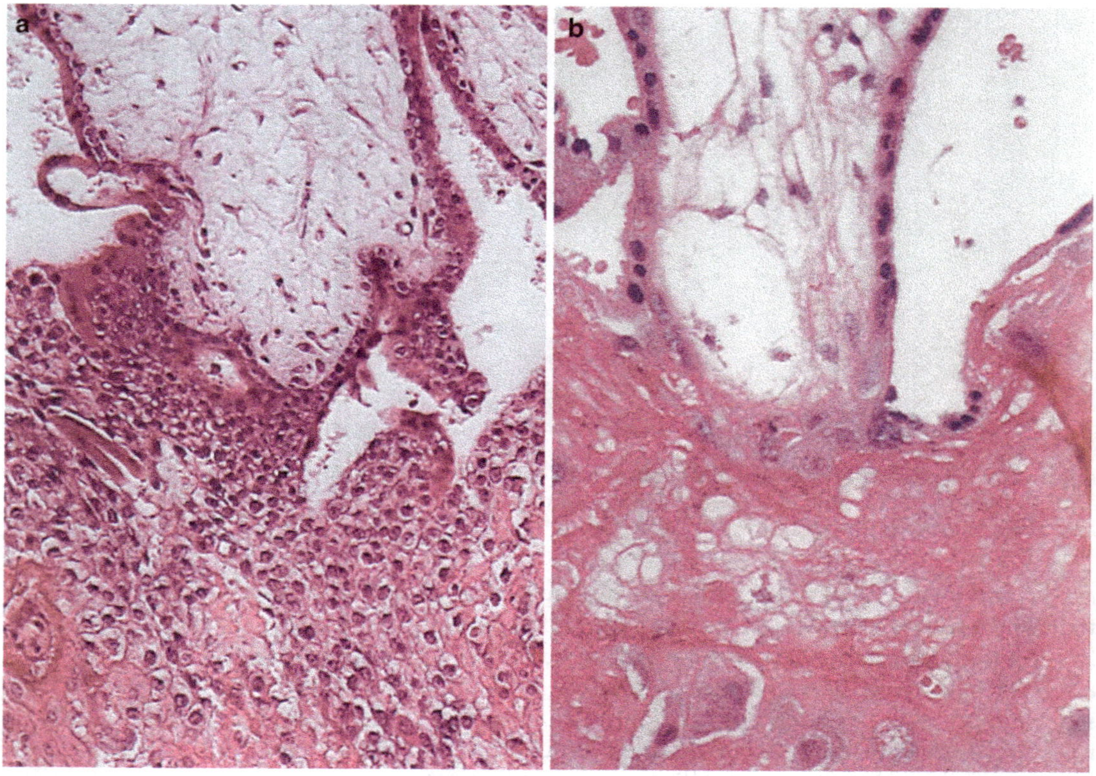

Figure 7.9. Cell columns at the sixth week (**a**) and 20th week (**b**). Note the cluster of cells in the cell column from the early pregnancy as compared to term in which they are mostly replaced by fibrinoid. H&E ×300.

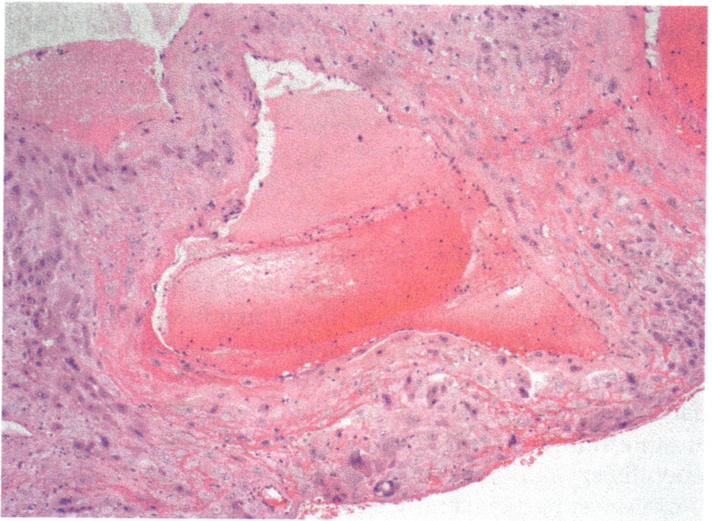

Figure 7.10. Extravillous trophoblastic cells (*dark* cells) in decidua basalis of a near-term placenta. A converted decidual vessel is present. H&E ×240.

The **inner surface** of the basal plate faces the intervillous space. It shows the *residual syncytiotrophoblastic lining* present only in small patches, and *maternal endothelium* lines the intervillous surface of the basal plate. Where syncytiotrophoblast and maternal endothelium are absent, the basal plate is covered by Rohr's fibrinoid. This superficial fibrinoid layer is an *incomplete and irregularly structured layer* (Fig. 7.10). In some areas, it engulfs attached villi, and here it is continuous with perivillous fibrinoid.

The **principal layer** is highly variable in composition and measures from 50 µm to 1 mm in thickness. It is composed of *extravillous cytotrophoblast, fibrinoid, loose connective tissue, decidual cells, remnants of encased anchoring villi, and "buried" cell columns*. Most of the connective tissue of this region is of maternal origin. Trophoblastic and decidual cells may be intensively admixed but do not have direct contact, as they are separated by fibrinoid, the external lamina of the decidual cells, or both.

In the last trimester, **anchoring villi** (Fig. 7.2i) become less prominent but *are still connected to the basal plate or to septa* by **cell columns**. As the proliferative activity of the cell columns slows down, the cells are rarified to one layer that is sometimes incomplete or even replaced by fibrinoid. Some *cell columns maintain their proliferative activity and thus continue to act as growth zones for the anchoring villi and basal plate*.

Nitabuch's fibrinoid layer, also called *uteroplacental fibrinoid* (Fig. 7.11), is located in the immediate maternofetal "battlefield" of the junctional zone. It is a more or less uninterrupted layer that varies from 20 µm to more than 100 µm in thickness. In the most complete areas, Nitabuch's fibrinoid separates trophoblastic cells from decidual cells and marks the *exact maternofetal border*. In many places, the layer may split and rejoin, with trophoblast, decidual cells, and endometrial connective tissue interposed. Mixed populations of the two cell types on one or both sides of this layer are the most typical finding.

Placental separation at delivery occurs in the decidua, which is the **separation zone**. This zone also contains extravillous trophoblast. The deeper tissue layers of the placental site, which remain in utero and are later discharged as lochia, show a similar cellular admixture and are referred to as the **placental bed**. In situ, the placental bed and basal plate cannot be delimited from each other because the separation zone becomes visible only shortly before delivery. Together they comprise the **junctional zone**. The term *basal plate is applicable only to the delivered placenta*.

Marginal Zone

The **marginal zone** is not precisely defined and consists of the *transitional zone between the chorionic plate, the basal plate, and the membranes*. It has characteristics of all three regions. The outer margin is the grossly visible transition from placenta to membranes. At this point, the intervillous space is occluded by fusion of the chorionic plate with the basal plate. Macroscopically, the marginal zone is often represented by a slightly prominent *opaque ring in the subchorionic region*, called the

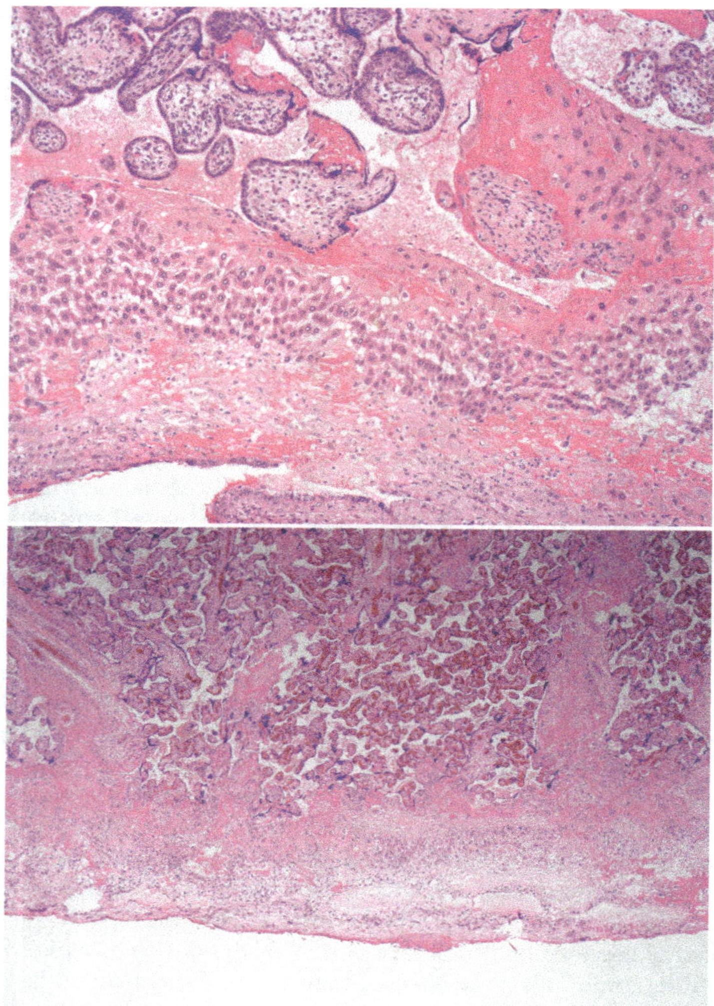

Figure 7.11. Developmental stages of the basal plate. At the 23rd week PM (*top*), the basal plate is composed of a dense mixture of extravillous trophoblastic and decidual cells, intermingled with a few trophoblastic giant cells. There is little fibrinoid. H&E ×160. At term (*bottom*), the typical layering of the basal plate is evident. Facing the intervillous space, it is covered by an interrupted layer of Rohr's fibrinoid, followed by an incomplete layer of extravillous cytotrophoblast. The latter is somewhat separated from the decidua cells by a loose layer of Nitabuch's fibrinoid. H&E ×40.

subchorionic closing ring. It measures about 1 cm in width. The opacity of the subchorionic closing ring is due to an increased number of extravillous trophoblastic cells and decidual cells. The presence of the subchorionic closing ring nearer to the center of the placenta is referred to as a **circumvallate placenta** (see Chap. 13).

Large uteroplacental veins present near the placental margin open into the intervillous space and comprise the **marginal sinus**. The border between the maternal veins and the intervillous space is difficult to define because maternal endothelial cells spread from the venous lumina to the intervillous surfaces of the basal and chorionic plates in the entire marginal zone. The initial portion of the marginal uteroplacental veins is largely replaced by fibrinoid with surrounding cellular degeneration. It is likely that the thin peripheral decidual cover in this region is responsible for the occurrence of the so-called marginal sinus hemorrhage.

Anatomy of the Intervillous Space

After leaving the spiral arteries, maternal blood circulates through the intervillous space, flowing directly around the villi outside the confines of the maternal vascular system. At delivery, much of this blood is lost, and, therefore, on histologic examination the usual appearance of the intervillous space is that of a system of narrow clefts. The inlets of the spiral arteries are near the centers of the villous trees, while the venous outlets are arranged around the periphery. Therefore, each fetomaternal circulatory unit is composed of one villous tree with a corresponding, centrifugally perfused portion of the intervillous space (Fig. 7.12). Most of these 40–60 "placentones" are in contact with each other and overlap. The placentone ranges in diameter from 1 to 4 cm, and therefore the entire unit may not be well represented in histologic sections. In addition, placentones from different locations may show varying degrees of maturation.

Calcification, Mineralization, and Pigment

The mature placenta often has fine deposits of calcium salts, which appear as *irregularly distributed, yellow, and stippled deposits on gross examination*. They have a gritty sensation when a knife passes through the placenta on sectioning. Calcium deposits are blue in H&E preparations and occur *most commonly in the fibrinoid in the basal plate and the placental septa* (Fig. 7.13). The amount of calcification present does not appear to have any clinical significance, as excessive calcification has not been associated with any significant clinical abnormalities in the mother or infant.

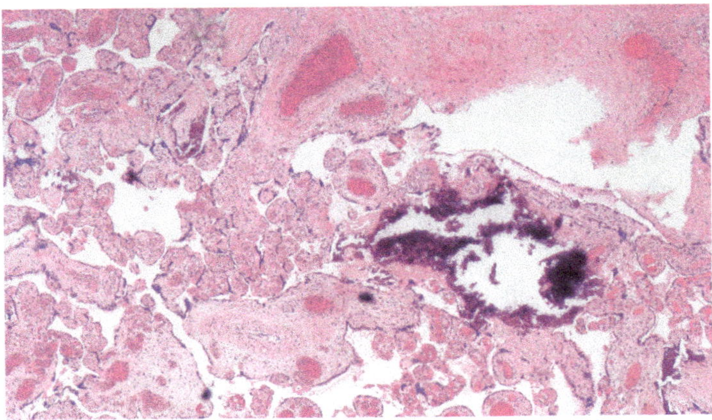

Figure 7.12. Irregular calcification (*dark black*) in mature placenta. H&E ×160.

One may find microscopic granular purple deposits lining the *villous basement membranes* (see Fig. 20.13). These **villous microcalcifications** are most common in abortion specimens and probably include deposits of minerals in addition to calcium. Other conditions associated with this mineralization of the trophoblastic basement membrane include *hydramnios, fetal vascular thrombosis, anencephaly, trisomy 21, Bartter syndrome, and congenital nephrotic syndrome.* These deposits are probably caused by deficient transport through the trophoblast, which are not consumed by the fetus due to cessation of capillary flow.

Melanin has also been demonstrated in the basement membranes of villi and in Hofbauer cells. It is present as often in Caucasians as in African-Americans. These deposits occur more frequently in association with chronic skin lesions, and the condition has been called "dermatopathic melanosis of the placenta." Melanin-containing macrophages in the amnion have also been found in cases of prolonged amnion

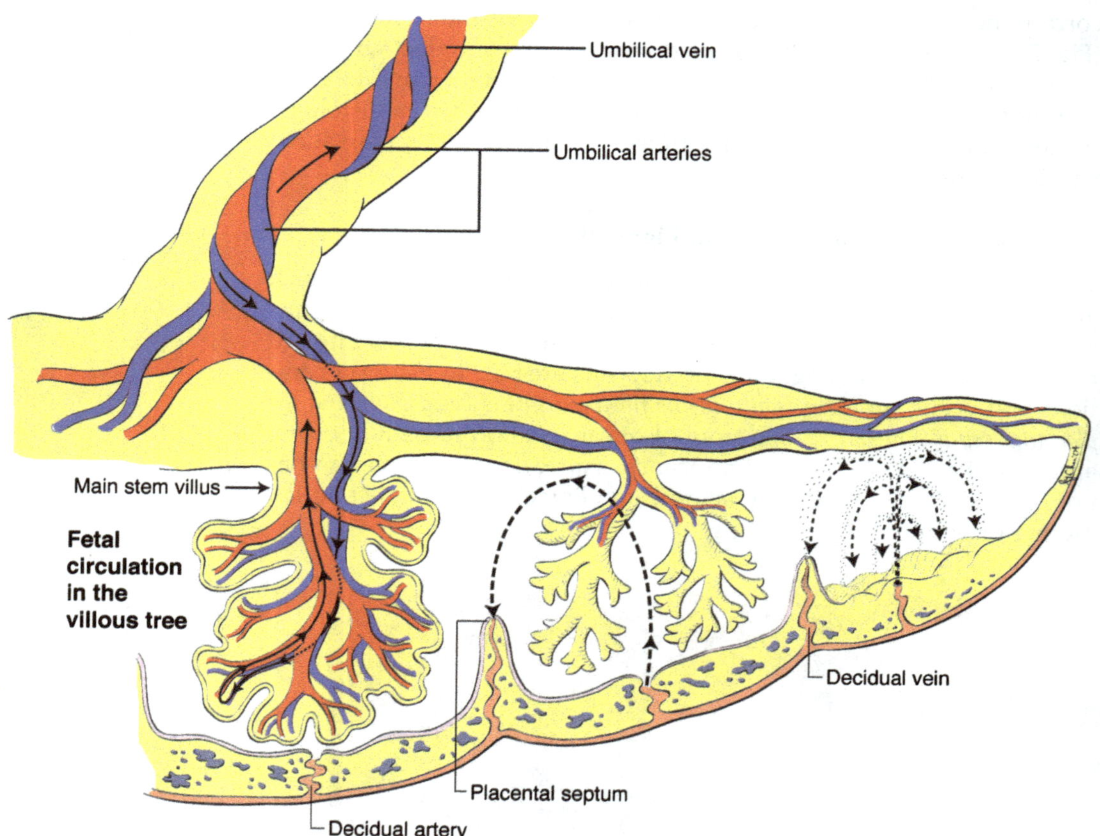

Figure 7.13. Typical spatial relations between villous trees and the maternal bloodstream. According to the placentone theory, a placentone is one villous tree together with the related part of the intervillous space. In the case of typical placentones that prevail in the periphery of the placenta, the maternal blood (*arrows*) enters the intervillous space near the center of the villous tree and leaves near the clefts between neighboring villous trees. One or only a few villous trees occupy one placental lobule (cotyledon). In the central parts of the placenta, the villous trees, because of size and nearby location, may partly overlap so that the zonal arrangement of the placentone disappears.

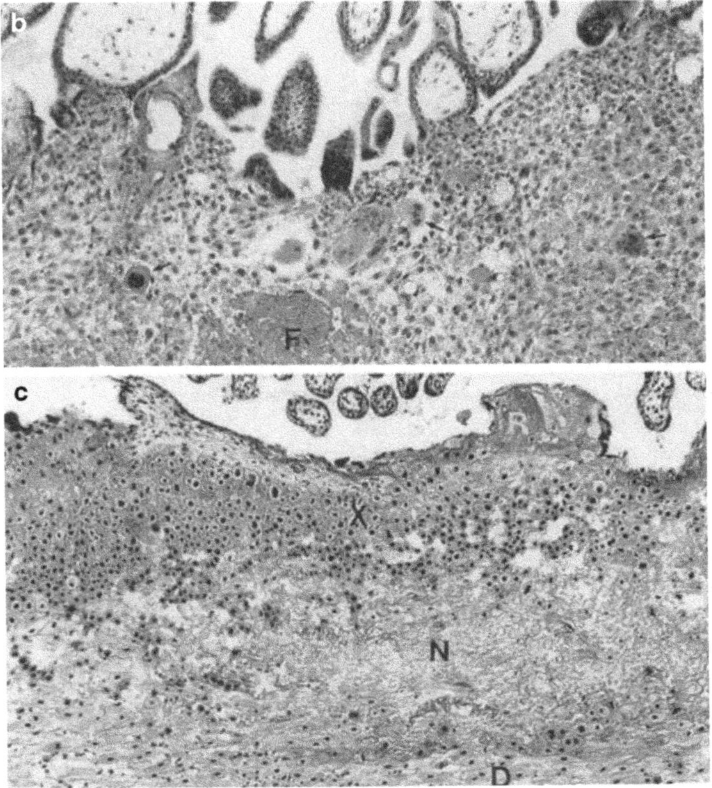

Figure 7.13. (continued)

rupture. **Lipofuscin**, or "aging pigment," has been also demonstrated in placentas beyond 32 weeks, although it is generally accepted that only maturation, not aging, occurs in placental tissue.

Fetal Membranes

The term **membranes** is usually taken to be synonymous with the **amnion** and the **chorion laeve** of the extraplacental membranes. They are distinct from the **chorion frondosum**, which refers to a specialized, thickened part of the membranes, otherwise known as the placental disk. Their structure and function include *turnover of water and enzymatic activity during the initiation of labor*. The structure of the membranes remains constant from the fourth month until term. After birth, the following layers can be seen histologically (Fig. 7.14):

- **Amnion**
- **Amnionic epithelium**
  - **Basement membrane**
  - **Amnionic mesoderm**
    - **Compact stromal layer**
    - **Fibroblast layer**

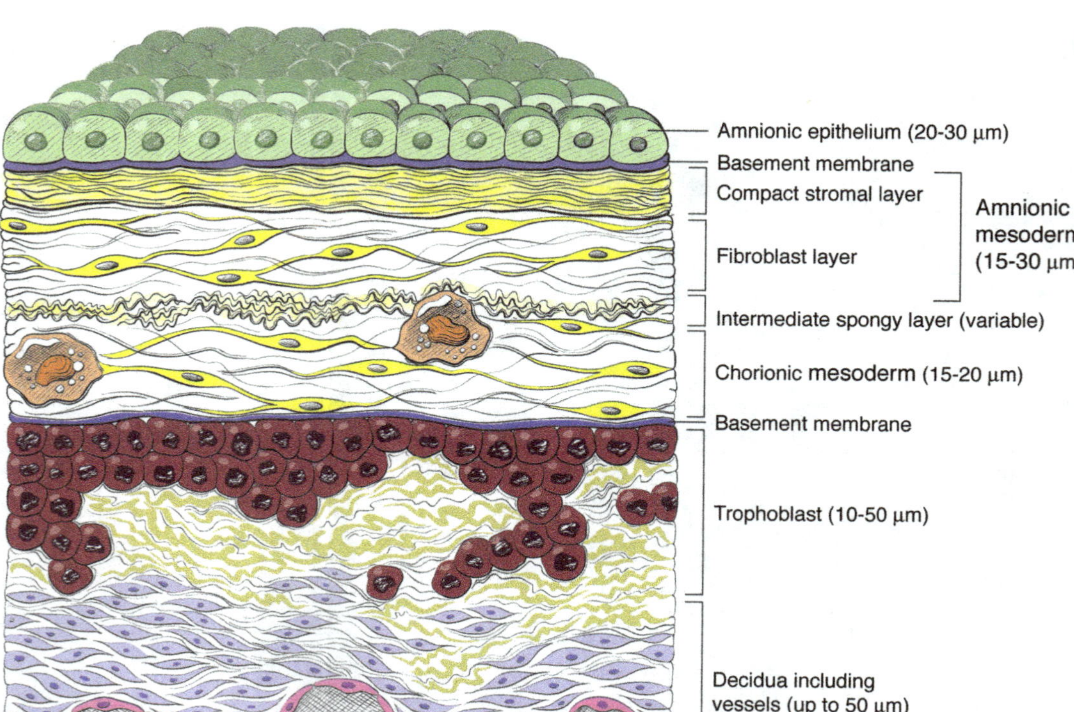

Figure 7.14. Detailed drawing depicting the layers of the fetal membranes. Drawing is not to scale.

- **Intermediate spongy layer (highly variable in thickness)**
- **Chorion laeve**
  - **Chorionic mesoderm**
  - **Chorionic vessels (in chorionic plate)**
- **Trophoblast (10–50 mm)**
- **Decidua capsularis (up to 50 mm)**

Amnion

Macroscopically, the **amnion** is a translucent structure, easily separated from the underlying chorion. It *never truly fuses with the chorion,* as it is only passively attached by the internal pressure of the amniotic fluid. The amnion does not possess its own blood vessels and obtains its nutrition and oxygen from the surrounding amniotic fluid and fetal surface vessels. *The amnionic epithelium is derived from the fetal ectoderm and is thus contiguous over the umbilical cord and fetal skin.* The epithelium is composed of a *single layer of flat, cuboidal to columnar cells.* Taller, columnar cells are usually present near the insertion of the membranes at the placental margin, whereas flatter cells are generally present in the periphery. The amnionic epithelium rests on a basement membrane, which is connected to the **amnionic mesoderm**, a thin connective tissue layer (Fig. 7.14). The latter consists of a **compact stromal layer** and a **fibroblast layer**. These separate layers are difficult to distinguish on histologic section.

The amnion has multiple functional roles in the placenta. It is essential for the *structural integrity and junctional permeability of the membranes, and has a role in the turnover of amniotic fluid as well as maintenance of amniotic fluid pH*. It is also thought to have a role in the onset of labor, including the initiation and maintenance of uterine contractions.

Chorion Laeve

The **amnion** and **chorion** are easily separated and will readily slide along one another. This is due to the existence of the spongy layer which is composed of *loosely arranged bundles of collagen fibers with a few scattered fibroblasts*, separated by a communicating system of clefts (Fig. 7.14). The collagen composition of both amnion and chorion contributes to the mechanical stability and tensile properties of the membranes. The next layer, the **chorionic mesoderm** consists of a *coarse network of collagen bundles intermingled with finer argyrophilic fibrils*. Fibroblasts, myofibroblasts, and macrophages are also regular findings (Fig. 7.14). Chorionic vessels are present only in the mesoderm of the chorionic plate and not in the chorion laeve. Remnants of atrophied chorionic villi appear as round "balls" of loose connective tissue, without a trophoblastic cover (Fig. 7.15).

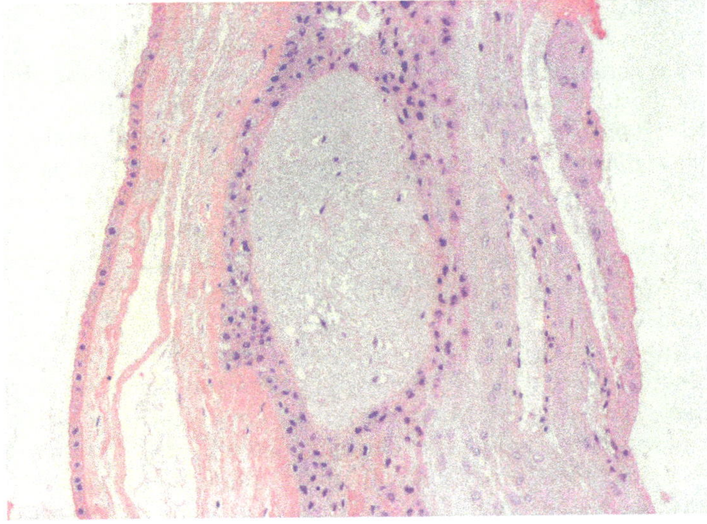

Figure 7.15. Extraplacental fetal membranes. The amnionic epithelium (at the *left*) sits on a thin layer of connective tissue that is not easily discernible from the chorionic connective tissue in histologic section. The following layer of extravillous trophoblastic cells contains an atrophic or "ghost" villus. At the right of the figure is the decidua capsularis with visible maternal vessels. H&E ×200.

Trophoblast Layer

A highly variable layer of **extravillous trophoblastic cells** persists until term. They constitute a population of cells that are not involved in implantation, commonly referred to as migratory trophoblast (see Invasive Phenotype in Chap. 8). With advancing gestation, some of these cells may show degenerative change and foci of fibrinoid between the cells (see Chap. 8). Toward the uterine wall, the trophoblast interdigitates intensely with the decidua.

Decidua

The **decidual layer** is the *only maternal component of the membranes.* The decidual tissue attached to the membranes after birth is largely derived from the **parietal and capsular decidua** (see Fig. 5.3). Whether the individual cells are derived from one or the other layer cannot be distinguished. The deeper layers of decidua, which remain in utero, are richly supplied with maternal blood vessels (Fig. 7.15), although decidual vessels are often present in the decidua capsularis. *Macrophages, lymphocytes, and other inflammatory cells may also be present.* At the edge of the placenta, the decidua capsularis is contiguous with the decidua basalis and delimits the "marginal sinus."

Structure and Histology of the Umbilical Cord

The **umbilical cord** contains *two arteries and a vein suspended in Wharton's jelly.* The surface of the cord consists of a layer of **amnionic epithelium**, which is contiguous with the surface of the placenta and the fetal skin. The amnionic epithelium, near the umbilicus, is largely *unkeratinized, stratified squamous epithelium.* This layer provides a transition to the keratinized stratified squamous epithelium of the abdominal wall. Farther away from the umbilicus, the epithelium becomes *stratified columnar epithelium* (two to eight cell layers) and finally *simple columnar epithelium as it continues onto the fetal surface.* The basal cells of the stratified portions resemble the epithelium of the membranes, whereas the superficial cells sometimes are squamous and are occasionally pyknotic. Unlike the amnion of the membranes, the amnion of the cord grows firmly into the central connective tissue core and cannot be dislodged.

The **connective tissue** of the cord is derived from the extraembryonic mesoblast. The jelly-like material of **Wharton's jelly** is composed of *ground substance (collagen, laminin, heparan sulfate, hyaluronic acid, carbohydrates with glycosyl, and mannosyl groups) distributed in a fine network of microfibrils.* Extracellular matrix molecules are often accumulated around "stromal clefts." The stromal spaces together with the surrounding meshwork of contractile cells serve as a mechanism for turgor regulation of the cord, avoiding compression of umbilical veins and counteracting bending or kinking of the cord. The cord is sparsely cellular and contains abundant water, which is also advantageous to prevent compression of umbilical vessels (Fig. 7.16). There

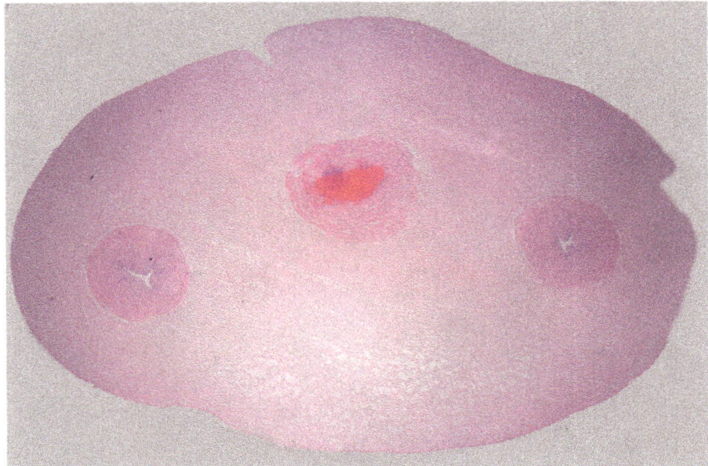

Figure 7.16. Cross section of mature umbilical cord, near its placental insertion showing a sparsely cellular Wharton's jelly, an umbilical vein and two arteries. H&E ×20.

are a few macrophages and somewhat greater numbers of mast cells. Myofibroblasts are present around vessels and underneath the cord surface.

Umbilical Vessels

There are normally **two arteries and one vein** in the human umbilical cord (Fig. 7.16). Originally, two veins are present, but the second normally atrophies during the second month of pregnancy. The mean intravital diameter of the arteries is around 3 mm, and the venous diameter is around twice this size. *The muscular coat of the arteries consists of crossing spiraled fibers. The venous muscular coats are thinner than those of the arteries and are composed of separate layers of longitudinal or circular fibers.* Each umbilical vessel is surrounded by crossing bundles of spiraled collagen fibers that form a kind of adventitia. The arteries possess no internal elastic membrane and have much less elastica than in other similar caliber arteries. The vein, on the other hand, has an elastic subintimal layer (Fig. 7.17). The umbilical vessels in the placenta also lack vasa vasorum. In general, no nerves traverse the umbilical cord from fetus to placenta and the placenta has no neural supply.

Selected References

PHP5, pages 16–29 (Microscopic Survey), pages 160–164 (Intervillous Space), pages 236–248 (Chorionic Plate, Marginal Zone, Basal Plate), pages 261–268 (Septa, Cell Islands and Cell Columns), pages 321–338 (Anatomy of the Fetal Membranes), pages 380–385 (Anatomy of the Umbilical Cord).
Bourne G. The human amnion and chorion. London: Lloyd-Luke, 1962.
Bourne G. The microscopic anatomy of the human amnion and chorion. Am J Obstet Gynecol 1960;79:1070–1073.

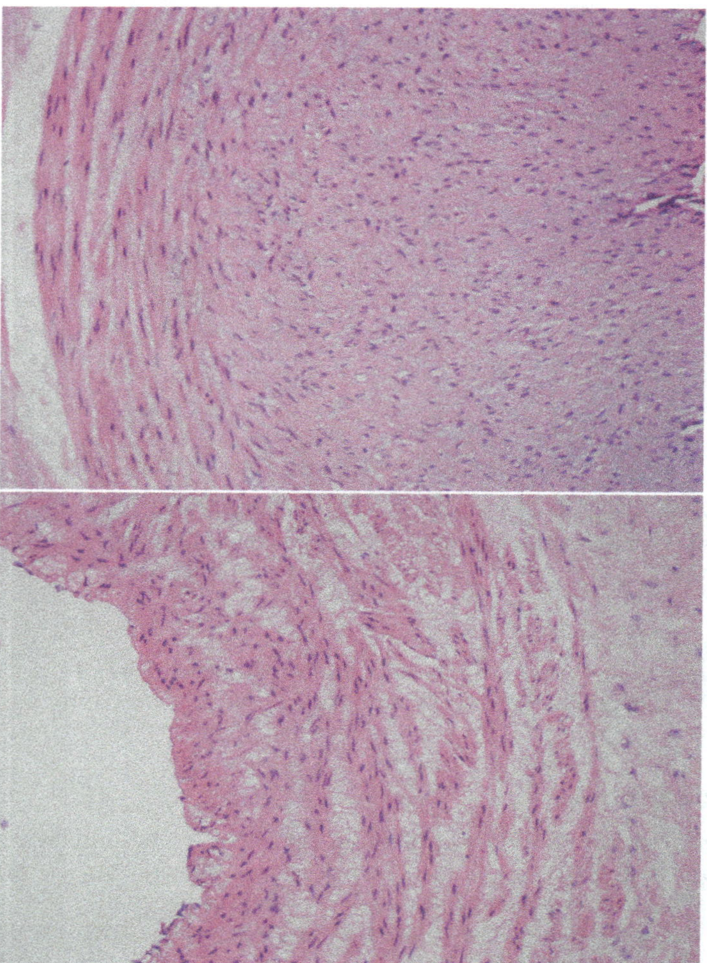

Figure 7.17. Umbilical cord sections of one umbilical artery (*top*) and a vein (*bottom*). In these sections, one may observe the presence of a delicate subendothelial elastica only in the vein at left. H&E ×200.

Bourne GL, Lacy D. Ultrastructure of human amnion and its possible relation to the circulation of amniotic fluid. Nature 1960;168:952–954.

Boyd JD, Hamilton WJ. The human placenta. Cambridge: Heffer & Sons, 1970.

Nanaev AK, Kohnen G, Milovanov AP, et al. Stromal differentiation and architecture of the human umbilical cord. Placenta 1997;18:53–64.

Takechi K, Kuwabara Y, Mizuno M. Ultrastructural and immunohistochemical studies of Wharton's jelly umbilical cord cells. Placenta 1993;14:235–245.

Wigglesworth JS. Vascular anatomy of the human placenta and its significance for placental pathology. J Obstet Gynaecol Br Commonw 1969;76:979–989.

Chapter 8

Extravillous Trophoblast, Trophoblastic Invasion, and Fibrinoid

General Considerations

The nonvillous parts of the placenta include the **chorionic plate, cell islands, cell columns, placental septa, basal plate, marginal zone, and fibrinoid deposits** (Fig. 8.1). These structures do not participate in maternofetal exchange, but have mechanical and metabolic functions. Irrespective of their location and structure, the nonvillous parts of the placenta have the same three basic components, which structurally and functionally do not vary from one area to the next:

- **Extravillous trophoblast,**
- **Fibrinoid**, and
- **Decidua**

Extravillous Trophoblast

Among placental biologists, the term **extravillous trophoblast** is in general use, whereas among gynecologic pathologists the term **intermediate trophoblast** is widely applied. Unfortunately, this latter term is misleading. It had originally been used to designate villous trophoblastic

R.N. Baergen, *Manual of Pathology of the Human Placenta,*
DOI 10.1007/978-1-4419-7494-5_8, © Springer Science+Business Media, LLC 2011

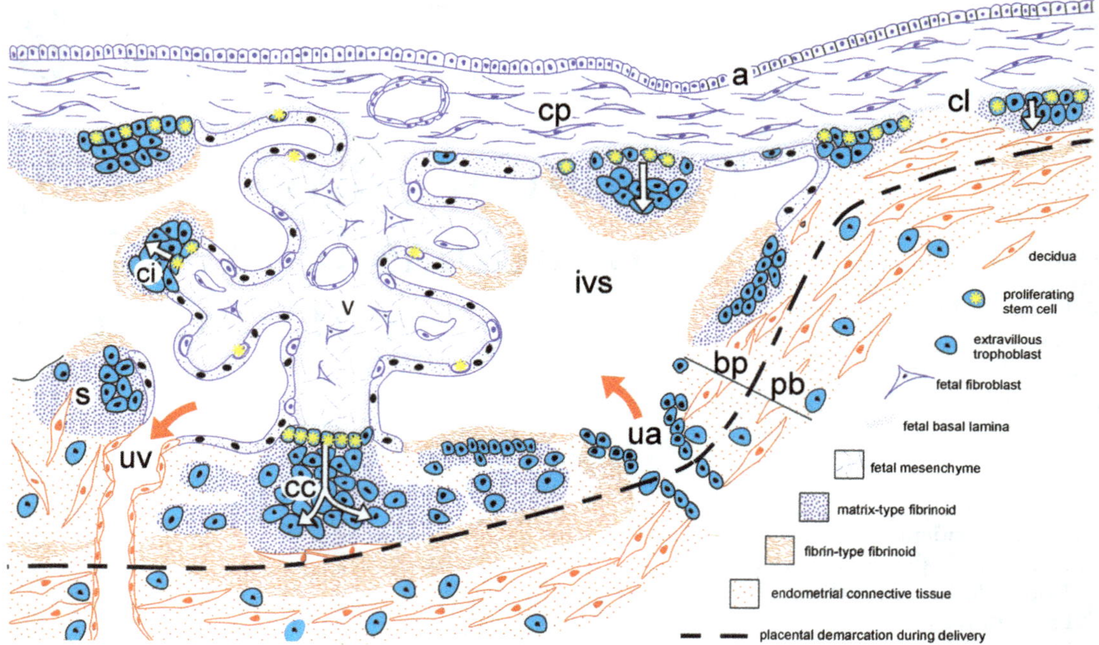

Figure 8.1. Schematic drawing of the distribution of the various trophoblast populations (*blue*) of the human placenta. Trophoblastic cells that rest on the trophoblastic basal lamina of the membranes, chorionic plate, villi, cell columns, and cell islands represent the proliferating trophoblastic stem cells (Langhans' cells). Those close to the intervillous space (ivs) differentiate and fuse to form the syncytiotrophoblast, which usually takes place in the placental villi (v). Without contact to the intervillous space, the daughter cells of the proliferating stem cells (marked by *asterisks*) do not fuse syncytially but rather differentiate and become extravillous trophoblastic cells. Their routes of invasion or migration are symbolized by *arrows*. Extravillous trophoblastic cells can be found in cell columns (c), cell islands (ci), chorionic plate (cp), chorion laeve (cl), septa (s), basal plate (bp), and uteroplacental arteries (ua). Fibrinoid (matrix-type fibrinoid) is *point-shaded*; fibrin (fibrin-type fibrinoid) is *line-shaded*.

cells that were *transitional* between villous cytotrophoblast and syncytiotrophoblast, cells that were in the process of donating their nuclei to the syncytium. The implication was that "intermediate trophoblast" was intermediate between cytotrophoblast and syncytiotrophoblast and therefore a type of *villous trophoblast*. However, the term "intermediate trophoblast" is currently used by many pathologists to indicate those cells in extravillous sites such as the implantation site, chorion laeve, chorionic plate, and so on, roughly equivalent to the traditional term **extravillous trophoblast.** However, the term "villous intermediate trophoblast," has also been used, and implies an "extravillous," "villous" trophoblast, which is essentially meaningless and its use should be discouraged. These distinctions are important in understanding the derivation and differentiation of trophoblastic tumors (see Chap. 25).

Although extravillous trophoblast is present in a variety of locations, its general structure and function are surprisingly homogeneous. Histologically, extravillous trophoblastic cells are *round to polygonal cells* that are present singly or in groups. They are usually associated with

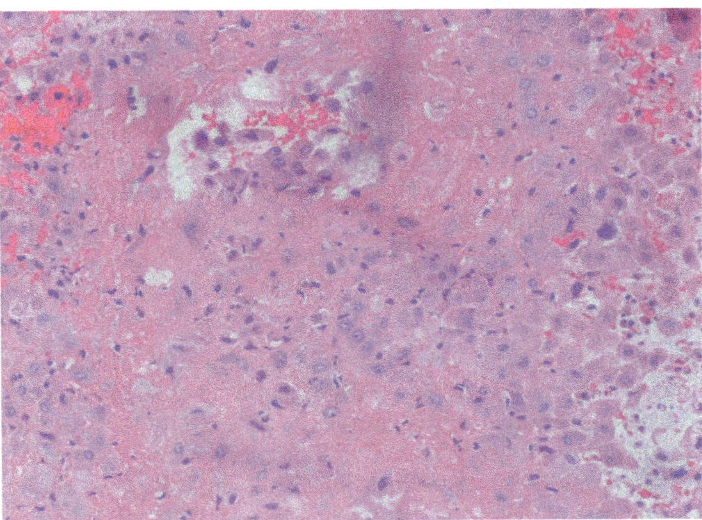

Figure 8.2. Implantation site with extravillous trophoblastic cells intermixed with decidual cells. Note that the trophoblast have hyperchromatic, irregular nuclei and the decidual cells have regular, rounded nuclei with fine chromatin and well defined cell border. H&E ×200.

fibrinoid, a type of extracellular matrix material (see below). They tend to have *pleomorphic, hyperchromatic, or irregular nuclei* (Fig. 8.2) and cytoplasm, which is usually *amphophilic* but occasionally eosinophilic. They are predominantly mononuclear, but binucleate, trinucleate, and multinucleate cells are also seen. Extravillous trophoblast in the chorionic plate and chorion laeve is often smaller and less pleomorphic than that present in the implantation site but has the same general characteristics.

Trophoblastic Stem Cells

Populations of **trophoblastic stem cells** include the *villous cytotrophoblast, the basal layers of the cell columns, the cell islands, the chorionic plate, and the chorion laeve*. It can be seen that, although these cells are in different sites, they all are in contact with the basal lamina of the fetoplacental stroma. The future fate of these stem cells, whether they acquire a villous phenotype or an extravillous phenotype, depends on the surrounding environment, that is, contact with extracellular matrix molecules (Fig. 8.1). *Transformation to extravillous trophoblast occurs on exposure to maternal blood or maternal extracellular matrix. Transformation to villous trophoblast occurs with contact to the syncytiotrophoblast.* Accordingly, the stem cells of the cell columns have a double function, contributing trophoblast for subsequent invasion *and* acting as a growth zone for villous trophoblast of the anchoring villi. Other populations of stem cells have the capacity to differentiate along both pathways but primarily contribute to either the villous or extravillous pathway.

Proliferative Phenotype

Extravillous trophoblast in the proximal portion of the cell columns is **proliferative** and will stain positively with proliferation markers such as MIB-1 (Ki-67). These proximal **proliferating extravillous trophoblastic cells** are *either in immediate contact with the basal lamina* or *separated from it by other proliferating trophoblastic cells*. These cells represent the *stem cells of the extravillous pathway of differentiation* (Figs. 8.1 and 8.3) and are said to have a proliferative phenotype.

Invasive Phenotype

Further differentiation of extravillous trophoblast results in a switch from a proliferative to an **invasive phenotype** (Fig. 8.3). In normal placentation, proliferation and invasion do not coexist in one and the same cell. *Thus, temporal and spatial separation of proliferation and invasiveness limits the depth of trophoblastic invasion.* This separation is thought to embody the major difference between "normal" trophoblastic invasion in pregnancy as compared to "malignant" invasion in tumors,

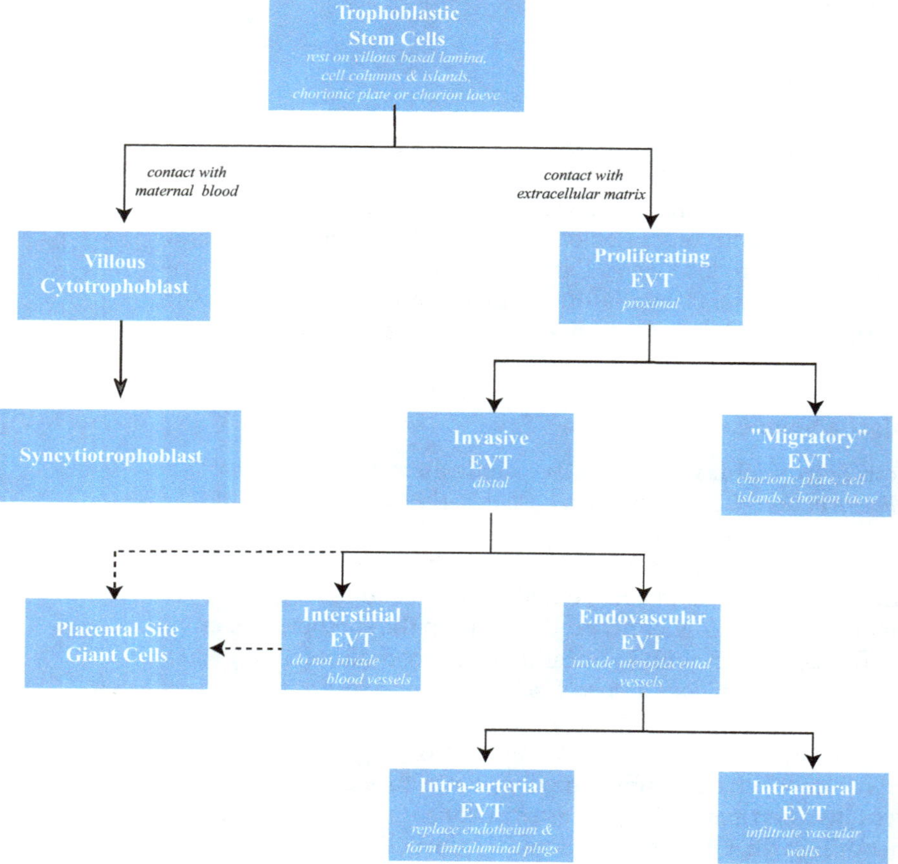

Figure 8.3. Diagram of trophoblastic differentiation. *Dotted lines* indicate possible routes. See text for discussion. *EVT* extravillous trophoblastic cells.

the latter being characterized by temporal and spatial coincidence of proliferation and invasion. Differences between the proliferative and invasive phenotypes are shown in Table 8.1.

A variant of the invasive type is the extravillous trophoblast of the chorion laeve chorionic plate and cell islands, which do not show true invasive behavior. This phenotype is often called "**migratory**." This is likely a quantitative rather than a qualitative difference as a result of downregulation by local factors in the normal intrauterine milieu. In an abnormal environment in which there is locally deficient decidualization, such as ectopic pregnancy and placenta accreta (see Chap. 12), abnormally invasive implantation occurs.

Interstitial Phenotype

The invasive extravillous trophoblast further differentiates into either an **interstitial phenotype** or **endovascular phenotype** (Fig. 8.3). *Interstitial trophoblast does not invade blood vessels, while endovascular trophoblast invades the walls and lumens of uteroplacental vessels* (Fig. 8.4). In contrast to normal epithelial cells, **interstitial extravillous trophoblast** secretes extracellular matrix in an **apolar** fashion, a feature usually only seen in mesenchymal cells. Matrix molecules accumulate extracellularly in large, three-dimensional patchy aggregates called fibrinoid, which completely embed the extravillous trophoblast (see below). Typically, this apolar matrix is secreted in the direct vicinity of maternal tissues, namely facing the maternal blood (e.g., cell islands, intervillous surface of the chorionic plate, placental septa) or maternal decidua (basal plate with cell columns, chorion laeve). As a consequence, fibrin from

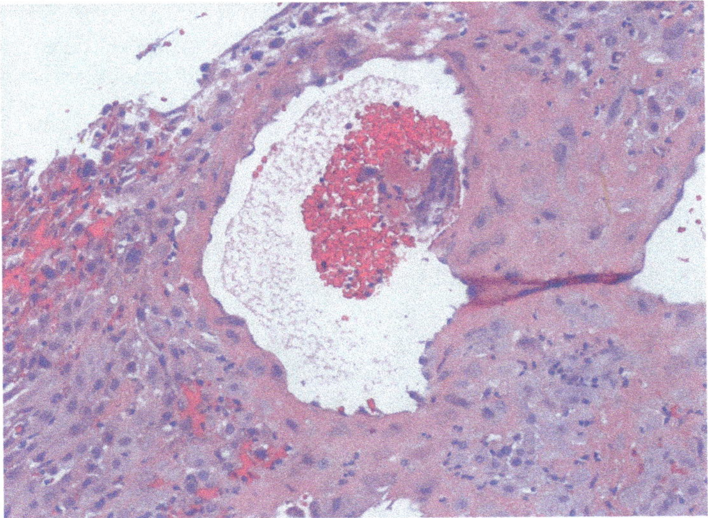

Figure 8.4. Physiologic conversion of the decidual vessel into a uteroplacental vessel by invading extravillous trophoblast. Note the fibrin in the wall, whose muscular coat is destroyed. The paler cells are decidual stromal cells, while those with dark, hyperchromatic nuclei are extravillous trophoblast. H&E ×200.

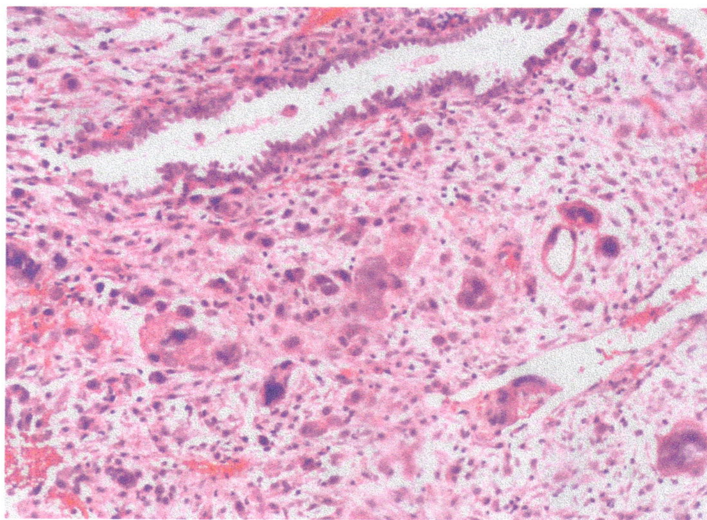

Figure 8.5. Multinucleated placental site giant cells present in the implantation site. H&E ×200.

maternal blood and decidual secretory products are added to the extra-cellular matrix.

The endovascular extravillous trophoblast further differentiates into **intramural extravillous trophoblast** and **intraarterial extravillous trophoblast**. The intramural trophoblast infiltrates the walls of uteroplacental vessels and therefore is essential to the conversion of decidual vessels into uteroplacental vessels. The intraarterial trophoblasts replace the endothelium, and as they do, they undergo "pseudovasculogenesis," in which they achieve an endothelial phenotype. Early in gestation, intraluminal plugs of these cells are present. However, later in pregnancy, they are an abnormal finding, often associated with other abnormalities of implantation and the decidual vessels (see Chap. 18).

Multinucleated Extravillous Trophoblast

Giant multinucleated extravillous trophoblastic cells in the implantation site and superficial myometrium are called **placental site giant cells**. Placental site giant cells tend to be *vacuolated and degenerative* (Fig. 8.5) and are occasionally found in association with fibrinoid deposits. They are thought to be highly differentiated extravillous trophoblastic cells that have *reached the end of the differentiation pathway*. Because surprisingly few invasive trophoblasts undergo apoptosis, local syncytial fusion at the end of the invasive pathway is an alternative mechanism for reducing the number of invasive trophoblast.

Decidua

The changes that occur in the human endometrium in response to the physiologic stimuli of pregnancy and implantation of the blastocyst are called *decidualization*. If the stimulus is a physiologic one, the resulting tissue is the **decidua**, but if the stimulus is experimental or artificial, the tissue is called **pseudodecidua**. Decidualization is characterized by the enlargement of endometrial stromal cells, which eventually assume an epithelioid appearance. They become *round to polygonal, with sharply defined cell borders and a single round nucleus containing a small but prominent nucleolus* (Fig. 8.6a). The nuclei undergo endomitosis, become polyploid, and are sometimes atypical, acquiring the morphologic features known as the **Arias-Stella change** (Fig. 8.6b). Most of the glands atrophy but occasional remnants may be found in the basal plate or decidua capsularis. Within the decidual tissue are considerable numbers of hematopoietic cells including **macrophages,**

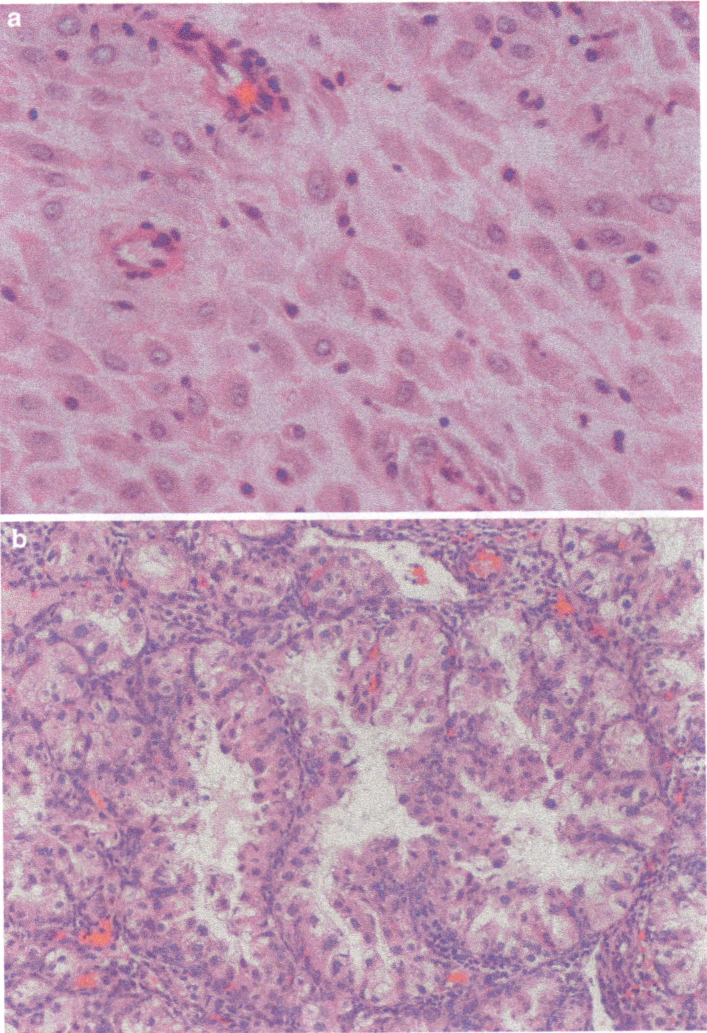

Figure 8.6. (a) Decidualized endometrial stromal cells showing abundant cytoplasm and vesicular nuclei H&E ×200. (b) Arias-Stella reaction of the decidua. Note the marked nuclear atypia and pleomorphism. H&E ×200.

T lymphocytes, granulocytes, and **large granular lymphocytes** (endometrial natural killer [NK] cells, endometrial NK cells, or "endometrial granular cells").

Fibrinoid

Fibrinoid is one of the most prominent components of the human placenta. It is a nonfibrous, acellular, relatively homogeneous material *derived from cellular secretion, cellular degeneration,* and other sources as yet unknown. Its light microscopic appearance varies from *glossy and homogeneous to lamellar, fibrous, or reticular* (Fig. 8.7). In routine sections, the color of fibrinoid varies from slightly pink to intense red. When Mallory's trichrome stain is used, the color is a light blue but may vary from dark blue to lilac or even red. *Because fibrin, blood clot, and secretory products are usually deposited in proximity and cannot be easily discriminated, the general term fibrinoid, rather than fibrin, is used.*

Fibrinoid is found throughout the placenta including the **subchorionic region** (Langhans' stria) (Figs. 8.1 and 8.7), **intervillous space** (perivillous), **chorionic villi** (intravillous), **placental septa, cell islands, cell columns, superficial basal plate** facing the intervillous space (Rohr's stria), **deep basal plate** (Nitabuch's stria), **uteroplacental arteries and veins** (intramural), and **fetal membranes** (chorion laeve) (see also Figs. 7.1, 7.2, and 7.4 in Chap. 7). Detailed histochemical, biochemical, immunohistochemical, ultrastructural, and experimental studies

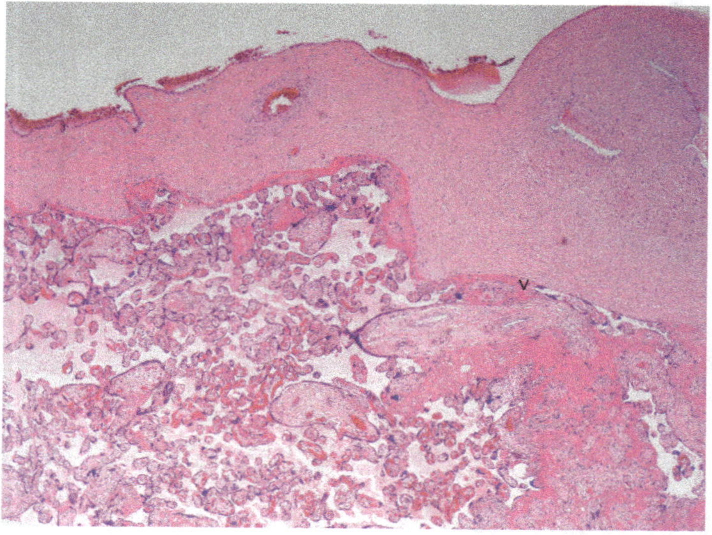

Figure 8.7. Section of the chorionic plate at the 40th week postmenstruation. There is deposition of Langhans' fibrinoid below the chorionic plate, particularly near the stem villi, near term. Clusters of extravillous trophoblast cells and residues of buried villi (V) are typically incorporated into mature Langhans' fibrinoid. ×85.

have revealed that fibrinoid is composed of two histologically similar types that differ in their origin and composition. **Fibrin-type fibrinoid is derived from the coagulation cascade and is mainly composed of fibrin, likely derived from maternal blood and fetal plasma. Matrix-type fibrinoid** is a secretory product of extravillous trophoblastic cells and decidual cells and is mainly composed of collagen IV and glycoproteins of the extracellular matrix. These two types are indistinguishable on H&E sections. As a general rule, **fibrin** *lines the intervillous space in all those locations where the syncytiotrophoblast layer is interrupted and is always interposed between fibrinoid and maternal blood.* **Fibrinoid** *embeds the extravillous trophoblastic cells and is found where trophoblastic migration or invasion takes place.*

Uteroplacental Vessels and Physiologic Conversion

The **uteroplacental arteries** derive from the distal segments of the uterine spiral arterioles. Trophoblastic invasion of these vessels and the subsequent alterations have been designated **physiologic conversion.** Physiologic conversion is characterized by a *loss of elastic fibers and smooth muscle cells* due to proteolytic activities of the invasive endovascular trophoblastic cells, replacement of the vessel walls by *intramural fibrin and fibrinoid*, and a considerable *increase in the luminal diameter* (see Fig. 8.4). These changes transform the originally flexible vessels into rigid channels, which are incapable of constricting. Thus the nutrient supply to the placenta will not be reduced despite changes in blood pressure in the mother. **Intraarterial trophoblastic cells** invade the spiral arterioles and *achieve an endothelial phenotype* and thus become difficult to distinguish from maternal endothelial. The majority of cells lining the lumens of uteroplacental arteries in the endometrium and inner myometrium are intraarterial trophoblast.

Table 8.1 Differences between the proliferative and invasive phenotype of extravillous trophoblast.

	Proliferative phenotype	Invasive phenotype
Invasion	−	+
Proliferation	+	−
Contact on or near fetal stromal basal lamina	+	−
Expression of proliferation markers	MIB-1, EGFR (c-erbB-1)	c-erbB-2
Integrin expression	Epithelial types ($\alpha6\beta4$, $\alpha3\beta1$)	Interstitial types ($\alpha5\beta1$, $\alpha1\beta1$, $\alpha v\beta3$, $\alpha v\beta5$)
Secretion of extracellular matrix	Polar	Apolar

Selected References

PHP5, pages 191–235 (Nonvillous Parts, Extravillous Trophoblast, Decidua, Fibrinoid, Trophoblast Invasion), pages 249–260 (Uteroplacental Vessels).

Arias-Stella J. Gestational endometrium. In: Norris HJ, Hertig AT, Abel AT, Abel MR (eds) The uterus. Baltimore: Williams & Wilkins, 1973:183–212.

Boyd JD, Hamilton WJ. The human placenta. Cambridge: Heffer & Sons, 1970.

Brosens I, Robertson WB, Dixon HG. The physiological response of the vessels of the placental bed to normal pregnancy. J Pathol Bacteriol 1967;93:569–579.

Enders AC. Fine structure of anchoring villi of the human placenta. Am J Anat 1968;122:419–452.

Fisher SJ, Librac C, Zhou Y, et al. Regulation of human cytotrophoblast invasion. Placenta 1992;13:A.17.

Grünwald P. The lobular architecture of the human placenta. Bull Johns Hopkins Hosp 1966;119:172–190.

Hunt JS. Immunobiology of the maternal-fetal interface. Prenat Neonat Med 1998;3:72–75.

Kaufmann P, Castellucci M. Extravillous trophoblast in the human placenta. Trophoblast Res 1997;10:21–65.

Kaufmann P, Huppertz B, Frank HG. The fibrinoids of the human placenta: origin, composition and functional relevance. Ann Anat 1996;178:485–501.

Loke YW, King A. Human implantation: cell biology and immunology. Cambridge: Cambridge University Press, 1995.

Pijnenborg R, Dixon G, Robertson WB, et al. Trophoblastic invasion of human decidua from 8 to 18 weeks of pregnancy. Placenta 1980;1:3–19.

Section III

Multiple Gestation

This section is concerned exclusively with the placentas of twins and multiple births. Chapter 9 covers basic issues in twin placentation, such as incidence and zygosity, discusses the types and origins of twin placentation, and covers aspects of the gross examination that are particular to twin placentas. Diamnionic-dichorionic, diamnionic-monochorionic, and monoamnionic-monochorionic placentation are specifically addressed in this chapter. Chapter 10 continues with specifics of pathogenesis, pathology, and clinical features of twin variants such as fetus papyraceous, conjoined twins, and acardiac twins as well as twin-to-twin transfusion. Chimerism, mosaicism, sacrococcygeal teratoma, and epignathus are also discussed, as these topics have significance in the study of multiple gestations.

Chapter 9

Multiple Gestation: General Aspects

General Considerations

There is no doubt that the complexity of human twinning cannot be understood without knowledge of placentation and that placental examination is vital to this endeavor. Examination of the placenta contributes to the determination and confirmation of zygosity as well as an understanding of abnormal events. With the advent of assisted reproductive technology, twins and higher multiple gestations are becoming more common. Since multiple gestations represent a disproportionate portion of complications with *higher rates of prematurity, perinatal morbidity, perinatal mortality, and malformations than singletons*, placental examination has become especially important.

R.N. Baergen, *Manual of Pathology of the Human Placenta*,
DOI 10.1007/978-1-4419-7494-5_9, © Springer Science+Business Media, LLC 2011

Zygosity

With regard to zygosity, there are generally two types of twins, "fraternal" or **dizygotic (DZ) twins** and "identical" or **monozygotic (MZ) twins**. In higher multiple births, these types are often admixed. *MZ twins arise from fertilization of one ovum by one sperm with subsequent division of the zygote into two genetically identical individuals. DZ twins arise from fertilization of two ova by two sperm resulting in two nonidentical individuals.* MZ twins by definition are identical genotypically and phenotypically and are of like sex, although rare exceptions occur. If one of a 46XY male MZ pair loses the Y chromosome, the twins will have a male and female (Turner's phenotype) and thus appear to be of different sex. DZ twins often have significant phenotypic similarity due to their relationship as siblings and may be of different or like sex. An interesting, but as yet unexplained, observation is that among DZ twins there is an excess of like-sex pairs.

Incidence

The overall spontaneous twinning rate is approximately 1 in 80 births, of which about 28% are MZ. The occurrence of higher multiple births, such as triplets, quadruplets, etc., has commonly been estimated by the "Hellin–Zeleny" hypothesis. This useful approximation says that if twins occur with a frequency of $1/N$, then triplets have a frequency of $(1/N)^2$, quadruplets have a frequency of $(1/N)^3$, and so on. The *DZ twinning rate varies with ethnicity, race, and geographic location*, and varies from 1.4 to 49.0 per 1,000 births. This only applies to spontaneous conceptions. In contrast, *the MZ twinning rate is nearly constant in all populations* at about 3.5 per 1,000 births. The sex proportion of all MZ twins is 0.487 (male/female), while DZ twins have a proportion of 0.518. In other words, MZ twins are more commonly female. Conjoined twins and acardiac twins (see Chap. 10) are also more commonly female, while abortuses are more often male. Theories abound to explain these phenomena, but at present the cause is unknown.

Twin Placentation

There are three types of twin placentation: **diamnionic–dichorionic (DiDi)**, **diamnionic–monochorionic (DiMo)**, and **monoamnionic–monochorionic (MoMo)**. This nomenclature is based on which of the fetal membranes the twins share (Fig. 9.1). In DiDi placentas, each twin has its own chorion and amnion; in DiMo placentas, twins share the chorion but have separate amnions, and in MoMo placentas, both amnion and chorion are shared and the twins reside in the same amniotic cavity. *Monochorionic placentas **always** come from MZ (identical) twins. Dichorionic placentas, however, may occur with both DZ and MZ twins.* Close to 20% of twin placentas are DiMo (and thus MZ), and overall, 28% are MZ. These relationships are shown in Fig. 9.2.

Dizygotic Twins　　　　　　　　　**Monozygotic Twins**

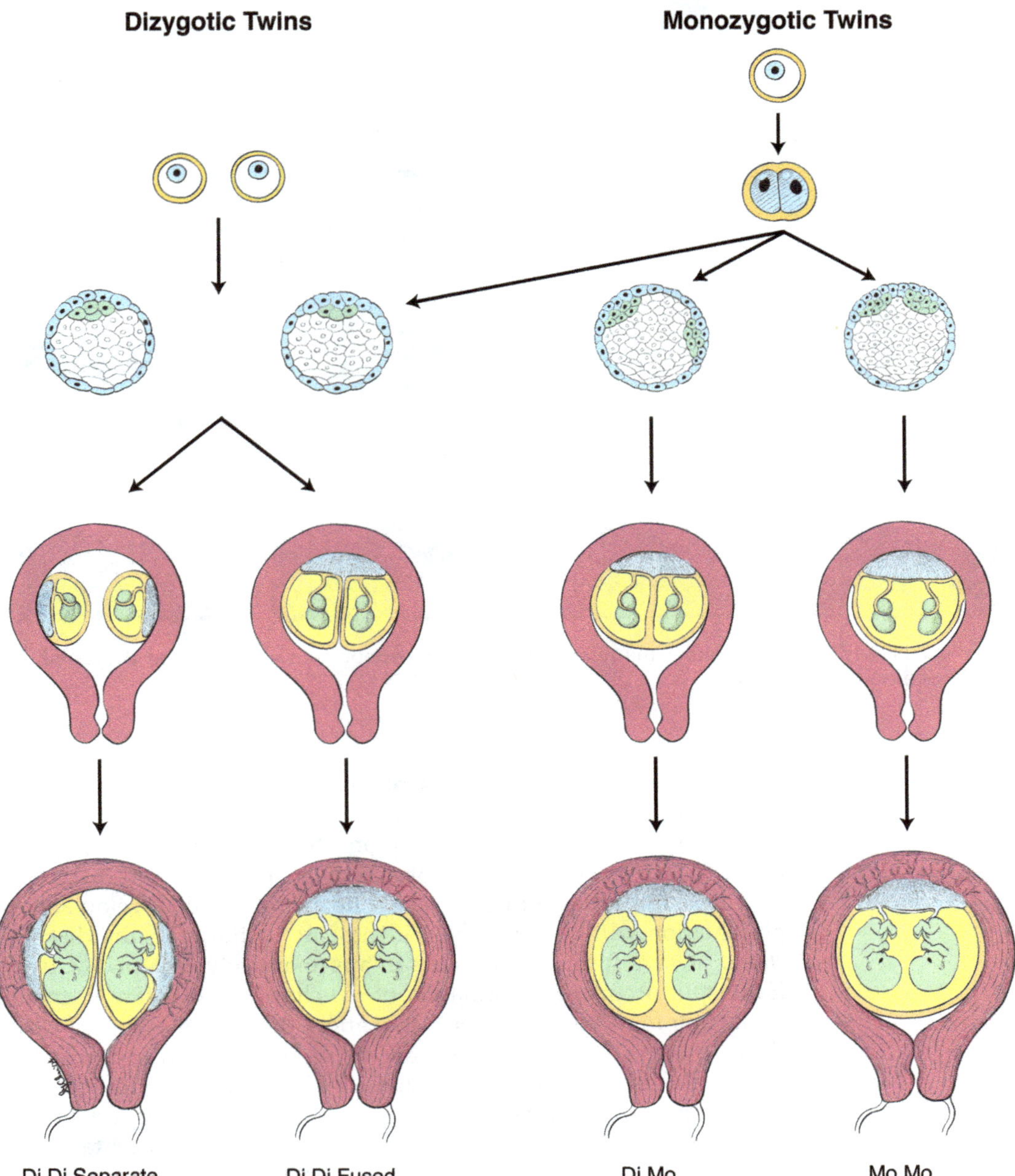

Figure 9.1. Diagram of types of placentation in dizygotic and monozygotic twins. Dizygotic twinning results in two zygotes. If these implant close together, a fused placenta results, and if they implant far apart, separate placentas result. Depending on which the embryonic split occurs, monozygotic twinning may result in fused or separate diamnionic–dichorionic placentation (DiDi), diamnionic–monochorionic placentation (DiMo) or monoamnionic–monochorionic placentation (MoMo).

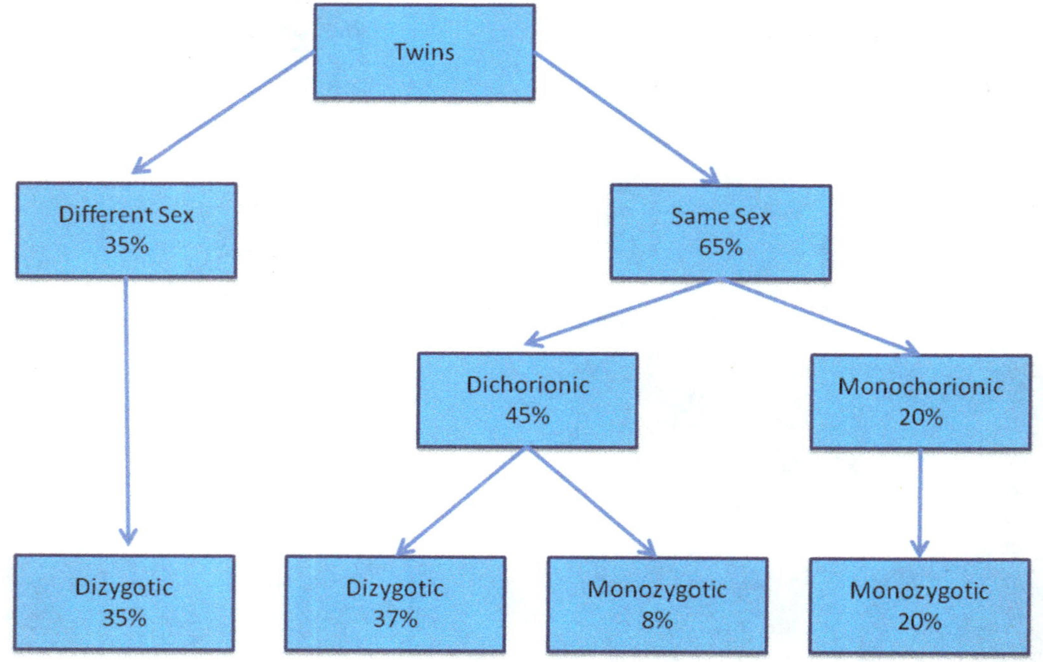

Figure 9.2. Flow diagram depicting the relative frequencies of monozygotic (MZ) and dizygotic (DZ) twins. Based on historical data.

In MZ twins, different types of placentation and twinning occur depending on when the split occurs. They may be DiDi, DiMo, or MoMo, and the later the split, the more structures they share (Fig. 9.3). If the split occurs before the formation of the blastocyst in the first 5–6 days after fertilization, two separate chorions will develop and the placentation will be DiDi. Even if they are dichorionic, the disks are *almost* always fused. This occurs in approximately 25% of MZ twins. If the split occurs after formation of the chorion but before formation of the amnion, 7–8 days after fertilization, the placenta will be DiMo. This is the most common type of MZ twins, occurring in approximately 75%. If the split occurs after formation of the amnion, but before the formation of the embryonic axis, from 9 to 15 days after fertilization, there will be one amnion and one chorion and the placenta will be **MoMo**. It is generally thought that later splitting will result in varying degrees of **conjoined twins**; however, this etiology has come into question. The etiology of conjoined twins is discussed in more detail in Chap. 10. The MoMo placenta is rare, occurring in less than 1% of MZ twins. It is also associated with the highest perinatal morbidity and mortality in twins.

Twin placentas from DZ twins are always DiDi, but may have different configurations depending on where the two zygotes implant (Fig. 9.1). If the zygotes implant close together, the placental disks will become fused as they grow, forming a **fused DiDi placenta**. If they implant further from each other, they will became **separate**

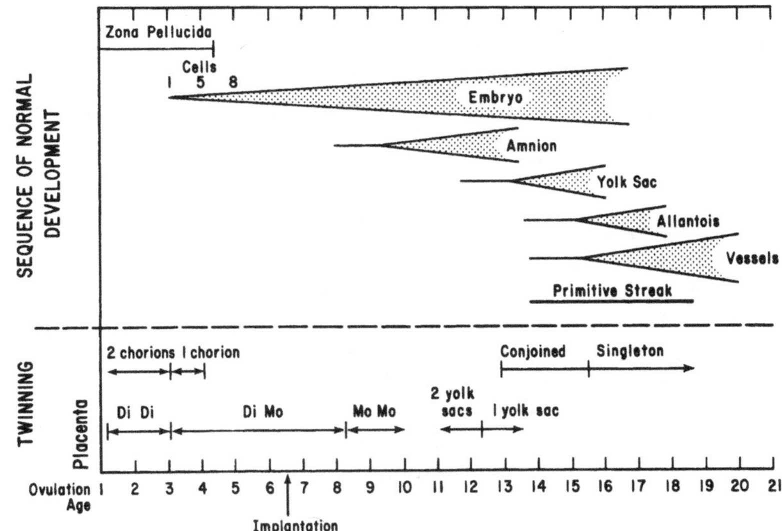

Figure 9.3. Interpretation of early events in MZ twinning. Embryonic events are depicted in the *upper portion*. The *bottom portion* suggests that certain placental structures result if twinning occurs at certain times. It is also assumed that with later development (after day 8) MZ twinning becomes ever more difficult. Once the primitive streak is formed, conjoined twins may develop at first. Soon, however, the presumed twinning "impetus" is ineffective.

DiDi placentas. At times, the placental disks may be separate but the membranes may be "fused." Generally speaking, **DiMo** placentas will be fused.

Pathogenesis

A fundamental difference exists in the respective etiologies of DZ and MZ twins. DZ twins (and higher multiples) are the result of *polyovulation, a process that is familial, likely hereditary, and related to ethnicity, race, and maternal age*. Polyovulation may be related to increased follicle-stimulating hormone (FSH) production, increased gonadotropin-releasing hormone (GnRH) production, or greater follicle sensitivity to FSH. Polyovulation can be induced by the administration of gonadotropins and other hormones as is evident from their use for stimulation of ovulation in infertility patients. FSH and, to a lesser extent, luteinizing hormone (LH) and estradiol are elevated in twin-bearing mothers, suggesting that the genesis of DZ twins is at least partially due to excess production of FSH. Genes responsible for higher FSH levels may explain why DZ twins run in families and why racial differences in DZ twinning rates exist. There is a steady rise in DZ twinning up to the maternal age of 35, and then after that a sharp decline.

While DZ twinning is familial, it is not so for MZ twinning. The incidence of *MZ twinning* is nearly the same throughout the world and appears to be a *sporadic event, unrelated to heredity*. Interestingly, although multiple births after gonadotropin stimulation are generally multizygotic, there is often an admixture of DZ and MZ infants.

In vitro fertilization has 12 times the expected MZ twinning rate compared to single sperm injection fertilization. The actual cause of MZ twinning is not fully understood but it appears that *MZ twins originate from the spontaneous separation of the blastomeres occurring at random during the early embryonic period*. Recent reports have suggested, however, that splitting in MZ twins does not occur equally. That is to say, when splitting occurs, one twin will receive more cells than the other. Since this unequal splitting may also involve trophoblastic cells, it could lead to unequal placental sharing as well. Therefore, discordant fetal growth, sometimes referred to as "selective intrauterine growth restriction (SIUGR)," may be due to the embryo having intrinsically fewer cells or due to diminished growth from a smaller placenta and thus decreased placental perfusion.

Clinical Features and Implications

The incidence of **congenital anomalies** in twins in higher than in singleton gestations. *Anomalies occur with a frequency of approximately 10% in twins, three times the singleton rate*. Discordance for anomalies between twins is common, and the discordance is higher in MZ compared to DZ twins, reaching 80%. Triplets and higher multiples share this discordance as well. Certain anomalies are much more common in twins; for instance, sirenomelia is increased 100-fold in twins versus singletons. Some anomalies, such as anencephaly, occur in DZ twins with the same frequency as in singletons, but are increased in MZ twins. Other anomalies such as porencephaly and visceral ischemic lesions are much more commonly seen in MZ as they are *related to the vascular anastomoses in the placentas* of these twins (see below). Most anomalies in twins have no evidence of a genetic component even though anomalies with a strong genetic etiology, such as cleft lip and cleft palate, are frequently discordant in MZ twins. Possible explanations for the increased incidence of anomalies and the discordance include adverse placentation [e.g., velamentous insertion of cord or single umbilical artery (SUA)] or unequal splitting.

Umbilical cord abnormalities are much more common in multiple gestations, and this includes **velamentous cord insertion, marginal cord insertion, SUA,** and **hypocoiled umbilical cords** (see Chap. 15). Velamentous insertion is nine times more common in twins than in singletons. Marginal insertions are found twice as often in twins, and both velamentous and marginal insertions are found twice as frequently in monochorionic placentas compared to dichorionic placentas. Membranous umbilical vessels are susceptible to *compression, thrombosis, and rupture,* and if membranous vessels are present over the cervical os (vasa previa), they may rupture during delivery and lead to fetal exsanguinations. Cord prolapse may also occur. Abnormal cord insertions and SUA in turn are often associated with *preterm delivery, premature rupture of membranes, fetal anomalies, and fetal growth restriction*. Growth discrepancies are seen quite commonly in monochorionic twins with velamentous insertions.

The mortality of twins is also much greater than that of singletons, being approximately 10%. Prematurity is one of the most important factors in determining outcome, and this is significantly increased in multiple gestations. In addition, monochorionic twins generally deliver earlier than dichorionic twins. *Monochorionic twins have a higher mortality than that of dichorionic twins and the mortality of monoamnionic twins is the highest.* The higher incidence in DiMo twins is predominantly due to the consequences of vascular anastomoses. MoMo twins have a high mortality predominantly due to entanglement of their umbilical cords. Perinatal mortality increases exponentially with each higher multiple offspring, being approximately 16% in triplets, 21% in quadruplets, and 41% in quintuplets. This is one of the prime motivators for the practice of "fetal reduction" during early pregnancy in which triplets are "reduced" to twins or quadruplets are reduced to triplets or twins, and so on.

Numerous maternal complications are associated with multiple gestation as well. These include *premature delivery, preeclampsia, polyhydramnios, placenta previa, abruptio placentae, uterine atony, and postpartum hemorrhage.* Placental abnormalities often mirror these events. Hydramnios in twin pregnancies is most commonly due to the transfusion syndrome, but may also be secondary to fetal or placental anomalies. Uterine atony and postpartum hemorrhage are most likely due to increased uterine distention from multiple pregnancy.

Examination of the Placenta in Multiple Gestation

Gross Examination

Examination of the placenta in multiple gestations involves all the aspects of examination of the singleton placenta. There is then the added complexity of the relationship of the placentas to each other and the relationship between the placentas and the fetuses. In order to derive benefit from the study of twin or multiple births, it is mandatory that the umbilical cords be labeled in the order they are delivered for identification of the infants with their respective placentas. This must be done in the delivery room, and a standard protocol for identification of multiples should be used. For example, ties or clamps may be placed around the placental cut ends of the cords and optimally around individual cord fragments. The first placenta and infant, "A" should be labeled with one tie or clamp, "B" with two ties or clamps, "C" with three, and so on. It is recommended that this be standardized for each institution and that this also be indicated on the requisition form so that there is no confusion.

In addition to the usual placental examination, there are several additional features than need to be evaluated:

- Examination of the relationship of the placental disks:
- If separate, the placentation is **DiDi separate.**
- If separate but connected only by membranes, the placentation is also **DiDi separate.**
- If fused, the placentation is **DiDi fused, DiMo, or MoMo.**
  - o **MoMo** placentas will have only one disk and **no** dividing membranes.

- Examination of the nature of the dividing membranes:
  ○ Sections should be taken of the dividing membranes, either by excising and rolling a square of these dividing membranes as is done for the individual placentas, or taking a section from the site where the membranes insert on the surface the so-called "T zone" or "T section."

The experienced examiner may make the diagnosis of DiMo versus DiDi twin placentation by macroscopic inspection using the following criteria:

- The dividing membranes of DiMo placentas, with only two amnions, are usually *translucent, thin, and contain no blood vessel remnants* (Fig. 9.4). In addition, the chorionic plate between the two placental

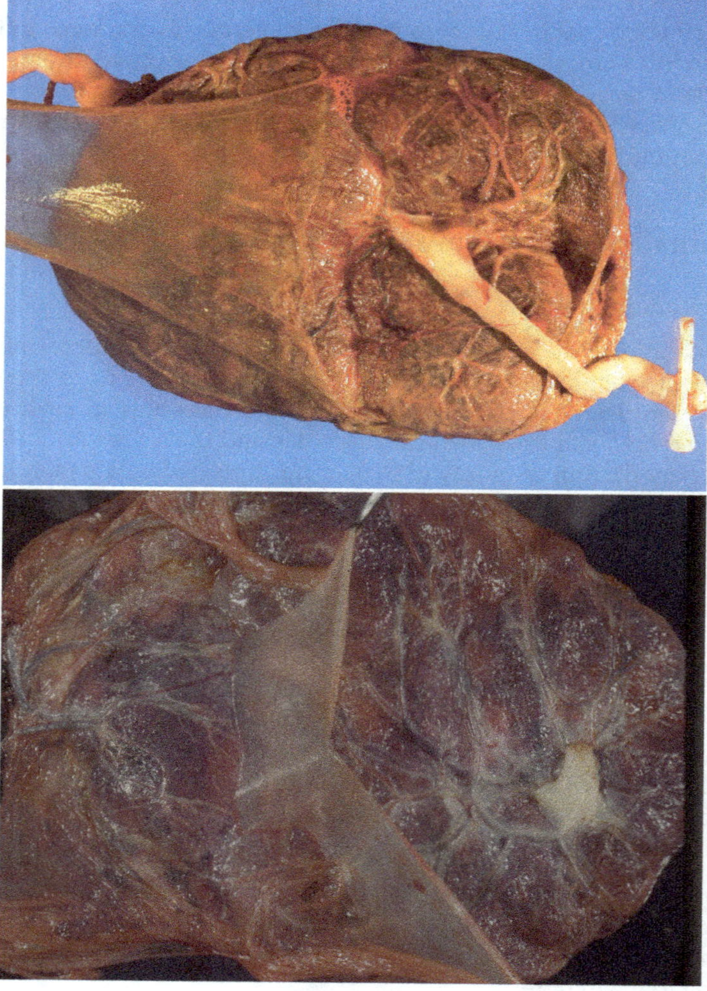

Figure 9.4. Diamnionic–monochorionic twin placentas. The dividing membranes are held up, to disclose their transparency. Note that the fetal surface of the placenta is completely continuous and that numerous vessels (anastomoses) cross from one placenta to the other (see Fig. 9.5 for contrast with DiDi placenta).

vascular territories is flat without the fibrin ridge seen in DiDi placentas (Fig. 9.4).

- DiDi membrane partitions, with two amnions and chorions, are more *opaque, containing remnants of vessels* that are grossly visible as fine branching streaks (Fig. 9.5).
- The fetal surface of DiDi placentas show a white, slightly elevated *ridge of fibrin* not present in DiMo placentas (Fig. 9.5). This is the **twin peak** sign seen by sonography.
- The area of fusion between the two placentas, the **vascular equator** will show an abrupt termination of the surface vessels from each placenta in a DiDi placenta, while in the DiMo placenta, vessels will cross, intermingle and anastomose (Fig. 9.4). It is important to note that the vascular equator most often *does **not** run along the dividing membranes.*

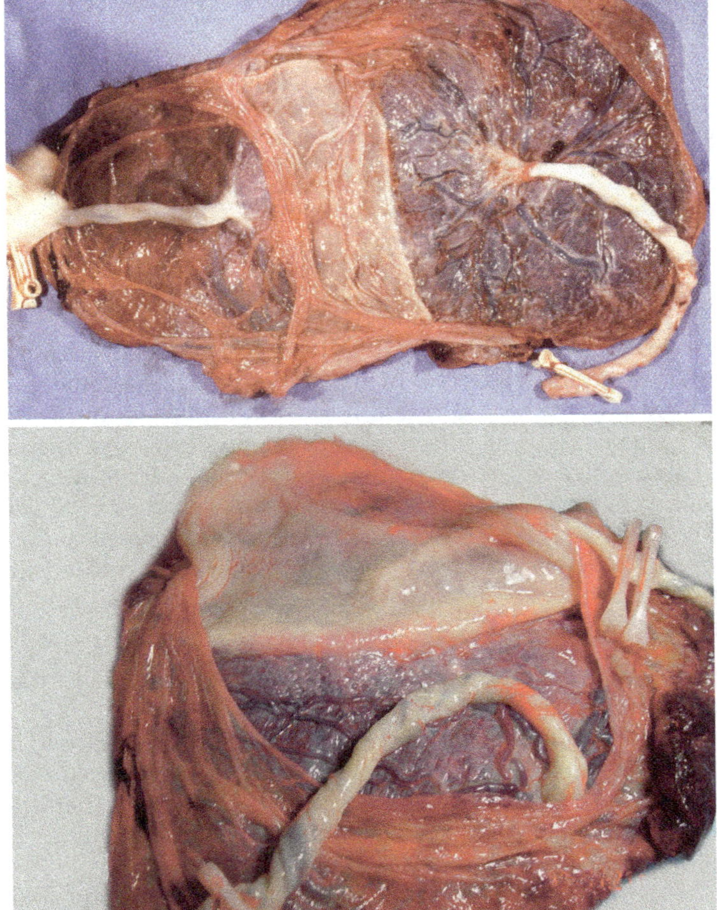

Figure 9.5. DiDi fused twin placenta with visible ridge on the fetal surface at the dividing membranes. The latter appear opaque and thicker than those seen in Fig. 9.4 and show thin streaks, which are the remnants of vessels in the chorion. The fibrin ridge on the chorionic plate at the site of the dividing membranes between the two placentas can be clearly seen.

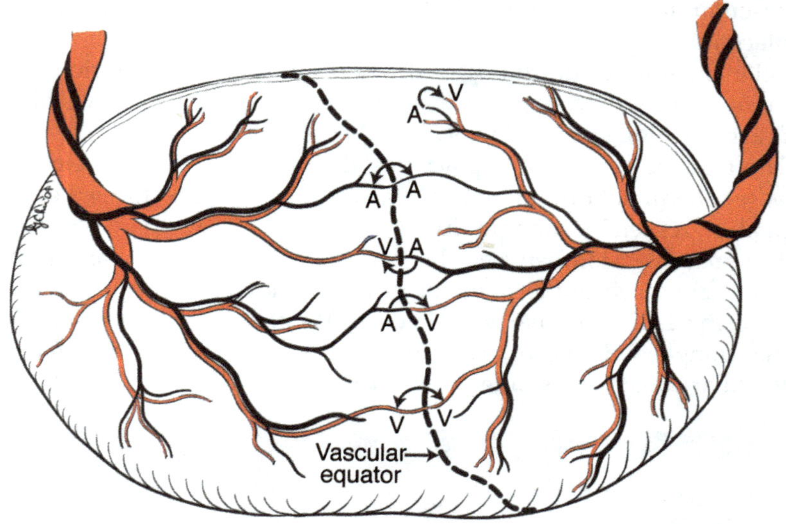

Figure 9.6. Diagram of a monochorionic twin placenta showing the vascular equator and multiple types of anastomoses including A–A, V–V, and A–V anastomoses. The normal pairing of artery and vein derived from one twin is also depicted where one artery extends towards the periphery and is paired with a vein coming back to the cord. *A* artery, *V* vein. Note that when there are anastomoses, the vessel coming from one twin is unpaired, with no vessel coming back.

Examination of Vascular Anastomoses

Monochorionic placentas virtually always have blood vessel connections or anastomoses between the two placentas. Vascular anastomoses may be arteriovenous (either from A to B or from B to A), vein to vein, or artery to artery (Fig. 9.6). Injecting fluid in one vessel and documenting its appearance in the circulation of the other placenta facilitates examination of the vascular anatomy. *General examination of the placenta should be completed first, but samples for histologic study should only be removed after injection has been done.* **Milk, water, any colored liquid,** or even **air** may be used for injection. The following procedure is recommended:

* The umbilical cords should be cut near the placental surface to reduce vascular resistance.
* The amnion should be stripped from the chorionic surface to better expose the vessels (with portions reserved for routine sectioning).
  * Arteries and veins can be distinguished by the fact that **arteries cross over veins**. A ratio of 1:1 is usually found in the final vascular ramifications.
* The major vessels may be followed to their ends visually, and it is usually quite clear which vessels are likely to have communications between the two fetal circulations.
* A–A and V–V anastomoses will appear as direct connections between vessels from one placenta to the other. A–A is the most

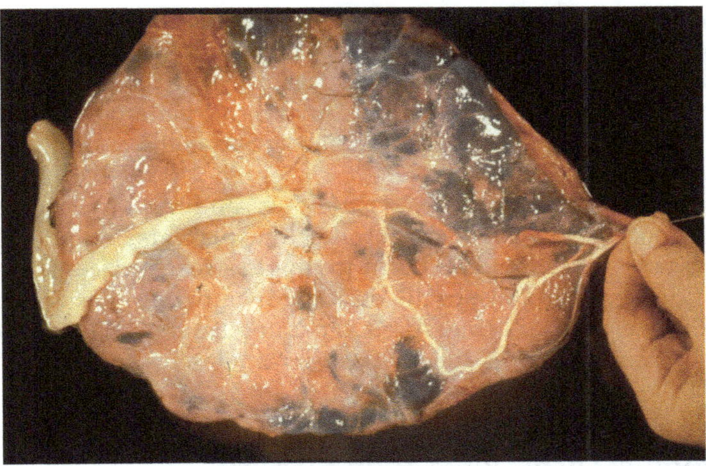

Figure 9.7. Injection technique for demonstration of A–V anastomosis. Fluid is injected while holding the vessel around the needle to prevent leakage. The fluid is easily visible filling the vessel.

common type and V–V is the least common type. *To demonstrate these anastomoses, it is often sufficient to stroke the blood back and forth through the vessels.*

- A–V anastomoses are more difficult to demonstrate. Normally, the fetal arteries terminate in the periphery, dip into the villous tissue, and emerge as nearby veins, which then course back toward the umbilical cord. Injection may be used to conclusively demonstrate these anastomoses (Figs. 9.6 and 9.7).
  - Injection of deep A–V anastomoses.
    - These perfuse a shared cotyledon.
    - A needle is inserted into a vessel near the point of presumed anastomosis and then, holding to needle to prevent back pressure, the liquid is gently injected (Fig. 9.7). Alternatively, an umbilical vessel may be injected.
    - One cotyledon will distend as the fluid is accumulated. After a short time, the fluid will emerge from a vessel in the other placenta.
- It is suggested that the vascular relationships be *recorded in a drawing,* if complicated.

Although the preceding procedure is used to definitively identify anastomoses, particularly of the A to V type, with experience most anastomoses can be identified by visual inspection. As stated previously A–A and V–V anastomoses can be identified by the presence of *an artery or vein crossing the vascular equator in a continuous manner from the umbilical cord of one twin to the other.* A–V anastomoses are somewhat more difficult to identify but can be recognized by the presence of an **unpaired artery or vein.** Normally, each artery that branches out from the umbilical cord has a paired vein returning blood back to the same cord and vice versa. With an A–V anastomosis, an artery branches out from one umbilical cord and does **not** have a paired vein returning to the same umbilical cord but rather has a vein returning to the opposite umbilical cord. Identification of this pattern of unpaired vessels is indicative of an A–V anastomosis and is the easiest way to identify them.

Following examination of anastomoses and examination and sectioning of the dividing membranes, the placentas should then be examined. Care should be taken to divide a fused placenta along the vascular equator and **not** the dividing membranes. Each portion should be weighed and measured separately, and routine sections of each placenta should then be taken separately as outlined in Chap. 3.

Diamnionic–Dichorionic Twin Placenta

The DiDi twin placenta is the most common type of twin placenta. Sections of the dividing membranes in fused DiDi placentas will easily demonstrate the presence of two amnions and two chorions (Figs. 9.8 and 9.9). DiDi placentas share with the other types of twins an *increased frequency of marginal and velamentous insertion of the umbilical cord and SUA*. With rare exception, DiDi placentas have no vascular anastomoses. A very common feature of DiDi twin placentas is the phenomenon of **irregular chorionic fusion** (Fig. 9.10). Here, the membranes do not meet over the areas perfused by the individual fetuses, and a portion of one may be covered by the membranes of the other. This develops when the intraamniotic fluid pressure of one cavity expands its sac and pushes the other away. It is not unlike the process of lifting the marginal chorion in cases of circumvallate placentation (see Chap. 13). As a result, the "vascular equator" is usually **not** in the same location as the dividing membranes. This is particularly important in the determination of the weights of the respective placentas. *One must always separate twin placentas along the vascular equator and not along the dividing membranes.* The irregular fusion has no influence on fetal well-being and no vascular fusion takes place in the areas of overlap.

Diamnionic–Monochorionic Twin Placenta

The DiMo twin placenta is the most common placentation in MZ twins. Both twins reside in the same chorionic sac, but each twin is enclosed in its own amniotic sac. The "dividing membranes" are composed of two amnions only (Figs. 9.8 and 9.9). Similar to DiDi twins, the membranes may move over the surface before birth, and the dividing membranes are often at a place that does not correspond with the vascular equator (see above). The cord insertion is often marginal or velamentous, and a SUA in one or both twins is much more common than in singletons.

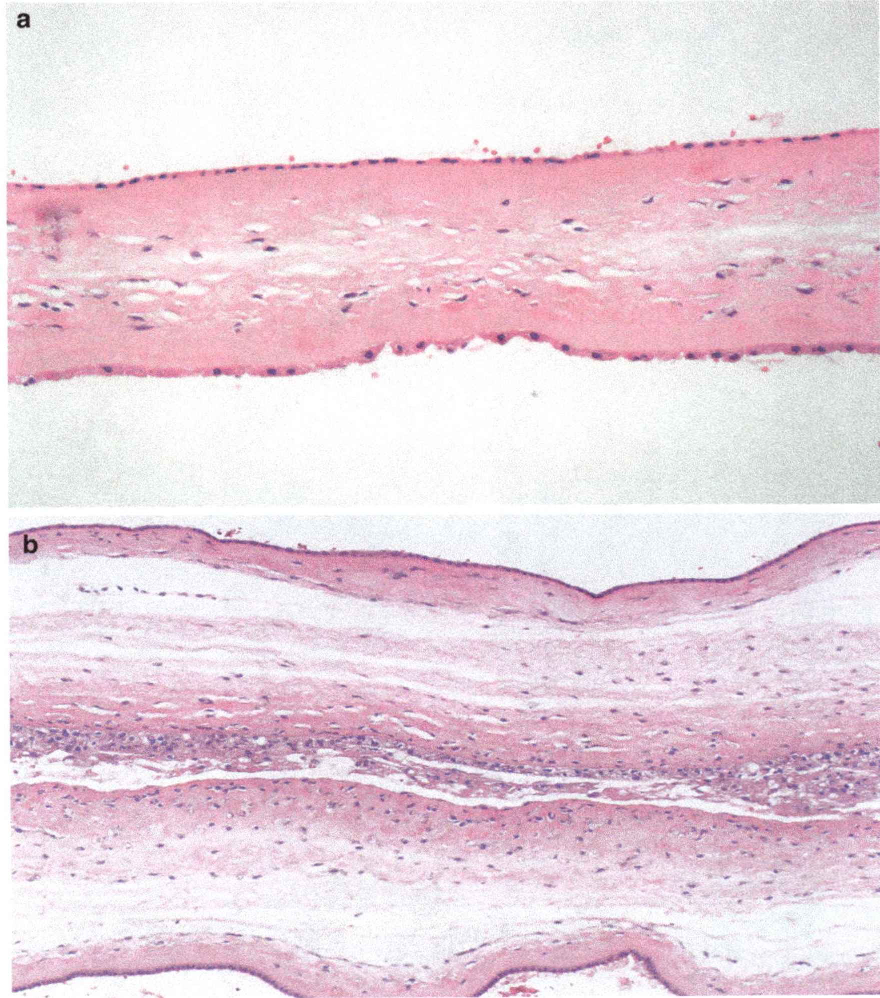

Figure 9.8. (a) Diamnionic–monochorionic dividing membranes of identical (MZ) twins. There is always a space between the two amnions. The amnion usually consists of single layer of cuboidal epithelial cells and scant connective tissue. (b) Diamnionic–dichorionic dividing membranes. In addition to the layers as indicated above, there are trophoblastic remnants in between the membranes, which appear to have fused. H&E ×100.

Monoamnionic–Monochorionic Twin Placenta

The MoMo twin placenta is the least common type and occurs only once in 10,000–16,000 pregnancies or once in 100 sets of twins. The fetal surface of MoMo twin placentas usually has a continuous sheet of amnion without ridges or folds between the cord insertions. By definition, there are no dividing membranes. The umbilical cords usually *insert close to each other on the placental surface* (Figs. 9.11 and 9.12). There may also be a *single fused cord or a forked cord* (Fig. 9.13). Since the yolk sac develops around day 11, MoMo twin placentas may have a partially divided yolk

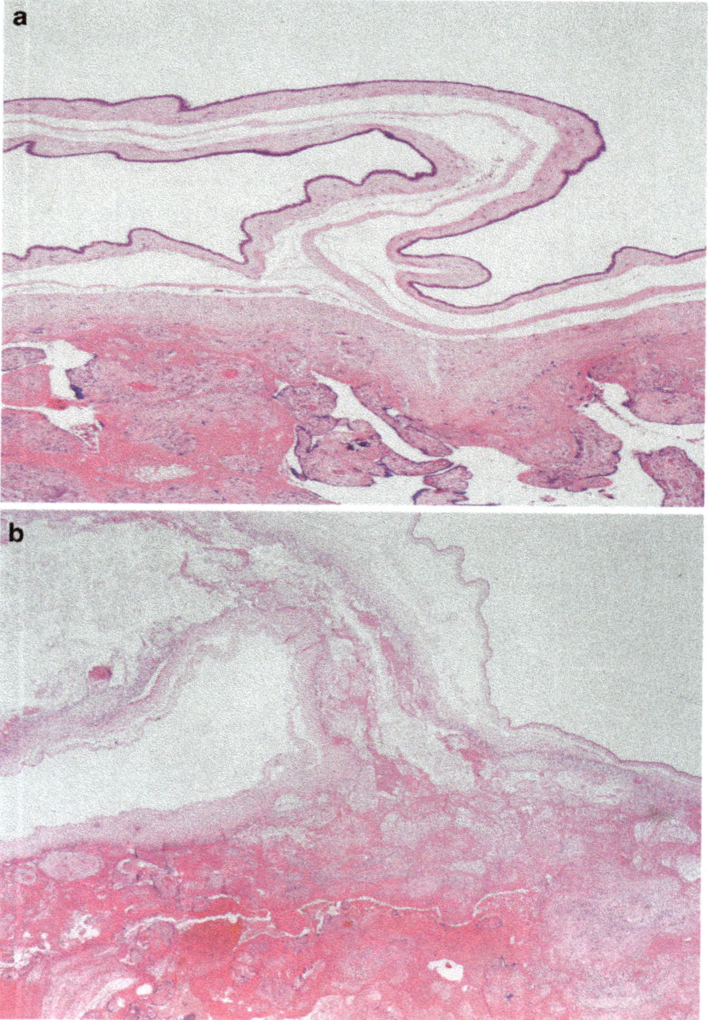

Figure 9.9. (a) T section of dividing membranes of DiMo twins. Note the contiguity of the chorion over the surface of the placenta at bottom. (b) T section of a DiDi twin placenta. There are trophoblastic remnants between the two chorionic membranes and sometimes atrophic villi. The two chorions appear to have fused. H&E ×40.

c or two yolk sacs. Anastomoses of fetal blood vessels are even more common in MoMo placentas than in DiMo twin placentas and are often large (Fig. 9.14), this perhaps being the reason for the rarity of the twin-to-twin transfusion syndrome in MoMo twins (see Chap. 10).

When examining the apparent MoMo placenta, one must be mindful of artifacts causing a **"pseudomonoamnionic" placenta**. Disruption of the membranes during delivery may cause the dividing membranes to be pulled away from the fetal surface, giving the erroneous impression of a MoMo placenta. The intertwin membranes may spontaneously

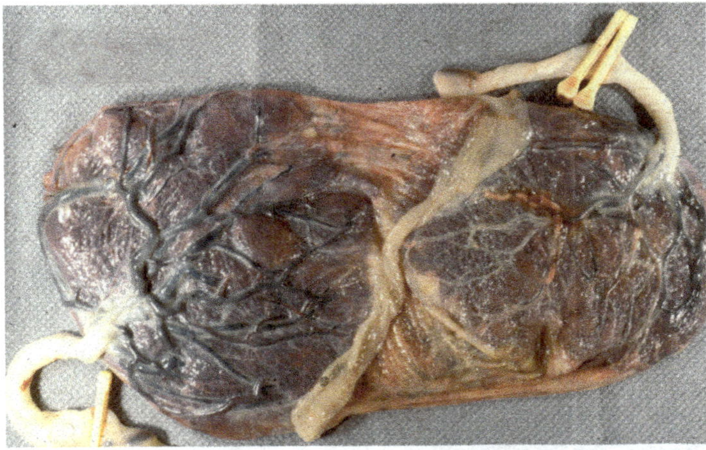

Figure 9.10. DiDi twin placenta with "irregular chorionic fusion." The chorion laeve of both placentas overlap the other. There is no vascular fusion or anastomoses.

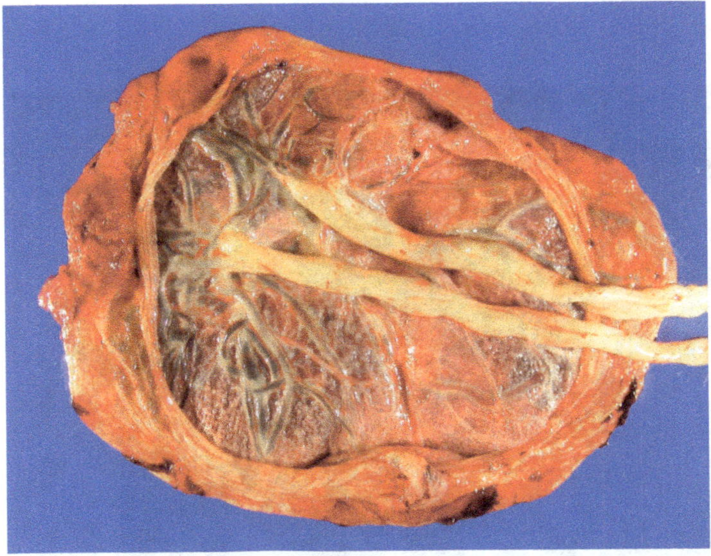

Figure 9.11. MoMo twin placenta, slightly immature, with cords inserting close to each other on the fetal surface.

rupture prenatally or there may be intentional rupture of the membrane for therapeutic purposes such as amniocentesis, funipuncture, or treatment for twin-to-twin transfusion syndrome (see Chap. 10). These events may make it impossible to differentiate a DiMo from a MoMo placenta. The position of the cords may be helpful, since in true MoMo placentas the cords usually insert very close to each other. Clinical history is also essential, as it is unlikely that the clinicians would be unaware of a MoMo placenta prior to delivery. Note, though, that even in situations

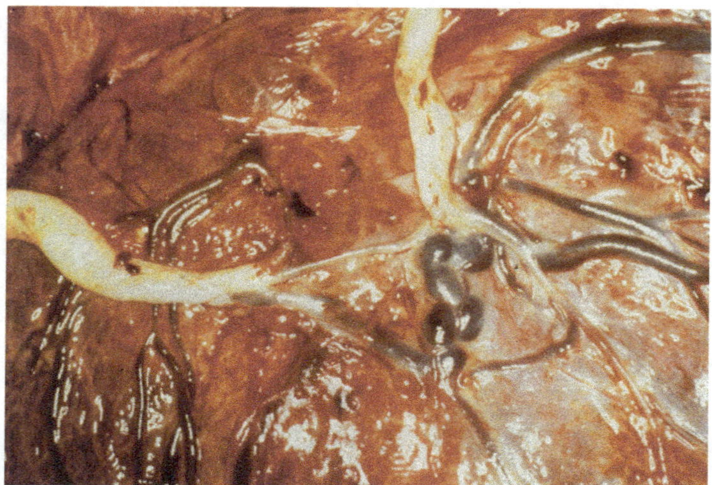

Figure 9.12. MoMo twin placenta with amnions removed. The cords insert next to each other, adjacent to major anastomoses visible on the surface.

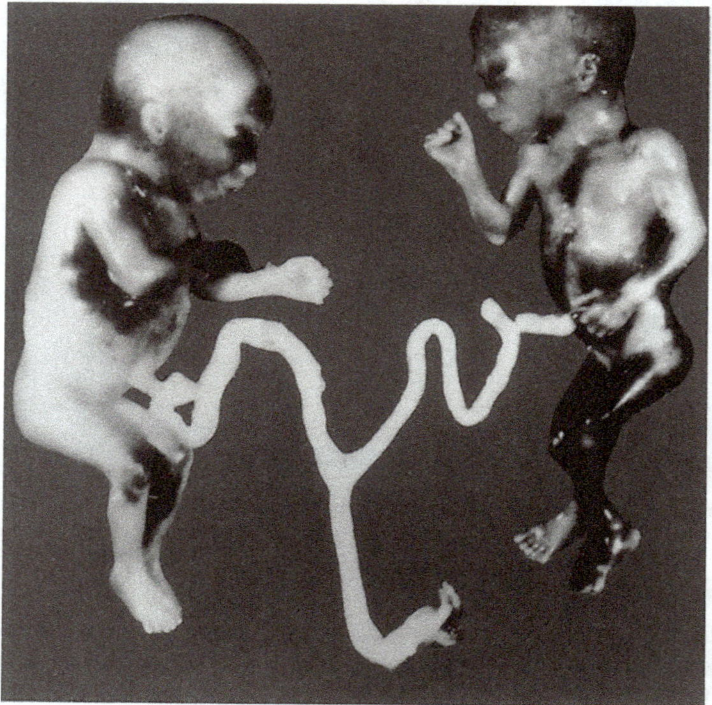

Figure 9.13. Forked umbilical cord of MoMo twin abortuses at 17 weeks' gestation. The smaller twin (*right*) had a single umbilical artery but no other anomalies (courtesy Dr. Marilyn Jones, San Diego).

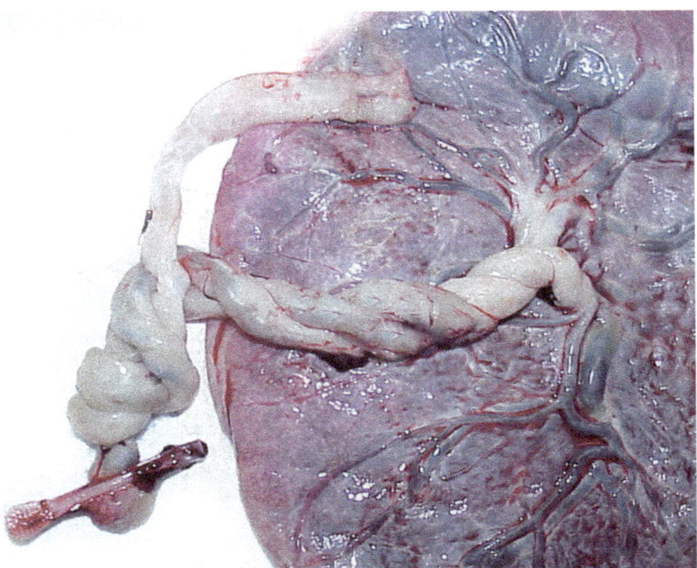

Figure 9.14. MoMo twin placenta with entanglement of umbilical cords. The cords are twisted around each other before becoming knotted. These twins had fetal distress during labor but did well in the neonatal period.

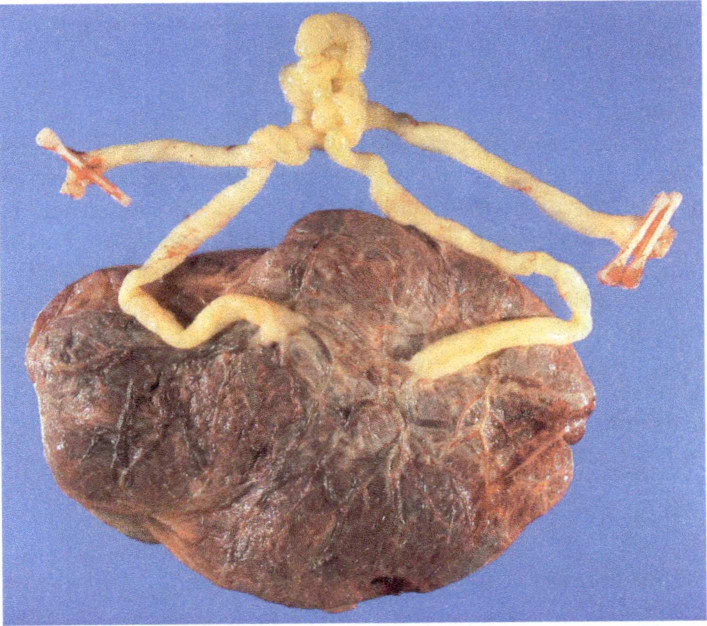

Figure 9.15. MoMo twins with cords entangled in a complex knot, which ultimately caused the demise of both twins in utero.

of a pseudomonoamnionic placenta, if the dividing membranes are disrupted **prior** to delivery, morbidity and mortality may occur from cord entanglements just as with true MoMo twins (see below).

The perinatal mortality of MoMo twins has been reported to reach 40% in some series. Fetal death most commonly occurs due to entanglement of the umbilical cords from fetal movement, resulting in venous obstruction (Fig. 9.15). Knotting of the cords is unpredictable and is often found in very young pregnancies with early abortion ensuing. If fetal demise does occur, it usually happens before 24 weeks, when there is still enough room for fetal movement, and entanglement is still possible. Few deaths occur after 30–32 weeks, presumably for this reason.

Suggestions for Examination and Report
(Twin Placenta)

Gross Examination: In DiMo twins, vascular anastomoses should be documented. In all twins with fused placental disks, the dividing membranes should be submitted. The disks should be separated along the *vascular equator* and then weighed and examined separately. See section above on gross examination for additional details.

Comment: Possible diagnoses are Diamnionic–Dichorionic (fused or separate) twin placenta, Diamnionic–Monochorionic twin placenta, or Monoamnionic–Monochorionic twin placenta. A comment on the nature of the vascular anastomoses should also be included. For example, when a single dominant A–V anastomosis is present, the possibility of twin-to-twin transfusion syndrome should be entertained. If multiple anastomoses of various types are present, a comment to that effect should be made. As previously stated, a drawing of the vascular connections can be helpful in many cases. In higher multiples in which complicated relationships occur, the overall placentation should be mentioned along with specific monochorionic pairs. For example, in a triplet placenta with one MZ pair, the diagnosis would be Triamnionic–Dichorionic triplet placenta, Diamnionic–Monochorionic for triplet A and C. The same can be applied for higher multiples. A drawing of the relationships of higher multiples is suggested as the dividing membranes can be quite complicated. See Chap. 10 for more information on triplets and higher multiples.

Selected References

PHP5, pages 877–919 (Multiple Pregnancies- Zygosity, Causes and Incidence, Vascular Anatomy of Twin Placentas, Monoamnionic-Monochorionic Twin Placenta, Diamnionic-Monochorionic Twin Placentas, Diamnionic-Dichorionic Twin Placentas).

Baldwin VJ. Pathology of multiple pregnancy. New York: Springer-Verlag, 1994.

Benirschke K. Twin placenta in perinatal mortality. N Y State J Med 1961;61: 1499–1508.

Bulmer MG. The biology of twinning in man. London: Oxford University Press, 1970.

Cameron AH. The Birmingham twin survey. Proc R Soc Med 1968;61:229–234.

Carr SR, Aronson MP, Coustan DR. Survival rates of monoamniotic twins do not decrease after 30 weeks' gestation. Am J Obstet Gynecol 1990;163:719–722.

Coulton D, Hertig AT, Long WN. Monoamniotic twins. Am J Obstet Gynecol 1947;54:119–123.

Eberle AM, Levesque D, Vintzileos AM, et al. Placental pathology in discordant twins. Am J Obstet Gynecol 1993;169:931–935.

James WH. Twinning rates. Lancet 1983;1:934–935.

MacGillivray I, Campbell DM, Thompson B, eds. Twinning and twins. Chichester: Wiley, 1988.

Nikkels PGJ, Hack KEA, vanGemert MJC. Pathology of twin placentas with special attention to monochorionic twin placentas. J Clin Pathol 2008;61:1247–1253.

Ramos-Arroyo MA, Ulbright TM, Christian JC. Twin study: relationship between birth weight, zygosity, placentation, and pathologic placental changes. Acta Genet Med Gemellol 1988;37:229–238.

Sherer DM. Adverse perinatal outcome of twin pregnancies according to chorionicity: review of the literature. Am J Perinatol 2001;18:23–37.

Spellacy WN, Handler A, Ferre CD. A case-control study of 1253 twin pregnancies from 1982–1987 perinatal data base. Obstet Gynecol 1990;75:168–171.

Steinman G. Mechanisms of twinning. VI. Genetics and the etiology of monozygotic twinning in in vitro fertilization. J Reprod Med 2003;48:583–590.

Victoria A, Mora G, Arias F. Perinatal outcome, placental pathology and severity of discordance in monochorionic and dichorionic twins. Obstet Gynecol 2001;97:310–315.

Chapter 10

Multiple Gestation: Twin Variants and Related Conditions

Vanishing Twin and Fetus Papyraceous

Clinical Features and Implications

The phenomenon of a **vanishing twin** occurs *when a multiple pregnancy is identified sonographically during the first 15 weeks of pregnancy, but the outcome is a single fetus*. Specifically, the term *vanishing twin* is used when there is no evidence of the fetus at the time of delivery. When the diagnosis of twins is made prior to 10 weeks, the rate of disappearance is 71%. When the diagnosis is made between 10 and 15 weeks, the disappearance rate is 62%. When there is documentation of twins after the 15th week and subsequent loss of one fetus, a fetus papyraceous usually develops. These can clearly be documented on pathologic examination (see below). A clue to the presence of a vanished twin or fetus papyraceous may be an elevation in maternal α-fetoprotein (AFP) or acetylcholinesterase, which occasionally may pose clinical problems, as these elevations are associated with other conditions such as fetal anomalies. When there is a vanished twin or fetus papyraceous, there are no apparent clinical implications or adverse effects on the mother or the remaining fetus.

R.N. Baergen, *Manual of Pathology of the Human Placenta,*
DOI 10.1007/978-1-4419-7494-5_10, © Springer Science+Business Media, LLC 2011

Pathogenesis

As indicated above, if one twin dies early in gestation and the pregnancy continues undisturbed, the fetus may become a **fetus compressus** or **fetus papyraceous.** The fetus may become macerated, lose much of its fluid and become *flattened, misshapened, and paper-like,* hence the name. This is most common when death occurs during the second trimester. Previously, a fetus papyraceous was a rare finding but now is quite routine. It is well known that assisted reproductive technology (ART) has led to an increase in multiple gestations and due to the increased morbidity and mortality associated with higher multiples, the practice of "fetal reduction" is now often used after fertilization by ART.

Pathologic Features

A fetus papyraceous may be so small and compressed that it is difficult to identify on gross inspection. They may appear as a *flattened disk of macerated tissue in the membranes* of the remaining twin (Fig. 10.1). Occasionally, just a thin plaque is identifiable with a pigmented macule representing the eye as the only clue to the diagnosis (Figs. 10.2 and 10.3). At times, radiographs or histologic sections may be necessary to document their nature (Fig. 10.4). The associated placenta, which is usually atrophic and thus appears completely infarcted, may also be difficult to identify, as it often persists as only a crescent of atrophied tissue at the periphery of its twin. When maceration is advanced, the fetus may become a **lithopedion**. This feature is more common when a fetus is retained for months beyond the expected gestation and need not be a twin.

Suggestions for Examination and Report
(Fetus papyraceous)

Gross Examination: Careful examination of membranes is sometimes necessary to identify a fetus papyraceous. Dissection of the dividing membranes between the fetus papyraceous and the other placenta(s) should also be undertaken if possible. Even in cases of ART, the zygosity is not always clear and the number of embryos implanted may not result in the same number of fetuses and/or infants. Monozygotic twinning is increased in ART and so some may split while others may have become a "vanished" twin. Histologic sections of the fetus papyraceous and the associated placenta should be submitted to document their presence.

Comment: The final report should contain a comment about the placentation and zygosity (if possible) along with the diagnosis of a fetus papyraceous. Since the advent of ART, more than one fetus papyraceous may be present and some discussion has occurred on the subject of how to indicate the plural of fetus papyraceous. It is safe to say that there is not clear consensus but it is suggested that "fetuses papyraceous" be used.

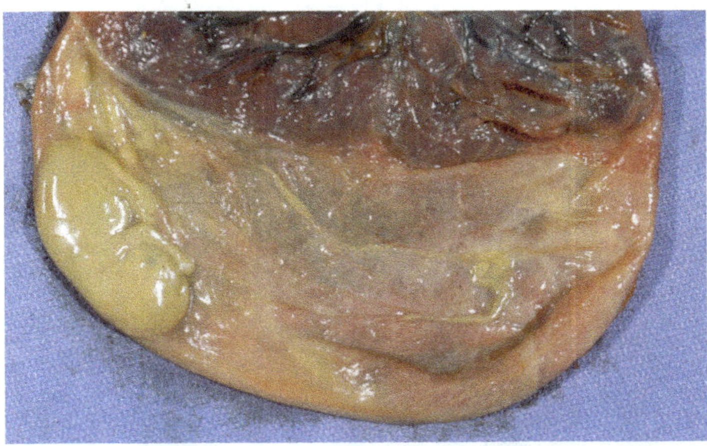

Figure 10.1. Fetus papyraceous (on the *left*) in the fetal membranes of a placenta.

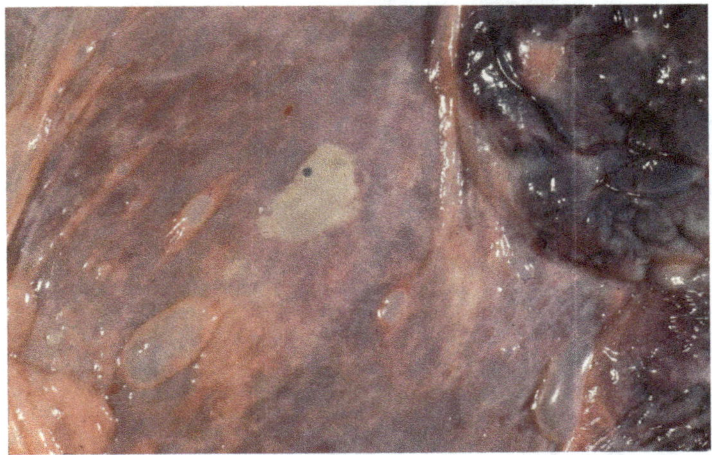

Figure 10.2. Term placenta with a fetus papyraceous in the membranes. It presents as a thin, flattened mass that is almost unrecognizable but the ocular pigment is readily seen. No placental remains could be identified.

Acardiac Twins

An **acardiac** fetus is one of *MZ twins or higher multiples that has the absence of a heart or a severely malformed heart.* **Acardiac twins** are the most severely malformed fetuses that one can imagine. They range from a small, teratoma-like mass to larger more well-formed fetuses with a great variety of anomalies. The incidence of acardiac pregnancies is difficult to ascertain. Even though well over 600 cases have been reported, most are not reported. A reasonable estimation of their **incidence** is 1 in 35,000–48,000 births. Acardiacs are more common in higher multiple births than in twins and occur most commonly

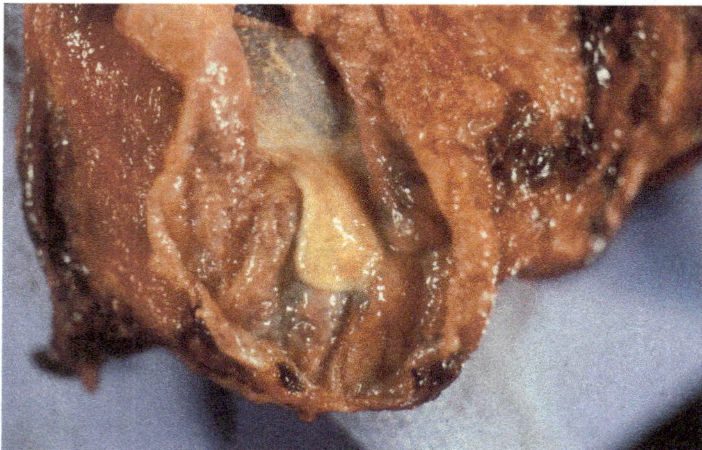

Figure 10.3. Another example of a fetus papyraceous that is difficult to recognize. The second amniotic sac is opened here and an ill-formed nodule of tan to yellow tissue is identified within representing the fetus papyraceous. Note the yellow nodules and plaques on the fetal surface of the placenta representing amnion nodosum (see Chap. 14).

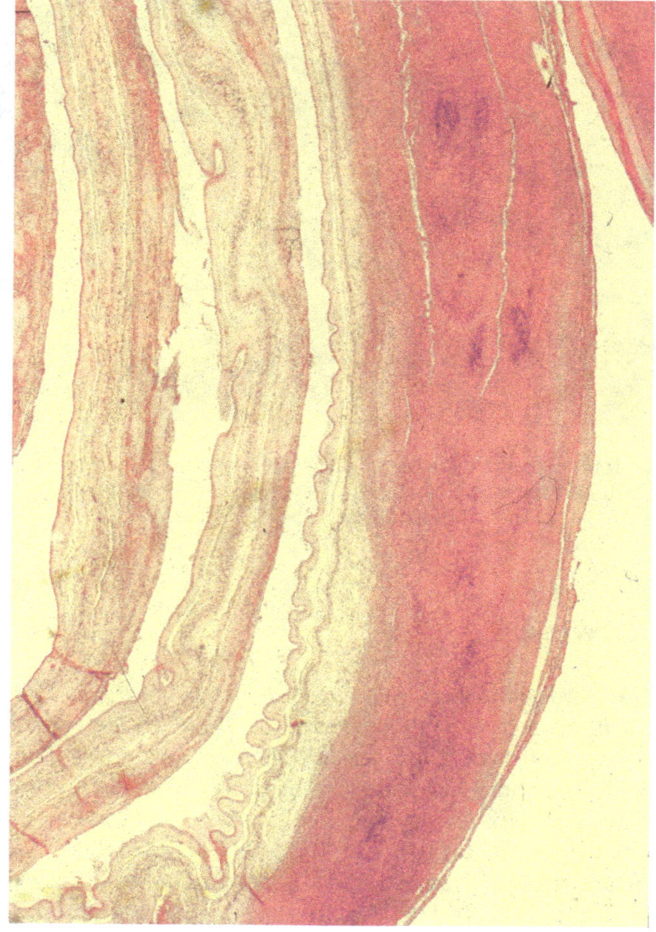

Figure 10.4. Membrane roll of fetus papyraceous with macerated embryonic structures. H&E ×16.

associated with MoMo placentas but occasionally have been reported associated with DiMo placentas.

Pathogenesis

The acardiac develops due to the presence of *two dominant anastomoses in the monochorial placenta. An artery-to-artery anastomosis brings blood from a usually normal co-twin to the monster, and a vein-to-vein anastomosis returns the blood* (Fig. 10.5). The normal twin provides the cardiac flow to the monster but in a reversed fashion, and this reversal of blood flow has been proved to exist with the use of Doppler sonography. The presence of the placental anastomoses has been considered to be the fundamental cause of the acardiac dysmorphism, and therefore dichorionic (and DZ) human twins cannot develop into acardiacs as they lack these communications. *Vascular reversal nourishes the acardiac, and this vascular reversal can lead to suppression of cardiac development.* In fact, much of the failure of organ system development is considered to be from the deficient circulation, as blood arrives deoxygenated and at a reduced pressure. The fact that the lower limbs of acardiacs are usually better formed than the arms has been considered to result from preferential perfusion of the legs, as they are closest to incoming reversed arterial flow. The term **twin reversed arterial perfusion (TRAP)** has been applied to this syndrome. Although this etiology has been accepted in the past, another theory of development that has recently been introduced also has merit. As indicated in the previous chapter, during MZ twinning, unequal distribution of cells may occur. If the inequality is of major proportions, an acardiac twin could develop by this mechanism.

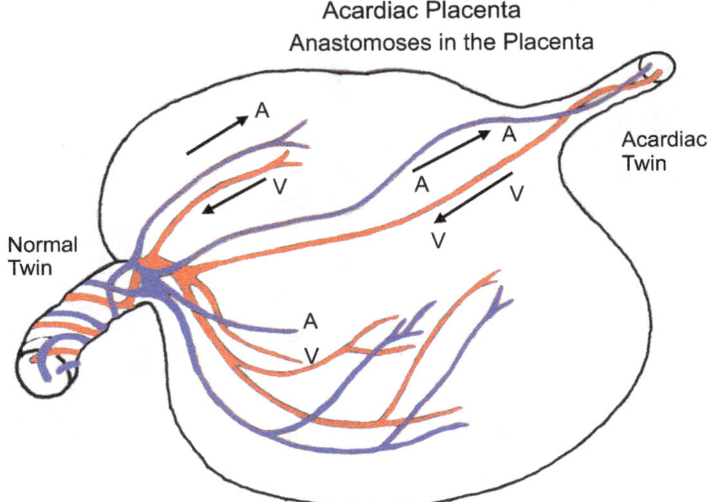

Figure 10.5. Usual pattern of vascular anastomoses in acardiac twins. *A* artery, *V* vein. There is an artery-to-artery and a vein-to-vein anastomosis. Blood flows from the artery of the "pump" twin to the artery of the "acardiac" twin and then returns via a vein from the "acardiac" back to the "pump" twin.

Furthermore, we believe that many of the previously described placental teratomas are really acardiac fetuses that lacked the development of a defined or recognizable umbilical cord. The presence of an umbilical cord is usually considered a prerequisite for the diagnosis of acardiac fetus, but the presence of axial skeleton as a criterion is preferred.

Pathologic Features

There is a *wide spectrum of appearance of acardiacs,* ranging from a total absence of most organs to the presence of well-formed organs including hearts, lungs, and gonads (Figs. 10.6–10.8). They may appear similar to an inside-out teratoma with little resemblance to a fetus. They may have a relatively well-formed lower trunk and legs with a misshapen upper body or they may even have remnants of a face and arms. The only organ that has not been described in acardiacs is the liver. For the study and diagnosis of acardiacs, it is usually best to obtain a radiograph of the specimen before dissection, as it gives some idea of the complexity of the abnormality, enables better classification, and delineates if a skull is present. *Most acardiacs have a MoMo placenta, though some in DiMo placentas have also been described.* Most, but not all, acardiac fetuses have a *single umbilical artery.*

Clinical Features and Implications

Acardiacs occasionally have great mobility and may die from cord entanglement. In cases of a DiMo placenta, *amnion nodosum is usually present in the acardiac* because of its deficient or absent urine production. Acardiacs often develop *hydrops,* and the pregnancy is thus frequently complicated by polyhydramnios. This problem may result from hypoproteinemia or heart failure of the donor twin. Plethora is also frequently observed in acardiacs and probably

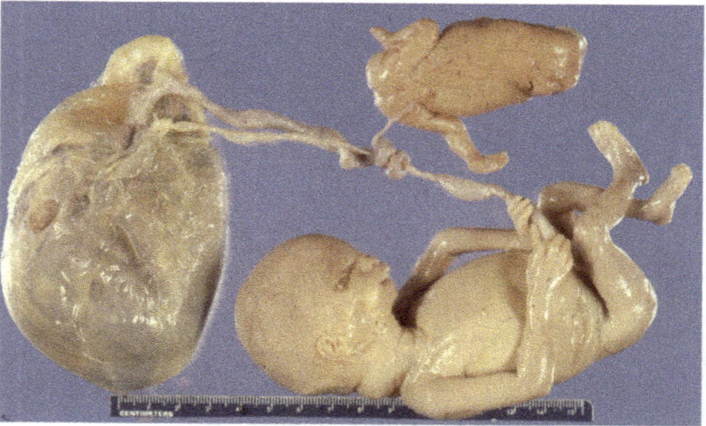

Figure 10.6. Macerated MoMo twins, one an acardiac (150 and 20 g). The twins died because of entangling of cords. The acardiac had a remnant of heart with calcification in the remaining muscle fibers. (Courtesy Dr. S. Kassel, Fresno, CA.).

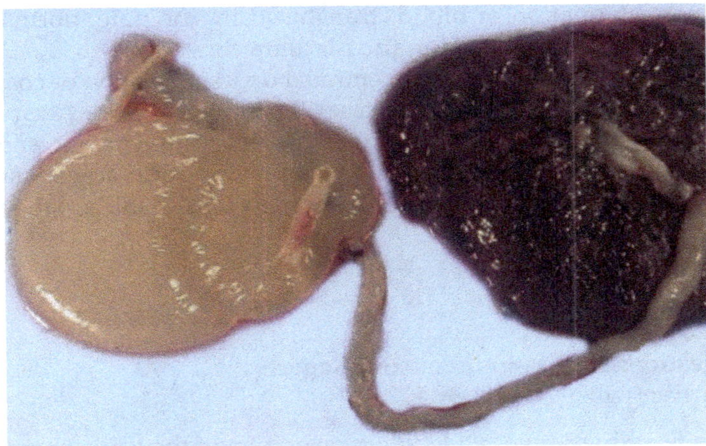

Figure 10.7. Acardiac twin with minimal development.

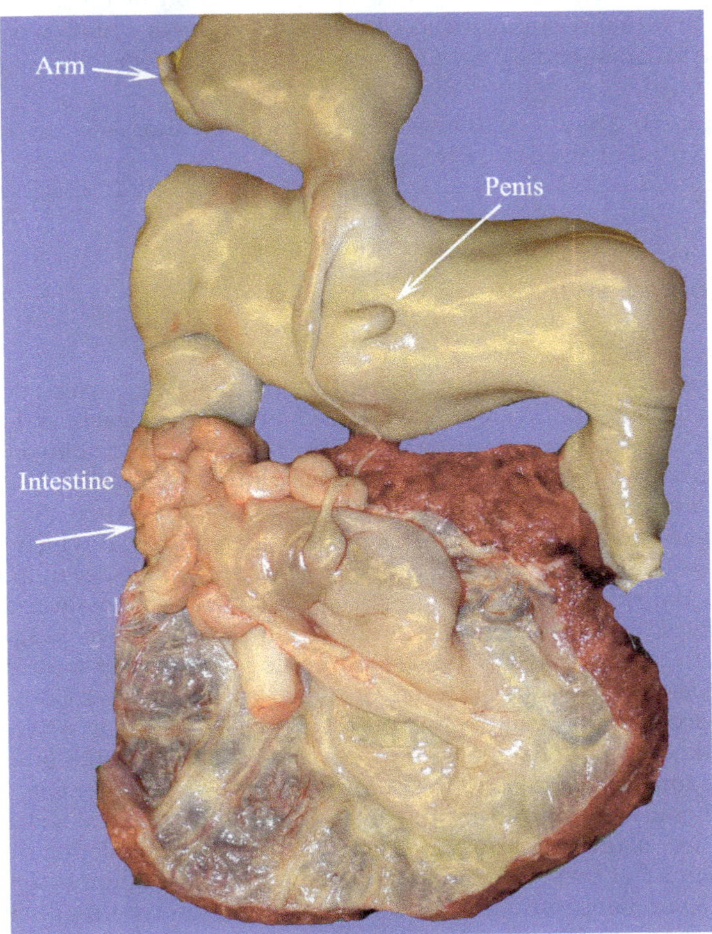

Figure 10.8. Unusual acardiac twin whose abdominal contents were embedded on the placental surface. (From Emery et al. Pediatr Dev Pathol 2004;7:81–85.).

represents stagnation of blood, transfused by the pale, normal co-twin. This is often reflected in the placenta as well.

Treatment of acardiacs has concentrated on laser ablation or coagulation of anastomoses and in some cases the umbilical cord. At present, this is the treatment of choice in documented acardiac twins and has had relative success. However, as stated previously, in acardiacs with MoMo placentation, umbilical cord entanglement is still a danger for the "normal" twin.

Suggestions for Examination and Report
(Acardiac twins)

Gross Examination: Detailed documentation of the fetal anomalies of the acardiac should be performed as well as identification of the type placentation and the type of anastomoses (see Chap. 9). Due to the marked variation in phenotypes, dissection of the acardiac cannot be easily summarized. However, clear documentation of the presence or absence of each organ is essential. Photographs are also suggested.

Comment: The vascular anastomoses and fetal anomalies are usually typical of acardiac twinning.

Conjoined Twins

Pathogenesis

Incompletely separated or **conjoined twins** (Siamese, x-pagi, double monsters) take their origin after day 13 of embryogenesis and arise from MZ twins. The precise manner of the formation of conjoined twins is uncertain, with theories of incomplete splitting and partial fusion of embryonic precursors both having proponents. However, there are numerous anatomic types of conjoined twins reported in which there is no possible way fission can explain the malformations, even in light of unequal splitting, including cases of one phenotypic male and one phenotypic female. Therefore, more recent theories have suggested fusion to two existing embryos as the etiology for at least some cases. Fusion also explains the rare cases of chimerism (see below). Conjoined twins occur in approximately 1 of 50,000 births, or in 1 of 600 twins. For unknown reasons, they are much more common in the Japanese population, in Nigeria, and in South Africa, and 70% are female. They are generally designated by the areas of the fetus that are shared or fused; for example, those joined at the chest are thoracopagus, and those joined at the chest and abdomen are thoracoabdominopagus or thoracoomphalopagus. These are the most common type representing 28% of the total. However, they may be joined in an infinite number of configurations, and conjoined siblings in higher gestations have also been reported (Figs. 10.9 and 10.10).

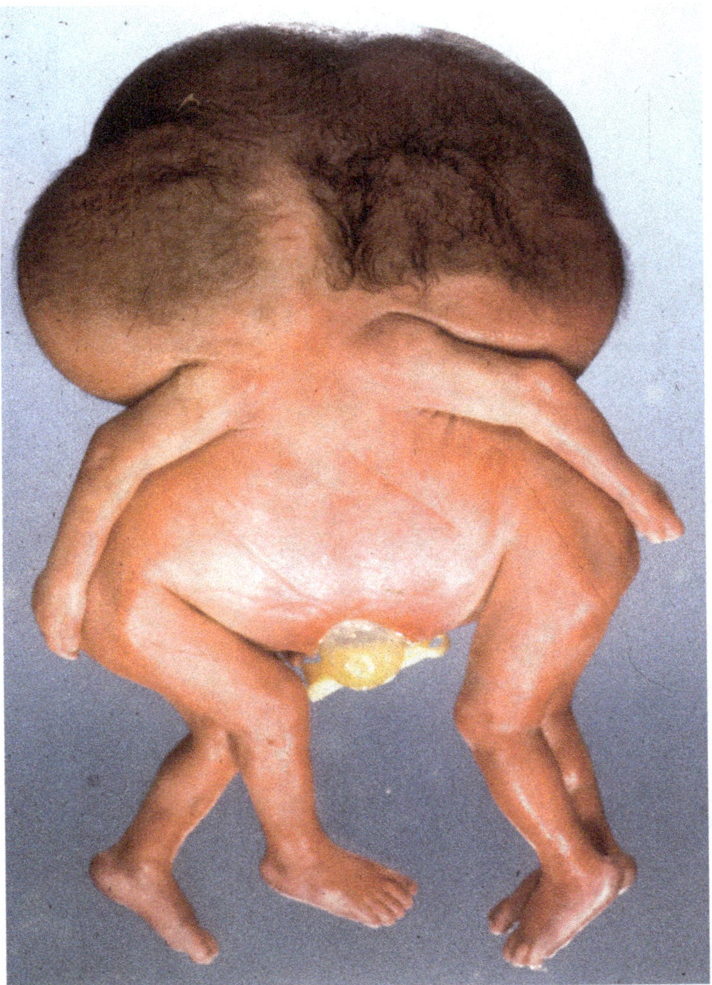

Figure 10.9. Conjoined twins with fusion of anterior portion of the head, chest, and upper abdomen.

Pathologic Features

The placenta of conjoined twins is almost always MoMo; however, separate placental disks and rare cases of DiMo placentas have been reported. *The structure of the umbilical cords varies widely.* There is usually one umbilical cord and in only about 6% there are two cords. Anastomoses occur very frequently as might be expected. When the cord is fused, it has a variable number of umbilical vessels (Fig. 10.11). As few as three and up to eight vessels have been reported; the latter case had six arteries and two veins. *Single umbilical cord is also found quite commonly in conjoined twins.* Some cords are separate at their insertion onto the placental surface but are fused along their length and their insertion into the abdomen. There is no apparent association of cord vasculature and structure with the type of conjoined twin.

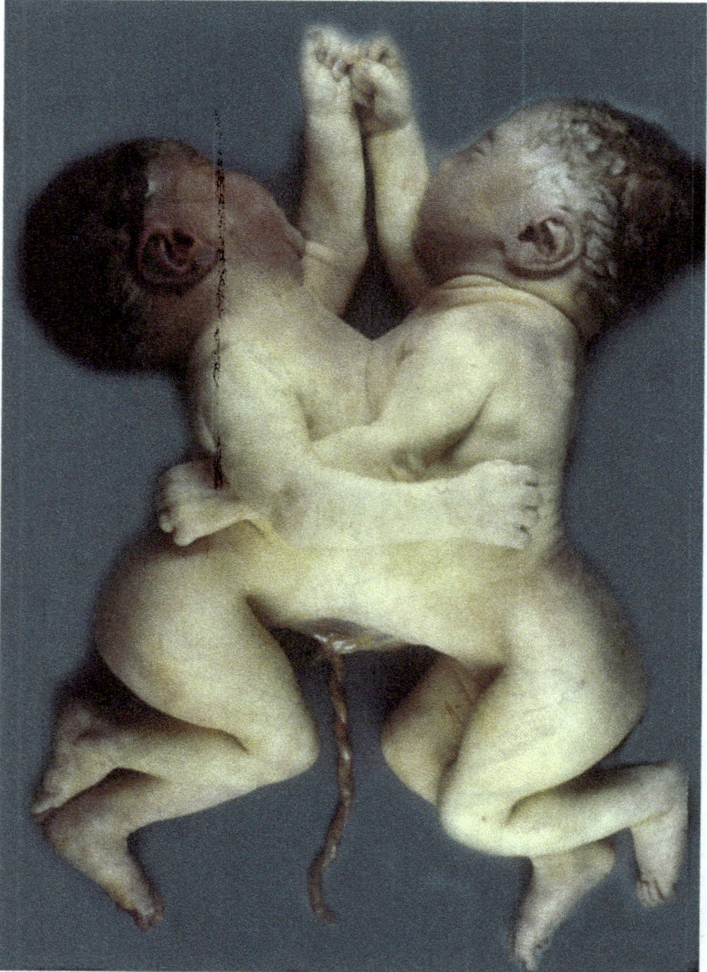

Figure 10.10. Conjoined twins (thoracoabdominopagus).

Suggestions for Examination and Report
(Conjoined twins)

Gross Examination: Documentation of placentation and cord abnormalities should be undertaken as with any monochorionic twin placenta. Evaluation of the anomalies and shared structures is usually done by pediatricians concerned with future viability and possible surgical separation.

Comment: No additional comments are usually necessary.

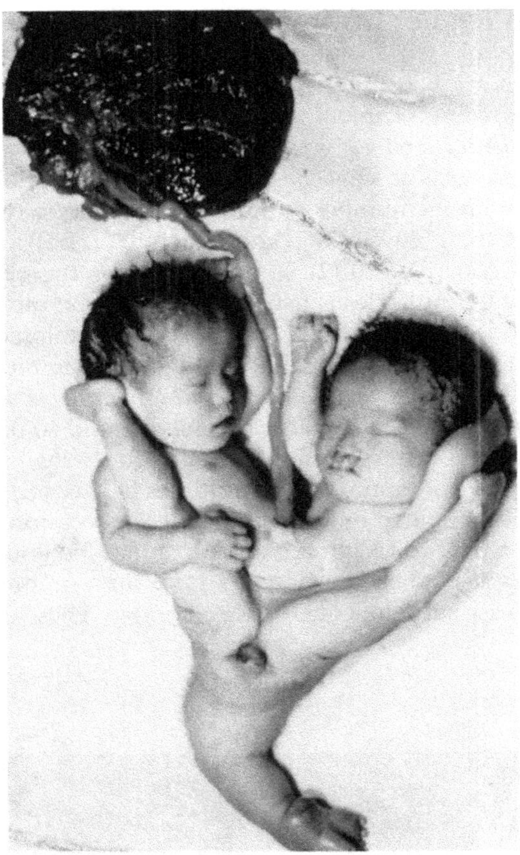

Figure 10.11. Conjoined twins (ischiopagi) with a MoMo placenta, a single velamentous umbilical cord, and a single umbilical artery (SUA). They were delivered at 40 weeks' gestation. One had a cleft face and microcardia. There were two female genital tracts. (Courtesy Dr. S. Sekiya, Tokyo.)

Twin Variants

DZ and MZ twinning are the most common types of twinning, but other unusual variants have been described. In what has been called the **third type of twin,** *the ovum and polar body are fertilized separately by two different sperm.* Thus, the twins have the same maternal genetic contribution but two different paternal contributions. Therefore, the twins are intermediate in their genetic configuration between MZ and DZ twins. This type of twinning occurs in less than 1% of twins and likely develops in situations when the polar body is of similar size to the oocyte. It has been recognized by the finding of one corpus luteum in cases of presumed DZ twins. *The placentation is DiDi and the placentas will usually be fused.* Another unusual variant of twinning occurs in **super-fecundation,** where two ova are fertilized by sperm from two different fathers. **Superfetation,** on the other hand, is when fertilization occurs at different times, resulting in twins of different gestational ages.

Triplets and Higher Multiple Births

Multiple births are becoming more common, and presently nonatuplets hold the record. Triplets and higher plural births are not only *smaller than expected for their gestational age; they also commonly deliver much earlier than twins or singletons*. Morbidity and mortality increases exponentially with the number of multiples. Triplets may be any combination of MZ and DZ twins and chorionicity, i.e., TriTri, TriDi, TriMo, DiMo, and MoMo (Fig. 10.12). Terminology for the chorionicity of triplets and higher multiples is usually based first on the total number of chorions and amnions. For example, quadramnionic-trichorionic describes quadruplets with four chorions and three amnions. The diagnosis would then read *quadramnionic-trichorionic quadruplet placenta, diamnionic-monochorionic for quadruplets B and C*, and so on. Otherwise, examination and reporting are similar to that for twins.

Uneven numbers of monozygotic multiples (such as triplets or quintuplets) may be explained by assuming that, on occasion, one embryo may not have survived. Alternatively, there may be one division initially and then a secondary division occurs, or three or more embryonic centers might arise simultaneously instead of two. These divisions then

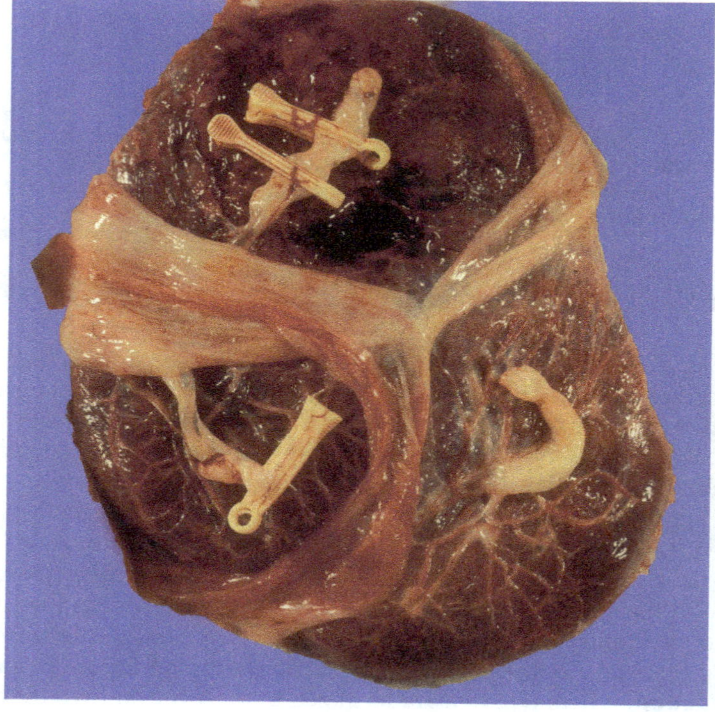

Figure 10.12. Triplet placenta – triamnionic-trichorionic (TriTri). Note the fibrin ridges and the opaque membranes, indicating two amnions and two chorions where the placentas fuse.

are likely unequal. Because plural gestations generally have poor outcomes, their early diagnosis and the selective reduction of some cases are currently relatively common.

> **Suggestions for Examination and Report**
> (Triplets and higher order multiples)
>
> **Gross Examination:** Examination should be along the same lines as that for twins, i.e., documentation of the vascular anastomoses, separation of fused disks along the vascular equator and separate examination of each placenta. In complex arrangements a drawing of the relationships may be helpful.
>
> **Comment:** As noted above, the number of amnions and chorions should be included in the diagnosis. The specifics of individual relationships may be added, for example, "triamnionic-dichorionic triplet placenta (diamnionic-monochorionic for triplets A and B)."

Twin-to-Twin Transfusion

Chronic Twin-to-Twin Transfusion

Pathogenesis
The **twin-to-twin transfusion syndrome (TTTS)** is a specific entity caused by the *unidirectional, prenatal transfusion of blood through arteriovenous (A-V) anastomoses in the monochorionic twin placenta* (Fig. 10.13). Thus, one twin is a **donor,** and the other is the **recipient.** Usually, there is a *discrepancy in size and development of the twins, particularly with respect to amniotic fluid and fetal fluid status.* The donor will then be pale, anemic, and small, with small organ weights as well as oligohydramnios. The recipient will be phlethoric, possibly polycythemic, much larger than the co-twin, and associated with polyhydramnios. The syndrome is variable in its consequences because the A-V anastomoses may be single or multiple, of varying size, and may or may not be associated with artery-artery (A-A) or vein-vein (V-V) anastomoses. However, generally speaking there is usually a dominant A-V anastomosis and few other anastomoses. When a simultaneous large anastomosis coexists, often the most severe aspect of the syndrome is prevented due to equalization of blood flow between the twins. The twins reach greater gestational maturity or may not even develop TTTS.
Prenatal diagnosis is usually made when one monochorionic twin shows oligohydramnios and the other shows polyhydramnios. The twins may also show a significant weight discrepancy. This has led to use of the term *twin oligohydramnios polyhydramnios sequence* (TOPS), a practice with which we strongly disagree. Use of this term ignores the etiology, which lies in the placental anastomoses. Grading of the

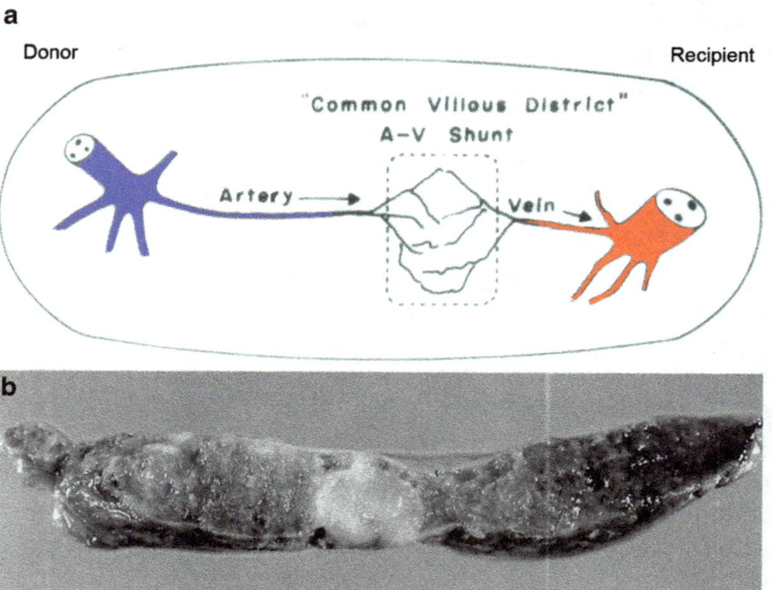

Figure 10.13. (a) Vascular anastomoses in chronic twin-to-twin transfusion syndrome. The predominant anastomosis is an artery-to-vein anastomosis from the donor (*left*) to the recipient (*right*). (b) Cross section of a monozygotic placenta after injection of shared cotyledon has been injected with water and shows marked pallor.

severity of TTTS is often done with information from ultrasound examination based on fluid in the amniotic cavity, bladder, and so on.

Pathologic Features

The prenatal unidirectional exchange of blood results in deprivation of nutrients from the **donor** twin and excessive development of the **recipient**. The twins may be remarkably discordant (Fig. 10.14) and there is a high degree of brain-sparing growth restriction in the smaller twin. *Typically, one twin is dehydrated and anemic, possessing organs much smaller than expected. The recipient is often plethoric and has enlarged organs.* The discrepancy is particularly striking in the hearts, and this is one of the most important means for the diagnosis of the transfusion syndrome when the twins die and autopsy examination is performed. After birth or demise of one twin, rapid blood shifts may occur between the twins, which change the hematologic values. However, a marked discrepancy between the donor's and recipient's hematocrit is an important confirmatory clue to diagnosis. The remarkable pallor of the donor twin's placental portion and congestion of the recipient's placenta may also be quite striking (Fig. 10.15). The histologic structure of the villi can differ substantially as well (Fig. 10.16), with enlarged, edematous villi in the donor and congested villi in the recipient. Both usually contain markedly increased nucleated red blood cells.

A number of studies on the treatment of TTTS have shown success with use of intrauterine laser coagulation of the anastomoses to prevent the potentially dire consequences (see below). Twin placentas that have

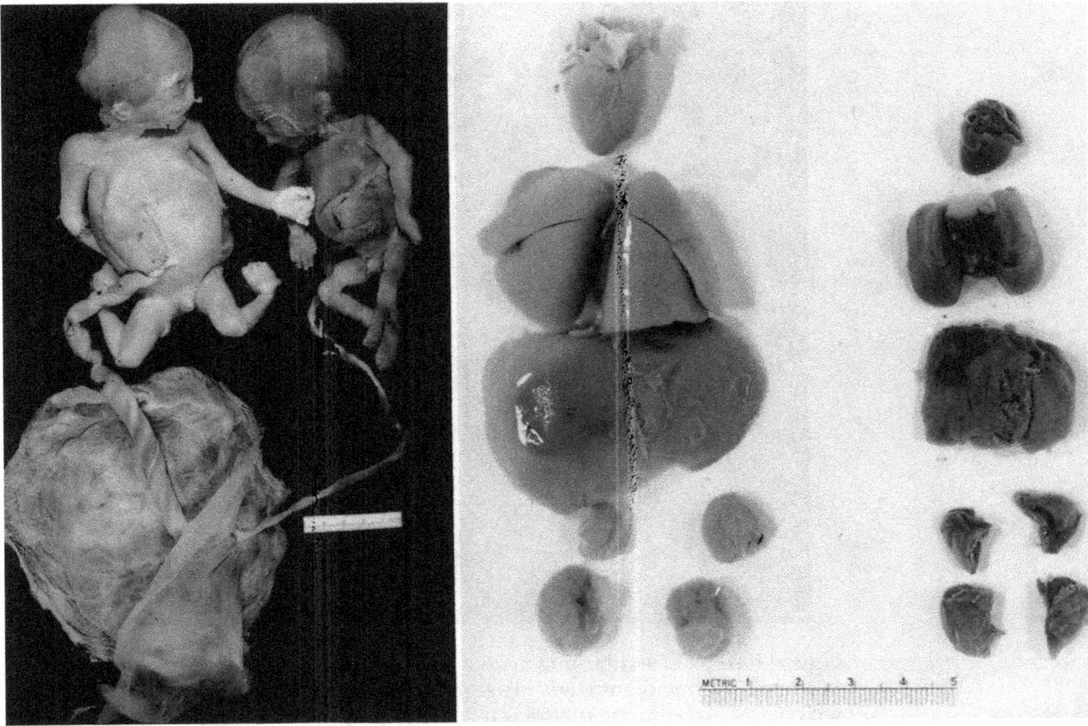

Figure 10.14. DiMo twins with chronic transfusion syndrome at 28 weeks' gestation. The donor (*right*) is plethoric; the recipient (*left*) is edematous and pale. Recipient: 285 g; 15 cm crown–rump (CR) length; heart 3 g; lungs 10 g; liver 17.5 g; kidneys 1.5 g. Donor: 189 g; 13 cm CR length; heart 0.7 g; lungs 3 g; liver 4 g; kidneys 1 g. The plethora of donor is thought to be due to other twin's earlier death, with exsanguination from the recipient to the donor (acute twin–twin transfusion).

been treated in this way will show coagulation of the anastomotic vessels, often with fibrin collection underneath the fetal surface and infarction of the underlying shared cotyledon or cotyledons (Fig. 10.17). It is thought that the entire thickness of the placenta is originally infarcted, but over time vascular connections develop deep to the laser ablation injury, resulting in a predominantly superficial infarct.

Clinical Features and Implications

The frequency of the transfusion syndrome is difficult to determine but it is estimated to occur in *5–30% of monochorionic twins*. Observations suggest that it may be more common. The various definitions used to make the diagnosis and the wide spectrum of severity makes assigning a precise frequency and assessing therapeutic efficacy, difficult. For unknown reasons the syndrome is much more common in female twins. Typically, the transfusion syndrome is first recognized by the finding of *polyhydramnios*. It usually develops around midgestation, but has been diagnosed as early as 12 weeks. The donor twin has oligohydramnios and may move much less than the recipient, so the term *stuck twin* has been applied to this feature. Size discrepancy of the two twins was previously included as part of the clinical diagnosis of TTTS. However, in many cases, the size discrepancy is small or not significant, and so this

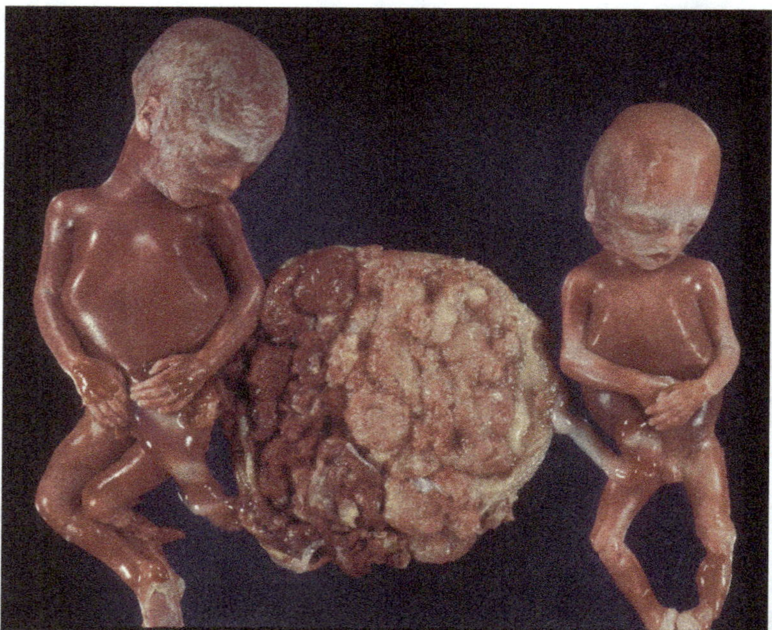

Figure 10.15. DiMo placenta at 26 weeks with chronic TTTS. Both fetuses died in utero. The recipient (*right*) is significantly larger than the donor (*left*). The recipient's placenta (*right*) and is markedly congested, while the donor's (*left*) is pale. There is also a disparity in the diameter of the umbilical cords.

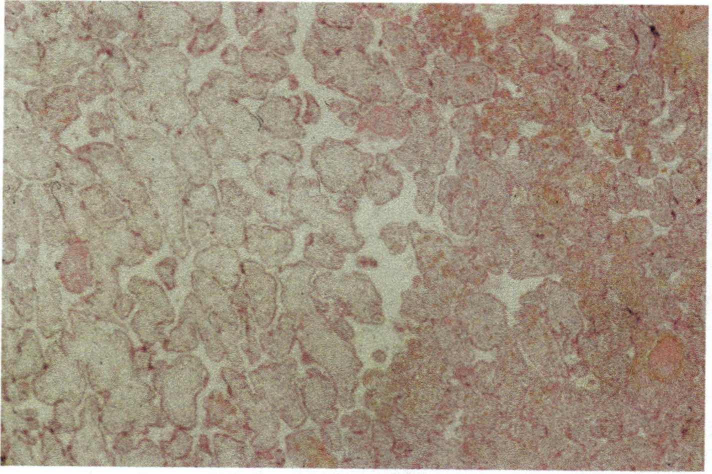

Figure 10.16. Histologic appearance of DiMo placenta depicted in Fig. 10.15. The section has been taken through the vascular equator of the two placental portions. The donor's placenta is on the *left* and the recipient's is on the *right*. Note that the chorionic villi of the donor are larger, more immature-appearing with edematous stroma. The recipient's villi are smaller, more mature, and more congested.

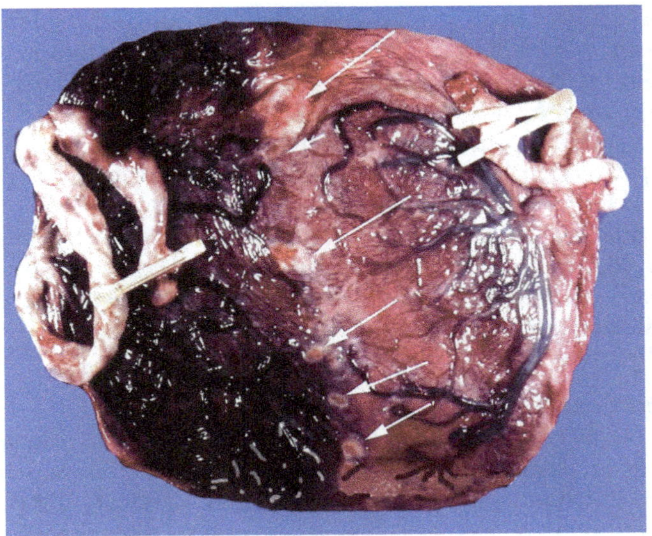

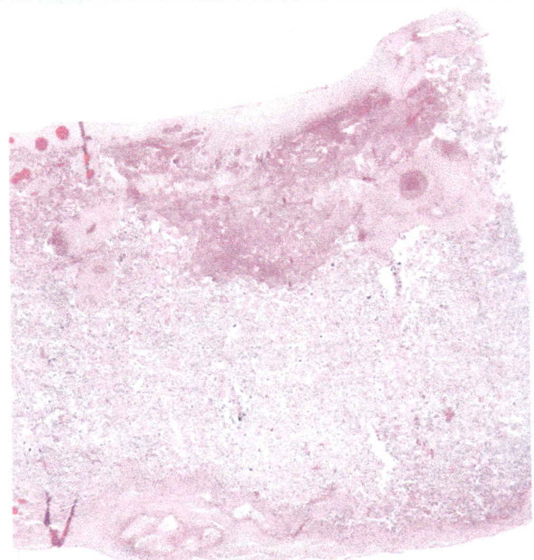

Figure 10.17. DiMo placenta with twin-to-twin transfusion syndrome in which laser ablation has been performed. Gross examination of the placenta (*top*) shows the presence of fibrin and infarcted villous tissue under the chorionic plates (*arrows*). The *bottom portion* of the figure shows a microscopic view of a laser-induced infarct with infarction of the subchorionic villous tissue but preservation of the deep villous tissue. (Courtesy of Kurt Benirschke, MD.)

criterion is less often used. In general, the earlier clinical manifestations are present, the poorer the prognosis, although overall the prognosis is poor, particularly if untreated. When the condition is diagnosed before 28 weeks of gestation, the overall survival rate is as low as 21%.

The hydramnios often leads to preterm labor and premature rupture of the membranes, and delivery often occurs before the 30th week of gestation. Alternatively, one twin may die, in which case the hydramnios ceases nearly immediately and the pregnancy may reach term. *Morbidity and mortality are significant* in this syndrome. The donor often succumbs from hypovolemia and heart failure while the recipient may succumb from congestive heart failure. Other pathophysiologic consequences of the syndrome include *poor fetal growth, periventricular encephalomalacia, intracranial hemorrhage, intraventricular hemorrhage, polycythemia in the recipient, anemia in the donor, hypoglycemia, hyperbilirubinemia, skin necrosis resembling aplasia cutis, cardiac dysfunction, cardiac hypertrophy, and thromboses.* These sequelae can often be explained by fluid shifts between the twins through the placental anastomoses, a phenomenon that has been documented prenatally.

Treatment Considerations

It has now become possible to *obliterate the interfetal vascular connections by prenatal laser treatment.* It is hoped that this will result in improved outcome and normalization of the pregnancy, and presently has enjoyed relative success is less severe cases. Other modes of treatment that are less commonly used include *septostomy* (in the dividing membranes) and *amniocentesis* of the twin with polyhydramnios. In the future, mapping not only the anastomoses but also the character and location of ablated vessels is likely to be important in planning future treatment options.

Acute Twin-to-Twin Transfusion

Pathogenesis

Acute twin-to-twin transfusion may occur *with or without* chronic TTTS, and, although it is also caused by placental anastomoses, it is a different entity. It occurs to some degree in **all** *monochorionic twins when one twin dies in utero.* If placental anastomoses are small, little blood will be transferred and the placenta of the dead fetus gradually atrophies and becomes completely infarcted. If, on the other hand, there are large interfetal vascular communications, the placental half belonging to the dead fetus will continue to be perfused by the survivor. In addition, when one twin dies, the vascular bed of that twin is devoid of counter blood pressure and becomes a "sink" for blood flow through the placental anastomoses. Then, the surviving co-twin can bleed or even literally exsanguinate into the dead twin. Thus the result will depend on the size of the anastomoses and will vary from no significant effect on the survivor to severe brain damage and death. In summary, *when one twin of a DiMo pair dies, the survivor experiences some degree of acute blood loss into the dead twin's circulation through superficial large interplacental anastomoses,* and this is referred to as acute twin-to-twin transfusion. This is in contrast to previous theories suggesting that when one twin dies, thromboplastic material is somehow transported from the dead twin to the live twin over the ensuing days. Since the dead twin has no blood pressure, flow could not occur in this direction, and sonographically, reversal of blood flow in the umbilical cord has been observed after death of one twin. These facts essential disprove the "thromboplastic" theory. The shift or transfusion of blood leads to hypotension in the surviving twin and this occurs immediately, likely within minutes, after the co-twin dies.

Clinical Features and Implications

Cerebral palsy is five times more common in twins than in singletons and mostly affects MZ twins. When there is intrauterine fetal demise of one twin, cerebral palsy is particularly common in the surviving twin, and this is clearly due to acute twin-to-twin transfusion. Death of the surviving twin is also quite common. The presence of cerebral lesions, such as porencephaly, correlates well with the presence of vascular anastomoses in MZ twins and occurs even when there is not death of one twin. This is thought, in many cases, to be the result of irregular flow through placental anastomoses, particularly V-V anastomoses.

Acute on Chronic Twin-to-Twin Transfusion

In cases of TTTS, or chronic twin-to-twin transfusion, the clinical and pathologic picture can be complicated by acute transfusion when one twin dies as described above. Mortality is high in TTTS, and so intrauterine death of one twin is a relatively common outcome. Although either donor or recipient can die in utero, most often it is the donor. When this occurs there is actual reversal of the chronic transfusion of blood in that the recipient then becomes the donor and the donor becomes the recipient. In this case, the larger twin can be severely anemic rather than phlethoric, and the small, original donor can appear dark and congested, leading to some confusion in the original configuration.

Suggestions for Examination and Report
(Twin-to-twin transfusion)

Gross Examination: Documentation of vascular anastomoses is essential to the diagnosis of twin transfusion syndromes (see Chap. 9). In addition, careful attention to the color of the villous tissue (pallor of the donor and congestion of the recipient) and the vascular territories is recommended. If laser coagulation has been performed, the fetal surface can show fibrin deposition, coagulation of vessels, and infarction of villous tissue underlying the anastomotic vessel. These findings should always be noted and attributed to the intervention if possible.

Comment: The presence of a monochorionic placenta with a dominant artery to vein anastomoses is consistent with the diagnosis of chronic TTTS. Usually there are few or no other superficial anastomoses. With fetal demise of one twin, acute twin-to-twin transfusion should be considered as it occurs even in the absence of chronic TTTS. Both may lead to significant morbidity and mortality.

Chimerism and Mosaicism

Chimerism and mosaicism are related but different phenomena. **Whole-body chimerism** is when an *individual is composed of two populations of cells, the origin of which is two genetically different fertilization products*. It may develop in very early stages of development, when dizygotic twin embryos fuse to form a single individual. When *two spermatozoa fertilize an ovum and a polar body and then form a single embryo*, such individuals represent, genetically speaking, fraternal twins fused into one body. This is a variant of the **third type of twin** (see above). The fact that fusion of embryos has occurred in these cases lends credence to the concept that some conjoined twins develop from fusion rather than division. Whole-body chimeras are not necessarily clinically manifest, and therefore the incidence is likely underestimated. Most are discovered when the two populations of cells have different sex chromosomes (XX/XY), resulting in gonadal abnormalities, most common among which is **true hermaphroditism.** Whole-body chimeras may also be discovered during routine blood grouping tests, because of unusual phenotypic features, such as heterochromia (eyes of different color) or abnormal patches of the skin resulting from the irregular distribution of melanocyte precursors derived from different genotypes.

It is important to distinguish two pathogenetically different types of chimeras: blood chimeras and whole-body chimeras. **Blood chimeras** *develop from fused placentas with connections between the fetal vessels enabling blood exchange between DZ twins*. This has long been described in animals, but vascular connections between the placentas of human DZ twins are quite rare. *Study of these individuals' shows that they are blood chimeras but not whole-body chimeras.* Tissue samples are of one genotype while the blood elements consist of two genotypes. Chimeras are important to recognize particularly in the concept of organ and bone marrow transplantation.

Mosaics are different from chimeras as they are *individuals composed of different cell lines but derived from a single fertilization product*. Because of "lyonization" and X chromosome inactivation, all human females are thus mosaics as different cells express a different X chromosome. Not only may mosaics have different cell lines with different chromosome numbers, but, because of mutations, they may also have cell lines with different phenotypic expression.

Heterokaryotypic Monozygotic Twins

Heterokaryotypic MZ twins begin as MZ twins, and then nondisjunction of chromosomes in one twin gives them a different genetic makeup. Most commonly, this occurs with a sex chromosome resulting in karyotypes of 45XO and 46XY and MZ twins of different sex. Nondisjunction of autosomes may also occur, however. *These twins show mosaicism resulting from the simultaneous occurrence of twinning and somatic nondisjunction of chromosomes.* If the Y chromosome of a 46XY embryo is lost by nondisjunction during early development, male and female (45X0 and 46XY) MZ twins may be the outcome. Heterokaryotypic MZ twins may have varying degrees and types of mosaicism. Mosaicism may be present in certain cell types only, such as lymphocytes and other blood cells, in which case it would be directly due to the presence of placental anastomoses. Mosaicism of fibroblasts suggests the loss of a chromosome in one twin after splitting has occurred.

Sacrococcygeal Teratoma and Epignathus

Sacrococcygeal teratoma and **epignathus** (a tumorous mass affixed to the jaw) are, in our opinion, *malformed twins that are part of the spectrum of MZ twinning*, although some may take exception to this concept. Nevertheless, findings of perfectly formed extremities, digits, and other structures favor this view. At times, however, an apparently benign sacrococcygeal teratoma eventuates in a malignancy. An alternate etiologic point of view is that sacrococcygeal tumors and epignathi derive from misplaced germ cells that then develop neoplastic growths.

Placentomegaly has often been described to be a complication of sacrococcygeal teratomas, and the same is true of the placenta in epignathi. Other teratomas and acardiac twins may also be associated with hydramnios and fetal hydrops. These placental changes are likely the result of high output failure. In effect, the teratoma acts as an arteriovenous fistula. If there is hydrops, the placenta will be *exceptionally pale.* There may be *severe villous edema, and the villi may show increased cellularity and vascular congestion.* Numerous Hofbauer cells may be present as well as many nucleated red blood cells.

Selected References

PHP5, pages 893–1000 (Multiple Pregnancies-Superfetation and Superfecundation, Vanishing Twin Phenomenon, Fetus Papyraceous, Twin-to-Twin Transfusion Syndrome, Acardiac Twins, Conjoined Twins, Sacrococcygeal Teratoma and Epignathus, Cytogenetics and Heterokaryotypic Monozygotic Twins, Chimerism and Mosaicism, Triplets and Higher Births, Morbidity and Mortality).

Bajoria R, Wigglesworth J, Fisk NM. Angioarchitecture of monochorionic placentas in relation to the twin-twin transfusion syndrome. Am J Obstet Gynecol 1995;172:856–863.

Bejar R, Vigliocco G, Gramajo H, et al. Antenatal origin of neurologic damage in newborn infants. Part II. Multiple gestations. Am J Obstet Gynecol 1990;162:1230–1236.

Bendon RW. Twin transfusion syndrome: pathological studies of the monochorionic placenta in liveborn twins and of the perinatal autopsy in monochorionic twin pairs. Pediatr Pathol Lab Med 1995;15:363–376.

Benirschke K. Chimerism, mosaicism and hybrids. In: Human Genetics, Proceedings Fourth International Congress Human Genetics, Paris, Excerpta Medica, Amsterdam, 1971:212–231.

Benirschke K. Intrauterine death of a twin: mechanisms, implications for surviving twin, and placental pathology. In: Seminars in Diagnostic Pathology, WB Saunders, Philadelphia, 1993;10:222–231.

Benirschke K. The monozygotic twinning process, the twin-twin transfusion syndrome and acardiac twins. Placenta 2009;30:923–8.

Bieber FR, Nance WE, Morton CC, et al. Genetic studies of an acardiac monster: evidence of polar body twinning in man. Science 1981;213:775–777.

Costa T, Lambert M, Teshima I, et al. Monozygotic twins with 45X,46,XY mosaicism discordant for phenotypic sex. Am J Med Genet 1998;75:40–44.

De Lia JE. Surgery of the placenta and umbilical cord. Clin Obstet Gynecol 1996;39:607–625.

Emery SC, Vaux KK, Pretorius D, Masliah E, Benirschke K. Acardiac twin with externalized intestine adherent to placenta: unusual manifestation of omphalocele. Pediat Develop Pathol 7:81–85, 2004, with permission.

Fisk NM, Dun combe CJ, Sullivan MHF. The basic and clinical science of twin twin transfusion syndrome. Placenta 2009;30:379–390.

Jauniaux E, Elkazen N, Leroy F, et al. Clinical and morphologic aspects of the vanishing twin phenomenon. Obstet Gynecol 1988;72:577–581.

Machin GA. Some causes of genotypic and phenotypic discordance in monozygotic twin pairs. Am J Med Genet 1996;61:216–228.

Moore TR, Gale SA, Benirschke K. Perinatal outcome of forty-nine pregnancies complicated by acardiac twinning. Am J Obstet Gynecol 1990;163:907–912.

Nikkels PGJ, Hack KEA, van Gemert MJC. Pathology of twin placentas with special attention to monochorionic twin placentas. J Clin Pathol 2008;61:1247–1253.

Scheller JM, Nelson KB. Twinning and neurologic morbidity. Am J Dis Child 1992;146:1110–1113.

Spencer R. Conjoined twins: developmental malformations and clinical implications. Baltimore: Johns Hopkins University Press, 2003.

Yamamoto M, Ville Y. Twin-to-twin transfusion syndrome: management options and outcomes. Clin Obstet Gynecol 2005;48:973–980.

Section IV

Abnormalities of the Placenta

This section covers abnormalities and lesions of the placenta. Chapter 11 discusses abnormalities encountered in the early abortion specimen and the pathologic changes associated with chromosomal anomalies. Chapter 12 deals primarily with abnormalities of the implantation site and uterus that occur in the postpartum period, including uterine atony, endometritis, retained placental tissue, and placenta accreta. Chapter 13 discusses aberrations in placental shape, and as these aberrations are associated with abnormal implantation, theories of pathogenesis are briefly discussed. Placenta previa, as an abnormality in the location of implantation, has characteristics in common with these variants and so is discussed as well. Finally, pathologic lesions of the fetal membranes are presented in Chap. 14 and those of the umbilical cord in Chap. 15.

Chapter 11

Abortion and the Placenta in Chromosomal Anomalies

General Considerations

For purposes of the present discussion, an abortion will be defined as a conceptus expelled, removed or delivered before the 20th week of gestation. Local statutes and regulations, particularly state regulations, vary in the definition of what constitutes an abortion and thus viability, but 20 weeks is most commonly used. Furthermore, the definitions of abortion and the age of viability are vastly different from country to country, even reaching the level of 28 weeks in some countries, rendering the statistics on abortions, pregnancy loss, and neonatal and infant morbidity and mortality completely useless in comparing populations worldwide.

R.N. Baergen, *Manual of Pathology of the Human Placenta,*
DOI 10.1007/978-1-4419-7494-5_11, © Springer Science+Business Media, LLC 2011

The pathogenesis of pregnancy loss varies considerably depending on gestational age. Failure at less than 12 weeks is most commonly due to chromosomal or immune mediated phenomena. Loss between 12 and 20 weeks is uncommon and the etiology varies. Loss between 20 and 30 weeks is usually secondary to ascending infection and acute chorioamnionitis.

Abortions may be of several types, which are defined clinically as follows:

- **Induced** or voluntary, which include
  - **therapeutic** – electively terminated
  - **criminal** – illegally instrumented

- **Spontaneous** or involuntary, which include
  - **threatened** – uterine bleeding without cervical dilatation
  - **inevitable** – uterine bleeding with cervical dilatation or effacement
  - **incomplete** – all tissue has not yet passed
  - **missed** – intrauterine retention after embryonic death

- **Habitual/recurrent** – three or more consecutive spontaneous miscarriages

Induced, spontaneous and habitual abortion specimens are approached slightly differently, and each of these is discussed below. However, there are several goals in examination that should be addressed in all abortion specimens, and these are

- To document the presence of a **pregnancy**
- To rule out an **ectopic pregnancy**
- To identify suspected or unsuspected **abnormalities of the placenta or fetus**
- To rule out **gestational trophoblastic disease**

Induced Abortions

Clinical Features and Implications
Pregnancies may be terminated legally or illegally and both are termed **induced abortions**. There is little difference between the two from a pathologist's point of view, except that the latter type is more frequently followed by complications such as uterine infection and perforation. Induced abortions are performed by *dilatation and curettage, vacuum extraction, prostaglandin induction (with or without cervical laminaria), intraamnionic injection of hypertonic saline or urea solutions, and other means, although injection is rarely used.* Some induced abortions are performed because of the prenatal diagnosis of fetal anomalies, while others are presumably normal but "unwanted" pregnancies. Although in the latter case, the likelihood of anomalies is slight, occasionally abnormalities are identified on examination.

Complications of abortions, particularly "criminal" abortions, are rare but can include *uterine bleeding or hemorrhage, uterine perforation, infections, septic abortions, pulmonary embolism, disseminated intravascular coagulation, and other minor complications.* These occur in up to 13% of induced abortions. In **septic abortions**, microscopic examination often reveals *acute villitis, acute intervillositis, and bacterial colonies filling the fetal villous capillaries.* Depending on the organism, some cases may show little inflammatory reaction (see Chap. 16). With the exception of infections, the various complications do not usually reveal specific pathologic lesions in tissue submitted to pathology.

Pathologic Features

To document the presence of an intrauterine pregnancy, and thus rule out an ectopic pregnancy, one must identify *implantation site, trophoblastic cells, or chorionic villi.* Occasionally, no chorionic villi may be found. In this case, the presence of *decidua with infiltration by extravillous trophoblast and physiologic conversion of decidual arterioles, i.e., the implantation site,* is definitive proof of an intrauterine pregnancy (see Fig. 1.7 in Chap. 1). A few chorionic villi may be present without an identifiable implantation site. In these cases, caution is advised since, under rare conditions, a few chorionic villi may be transported from the fallopian tube in an ectopic pregnancy. Thus, the presence of chorionic villi alone does not always document an **intrauterine** pregnancy. The same can be said for the presence of scattered trophoblastic cells without chorionic villi or implantation site. If there are abundant chorionic villi, they are usually associated with the implantation site, and so the diagnosis of intrauterine pregnancy is straightforward. For cases without definitive implantation site and in which there are few chorionic villi, a cautionary comment in the report and communication with the clinician is suggested.

At times, it may be difficult to differentiate decidual cells from extravillous trophoblast, a necessary task if one wants to identify the implantation site. *Decidual cells have distinct cell membranes with lightly eosinophilic cytoplasm containing oval nuclei with dispersed chromatin.* In contrast, *extravillous trophoblasts are polygonal cells without distinct cell borders, which contain abundant amphophilic cytoplasm, and irregular, mildly pleomorphic, hyperchromatic nuclei* (Fig. 11.1). Another clue to the presence of extravillous trophoblast and the implantation site is the characteristic *fibrinoid deposition,* typically seen in the vicinity of extravillous trophoblast. If after histologic examination doubt still remains, immunohistochemistry may be used. Since trophoblast is epithelial in origin, *all trophoblastic cells stain strongly positive for cytokeratins, while decidual cells are always negative* (Fig. 11.2). Similarly, *decidual cells will stain for vimentin and trophoblast will be negative.* Cytokeratin staining is very sensitive for trophoblast but not specific, and so care should be taken when using this stain for other purposes such as the differential diagnosis of trophoblastic disease in which other stains are more appropriate (see Chaps. 23–25).

Although most tissue is normal in induced abortions, occasionally some abnormalities may be found. For instance, fetal death has been reported in approximately 2% of induced abortions, macroscopic anomalies in approximately 1%, and chromosomal abnormalities in

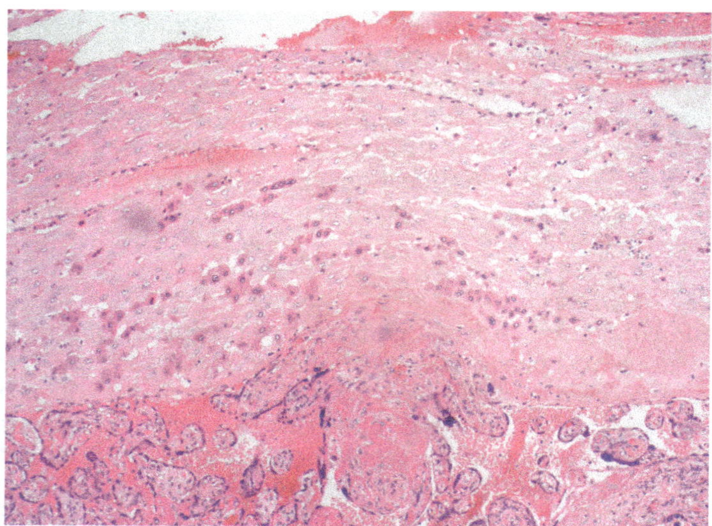

Figure 11.1. Implantation site showing extravillous trophoblast intermixed with decidual cells. The decidual cells have a more vesicular nucleus with pale eosinophilic cytoplasm and well-defined cell borders. The trophoblasts have more amphophilic cytoplasm and irregular, somewhat hyperchromatic nuclei. H&E ×200.

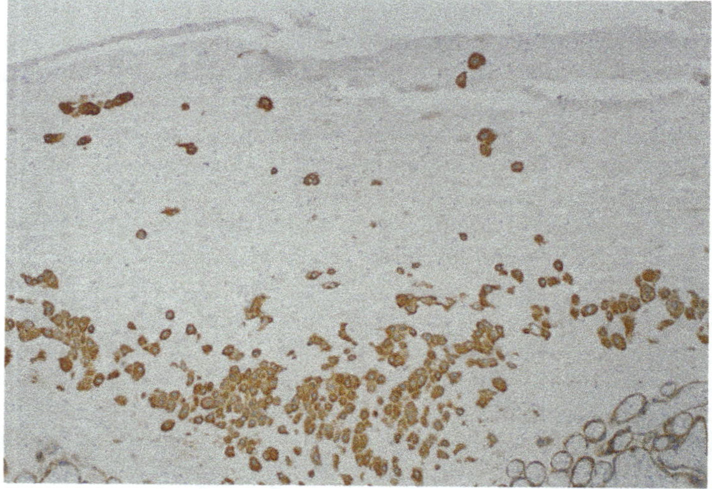

Figure 11.2. Cytokeratin stain of implantation site showing strong staining of the epithelial trophoblast and negative staining of decidual cells. Immunohistochemistry, cytokeratin 7. ×200.

5–6%. Rarely, unsuspected gestational trophoblastic disease may be diagnosed in an induced abortion (see Chap. 23). Normal implantation is often associated with *mild decidual necrosis and inflammation.* However, extensive inflammation or necrosis is an abnormal finding that should be reported as it may be associated with abnormalities of implantation and pregnancy loss. Although these findings may indicate an imminent pregnancy loss or an underlying problem, they are relatively nonspecific. Finally, abnormalities in the decidual vessels and the implantation site may be present in early abortion specimens. These include *lack of normal physiologic conversion, thrombosis, and marked vascular inflammation.* They are often associated with disorders of placental malperfusion (see Chap. 18).

When dilation and curettage (D&C) or suction curettage is performed, instrumentation of the cervix and uterus has occasionally led to misplacement of fetal tissues. Paracervical or endometrial masses consisting of **fetal skeletal parts** have been identified months to many years after the last preceding pregnancy. Incompletely removed fetal tissues may cause unexplained bleeding and have been incriminated in *causing infertility* because they may act similar to an intrauterine contraceptive device.

When abortions are induced by introduction of different substances into the amniotic cavity, certain pathologic changes may occur. Injection of **hypertonic saline** solution results in extensive fetal ion fluxes. This results in *hemorrhage and necrosis under the chorionic plate, intervillous thrombosis, amnion necrosis,* and occasional chorionic vascular obliteration. In addition, the villous tissue is often pale secondary to hemolysis. This type of abortion is now rarely performed. Introduction of hypertonic urea gives similar changes, although not so severe.

Spontaneous Abortions

A **spontaneous abortion,** a "miscarriage," is essentially the *spontaneous delivery of a fetus prior to viability.* This is important to state at the outset, as the pathologic features of failed pregnancies differ markedly from those specimens obtained later in gestation, which are considered **preterm** deliveries. In addition, the result of a pregnancy of less than about 20 weeks' gestation is usually considered an "embryo" and treated as a surgical specimen. At later than 20 weeks it is considered a "fetus," whose examination constitutes an autopsy.

As stated previously, statutes vary from state to state on the gestational age of viability and what constitutes a surgical specimen versus human remains. The definition is legal in this context and does not take into account cultural or religious beliefs about when "life" begins. Therefore, the pathologist may be confronted with complicated circumstances in which the desires of the patient and family are at odds with the legal definition. Frequently, although the law considers a fetus a "specimen" that may be examined without permission and disposed of with other surgical waste, the family may have objections to autopsy examination and may desire burial of the remains. Clearly, it is vital that the patient's wishes be communicated to the pathologist. Unfortunately, this does not always occur, leading to not only difficulties, but at times considerable angst on the part of the patient. There are many ways of handling this; at our institution, any fetus of 12 weeks' gestation or greater is not examined without autopsy consent, even though legally autopsy consent is not required. This ensures that no fetus will be examined when the patient objects. If the patient did want an autopsy, and the clinician did not obtain written permission, the fetal specimens are saved for a longer period than the routine surgical specimens so that the fetus can be later examined. Keeping the fetal specimens longer also ensures examination and proper disposal in the event the patient changes her mind. If private burial is requested at the time of examination or later, the fetus can be transported to the morgue for release to the funeral home. We request that the clinicians indicate on the surgical pathology requisition whether or not private burial is requested and whether autopsy is permitted in addition to requiring written consent. Although the clinicians may be unhappy with these extra steps, they ensure the patient's wishes are honored.

Pathogenesis

Most spontaneous abortions occur before 12 weeks of gestation and many are due to **chromosomal errors**. Chromosomal anomalies are present in 50% of all spontaneous abortions and in 70% of those occurring during the first 6 weeks. Increasing maternal age considerably increases the risk of spontaneous abortion, especially after the age of 35, and this correlates with an enhanced risk of fetal trisomies. However, the exact mechanism of the abortion in this situation is still disputed. Other less well-delineated *genetic defects* also make up a proportion of spontaneous abortions.

Endocrine disorders are a cause of a certain percentage of spontaneous abortions, and these include *luteal phase defects, polycystic ovary syndrome*, and *poorly controlled maternal diabetes*. Numerous physical factors have been associated with an increased incidence of abortions. *Uterine anomalies*, particularly *septate uteri*, have been implicated, and in the latter case, abortion likely ensues when implantation occurs on the septum. *Submucosal leiomyomas* and *trauma* have also been reported to increase spontaneous abortion as well. *Cervical incompetence* (see Chap. 16) is associated with preterm labor, preterm delivery and pregnancy loss. Other causes of spontaneous abortion are *multiple gestation* (see Chaps. 9 and 10), *antiphospholipid antibodies* (see Chap. 18), *drugs* (see Chap. 17), and *congenital malformations*. Relatively few spontaneous abortions occur in the period from 12 to 20 weeks' gestation. Between 20 and 30 weeks, spontaneous termination is primarily due to **ascending infection** (see Chap. 16). *Placental and fetal infections* that may lead to fetal infection and death in the first trimester are less common, but the causative organisms can include *Listeria, Cytomegalovirus, Toxoplasma, herpes simplex virus*, and *Coxsackie virus*.

Clinical Features and Implications

The incidence of spontaneous abortions is actually quite high. When prospective studies of complete populations are done on all pregnancies, including those that give few or no clinical symptoms of pregnancy, nearly 50% of conceptions terminate in abortion spontaneously. Some studies have quoted a higher figure of up to 65%.

There are also conceptuses that vanish even before implantation. Clinically recognized gestations end in abortion in approximately 15% of cases. Spontaneous abortions are usually accompanied by uterine bleeding and cramping with subsequent spontaneous passage of tissue. Often the embryo or fetus will pass first, followed by the placenta. Therefore, curettages done on women who have previously passed tissue often contain only decidualized endometrium and fragments of involuting implantation site.

Pathologic Features

Specimens will consist of embryonic tissue, decidua, and placental tissue, and each should be examined in turn. Specimens may have a *complete or incomplete embryo, have no embryo, or may contain an intact gestational sac.* If the embryo is present, it may be *grossly disorganized*, presenting as a nodular, cylindrical, stunted, or barely recognizable embryo (Fig. 11.3; see Chap. 2); it may show *focal, specific defects* such as spina bifida, cleft palate, etc., or it may be *without gross abnormalities*. The embryo may be macerated to a variable extent, and noting this may be helpful in assigning an estimation of intrauterine retention. Examination of abnormal fetuses is beyond the scope of this text; however, it is understood that with an abnormal embryo, as complete an examination as possible should be done.

Pathologic changes in the villous tissue may also be present. Unfortunately, in early abortion specimens, these changes often do not provide information on the cause of the pregnancy loss but rather

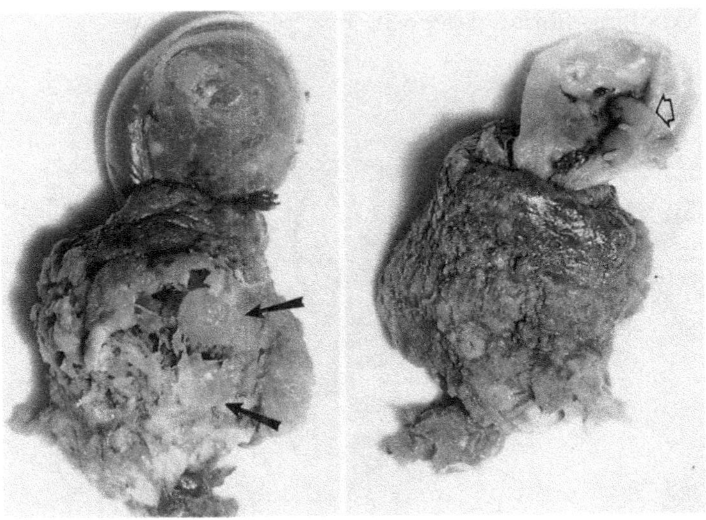

Figure 11.3. Spontaneous abortus at approximately 8 weeks' gestation. Note the opened sac at *right* with the nodular embryo at the *open arrow*. The hypoplastic placenta with hydropic degeneration is seen at the *arrows* (*left*). The decidua basalis is hemorrhagic.

on the presence of embryonic death. The few exceptions noted above include abnormalities of the implantation site vessels and excessive inflammation and necrosis. The pathologic changes in abortion speci- mens *are more often related to the timing of embryonic death and the age of the conceptus at the time of death than to the cause of the pregnancy failure.* The following is a list of the changes that generally occur after embry- onic death:

- Early embryonic death – menstrual age less than 7 weeks (Fig. 11.4)
  - Hydropic villi
  - Thinned trophoblastic cover
  - Lack of red blood cells and villous capillaries

- Embryonic death – menstrual age approximately 7–8 weeks (Fig. 11.5)
  - Focal villous hydrops
  - Focal villous stromal sclerosis
  - Villous capillaries with varying degrees of vascular obliteration
  - Nucleated red blood cells, which may be "naked" in the stroma
  - Increased syncytial knots
  - Thickened trophoblastic basement membrane

- Embryonic death – menstrual age approximately 8–12 weeks (Fig. 11.6)
  - Increasing villous fibrosis with collagenous stroma
  - Obliteration of villous vessels
  - Ratio of nucleated to nonnucleated red blood cells changes from 100 to 10%
  - Fine mineralization of trophoblastic basement membrane and villous stroma
  - Perivillous fibrinoid deposition

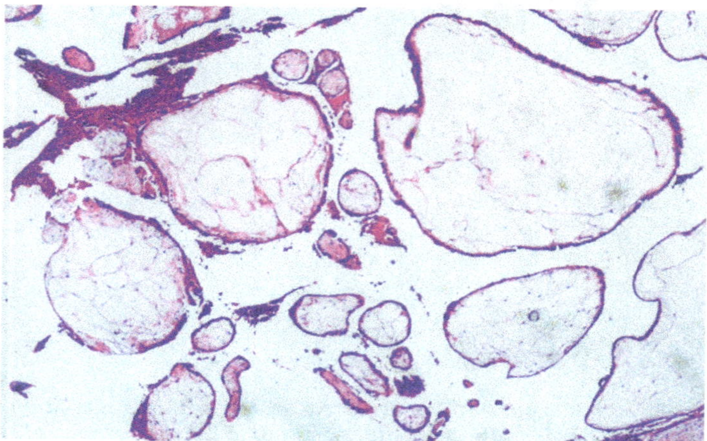

Figure 11.4. Early spontaneous abortion at about 6 weeks with prominent hydropic villi and no fetal capillaries or red blood cells. H&E ×40.

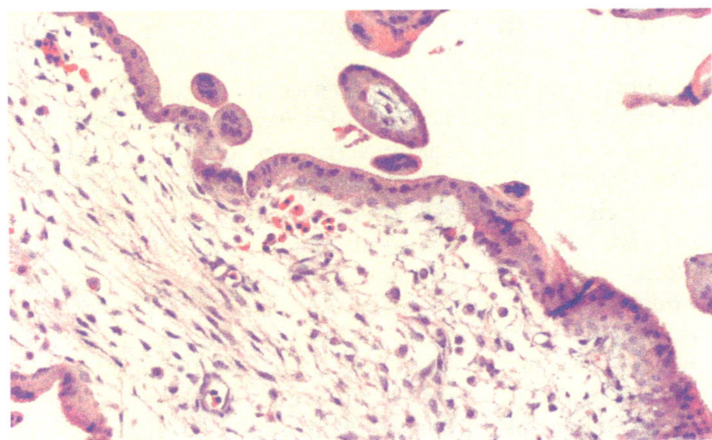

Figure 11.5. Early spontaneous abortion at about 7–8 weeks. This villus shows edema at the periphery and early fibrosis in the central region (*at the left*). Nucleated red blood cells are present "naked" in the villous stroma. H&E ×200.

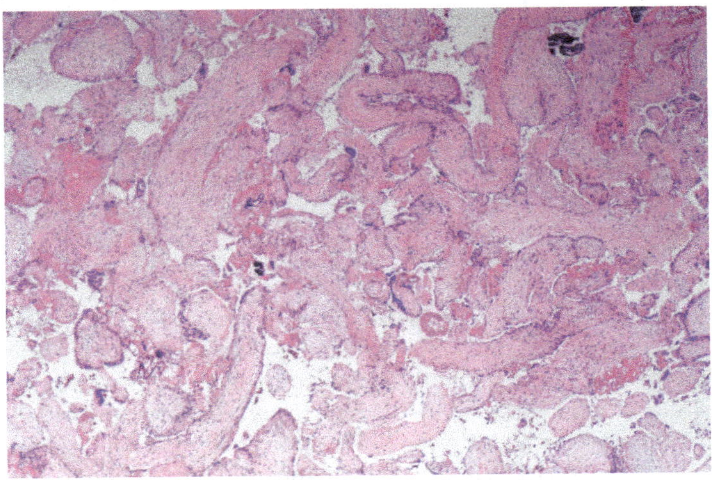

Figure 11.6. Spontaneous abortion with collagenous stroma and obliteration of blood vessels, at about 9 weeks. H&E ×20.

The reason for the preponderance of hydropic change in aborted specimens is not fully understood. It is generally believed that, following fetal death, the trophoblast continues to transport water from the intervillous space into the villi, where it cannot be removed by an absent fetal circulation; hence, the villi enlarge. Villous vascularization occurs at about 6.5 weeks menstrual age and so conceptuses reaching that age will show the presence of villous capillaries and nucleated red blood cells and will show less hydropic change.

Recurrent or Habitual Abortion

Habitual abortion is usually defined as a condition in which a woman has had *three or more consecutive spontaneous abortions*. Three consecutive losses is the preferred definition because after two consecutive spontaneous abortions, the chance of successful pregnancy is 80%. Known etiologies vary widely. There are many infectious causes (see Chap. 16) and a number of chronic maternal diseases such as *lupus erythematosus, maternal heart disease, thrombophilias, antiphospholipid antibody syndrome, and endocrine disorders* (see Chap. 17). *Recurrent villitis of unknown etiology, massive repetitive chronic intervillositis* (see Chap. 16), and *maternal floor infarction* (see Chap. 19) constitute another group of disorders that primarily placental in origin. The relation of *substance abuse* to spontaneous abortion and to abruptio placentae is difficult to evaluate, and the contribution of *maternal smoking* is also unclear. Many patients who smoke or use various toxic substances additionally consume alcohol, have various infections, and are prone to suffer misuse and trauma (see Chap. 17).

Parental chromosome aberrations and some *immunologic errors associated with placentation* are other well-studied causes of recurrent abortion. Some recurrent abortions are due to increasing maternal age with its increased chance of aneuploidy. Rarely, *balanced chromosomal translocations* of one parent have been the cause of habitual abortion. Therefore, it is suggested that in couples with recurrent abortions, the mother *and* the father be examined cytogenetically. The pathologist can contribute to a better understanding of the etiology by requesting cytogenetic evaluation of aborted specimens from recurrent aborters.

Chromosomal Anomalies

Some investigators have gone so far as to suggest that pathologic changes in chromosomally abnormal abortions are so characteristic that they enable chromosomal diagnosis from the morphologic findings of the villous tissue alone. When tested, experts and diagnostic pathologists are consistently unable to specifically label a given microscopic appearance with confidence. In general, *karyotyping is necessary to confirm the diagnosis*. The exception is the karyotypic abnormalities associated with hydatidiform moles (see Chap. 23). That being said, there are certain pathologic features that are commonly seen in aneuploid conceptuses as a group. One of the hallmarks of a **chromosomal anomaly** is the presence of *growth restriction of the fetus* and *an abnormally small and thin placenta*. Other histologic features that are often associated with chromosomal defects in general are *increased villous size, villous edema, trophoblastic inclusions or invaginations, irregular villous contour, and cytotrophoblastic giant cells*.

Trisomies

There are few specific findings that characterize a placenta with **trisomy**, but many abnormalities have been found sporadically. First, the

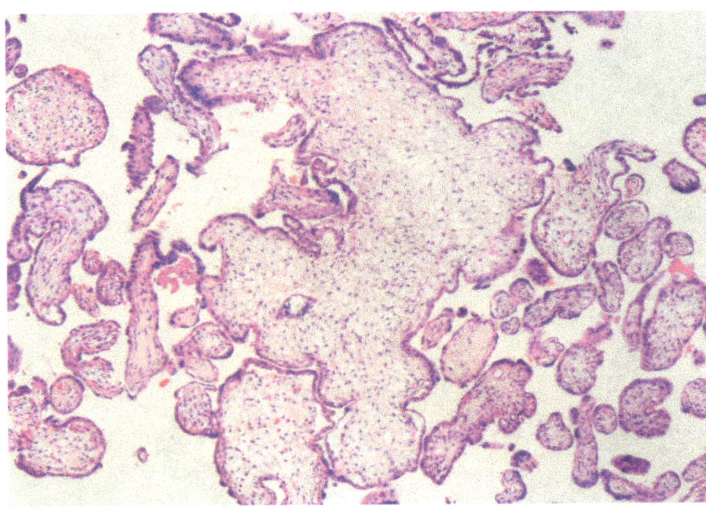

Figure 11.7. Spontaneous abortus with trisomy 13. There is scalloping of villi and trophoblastic "inclusions," most visible in the large villus in the center of the figure. H&E ×40.

incidence of *single umbilical artery* (SUA) is higher. Second, placentas tend to show *deficient vascularization* with a reduction in the number of small muscular arteries, decreased small muscular artery/villus ratio, and decreased numbers of capillaries. The villi are frequently *dysmature* with *trophoblastic inclusions or invaginations* (Fig. 11.7). Occasionally, *increased syncytial knots* and *increased cellularity of the villous stroma* are also found.

Trisomy 16 is one of the *commonest cytogenetic anomalies found in spontaneous abortion material*. The embryo is generally absent with a small, empty chorionic cavity. Histologically, the *villi and trophoblast are hypoplastic with decreased vascularization*. Some villi may be *hydropic*. Enlarged *cytotrophoblastic giant cells* are found in the stroma of up to 30% of villi (Fig. 11.8). The origin of these cells is unclear but they may be edematous stromal cells, enlarged Hofbauer cells, or cells derived from delaminating cytotrophoblast. In **trisomy 18**, *the chorionic villi are cystic and dilated, showing typical hydropic change*. Cysts may be large enough to be identified grossly (Fig. 11.9). There may also be *increased syncytial knots* (Fig. 11.10) or *increased cellularity of the villous stroma* (Fig. 11.11).

The abortions of **trisomies 6–12** have a variable morphology. The placenta is *less mature* than expected for gestational age. *Giant cytotrophoblastic cells* are found in 40% of villi (Fig. 11.8). In **trisomies 13–15** there is *variable placental maturation, decreased villous vascularity, and giant cytotrophoblast in 50% of villi. Occasionally, hydropic villi, scalloping, and trophoblastic inclusions may occur.* **Trisomy 21** is not accompanied by characteristic placental changes. Increased placental weight and size, however, have frequently been observed. There are even fewer characteristic patterns of the placentas of other trisomies, but *hydropic change is common and there is occasional atypical trophoblastic proliferation.*

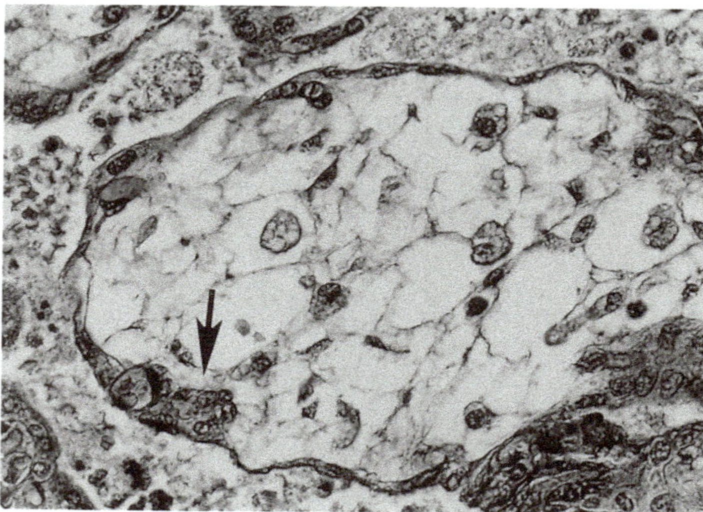

Figure 11.8. Villus with cytotrophoblastic giant cells in a spontaneous abortion. The much-enlarged cells in the villous core represent enlarged Hofbauer cells. Cystic lacunae are developing in the villus. H&E ×400.

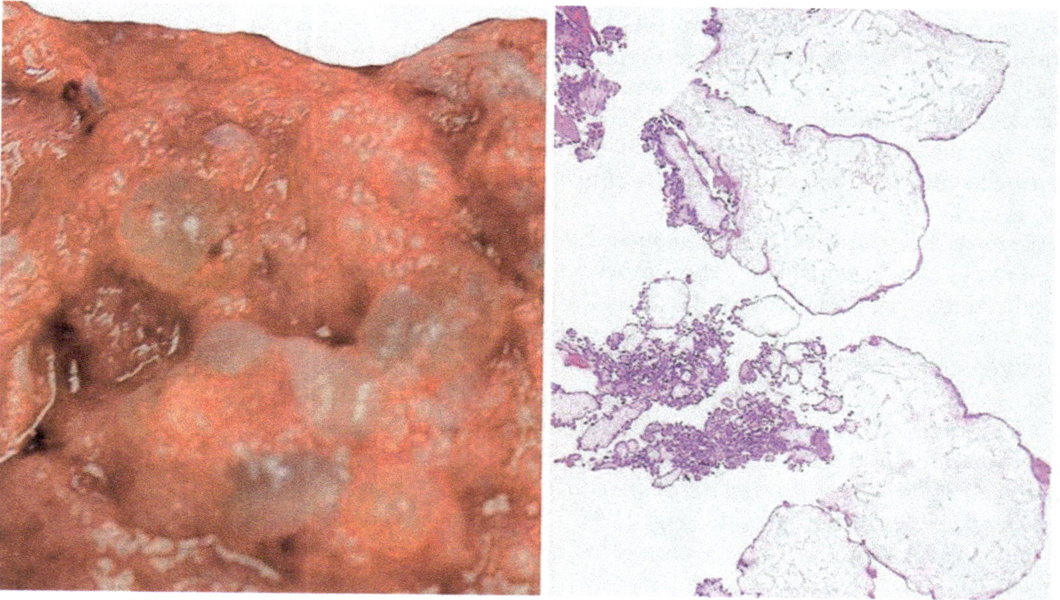

Figure 11.9. Premature trisomy 18 placenta. On the *left* is a gross picture of the hydropically enlarged villi. The *right* shows the histologic picture of hydropic villi and increased trophoblast, which may cause confusion with molar pregnancy. H&E ×160.

Other Chromosomal Anomalies

Triploid conceptuses may be either *dygynic* or *diandric*, with the extra chromosome set deriving from the mother and father respectively. Diandry results in partial hydatidiform moles. Triploidy due to dygyny

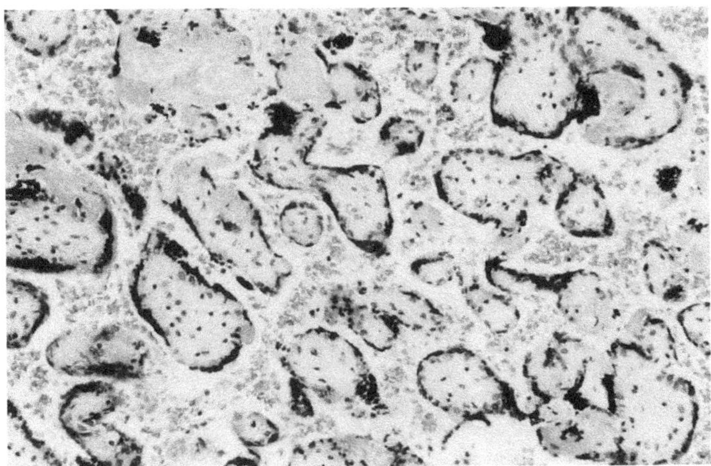

Figure 11.10. Villi of immature placenta (28 weeks' gestation) of a stillborn fetus with trisomy 18. There is increased syncytial knotting despite the absence of preeclampsia. Villi lack fetal vessels because of fetal demise, but many have hyalinized centers. H&E ×64.

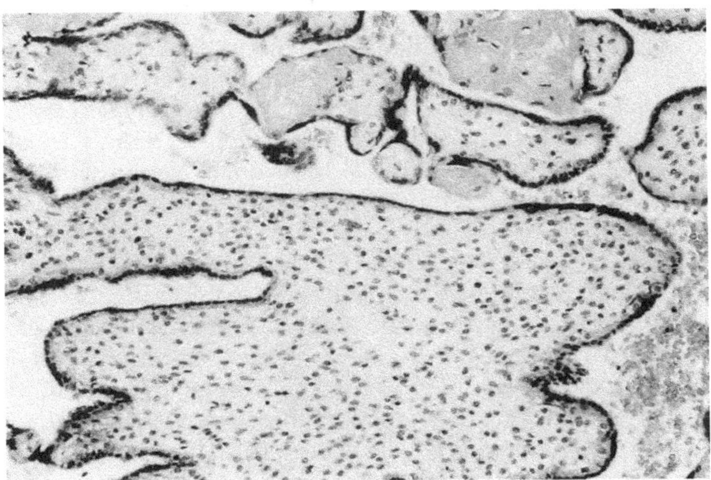

Figure 11.11. Trisomy 18 placenta with a marked increase in villous stromal cells. H&E ×160.

is much more common in older women in whom nondisjunction of chromosomes occurs more commonly. The fetus is usually *small for the expected age* and often has characteristic anomalous features such as *digital fusion; frequently the embryos are nodular and degenerating. SUA* is also common. Macroscopically, the placentas of triploids frequently show some degree of *hydropic change,* though not so prominent as seen with partial moles. Microscopically, some villi have *cavities or lacunae*

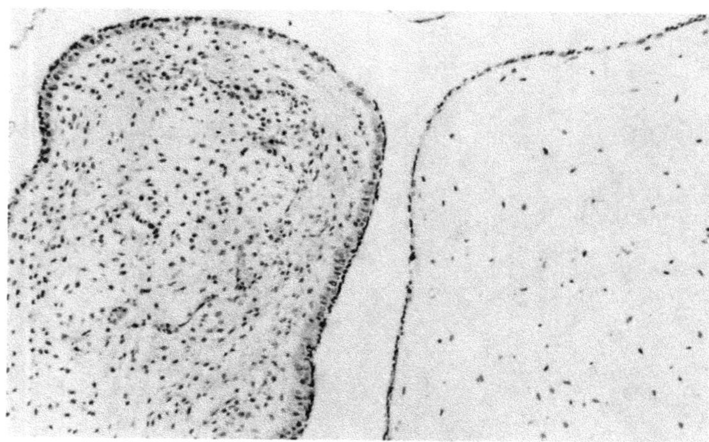

Figure 11.12. Two enlarged villi in a triploid abortus. One (*left*) is hypercellular, with faintly visible remnants of former fetal vessels; the other is hydropic. H&E ×160.

within the villi, which are smaller than the cisterns seen in molar pregnancies (see Fig. 23.4 in Chap. 23). Other villi may be disrupted or *compacted with increased cellularity* (Fig. 11.12), *and the trophoblast is variably hypoplastic.* There is characteristic *infolding or scalloping of trophoblast* into the villi, with trophoblastic nests occurring seemingly isolated in the villous stroma. A Breus' mole is occasionally found with triploid abortuses as well, although this is more common in monosomy X.

Tetraploid abortuses usually have an *empty cavity and voluminous, poorly vascularized villi.* They frequently have *severe decidual and villous hemorrhages,* and their villi are invariably somewhat cystic. Occasionally, massive hydropic change may be seen. The embryos and placentas of **monosomy X** often appear relatively normal with only *villous fibrosis* present. Frequently, only a cord remnant is found in a cavity that is small for gestational age. In some cases there are *intervillous thrombi* of the so-called Breus' mole type (see Chap. 14). The embryo may have nuchal hygroma and severe hydrops.

Ancillary Testing

In abortion specimens, the chromosomal errors are composed of trisomy in 50–60%, triploidy in 18%, monosomy X in 15%, and the remainder are double trisomies, tetraploidies, and individual chromosomal errors, such as rings, translocations, and mosaicism. The pathologist is occasionally asked to provide material for **cytogenetic study**. This is best done from embryonic tissue or from the chorionic surface when an embryo is not available or macerated. In some cases, due to lack of viable embryonic tissue, placental tissue may be the only tissue able to grow in culture. Caution is advised when only placental tissue is obtained due to confined placental mosaicism (CPM) (see below). Therefore, *if possible it is optimal to obtain both embryonic and placental tissue.* When sampling the placenta, it is best to cleanse the fetal surface, peel the amnion away, and then obtain chorionic tissue with sterile instruments.

Chorionic villus sampling (CVS) is the procedure by which a *small sample of villous tissue is obtained early in gestation for the purpose of chromosomal or DNA testing.* CVS is usually done at about 11 weeks' gestation. It has been suggested that CVS is a significant cause of fetal loss and limb reduction defects. However, only a 0.8% increase of fetal loss in CVS patients has been documented. The relationship between limb defects and CVS exists principally in the gestationally earlier CVS and not when CVS is done after 9 weeks.

Because hydropic villi are such a frequent finding in many placentas of spontaneous abortions, the differentiation from moles and partial moles may present difficulty. Therefore, use of **flow cytometry** is advocated as a *rapid means for the delineation of diploidy and triploidy.* Thus, triploid partial moles may be differentiated from complete diploid hydatidiform moles, and diploid abortuses may be distinguished from triploid partial moles (see Chap. 23).

The sera of pregnant women are often tested with the **triple screen** and more recently the **quadruple screen** or **quad test.** The triple screen includes measurements of *β-human chorionic gonadotropin (β-hCG), unconjugated estriol,* and *α-fetoprotein* in the maternal serum. The quadruple screen adds *dimeric inhibin A.* Abnormalities in one or more of these markers are associated with increased risk of neural tube defects and chromosomal anomalies, particularly trisomy 21 and 18. The abnormalities and their associated test results are summarized in Table 11.1.

New methodology is evolving that will make it feasible to describe the genetic defects more accurately, such as various **DNA studies,** the **polymerase chain reaction (PCR), fluorescence in situ hybridization (FISH)** of whole cells, and delineation of translocations by spectral color staining of chromosomes. Some of these tests are feasible even using fixed tissue and individual, selected cells from paraffin-embedded tissues. Ploidy analysis and routine karyotyping also are essential tools in diagnosis. Placental material also lends itself for *paternity diagnosis.*

In assisted reproductive technology, germinal vesicles of oocytes from older women may be implanted into enucleated eggs of younger women due to the increase in chromosomal errors in older patients. This is one of the reasons for the recently more widely practiced "preimplantation genetics," which seeks to avoid implanting chromosomally abnormal embryos or those afflicted with single gene mutations. In addition, prenatal diagnosis of X-linked diseases has been achieved by the study of male cells from maternal blood, and this is currently under active study.

> **Suggestions for Examination and Report**
> (Abortions)
>
> **Gross Examination:** If villi are grossly identified, one section in an induced abortion is sufficient, while two to three sections should be submitted in a spontaneous abortion. It is also suggested to submit a fragment of decidual tissue in addition to villous tissue as it often contains a portion of the implantation site. If villi are not grossly seen, consideration should be given to submission of the entire specimen, particularly if an ectopic pregnancy is suspected. If the clinical history indicates a habitual abortion, tissue should be sent for chromosome analysis if this has not already been completed. Embryonic tissue should be submitted to document its presence and to further clarify gross abnormalities.
>
> **Comment:** The tissues that are present including implantation site, decidua and chorionic villi, should be listed in the diagnosis if all are normal. Abnormalities such as lack of physiologic conversion, excessive inflammation should be listed separately. If features of chromosomal abnormalities are present, those should be listed and a comment may be made that the findings are suggestive of a chromosomal anomaly or, if clinical history is given, that the findings are consistent with the clinical history of a chromosomal anomaly.

Confined Placental Mosaicism, Uniparental Disomy, and Imprinting

In order to understand the concepts of confined placental mosaicism (CPM) and uniparental disomy (UPD), a few definitions are necessary:

- **Mosaicism** is when an organism has two genetically distinct cells lines derived from a single fertilization product or genotype.
- **Chimerism** is present when an organism has two genetically distinct cells derived from two different fertilization products or genotypes.
- **CPM** is present when the placenta has a different cell line than the fetus, both deriving from the same fertilization product or genotype.
- **UPD** is the presence of two chromosomes from one parent.
- **Imprinting** is the transcriptional silencing of a portion (paternal or maternal) of one parental genome.

The presence of CPM, UPD, mosaicism, and chimerism has caused discrepancies in chromosomal findings between results obtained via CVS, amniocentesis, and fetal lymphocyte culture. Although some of the discrepancy may be due to contamination with maternal tissue, other discrepancies may be due to the above conditions. The finding of mosaic cell lines may also reflect the differing origin of cells from the **inner cell mass (fetus)**, its **shell (placental trophoblast)**, the **amnion,**

chorion, or **connective tissue of the villi.** One must know which cells are found to be chromosomally abnormal in order to infer probable fetal genotype.

Confined Placental Mosaicism

CPM may manifest in different ways. An abnormal karyotype such as trisomy 18 might be found in the placenta while the fetus has a normal karyotype. The placenta will often be *grossly and histologically normal (although sometimes small),* while the fetus is *growth restricted.* It is postulated that an *aneuploid placenta functions less efficiently than a normal organ* and therefore produces fetal growth restriction. The genotypically normal fetus is thus small but shows no anomalies. CPM may also present as a trisomic fetus with a euploid placenta. *Fetuses with trisomy 13 and 18 who survive turn out to have placental karyotype mosaicism.* In these cases, the mosaicism appears to be confined to cytotrophoblast and not found in villous stroma, chorion, or amnion. The suggestion is that *trisomics with mosaic (aneuploid/diploid) placentas have a better chance of reaching maturity than those with truly trisomic placentas.*

CPM is also found more frequently in *unexplained stillbirths and unexplained growth restriction.* It is found three times more commonly in placentas with intrauterine growth restriction (IUGR) fetuses than normal fetuses. Moreover, 10% of gestations with CPM have fetal cytogenetic abnormalities. Regrettably, there is not yet much direct correlation with placental pathologic features in CPM. For the pathologist, it is important to realize that CPM occurs in the setting of unexplained fetal growth restriction or demise, and that *in order to document CPM, samples from multiple placental sites are necessary to make the diagnosis.* If resources allow, the placenta may be evaluated for CPM in cases of IUGR that have no other apparent cause.

Uniparental Disomy

In **UPD** there are *two chromosomes from one parent* rather than one from each parent. It is an occasional finding in *growth restricted newborns* and *stillborns* and appears to be linked to CPM. It is postulated to take its origin from a trisomic conceptus with the loss of one *trisomic chromosome leaving the fetus with a normal chromosome complement.* Depending on which chromosome is lost, the fetus may end up with two chromosomes from the same parent, resulting in UPD. There are several ways in which UPD may complicate CPM. A trisomic fetus that loses its extra chromosome becomes diploid and may have UPD. If the corresponding placenta remains trisomic, CPM results. On the other hand, the placenta may lose the extra chromosome and develop UPD.

Imprinting

A final aspect of this complex array of potential genetic events is the concept of **imprinting.** It is a reality affecting fetal and placental tissues as well as many disease states and is presumably accomplished via DNA methylation of specific genes. There is good evidence that some *pater-*

nal genes are silenced during embryonic development (maternal imprinting), while some maternal genes are silenced during placental development (paternal imprinting). Imprinting is important in understanding how different types of triploidy may result in the development of partial hydatidiform moles. Partial moles are generally triploid with one set of maternal genes and two sets of paternal genes. The excess of paternal genes acts similar to silence of maternal genes and leads to preferential development of trophoblastic tissues over fetal tissues. On the other hand, triploidy with two sets of maternal genes and one set of paternal genes does not lead to a molar pregnancy but results in a small placenta and a fetus, often with typical anomalies such as syndactyly.

Table 11.1. Maternal serum markers and risk of anomalies.

Abnormality	AFP	hCG	UE3	DIA
NTD	↑	–	–	–
Trisomy 21	↓	↑	↓	↑
Trisomy 18	↓	↓	↓	–

Note: Arrows indicate increase or decrease compared to normal results at that gestational age, results are reported as multiples of the median.
AFP α-fetoprotein, *hCG* human chorionic gonadotropin, *UE3* unconjugated estriol, *DIA* dimeric alpha inhibin, *NTD* neural tube defect.

Selected References

PHP5, pages 762–796 (Abortions, Placentas of Trisomies and Immunologic Considerations of Recurrent Reproductive Failure).

Bennett P, Vaughan J, Henderson D, et al. Association between confined placental trisomy, fetal uniparental disomy, and early intrauterine growth retardation. Lancet 1992;340:1284–1285.

Cohen J. Coming to term. Uncovering the truth about miscarriage. Boston and New York: Houghton Mifflin, 2005.

Cohen J. Sorting out chromosomal errors. Science 2001;296:2164–2166.

Jauniaux E, Burton GJ. Pathophysiology of histological changes in early pregnancy loss. Placenta 2005;26:116–123.

Kalousek DK, Barrett, I. Confined placental mosaicism and stillbirth. Pediatr Pathol 1994;14:151–159.

Kalousek DK, Barrett IJ, McGillivray BC. Placental mosaicism and intrauterine survival of trisomies 13 and 18. Am J Hum Genet 1989;44:338–343.

Moore GE, Ali Z, Khan RU, et al. The incidence of uniparental disomy associated with intrauterine growth retardation in a cohort of thirty-five severely affected babies. Am J Obstet Gynecol 1997;176:294–299.

Redline RW, Hassold T, Zaragoza M. Determinants of villous trophoblastic hyperplasia in spontaneous abortions. Mod Pathol 1998;11:762–768.

Rushton S. Examination of products of conception from previable human pregnancies. J Clin Pathol 1981;34:819–835.

Salafia CM, Burns JP. The correlation of placental and decidual histology with karyotype and fetal viability. Teratology 1989;39:478(P37).

Sermon K, Steirteghem A, van Liebars I. Preimplantation genetic diagnosis. Lancet 2004;363:1633–1641.

Stirrat GM. Recurrent miscarriage I: definition and epidemiology. Lancet 1990;336:673–675.

Stirrat GM. Recurrent miscarriage II: clinical associations, causes, and management. Lancet 1990;336:728–733.

Tycko B. Genomic imprinting: mechanism and role in human pathology. Am J Pathol 1994;144:431–443.

Warburton D, Stein Z, Kline J, et al. Chromosomal abnormalities in spontaneous abortions: data from the New York City study. In: Porter IH, Hook EB (eds) Human embryonic and fetal death. New York: Academic Press, 1980:261–287.

Chapter 12

Postpartum Hemorrhage, Subinvolution of the Placental Site, and Placenta Accreta

General Considerations

Postpartum hemorrhage, if severe, can be a major obstetrical emergency, which, if not treated promptly, may result in rapid exsanguination and demise of the mother. Specimens submitted to the pathology laboratory depend on the clinical situation and may include the *placenta, retroplacental curettings, other sampling from the endometrial cavity, the uterus, or, in some cases, no specimen at all.* Pathologic examination and diagnosis is facilitated by knowledge of the clinical situations and causes of postpartum hemorrhage such as:

- Injury from cervical lacerations or uterine rupture
- Coagulation defects
- Uterine atony
- Retained placental tissue
- Subinvolution of the placental site

R.N. Baergen, *Manual of Pathology of the Human Placenta,*
DOI 10.1007/978-1-4419-7494-5_12, © Springer Science+Business Media, LLC 2011

- Postpartum endometritis
- Placenta accreta
- Placental polyp

In the case of coagulation defects, specimens are rarely submitted. If they are, the findings usually consist only of hemorrhage and no specific pathologic lesion. If there is a rupture or laceration, whether or not it is repaired, with associated bleeding necessitating hysterectomy, documentation of the area of injury is essential. Since clinical history is sometimes missing, postpartum hysterectomy specimens should always be examined with the thought in mind that there might be this type of injury, and therefore documentation of any defect and whether there is surrounding hemorrhage should be done at minimum and sections submitted of the area. The remaining causes of postpartum hemorrhage usually result in pathologic lesions and will be discussed in the following sections.

Uterine Atony

Pathogenesis

After delivery of the placenta, cessation of blood flow through the endometrial vessels is largely accomplished by *contraction of the uterus*. **Uterine atony** is defined as the absence of normal uterine contraction. The most common underlying causes are:

- Overdistention from a large fetus, multiple pregnancy, or polyhydramnios
- Anesthetic agents
- Prolonged, augmented or rapid labor
- High parity

When the myometrium loses the ability to contract, the uterine vessels may bleed extensively and present a life-threatening situation necessitating hysterectomy. In general, uterine atony is a clinical diagnosis, but there are pathologic features that are seen in this setting that are relatively specific.

Pathologic Features

In normal circumstances, the postpartum uterus is *enlarged from myometrial hyperplasia and hypertrophy*. The uterine wall is usually markedly thickened but firm due to the contraction of the smooth muscle. If **atony** is present, the uterus will be *edematous and boggy*, and hemorrhage may be grossly evident. Usually this is a diffuse rather than focal change. Microscopically, the findings are relatively nonspecific and consist of typical hypertrophied myometrium with *diffuse, recent hemorrhage* often in the vicinity of large, open, dilated vessels. Groups of myometrial fibers will be *separated by edema fluid*, and these findings will be relatively diffuse throughout the uterus (Fig. 12.1). This is in contrast to what is

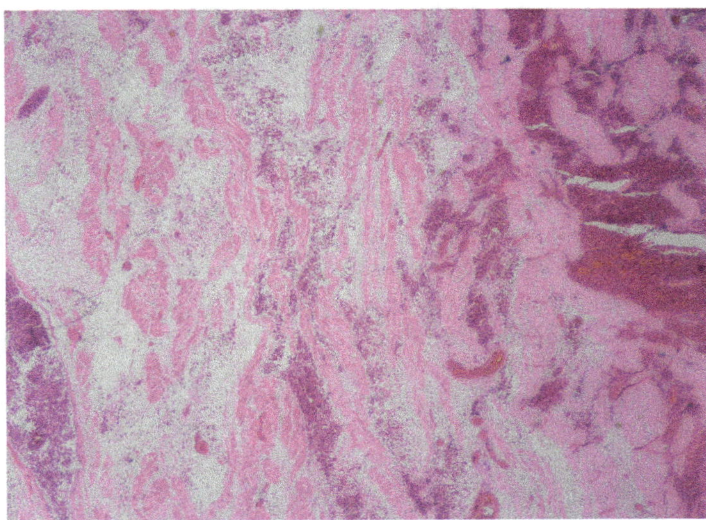

Figure 12.1. Microscopic appearance of the myometrium in a case of uterine atony. Muscle fibers are separated by edema fluid and there is focal recent hemorrhage. H&E ×20.

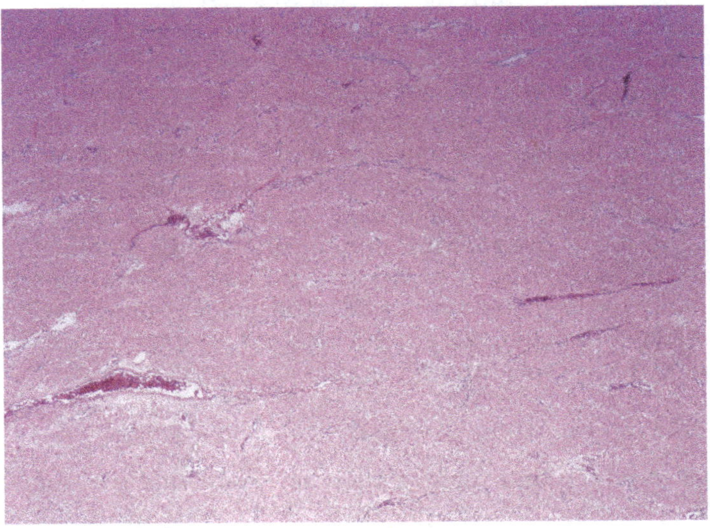

Figure 12.2. Normal postpartum uterus with hypertrophic but closely packed myometrial fibers, no significant hemorrhage and no edema. H&E ×20. Compare to Fig. 12.1.

present in a normally contracted postpartum uterus in which the muscle fibers appear tight against one another without separation by blood or fluid (Fig. 12.2).

> **Suggestions for Examination and Report**
> (Uterine atony)
>
> **Gross Examination:** Representative sections of the uterus should be submitted including the implantation site. The latter is usually a roughened, hemorrhagic area on the endometrial surface. Sections of the lower uterine segment and cervix, if present, should also be submitted. Attention should be given to the presence of lacerations, perforation or evidence of other injury, particularly in the cervix.
>
> **Comment:** Marked edema and hemorrhage are present, consistent with the clinical history of uterine atony. A comment may also be made about the absence of other pathologic findings, specifically addressing any clinical differential diagnoses.

Retained Placental Tissue and Involution of the Placental Site

It is often assumed that evaluation of the completeness of the maternal surface of the placenta will uncover the presence of missing placenta tissue that has been retained in the uterus. It is therefore interesting that many cases exist in which the placenta was described by experienced observers as "intact" and retained placental tissue was later found to be present. Thus, practically, one cannot be reassured by the integrity of the placenta postpartum, regardless of the experience of the examiner. On the other hand, when the maternal surface of the placenta is **not** intact, the likelihood of retention of placental tissue is heightened. Placental tissue may be retained for a number of reasons. It may be merely due to *inadequate removal of the entire placenta at delivery*. It also may occur due to endometritis, subinvolution of the placental site, or placenta accreta. When there is associated **postpartum hemorrhage**, particularly delayed postpartum hemorrhage, it is more likely to be associated with a pathologic process. Delayed postpartum hemorrhage may occur days, weeks, or even months after delivery.

Normal Involution of the Placental Site

In order to understand subinvolution, one must find understand the complex process of normal placental site involution. Unfortunately, pathologists rarely receive normal postpartum uteri that would enable detailed study of the involutional changes at the former site of implantation. The following is an overview of the events at the placental site following normal delivery. They are also summarized in Table 12.1.

The separation of the placenta from the uterus takes place within the decidua basalis, largely due to the *shearing action of the myometrium as it contracts against the incompressible placenta*. **Immediately following delivery**, contraction of the uterus clamps the arteries, preventing uterine bleeding. The endometrial surface becomes covered with *blood clot and fibrin*. Within minutes to hours, the blood vessels start to undergo *thrombosis* and thus are no longer completely patent. **Within the first postpartum day**, the walls of the arteries and veins in the

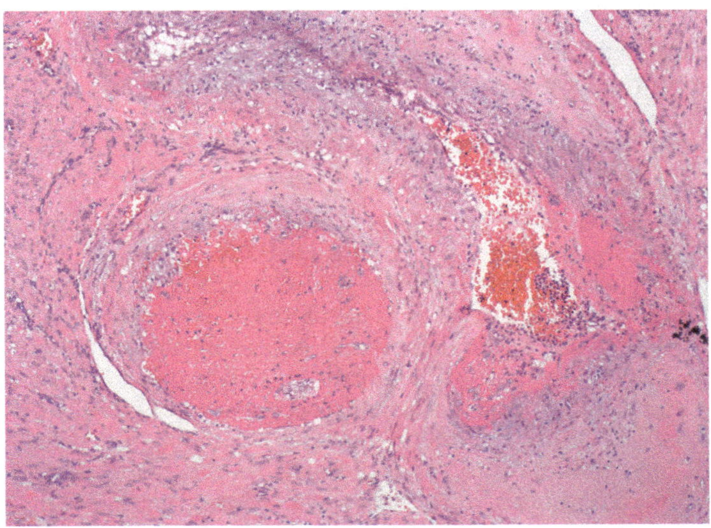

Figure 12.3. Normal involution of the placental site with thrombosed uterine vessels approximately 2 days after delivery showing thrombosis and early obliterative arteritis. H&E ×160.

implantation site *become hyalinized. Fibrinoid necrosis and inflammation* develop in the arteries. *The implantation site decreases in size*, from about 18 cm, the approximate diameter of a term placenta, to 9 cm. From **postpartum day 1 to day 3**, the *veins completely thrombose and the arteries develop obliterative endarteritis* (Fig. 12.3). There is early decidual necrosis and a modest neutrophilic and mononuclear infiltrate. From **day 3 to day 5**, *inflammation and necrosis* increase and reactive regenerating endometrial glands begin to appear. The thrombosed veins begin to organize, and the arteries show early intimal proliferation and continuing hyalinization. From **postpartum day 5 to day 8**, there is a *clear demarcation* of the necrotic decidua (which will be subsequently sloughed as the "lochia" or discharge) from the remaining endometrium. *Endometrial glands show pronounced reactive changes and are increased in number.* They regenerate by regrowth and extension of the adjacent endometrial glands and stroma. *Arteries are occluded* by endarteritis by this time. *Placental site giant cells are prominent* early in the involuting implantation site in the endometrium and superficial myometrium, but their numbers decrease over the ensuing weeks. **Three to four weeks** after delivery, *the endometrium at the implantation site is regenerated and inactive with scattered hemosiderophages.* Veins have mostly been recanalized, but *some residual vessels show hyalinization,* which may persist for many weeks even under normal circumstances.

The rapidity of the **involution of myometrial muscle mass** postpartum remains a mystery. *The average postpartum uterus weighs about 1,000 g and shrinks to less than 100 g in about 2 months.* The histologic changes are relatively minimal. Degenerative changes of the muscle occur within hours of delivery, and a mild chronic inflammatory infiltrate develops within the first 4 days and persists for up to 17 weeks. It is important to note that virtually *no myometrium repairs the incisional defect from cesarean* *sections and only a thin fibrous scar approximates the muscle layers.* Thus, in subsequent pregnancies the probability of dehiscence exists with possible **uterine rupture** or **placenta accreta** (see below).

Subinvolution of the Placental Site

Pathogenesis

When the uterus does not undergo normal involution, **subinvolution of the placental site** is said to occur. Here, there is *failure of the normal physiologic obliteration of the blood vessels in the placental site as well as delayed myometrial involution.* The uterus is somewhat boggy and edematous, but not to the degree that is seen in uterine atony. There may be delayed postpartum hemorrhage, which typically occurs 1–2 weeks after delivery, but occasionally occurs several months postpartum. This is in contrast to uterine atony in which hemorrhage occurs immediately after delivery and tends to be much more acute and severe. Subinvolution is, in fact, the most common cause of "delayed" postpartum hemorrhage. It is more common in *multiparous women and tends to recur in subsequent pregnancies.* Causes include *retained placental tissue, infection, placenta accreta, and idiopathic causes.*

Pathologic Features

Most patients with subinvolution have normal placentas at delivery. Later, bleeding occurs and the specimen most commonly submitted to the pathology laboratory is uterine curettings. On histologic examination of the endometrial tissue, large *dilated arteries filled with blood and partially organized thrombi* are seen. The arteries are often found in groups of three or four, adjacent to normally involuting vessels (Fig. 12.4). The

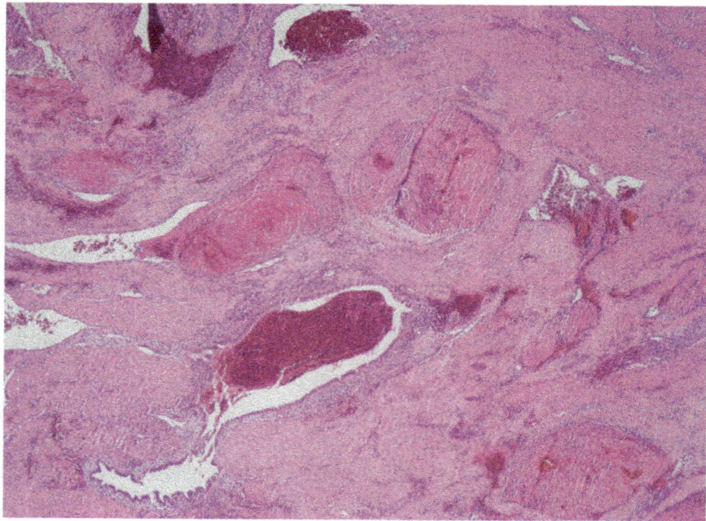

Figure 12.4. Subinvolution of the placental site. Note the enlarged, patent vessels with evidence of bleeding. The curettage was done 3 weeks after delivery and was accompanied by delayed postpartum hemorrhage. Involution is delayed, and the histologic picture is more consistent with what should be seen within the first day or two after delivery. H&E ×20.

histologic picture is often similar to normal involution, but the changes are delayed. Thus, clinical history is crucial in making the diagnosis, as the interval from delivery is necessary to evaluate whether normal involution has been delayed. Furthermore, in contrast to normal involution, where extravillous trophoblast is inconspicuous or absent, subinvolution is characterized by the *persistence of extravillous trophoblast*, particularly in a perivascular location. *Persistence of endovascular extravillous trophoblast* is also occasionally seen.

Suggestions for Examination and Report
(Subinvolution of the placental site)

Gross Examination: Subinvolution is most commonly seen in patients who present with postpartum bleeding. There are no specific gross lesions.

Comment: Subinvolution of the placental site is a common cause of postpartum hemorrhage, particularly delayed postpartum hemorrhage.

Postpartum Endometritis

Postpartum endometritis is an intrauterine infection that is classically caused by group A streptococci, but many other organisms, including anaerobes, have been implicated. It is an **acute endometritis** characterized by *pronounced acute inflammatory infiltrates within endometrial stroma and gland lumens* (Fig. 12.5) and may be associated with colonies of bacterial organisms. The inflammatory infiltrate should be in excess of the minimal acute inflammation associated with normal involution. Collections of neutrophils within gland lumina are an important diagnostic clue. Phlebothrombosis and a plasma cell infiltrate may also be present. Endometritis is often associated with subinvolution, and in this case the histologic features of subinvolution will also be present. Postpartum endometritis may lead to serious complications such as sepsis, pulmonary embolism, and even death. Treatment is usually curettage and antibiotics.

Suggestions for Examination and Report
(Postpartum endometritis)

Gross Examination: There is no specific gross appearance.

Comment: The diagnosis of acute endometritis postpartum, particularly if bacteria are present, may have serious clinical sequelae.

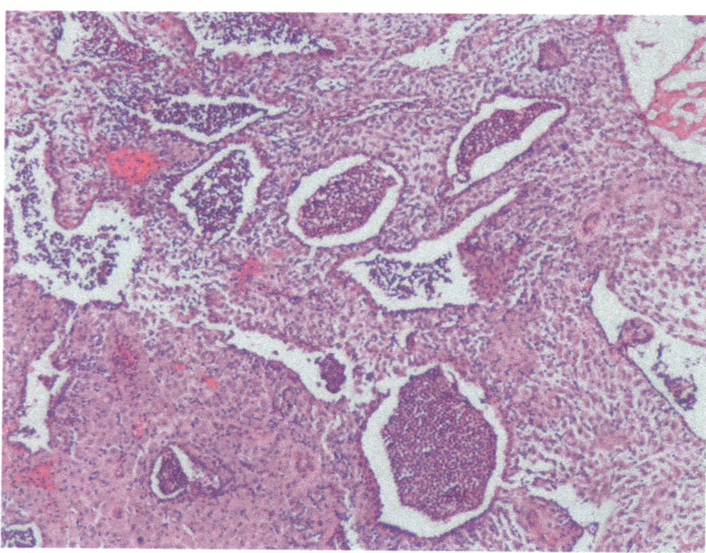

Figure 12.5. Postpartum endometritis showing an inflammatory infiltrate consisting predominantly of acute inflammatory cells. Note the large collections of neutrophils within the gland lumina H&E ×40.

Placenta Accreta, Placenta Increta, and Placenta Percreta

In normal implantation, the extravillous trophoblast invades the decidua in a controlled fashion and converts the spiral arterioles of the endometrium to uteroplacental vessels (see Chap. 8). In **placenta accreta**, there is a *failure of the normal decidua to form*, at least locally, because the endometrium is deficient and cannot decidualize. The trophoblast does not stop invading when it should, and chorionic villi penetrate into the myometrium. Traditionally, placenta accreta has been divided into **placenta accreta, placenta increta**, and **placenta percreta**, based on how deeply the trophoblastic tissues invade. In **placenta accreta**, *the chorionic villi are attached to myometrium without intervening decidua*, in **placenta increta** *the myometrium is invaded by the placental villous tissue*, and in **placenta percreta** *the villi penetrate through the entire uterine wall*. The underlying pathogenetic mechanisms and etiologies are likely to be the same, the only difference being a quantitative one, which, however, may be of considerable clinical importance, particularly in the case of placenta percreta.

Clinical Features and Implications

Placenta accreta is relatively rare, with an incidence of around one in 7,000 pregnancies. The incidence is higher in the setting of placenta previa, where it is estimated to be 1.18%. This has been termed "placental previa accreta" and develops due to deficient decidualization of the cervical stroma. The occurrence of placenta accreta has been steadily rising, and this is thought to be secondary to the increased cesarean section rate. The type of surgical closure after cesarean section is also thought to have an impact on the development of future placenta accreta. It is often detected after delivery *when the placenta fails to separate or is incompletely delivered.* Incretas and percretas more frequently manifest antepartum and earlier in gestation because of hemorrhage or uterine rupture. In 45% of cases, there is an elevation of maternal serum α-fetoprotein levels. Diagnosis by ultrasonography and magnetic resonance imaging (MRI) is possible, and cases have been reported as early as 14 weeks. Sonography of placenta accreta often displays *irregular lucencies in the villous tissue.* These "lakes" presumably derive from the abnormal implantation and an abnormal disposition of maternal spiral arterioles to the intervillous space.

Placenta accreta may be associated with *life-threatening hemorrhage that can lead to maternal and/or fetal death.* Maternal deaths occur in approximately 9.5% of cases and fetal death in a similar percentage. Placenta percreta may lead to uterine rupture, or it may invade the bladder, causing hematuria. Massive hemorrhage from perforation has also been described. Thus, when a placenta percreta or a deep placenta increta is identified by radiologic studies, delivery by cesarean section with hysterectomy is usually undertaken even in cases where the fetus is significantly premature. Although the usual treatment is hysterectomy, microembolization through the internal iliac arteries has been used to treat less severe cases of placenta accreta. Embolization is performed, and the placenta may be left within the uterus, to be followed by spontaneous expulsion several days later. Occasionally the placenta may be retained in these circumstances for months. Pathologic changes of uterine retention of the placenta are discussed below.

Pathogenesis

In **placenta accreta**, the villous tissues are anchored to muscle fibers rather than to intervening decidual cells due to a *deficiency of decidua.* Normally, the placenta separates from the uterine musculature in a plane just peripheral to Nitabuch's fibrinoid layer, within the decidua basalis. It is accomplished by the *shearing action of contracting myometrium against the stationary, noncontracting placenta and occurs in irregular planes of friable decidual cells.* Without this layer, uterine contractions do not dislodge the placenta or portions of the placenta, or the entire placenta is retained. Sometimes the area of adherence may be quite small, and retention of placental tissue in the uterus may not be immediately noticed.

Placenta accreta is a nice example of the *importance of endometrial decidualization for proper control of trophoblast invasion.* This correlation is further underlined by the fact that *absence of decidualization in tubal pregnancy also coincides with increased trophoblastic invasiveness,* and thus ectopic pregnancies are essentially tubal placenta accretas. They usually perforate the wall, becoming placenta percretas. Tubal rupture does not occur from distention of the tube but rather the penetration of the relatively thin muscular wall. A similar situation arises in the lower uterine segment and endocervix as decidualization is not fully developed in these areas. At present, the specific decidual characteristics responsible for control of invasiveness are still unknown.

Any condition that leads to the development of **deficient decidua** predisposes the patient to placenta accreta. *The most frequent predisposing condition is a history of previous cesarean section and/or curettage.* The risk for development of placenta accreta increases with a history of multiple cesarean sections and multiple surgeries. Other predisposing conditions include *placenta previa (see Chap. 13), submucosal leiomyoma, cornual implantation, placenta membranacea (see Chap. 13), and uterine anomalies.* In all these cases, there is the potential for deficient decidualization. Placenta accretas and particularly percretas are said to be increasing in frequency and this undoubtedly relates to the greater frequency of cesarean sections. In a surgical incision, reconstitution of a *normal* uterine wall is not possible. Therefore, in the subsequent pregnancy, the expanding uterus may dehisce at the former incision site. If the placenta implants over this previous scar, uterine expansion will cause the placenta to be implanted on very thin scar tissue and/or peritoneum.

Pathologic Features

In placenta accreta, the placenta is often disrupted during delivery and there may be *missing cotyledons.* However, completeness of the maternal surface cannot always be accurately evaluated. If the placenta is relatively intact, a **focal placenta accreta** may still be present. When histologic sections of such a placenta are made, the deficiency of endometrium that underlies placenta accreta is generally not evident. It may be possible to make the diagnosis of placenta accreta if curettings are done that include the myometrium, but it is very difficult as the tissue is often difficult to orient. If portions of the myometrium are removed with the placenta and remain attached to the floor (Fig. 12.6), the diagnosis may also be made.

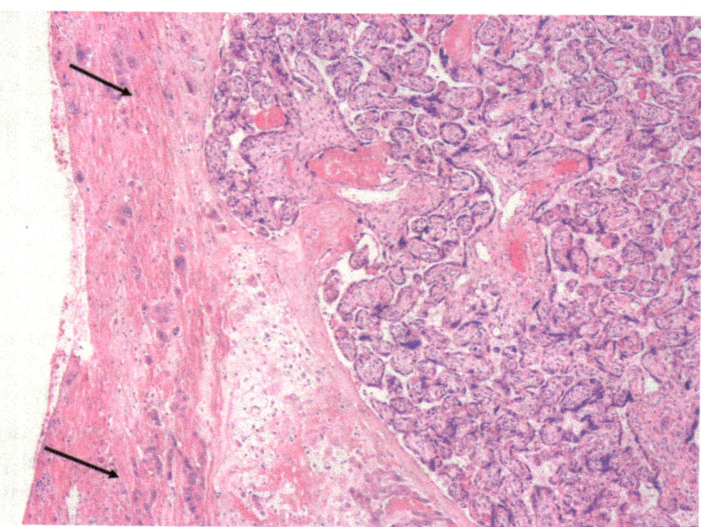

Figure 12.6. Section of the basal plate of a term placenta showing the presence of myometrial fibers (*arrows*) with intervening extravillous trophoblast but no decidua between the muscle and the chorionic villi indicative of at least focal placenta accreta. H&E ×40.

However, in the case of a placental specimen or curettings, the diagnosis of accreta can certainly not be ruled out. The diagnosis is much easier to accomplish when the entire uterus is available, which of course is the less acceptable outcome for the patient. Nevertheless, hysterectomy is a frequent sequel of placenta accreta.

The cesarean-hysterectomy specimen is often quite remarkable on gross examination (Fig. 12.7). If the diagnosis is known prior to delivery, the placenta may be left in situ in the uterus. Then, the true relationship of the placenta to the implantation site may be studied. The serosal surface of the uterus is often *congested and hemorrhagic, and may show nodular protrusions representing a thinned myometrium overlying placental tissue* (Fig. 12.7). As a cesarean section is performed prior to the hysterectomy, an anterior incision is usually evident, which may or may not have been sutured. Examination of the uterine cavity will show placenta implanted *over myometrium, which is markedly thinned, or even absent* (Fig. 12.7). At times, only a thin covering of peritoneum is present over the placenta. If the placenta is not left intact, retained placental tissue may still be visible firmly attached to the endometrium. In placenta percreta (Fig. 12.8), placental tissue may be visible perforating through the uterine serosa. Care must be taken to ensure that loss of

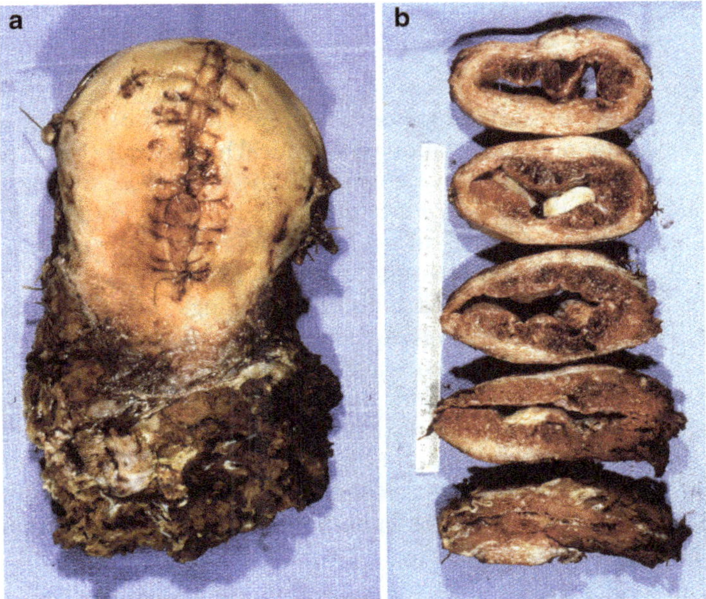

Figure 12.7. Cesarean-hysterectomy specimen with placental implantation over the cervical os leading to a placenta previa accreta. (**a**) Note the protrusion of hemorrhagic placental tissue in the lower segment. A *vertical* scar represents the incision made for the cesarean section, which was then sutured prior to the hysterectomy. (**b**) Same specimen as part (**a**). Serial transverse sections have been made with the most superior at the top and the most inferior at the bottom. Note that the myometrium becomes thinned to invisibility in the lower uterine segment. This was essentially a placenta previa percreta as it invaded through the lower uterine segment.

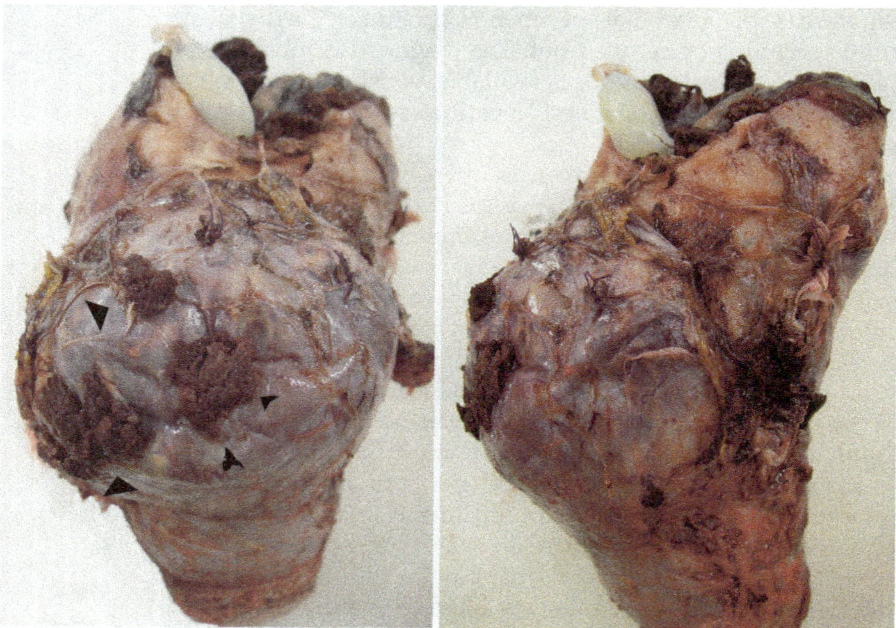

Figure 12.8. Photograph of cesarean-hysterectomy specimen with placenta percreta in which placental tissue can be seen protruding through the serosal surface (*arrowheads* at *left*).

integrity of the serosa is not due to rough handling of the specimen prior to examination. Correlation with clinical history may be helpful in these cases. On microscopic examination, one sees *villous tissue that has grown onto or into the myometrium without intervening decidua*. It is important to note that it is the **lack of decidua** that is diagnostic of this entity (Fig. 12.9). This point is discussed more fully in the next section.

There are several associated pathologic findings seen with placenta accreta. First, the normal *physiologic conversion of maternal vessels may be focally deficient*. This may be related to the abnormal invasiveness of trophoblast or to the general lack of availability of decidual vessels for implantation. There is also usually a *deficiency of placental septum formation*. When septa are present in a placenta accreta, they are composed of uterine muscle rather than decidua, extravillous trophoblast, and fibrinoid. This leads to abnormal flow patterns in the intervillous space, which may be appreciated on antepartum imaging.

Pitfalls in Diagnosis: There are several important pitfalls in the diagnosis of placenta accreta, partly due to confusion in distinguishing the populations of cells that make up the placental floor. The first difficulty lies in the fact that although the presence of chorionic villi attached to the myometrium is diagnostic of placenta accreta, *rarely are the chorionic villi present* **directly** *on the myometrium*. This is unfortunate because this is the most common definition of placenta accreta in textbooks and journal articles, and it is technically not quite correct. Villi implanted on the myometrium are really a fortuitous finding and are not required for

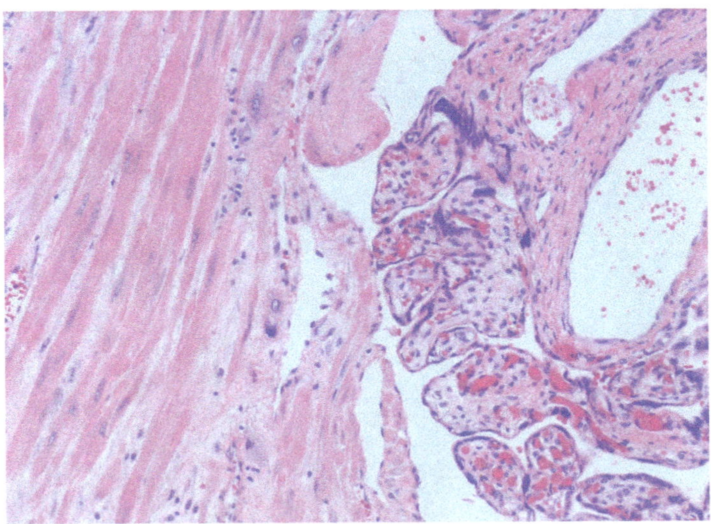

Figure 12.9. Placenta accreta showing "classic" picture with chorionic villi attached directly to the myometrium. H&E ×200.

diagnosis. The main defect in placenta accreta is the *deficiency of decidua*, and that is generally not discussed. In most cases, there is *fibrinoid and extravillous trophoblast in between* the myometrium and the villous tissue (Fig. 12.10a). The crucial point here is that the diagnostic feature of placenta accreta is the **lack of decidua and not implantation onto the myometrium**. Therefore, if villi are present adjacent to fibrinoid or extravillous trophoblast, which is **then** adjacent to myometrium, and there is no intervening decidua, the diagnosis of placenta accreta is made. Insistence on the demonstration of villous implantation on the myometrium will result in *underdiagnosis*.

The second cause of underdiagnosis is *confusion of extravillous trophoblast with decidua*. Extravillous trophoblasts are always present in the implantation site and are normally present adjacent to the myometrium and villous tissue. *If these trophoblastic cells are misinterpreted as decidual cells, the diagnosis will be missed* (Fig. 12.10a) and also result in underdiagnosis. If there is doubt about the true nature of cells in the implantation site, immunohistochemistry for cytokeratin can be extremely helpful, as trophoblastic cells are epithelial and are strongly positive for cytokeratins, while decidual cells are not.

Overdiagnosis of placenta accreta may also occur. In the normal implantation site, extravillous trophoblast and placental-site giant cells (see Chap. 8) are present in the basal portion of the placenta, the decidua, *and the myometrium*. Often, the presence of placental-site giant cells within the myometrium is interpreted as evidence of placenta accreta. However, the presence of these trophoblastic cells within the myometrium is *a normal finding and is not diagnostic of placenta accreta* (Fig. 12.10b).

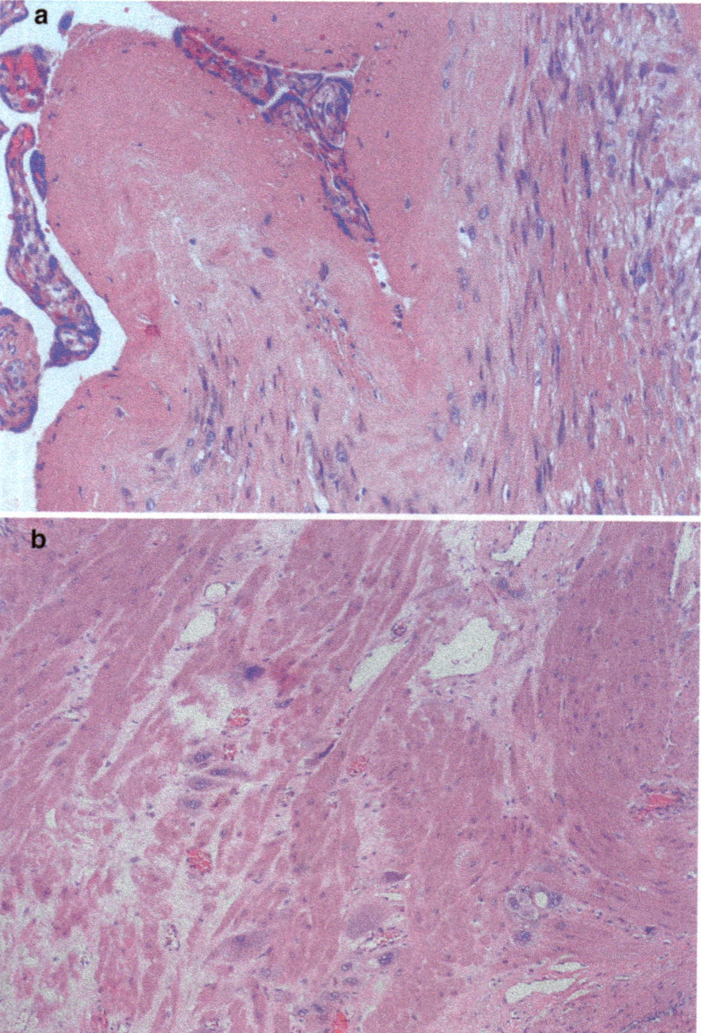

Figure 12.10. (**a**) Placenta accreta. Here, the chorionic villi implant on fibrinoid and extravillous trophoblast and not directly on myometrium (at the *right*), but with the absence of decidua is still diagnostic of placenta accreta. The extravillous trophoblast may be confused with decidual cells. H&E ×100. (**b**) Placental site giant cells present within myometrium, a normal finding of the implantation site that is not diagnostic of placenta accreta. H&E ×20.

Suggestions for Examination and Report
(Placenta accreta, placenta increta, and placenta percreta)

Gross Examination: If only the placenta is submitted, examination should involve careful inspection of the maternal surface for completeness and the presence of firm white tissue, which may represent attached myometrium. Retroplacental curettings should be completely submitted for microscopic examination. In a hysterectomy

(continued)

specimen, the area of accreta is often obvious, particularly if the placenta is left in situ. The myometrium will appear thinned on cut section. Sections should be taken to include placenta and myometrium in areas where *the myometrium is thinned or where there is firm placental attachment*. The anterior lower uterine segment is the most common place for placenta accretas associated with previous cesarean section. If the site of accreta is not obvious, or the placenta is not included, multiple sections should be submitted from the most likely areas to show accreta anteriorly – the lower uterine segment and cervix. The most hemorrhagic and roughened areas are the most likely to represent implantation site or retained placental tissue. One or two sections of normal implantation site should also be submitted along with a section without implantation site.

Comment: Comments should be directed to the location where the accreta was found and the extent of the accreta, e.g., depth and breadth. Usually a measurement is not necessary, but clinicians appreciate knowing whether it is only focal or extensive, where it is, and which side it involves. Other pathology that may be associated with increased risk of accretas should also be commented on, such as uterine scar, bicornuate uterus, etc.

Placental Polyp

Placental polyps are polypoid fragments of tissue consisting of degenerated chorionic villi that have become encased in fibrinoid and layered clot. They represent **focal placentas accretas**. Because of the degenerative changes associated with intrauterine retention of this tissue, the diagnosis may be difficult to verify. At times, however, some myometrial tissue is also present and one finds *villi directly attached to myometrium*. Placental polyps may be *seen in endometrial curettings for postpartum bleeding or may be spontaneously passed weeks or months after delivery* (Fig. 12.11). They are seen in up to 45% of women who present with delayed postpartum hemorrhage. When they are removed or spontaneously passed, the symptoms of bleeding usually abate. Rarely, failure to remove placental polyps has resulted in potentially life-threatening hemorrhage.

Suggestions for Examination and Report
(Placental polyp)

Gross Examination: Placental polyps are usually submitted as curettings or as an endometrial polyp in women with delayed postpartum bleeding. Unless unusually large, the specimen should be entirely submitted.

Comment: Placental polyps are usually indicative of a focal placenta accreta.

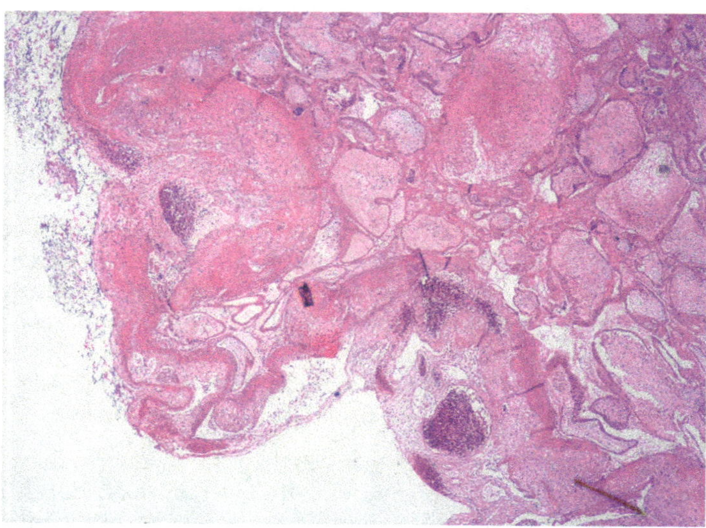

Figure 12.11. Placental polyp. Spontaneously passed tissue consisting of predominantly of degenerating chorionic villi enmeshed in fibrinoid and extravillous trophoblast. Although the implantation of this placental fragment is not present, the diagnosis of placenta accreta is presumed. H&E ×20.

Involution of a Retained Placenta

Placentas may be retained in utero after a fetal demise, when only one of a set of twins survives or when the placenta is not removed after delivery because of a placenta accreta. Since there is continued perfusion by maternal blood, the placental *tissue remains structurally intact for a long time*, particularly the trophoblastic cells. Initially there is *increased syncytial knotting*, followed by involution of the fetal vasculature, resulting in *avascular villi. Fibrinoid also accumulates in the intervillous space*. Eventually, the placenta atrophies and comes to resemble an infarct with marked calcification and villous hyalinization (Fig. 12.12). The more remote the fetal demise, the more likely the degenerative changes will mask any other pathologic lesions present.

Suggestions for Examination and Report
(Involution of a retained placenta)

Gross Examination: The placenta may appear grossly infarcted and is usually quite firm. The cord and membranes often are discolored red due to hemolysis. Routine sections should be submitted.
Comment: Increased syncytial knots, fibrinoid deposition, calcification, and degenerative changes are consistent with retention of placental tissue after delivery or fetal death.

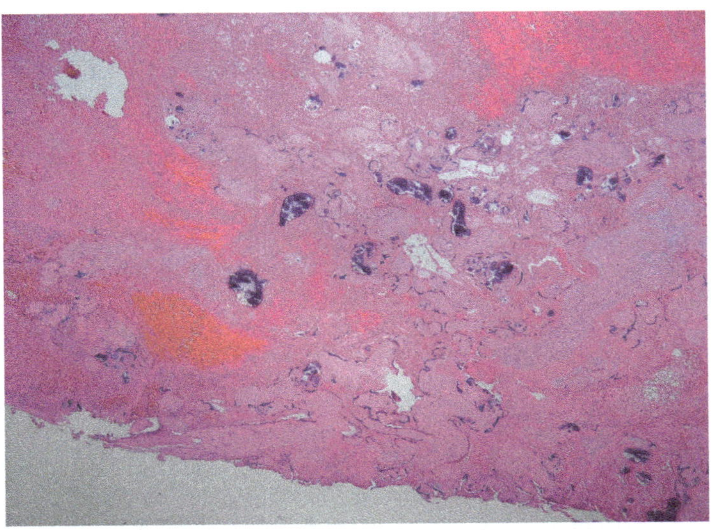

Figure 12.12. Involuting placenta in case of intrauterine fetal demise many weeks previously. Note the avascular, hyaline villi, fibrinoid and hemorrhage. H&E ×20.

Table 12.1. Histologic changes of normal placental site involution.

Time postpartum	Gross size (cm)	"Slough"	Glands	Decidua	Veins	Arteries
<1 day	From 18 to 9	Hemorrhage	Few, inactive	Viable	Hyalinized	Fibrinoid necrosis, minimal inflammation
1–3 days	7–8	Early necrosis	Mild reactive change	Necrosis and inflammation	Thrombosed	Obliterative endarteritis, hyalinization
3–5 days	6	Necrosis with inflammation	Regenerating glands, moderate reactive change	Increased necrosis and inflammation	Organizing	Hyalinization, intimal proliferation
5–8 days	4.5	Well demarcated	Marked reactive change, increased numbers of glands, placental site giant cells	Necrosis and inflammation	Organizing thrombi	Hyalinization
4–20 weeks	2.0	None	Inactive glands, hemosiderophages	None	Recanalized, hyalinized	Remnants of hyalinized vessels

Selected References

PHP5, pages 268–277 (Pathology of Trophoblast Invasion, Placenta Accreta, Placenta Increta and Percreta, Uterine Rupture), pages 313–320 (Involution of Placental Site, Retained Placenta).

Anderson WR, Davis J. Placental site involution. Am J Obstet Gynecol 1968;102:23–33.

Clark SL, Koonings PP, Phelan JP. Placenta previa/accreta and prior cesarean section. Obstet Gynecol 1985;66:89–92.

Cox SM, Carpenter RJ, Cotton DB. Placenta percreta: ultrasound diagnosis and conservative surgical management. Obstet Gynecol 1988;71:454–456.

Fox H. Morphological changes in the human placenta following fetal death. J Obstet Gynaecol Br Commonw 1968;75:839–843.

Fox H. Placenta accreta, 1945–1969. Obstet Gynecol Surv 1972;27:475–490.

Irving FC, Hertig AT. A study of placenta accreta. Surg Gynecol Obstet 1937;64:178–200.

Jacques SM, Qureshi F, Trent VS, et al. Placenta accreta: mild cases diagnosed by placental examination. Int J Gynecol Pathol 1996;15:28–33.

Khong TY. The pathology of placenta accreta, a worldwide epidemic. J Clin Pathol 2008;61:1243–1246.

Khong TY, Khong TK. Delayed postpartum hemorrhage: A morphologic study of causes and their relation to other pregnancy disorders. Obstet Gynecol 1993;82:17–22.

Khong TY, Robertson WB. Placenta creta and placenta praevia creta. Placenta 1987;8:399–409.

Lawrence WD, Qureshi F, Bonakdar MI. "Placental polyp": light microscopic and immunohistochemical observations. Hum Pathol 1988;19:1467–1470.

Rutherford RN, Hertig AT. Noninvolution of the placental site. Am J Obstet Gynecol 1945;49:378–384.

Williams JW. Regeneration of the uterine mucosa after delivery, with especial reference to the placental site. Am J Obstet Gynecol 1931;22:664–696, 793–796.

Chapter 13
Placental Shape Aberrations

General Considerations

Round or oval placentas are the predominant human placental form but many other shapes exist (Fig. 13.1). When the placenta is irregular, its shape is presumably determined by *location, atrophy, and perhaps the manner of original implantation*. Anomalies may develop from abnormal fetal genes expressed by the placenta, an abnormal maternal environment, or an abnormal fetal-maternal interaction. Interestingly, for each aberrant placental shape in humans, there is a counterpart in animals. Thus, the placenta membranacea is similar to the normally diffuse placenta in equines; the zonary placenta is typical of carnivores and so on.

R.N. Baergen, *Manual of Pathology of the Human Placenta*,
DOI 10.1007/978-1-4419-7494-5_13, © Springer Science+Business Media, LLC 2011

Abnormally shaped placentas are important to document as they can be associated with adverse outcome.

The Multilobate Placenta

The Bilobed Placenta

One of the most striking abnormalities is the **bilobed placenta** (placenta bilobata), in which *two roughly equal sized lobes are separated by a segment of membranes* (Figs. 13.1 and 13.2). It is present in 2–8% of placentas. The umbilical cord may insert in either of the lobes or in a velamentous fashion (see Chap. 15), in between the lobes, the latter being the most common arrangement. Even if the cord insertion is not velamentous, there *are always membranous vessels connecting the two lobes*. If one lobe is much smaller than the other, the placenta is said to have a **succenturiate** or **accessory lobe** (see below).

Succenturiate Lobes (Accessory Lobes, Placenta Succenturiata)

Succenturiate lobes have an incidence of approximately 5–6%. They may be single or multiple and differ from bilobed placentas only in the size and number of accessory lobes (Figs. 13.1 and 13.3). *Approximately one half are associated with infarction or atrophy of the succenturiate lobes*, much higher than the overall incidence of infarction, which is estimated to be 13%. As with bilobed placentas, membranous vessels are always present, connecting each lobe, and thus may be susceptible to damage. The umbilical cord most commonly inserts into the dominant lobe.

Pathogenesis
The pathogenesis of abnormally shaped placentas is thought to be due to **"dynamic placentation,"** in which the original implantation of the blastocyst is modified by placental expansion overlying poorly decidualized or vascularized regions of the uterus. This can result in local atrophy as growth occurs in other directions, leaving sections of the placenta "behind." A classic example is lateral implantation in between the anterior and posterior walls of the uterus with one lobe on the anterior and one on the posterior wall and atrophy in between. Other local factors leading to multilobation are implantation over *leiomyomas, in areas of previous surgery, in the cornu, or over the cervical os*. After implantation, there is preferential growth in areas of superior perfusion and atrophy in areas of poor perfusion. This process has also been called **trophotropism**. Indeed, intermediate forms exist in which there are two lobes, with partial or complete infarction of residual villous tissue between the lobes with thinning of these areas. This suggests that normal discoidal placentation was originally present, but local factors led to atrophy or infarction, resulting in multilobation.
The designation of multilobate placenta should only be invoked when there is only membranous tissue between lobes.

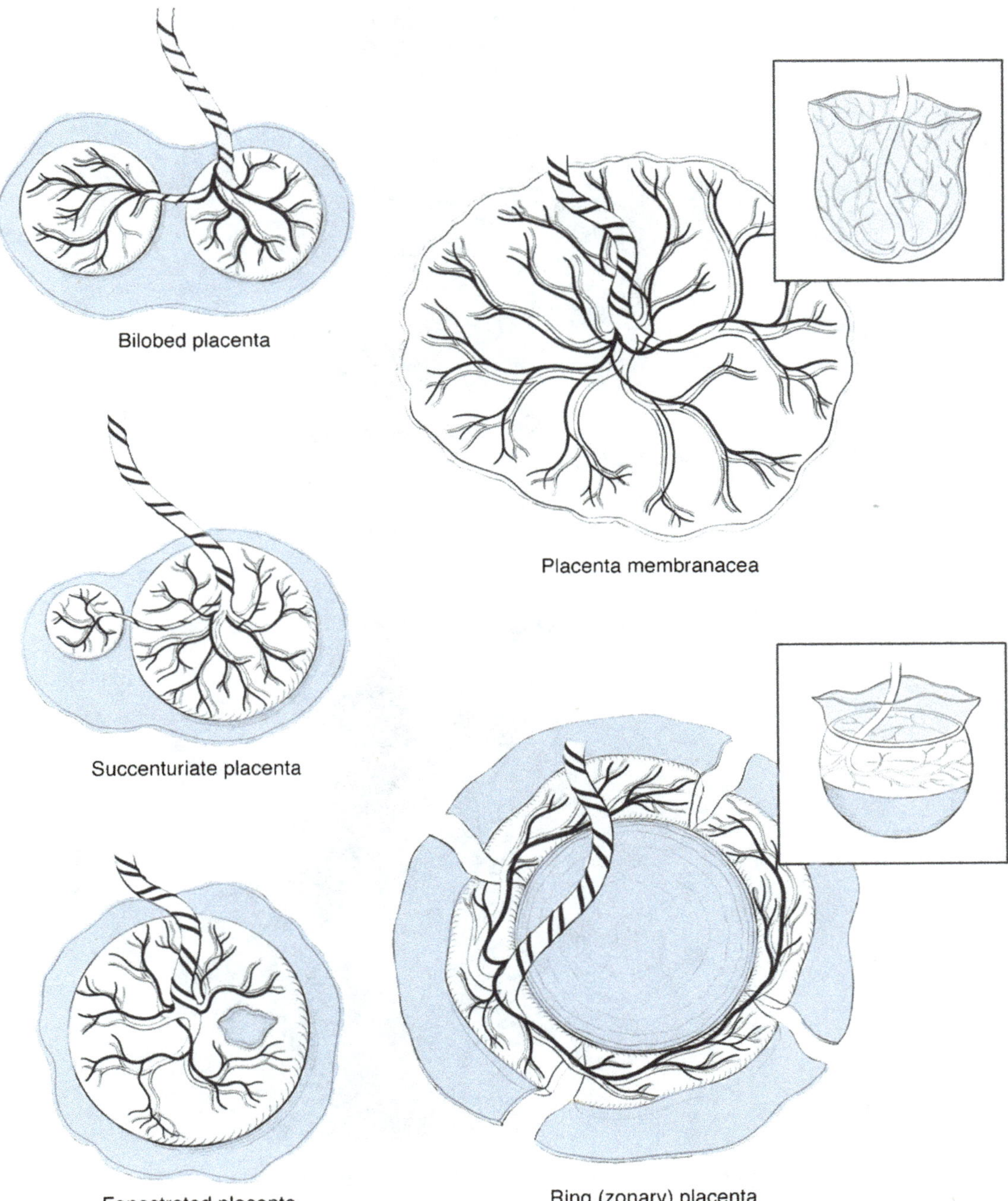

Figure 13.1. Diagram depicting placental shape abnormalities including multilobation (bilobed placenta and succenturiate placenta), placenta fenestrata, placenta membranacea, and ring or zonary placenta.

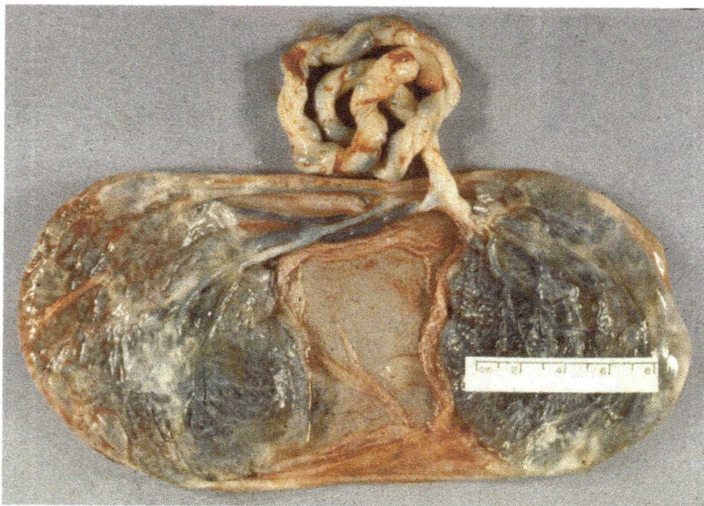

Figure 13.2. Bilobed placenta. Membranous vessels course from the velamentous cord insertion in between the two lobes.

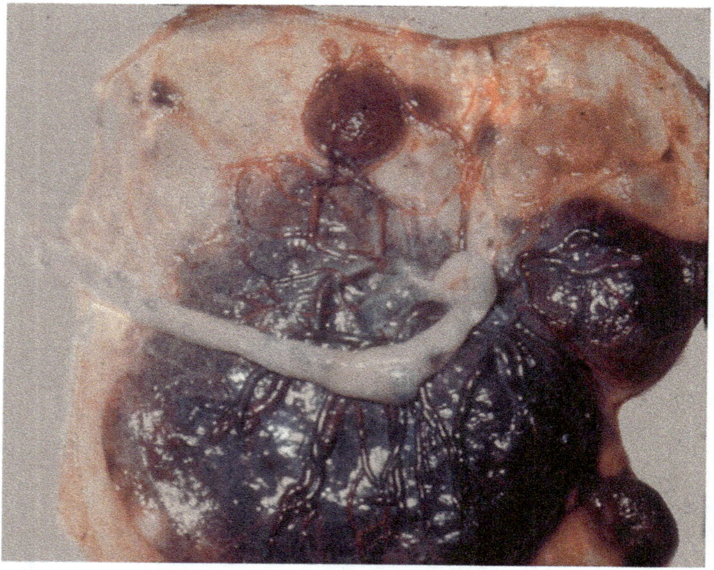

Figure 13.3. Succenturiate lobes in an immature placenta, with infarction of some of the lobes.

Clinical Features and Implications

There are **always** membranous vessels connecting the villous tissue between lobes. These membranous vessels, being devoid of the protection of Wharton's jelly, are susceptible to damage from *compression, rupture, or thrombosis.* They may occasionally present clinically as *vasa previa* with bleeding. Vasa previa occurs when the membranous vessels present "previous" to the delivering part of the baby (see Chap. 15).

Both bilobed placentas and succenturiate lobes are more common in twins and multiparas women and in placentas conceived via assisted reproductive technology. Complications associated with multilobed placentas include *non-reassuring fetal status, antenatal bleeding, postpartum hemorrhage, placenta previa, and retained placental tissue.*

Suggestions for Examination and Report
(Bilobed placenta and placenta with succenturiate lobes)

Gross Examination: Each lobe should be measured and weighed individually unless there are many small accessory lobes. The integrity of the membranous vessels connecting the lobes should be evaluated and it is recommended that sections be taken of the vessels. This is best accomplished by rolling the membranes containing the vessels creating a membrane roll with cross sections of these vessels. If the vessels are ruptured, show hemorrhage into the adjacent membranes or show gross thrombosis, photographs should also be taken.

Comment: It should be noted that accessory lobes are present and in the gross part of the part or a comment, that the membranous vessels are present and whether there is hemorrhage, disruption or thrombosis. If any of these are present, the possibility of fetal hemorrhage should be considered.

Circumvallate and Circummarginate Placentas

Pathologic Features

In **circumvallate** placentas, the membranes of the chorion laeve do not insert at the edge of the placenta but rather at some inward distance from the margin, toward the umbilical cord (Fig. 13.4). At the margin, one usually finds variable amounts of fibrin, recent clot, and old blood. In **complete circumvallates**, there is a complete circumferential ring that restricts the total surface of the chorion frondosum (Figs. 13.5 and 13.6). At the periphery, "naked" placental tissue protrudes. The fibrin that is present at the insertion of the membranes causes plication of the membranes, which is characteristic of circumvallates (Fig. 13.7). The amnion may follow the chorion into this plica, or most commonly it flatly covers the plica without infolding. When no plication of the membranes occurs, it is called a **circummarginate placenta** (Figs. 13.4 and 13.8). These two forms blend into each other, and partial forms are common.

Gross examination of the placenta *shows yellow-brown marginal fibrin* peripheral to the fibrin present at the membrane insertion. In cases where there is midtrimester hemorrhage and premature delivery, there may be substantial blood at the margin. Hemorrhage may undermine the margin of the placenta, thus imitating abruptio placentae. On microscopic examination, sections taken from the margin of the

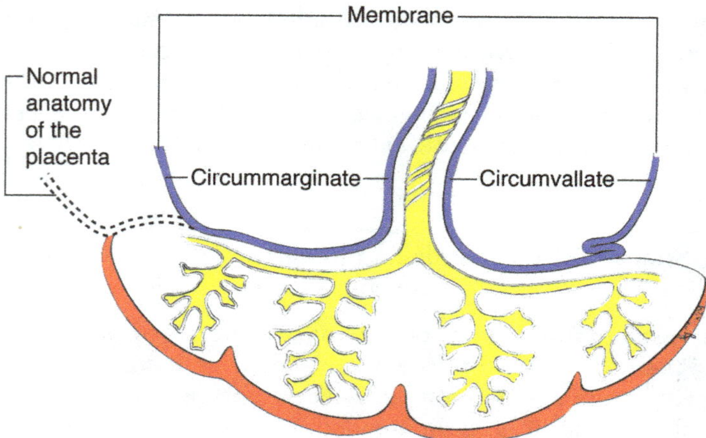

Figure 13.4. Diagram of circummarginate and circumvallate membrane insertion. In both, the fetal membranes do not insert at the edge of the placenta but rather at some point inwards. In circumvallation there is a plication of the membranes evident as a fibrin ridge on gross examination. In circummargination, the membrane insertion is flat and a ridge is not present.

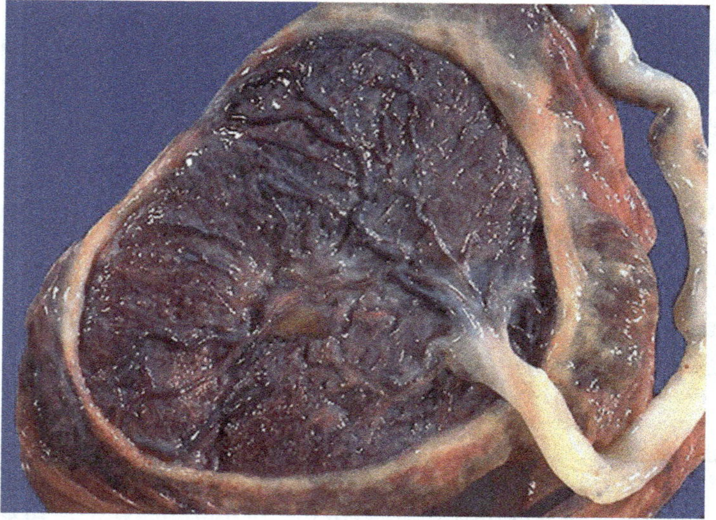

Figure. 13.5. Typical circumvallate placenta with prominent ridge of fibrin at the periphery.

placenta will show *absence of membranous covering peripherally with hemosiderin deposition and fibrin* (Fig. 13.7).

Clinical Features and Implications
The incidence of circumvallation is from 1.0 to 6.5% and the incidence of circummargination is up to 25% of placentas. They are rarely found in the first trimester. The most common complications of circumvallation are *antenatal bleeding and premature delivery.*

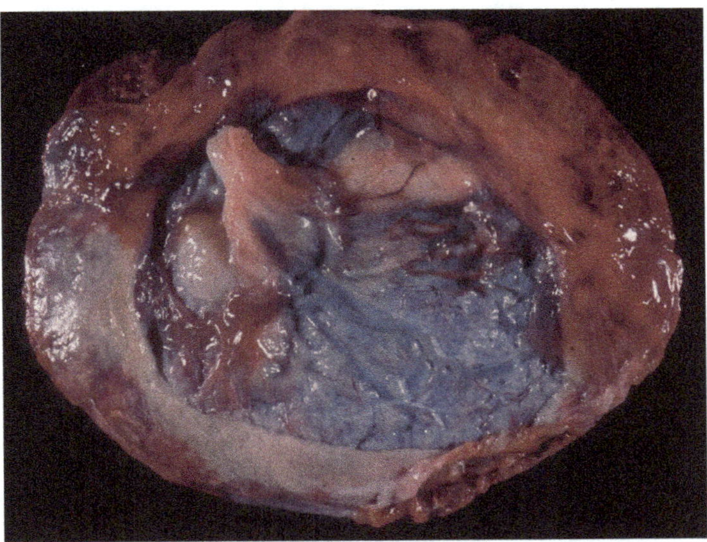

Figure 13.6. More extreme circumvallation with prominent subchorionic fibrin.

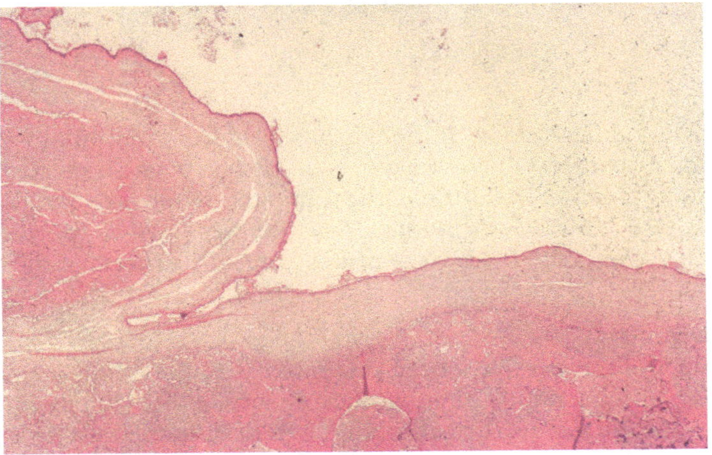

Figure 13.7. Margin of circumvallate placenta. The homogeneous material under the plica represents fibrin, atrophies villi and degenerated blood. H&E ×2.

Additional, uncommon associations include premature membrane rupture, oligohydramnios, non-reassuring fetal status, abruption, perinatal or intrauterine death, congenital anomalies, single umbilical artery, and intrauterine growth restriction. Cases with extensive hemorrhage and **marginal hematomas** may lead to significant clinical bleeding. Large hematomas may elevate the chorion laeve from its insertion site and cause disruption of the fetal vessels. Thus, the vaginal bleeding in these cases is frequently a mixture of

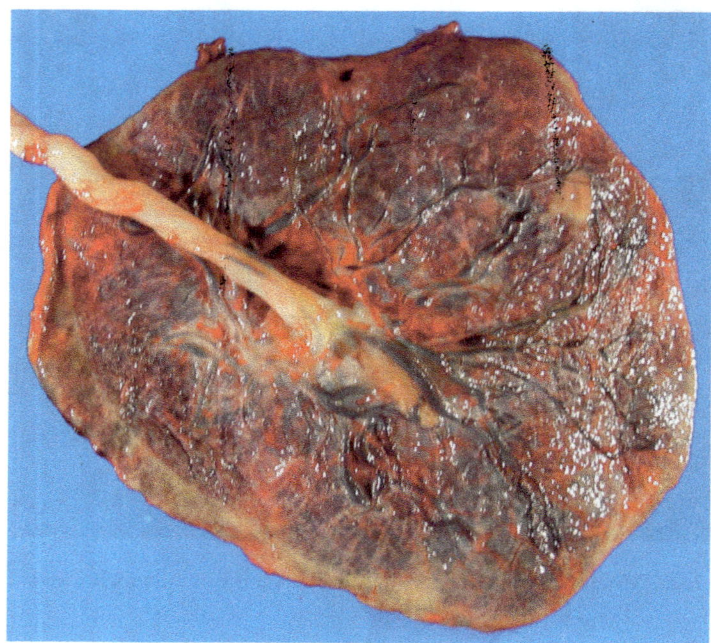

Figure 13.8. Sickle-shaped circummarginate placenta (*lower left*).

maternal and fetal blood. If there is bleeding from placental vessels, significant neonatal anemia may result. It has been suggested that circummargination has little clinical impact, while circumvallation has adverse clinical associations. Many studies have supported this view, but essentially these two entities are really aspects of the same process.

Pathogenesis

A number of theories have been presented as to the origin of circumvallation and circummargination. One theory is that circumvallation occurs due to marginal hemorrhage, which undermines the membranes and pushes them over the chorionic plate. Another theory is that circumvallates develop because the embryo implants too superficially and grows outward in a "polypoid" fashion, and yet another theory is that the embryo implants too deeply. It has also been suggested that there is a deficiency of amniotic fluid pressure necessary for growth resulting in a disconnection between growth of the amniotic cavity and fetus. Others have suggested that the etiology is poor development of the chorion frondosum and increased lateral growth of the placenta. The most recently favored theory is that marginal hemorrhage undermines the membrane attachment. The latter theory is supported by the fact that many of these cases show old hemorrhage around the periphery. However, it is likely that there may be different types and origins of circumvallation, and this issue is yet to be completely resolved.

Extramembranous Pregnancy

Pathogenesis

In **extramembranous** or **extrachorial pregnancy**, there is early rupture of both and the amnion and chorion, leading to escape of the fetus into the uterine cavity (Fig. 13.9). Evidence that the fetus must have escaped out of the membranes much earlier is manifested by the diminutive hole through the membranes, which may barely admit the umbilical cord, let alone the fetus (Fig. 13.9). It is a rare condition, and as with other conditions associated with early membrane rupture, such as amnionic bands (see Chap. 14), the etiology remains obscure.

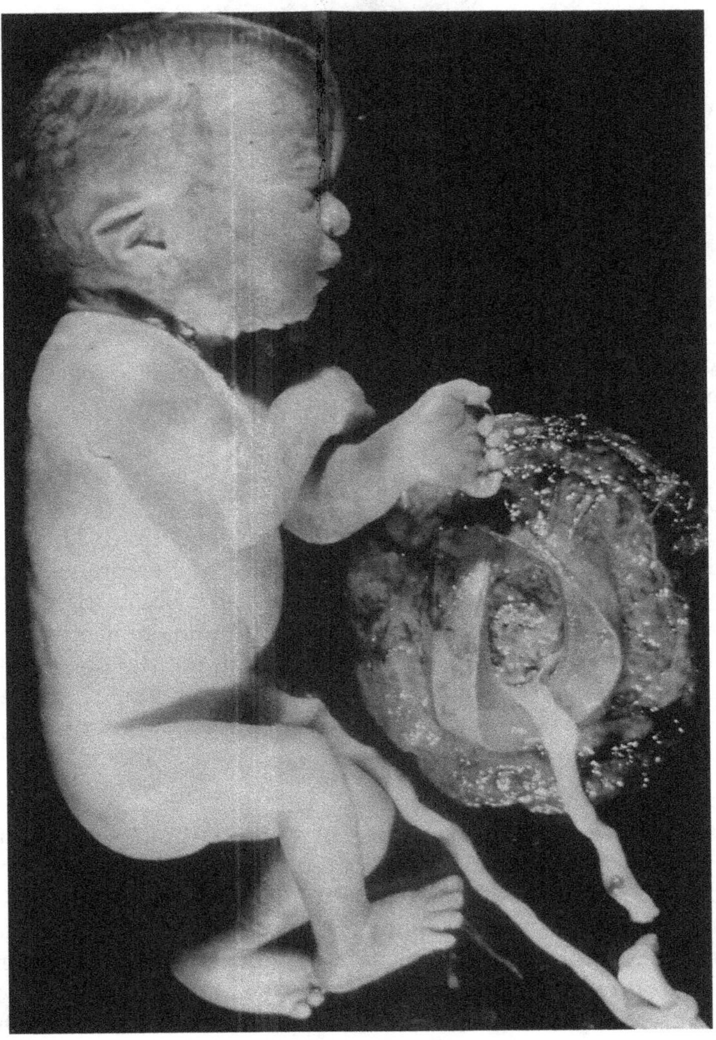

Figure 13.9. Extramembranous pregnancy with fetus. Note the size of fetus and the membrane opening. The placenta shows marked circumvallation.

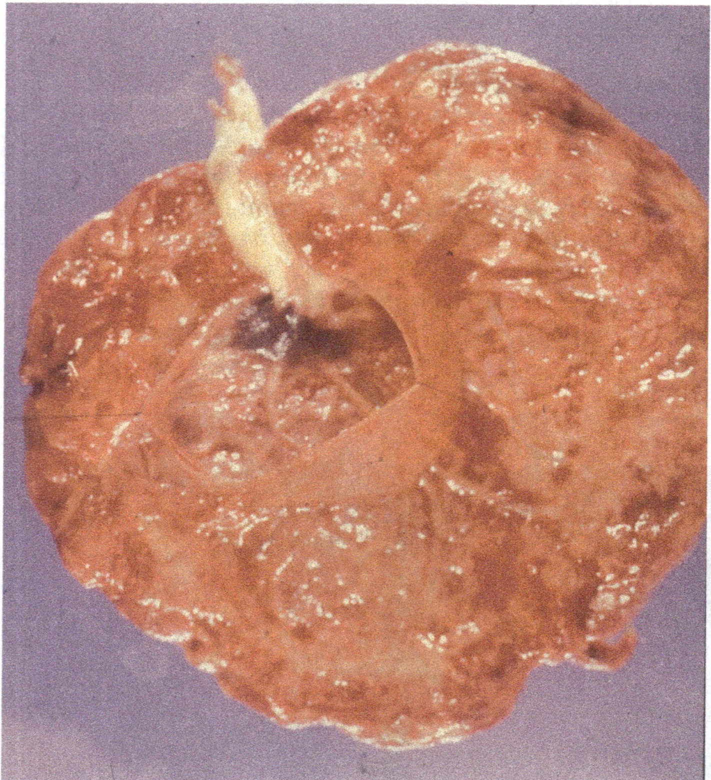

Figure 13.10. Extramembranous pregnancy with circumvallation and diminutive opening.

Pathologic Features

The placenta shows marked circumvallation (Fig. 13.10), the cord is usually short, and the fetal surface shows lack of membranous covering, being covered instead with fibrin and a brownish discoloration consistent with hemosiderin (Fig. 13.11). The remaining membranes are relatively normal. Microscopically, one finds substantial quantities of posthemorrhagic hemosiderin in the membranes. There also may be sparse amnion nodosum (see Chap. 14) over the placental tissue, but this is usually not striking.

Clinical Features and Implications

Due to membrane rupture and loss of amniotic fluid, extramembranous pregnancies are usually associated with prolonged amniorrhea due to periodic fetal urination. In addition, there are severe positional deformities of the fetus and pulmonary hypoplasia due to the oligohydramnios. Ascending infection is occasionally associated with extramembranous pregnancy, but this is not a constant finding. The majority of these pregnancies aborts or terminates prematurely and such fetuses only occasionally survive.

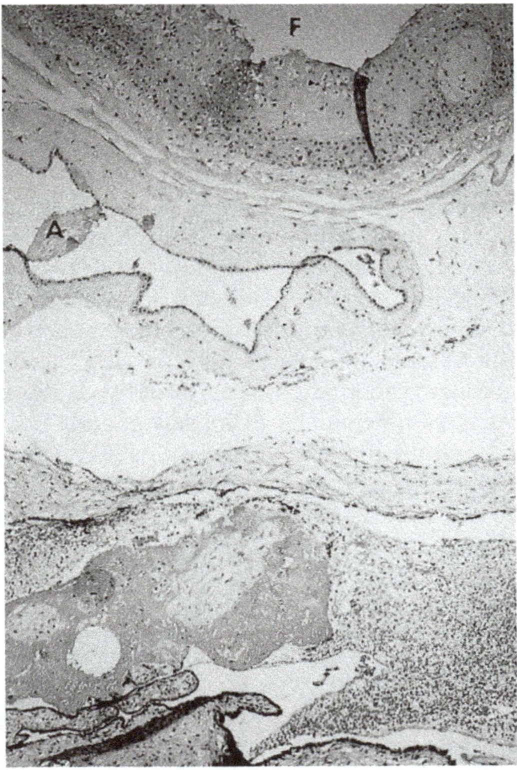

Figure 13.11. Membrane insertion in the extramembranous pregnancy shown in Fig. 13.9. *Below* is the villous tissue, membranes folded at *top right* and the fetus lay in space F. *A* amnion nodosum.

Suggestions for Examination and Report
(Circumvallate placenta, circummarginate placentas and extramembranous pregnancy)

Gross Examination: Extent of the circumvallation should be noted as well as a lack of amnion over the fetal surface and the presence of hemosiderin (brown discoloration) and fibrin. It should also be noted whether there is plication or the membranes (circumvallate) or not (circummarginate). The presence of extensive marginal hemorrhage (marginal hematoma) and disruption of fetal vessels should also be noted.

Comment: A comment is not necessary except when disrupted fetal vessels are present. In this case, the possible role of circumvallation in the etiology may be suggested. If extreme circumvallation and an extramembranous pregnancy are present, a comment may be made on the association with a history of chronic leakage of amniotic fluid prior to delivery, oligohydramnios, fetal positional deformities and pulmonary hypoplasia.

Placenta Membranacea (Placenta Diffusa)

Placenta membranacea is a rare abnormality of placental form in which all, or nearly all, of the circumference of the fetal sac is covered by villous tissue. The placental tissue is generally quite thin (approximately 1 cm), and is often disrupted (Figs. 13.1 and 13.12). Partial placenta membranacea can also occur. The etiology is not fully understood, but it seems obvious that those villi destined to atrophy and become the chorion laeve are retained while there is lack of growth of the villi destined to become the chorion frondosum. Underlying reasons postulated for lack of villous growth relate mostly to abnormalities of the endometrium, such as endometrial hypoplasia, poor vascular supply of the decidua basalis, endometritis, multiple curettages, adenomyosis, or atrophy of the endometrium. Placenta membranacea may manifest clinically as early bleeding and placenta previa. Affected pregnancies often terminate in premature delivery and placenta accreta is relatively common (see Chap. 12). Spontaneous abortion and second trimester fetal demise have also been reported.

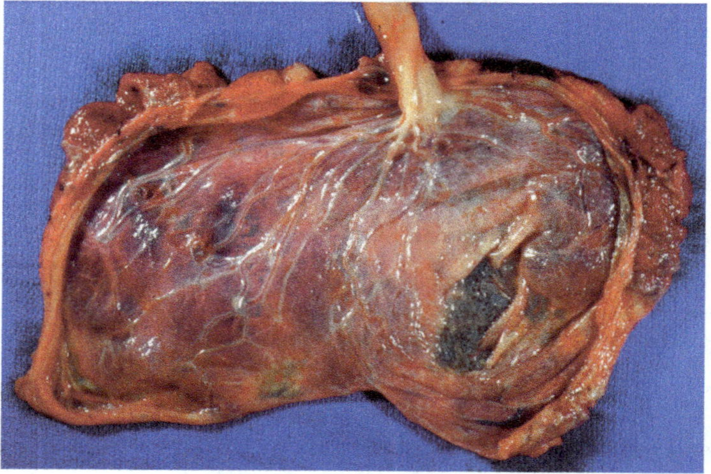

Figure 13.12. Placenta membranacea with virtually free membranes are seen; the placenta is very thin.

Suggestions for Examination and Report
(Placenta membranacea)

Gross Examination: Examination should include the usual measurements of placental dimension such that the increased diameter and excessive thinness of the placenta can be appreciated. As lack of chorion laeve or extraplacental membranes should also be noted.

Comment: Placenta membranacea is of unknown etiology and the clinical associations are vaginal bleeding, placenta previa, premature delivery and placenta accreta.

Miscellaneous Shape Abnormalities

In **placenta fenestrata,** a central area of the placenta is atrophied sufficiently to leave only membranes (Figs. 13.1 and 13.13). One must be careful to rule out the possibility of a missing cotyledon. The etiology is unknown, but it seems reasonable that it may often occur secondary to implantation over a leiomyoma or cornual tube orifice. **Zonary (annular) placentas** have a ring shape (Figs. 13.1 and 13.14). They are likely derived from a placenta previa with focal atrophy of the low-lying villous tissue covering the internal os, leaving a ring shape. Noting the shape and the presence of any membranous or velamentous vessels should be part of the examination of these specimens.

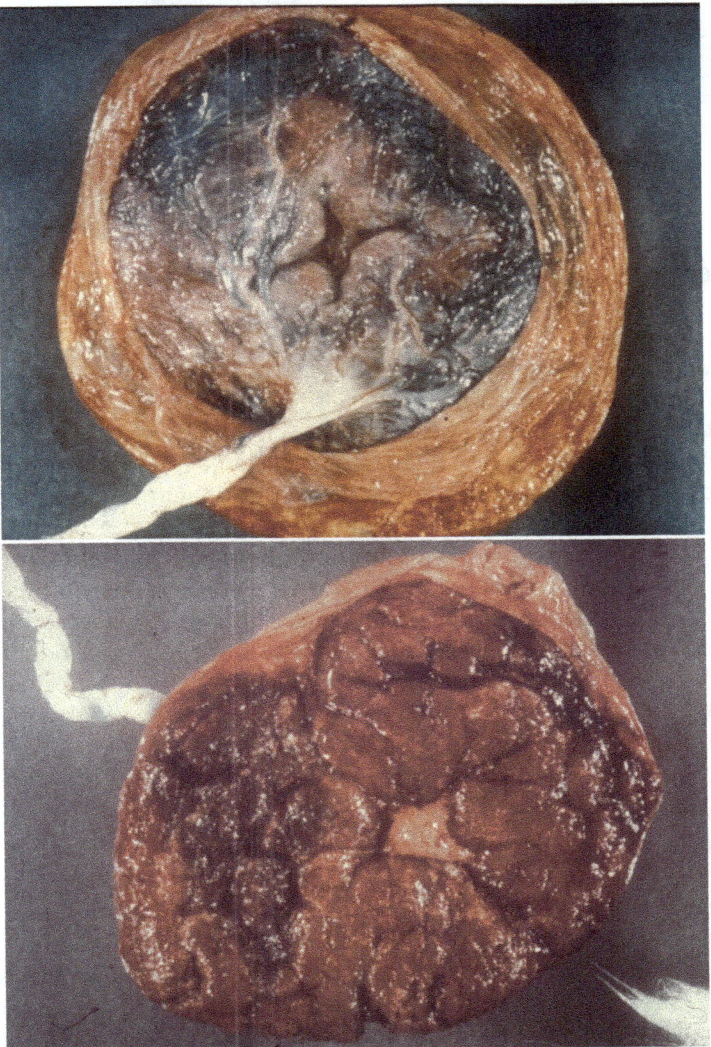

Figure 13.13. Placenta fenestrata. The central area of the placenta has a distinct defect, only chorionic membranes being present. (Courtesy Dr. L.F. Moreno, Caracas, Venezuela).

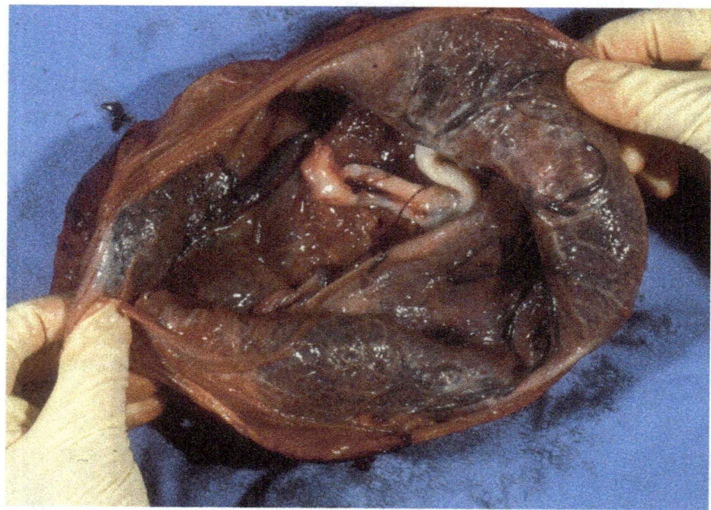

Figure 13.14. Zonary placenta showing a ring like shape. The placenta has been placed on its edge to demonstrate the unusual shape. The membranes ruptured and the infant delivered through the opening. Membranes were intact on the other surface and the cord inserted to the side (not seen in this picture).

Placenta Previa

Pathogenesis

The term **placenta previa** refers to the location of the placenta over the internal os. The placenta is thus "previous" to the delivering part of the baby. The overall incidence is somewhere between 0.3 and 1%. When, during early pregnancy, a placenta previa is unmistakably diagnosed, there is often conversion to a "marginal" or higher-lying placenta. The incidence at midtrimester is 5%, but over 90% of these "convert" to a nonprevia by term. Serial ultrasound examinations throughout pregnancy have shown that the placenta actually "wanders," a phenomenon referred to as **"dynamic placentation"** as referred to above. This placental movement is not accomplished by the placenta unseating and relocating itself, but rather through marginal atrophy on one side and growth and expansion on the other, a process called **trophotropism.**

Pathologic Features

It has become customary to subdivide placenta previa into several categories, such as **"central"** (total) and **"partial"** (lateral or marginal) placenta previa. The former generally poses the greater threat and requires early diagnosis. Vaginal delivery is usually permitted only in a marginal previa. In the vaginally delivered marginal placenta previa, the membranes will have no free margin, and the edge of the placenta will frequently be disrupted and hemorrhagic. There are often old clots at this site, varying from firm, laminated, and brown, to friable loose clots or partly necrotic material that is sometimes green or brown. The fetal vessels of the chorionic surface, when at the edge, may be also disrupted. Portions of placenta are occasionally either atrophied or infarcted.

Clinical Features and Implications

Placenta previa is more common in older women, and is also associated with multiparity, previous abortion, previous cesarean section, and male infants. Placenta previa is associated with a higher risk for abruptio, fetal malpresentation, postpartum hemorrhage, fetal and perinatal mortality, fetal growth restriction, fetal anomalies, prolapsed umbilical cord, and cesarean section. It is one of the principal causes of third trimester bleeding and often necessitates an emergency cesarean section, as both mother and fetus may experience life-threatening hemorrhage. Maternal hemorrhage may originate from the placental margin or from the disrupted intervillous space. Significant neonatal anemia may result from bleeding that occurs from disrupted placental villous vessels or fetomaternal hemorrhage (see Chap. 20).

Placenta previa is often associated with **placenta accreta** and then is called **placenta previa accreta** (see Chap. 12). In placenta previa there is implantation in the lower uterine segment and cervix where there is no normal endometrium and the mucosa does not respond well to the normal hormonal signals for decidualization. Thus, decidualization is deficient, which is the underlying mechanism in placenta accreta. Although placenta previa accreta and cervical pregnancy are relatively rare, the clinical consequences may be dire due to massive hemorrhage and other complications of blood loss.

Suggestions for Examination and Report
(Placenta previa)

Gross Examination: In a vaginal delivery, membrane rupture site **at** the placental margin is consistent with a marginal placental previa and should be recorded. However, since placenta previa is essentially a clinical term, it cannot be diagnosed by placental examination.

Comment: None.

Selected References

PHP5, pages 452–472 (Placental Shape Aberrations).

Ahmed A, Gilbert-Barnass E. Placenta membranacea. A developmental anomaly with diverse clinical presentation. Pediatr Dev Pathol 2003;6:201–202.

Benirschke K. Effects of placental pathology on the embryo and the fetus. In: Wilson JG, Fraser FC, eds. Handbook of Teratology. Plenum Press, New York, 1977;3:79–115.

Finn JL. Placenta membranacea. Obstet Gynecol 1954;3:438–440.

Fox H, Sen DK. Placenta extrachorialis. A clinico-pathologic study. J Obstet Gynaecol Br Commonw 1972;79:32–35.

Fujikura T, Benson RC, Driscoll SG. The bipartite placenta and its clinical features. Am J Obstet Gynecol 1970;107:1013–1017.

Mathews J. Placenta membranacea. Aust NZ J Obstet Gynaecol 1974;14:45–47.

Naeye RL. Placenta previa: predisposing factors and effects on the fetus and surviving infants. Obstet Gynecol 1978;52:521–525.

Perlman M, Tennenbaum A, Menash M, et al. Extramembranous pregnancy: maternal, placental and perinatal implications. Obstet Gynecol 1980;55:34S-37S.

Steemers NY, de Rop C, van Assche A. Zonary placenta. Intern J Gynecol Obstet 1995;51:251–253.

Suzuki S. Clinical significance of pregnancies with circumvallate placentas. J Obstet Gynaecol Res 2008;34:51–54.

Suzuki S, Igarashi M. Clinical significance of pregnancies with succenturiate lobes of placenta. Arch Gynecol Obstet 2008;277:299–301.

Torpin R. Human placental anomalies: etiology, evolution and historical background. Mo Med 1958;55:353–357.

Torpin R. Placenta circumvallata and placenta marginata. Obstet Gynecol 1955;6:277–284.

Chapter 14
Pathology of the Fetal Membranes

Cysts and Tumors

Pathologic Features

Localized edema with resultant cyst formation is occasionally seen on the fetal surface. Infrequently, such cysts represent **amnionic epithelial inclusion cysts**. These are simple cysts lined by a *single layer of amnionic epithelium* and usually contain clear fluid (Fig. 14.1). Rarely, an **epidermal inclusion cyst** or **epidermoid cyst** may be seen within the amnion lined by *keratinizing stratified squamous epithelium* (Fig. 14.2). **"Pseudocysts"** within the chorion of the extraplacental membranes

R.N. Baergen, *Manual of Pathology of the Human Placenta*,
DOI 10.1007/978-1-4419-7494-5_14, © Springer Science+Business Media, LLC 2011

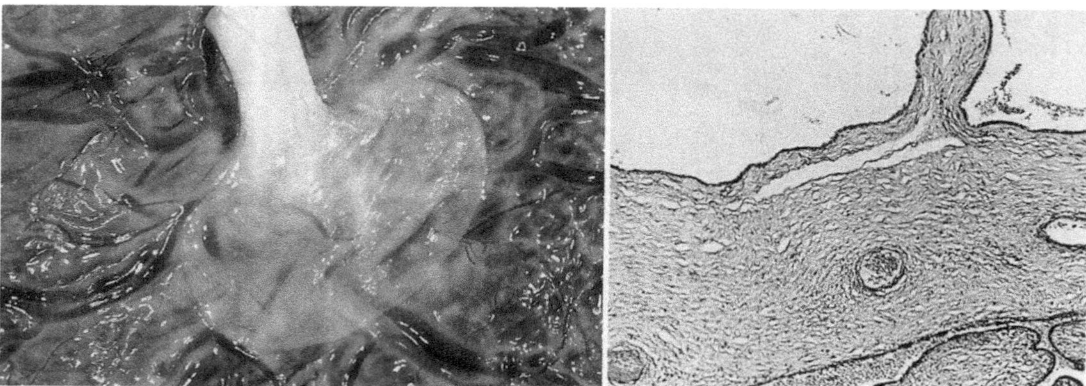

Figure 14.1. Amnionic cyst surrounding the umbilical cord. The cyst (**a**) contained 5 mL of clear fluid. Microscopic examination (**b**) revealed a single layer of amnionic epithelium. H&E ×160.

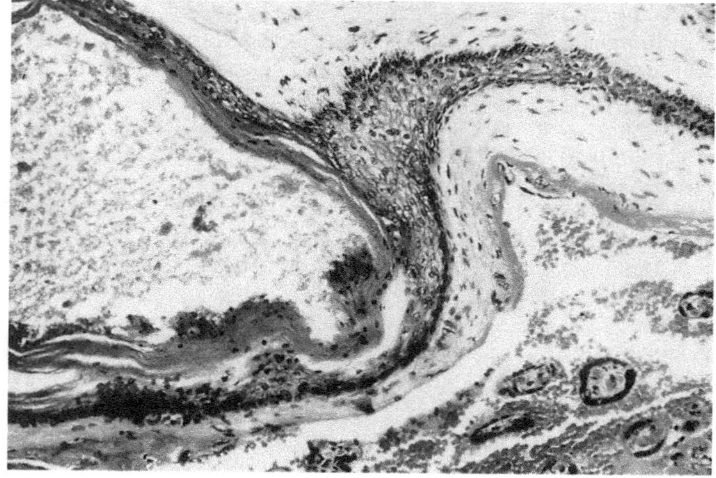

Figure 14.2. Subamnionic squamous epithelium lined cyst with keratinization. H&E ×160.

have also been described. These are lined by extravillous trophoblast and are morphologically similar to septal cyst and cysts of cell islands, which are present in approximately 14–17% of mature placentas. Being lined by trophoblastic cells, they actually represent true cysts and not pseudocysts (Fig. 14.3). These have been reported to have an increased incidence in placentas from mothers with *preeclampsia and diabetes mellitus*, and it has been suggested that they are a hypoxia-associated lesion. **Subchorionic cysts** of the chorionic plate have a similar morphology. They are quite common as they are found in 5–7% of mature placentas (Figs. 14.4 and 14.5) and are often multiple. They may be quite large; cysts as large as a fetal head have been described. The cyst content of these cysts is *viscid and mucus-like*, but does not contain true mucin. It

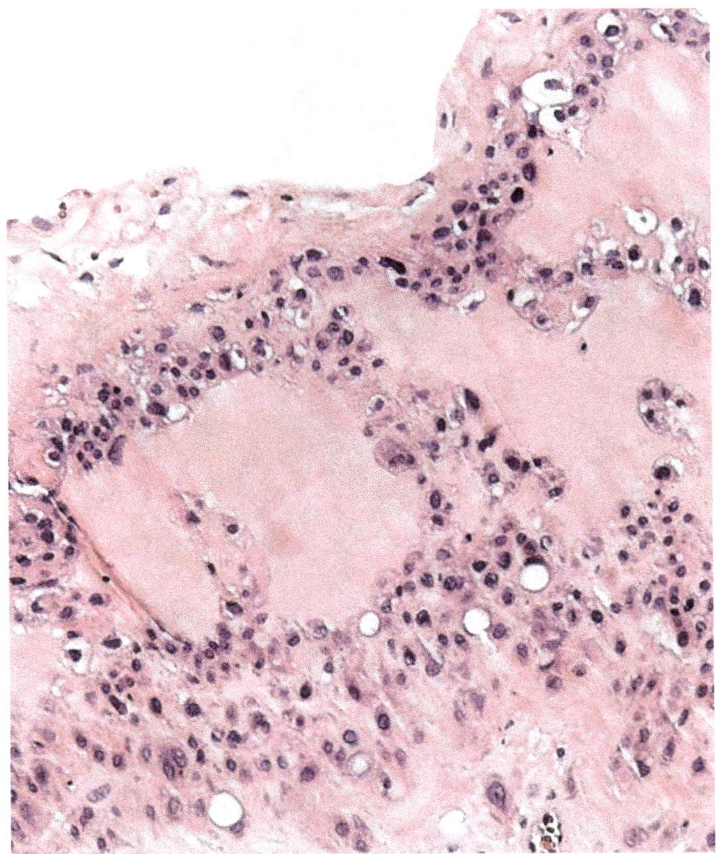

Figure 14.3. Chorionic cyst or "pseudocyst" in the fetal membranes. It is lined by extravillous trophoblast and contains secretions. H&E ×200.

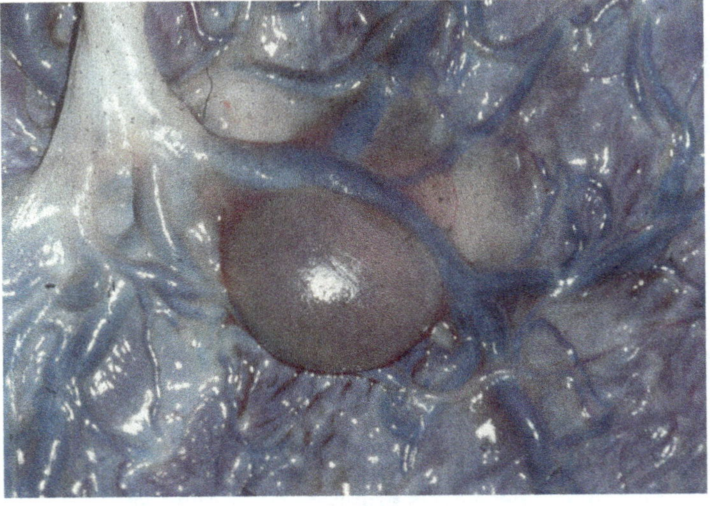

Figure 14.4. Single subchorionic cyst on the fetal surface of a mature placenta.

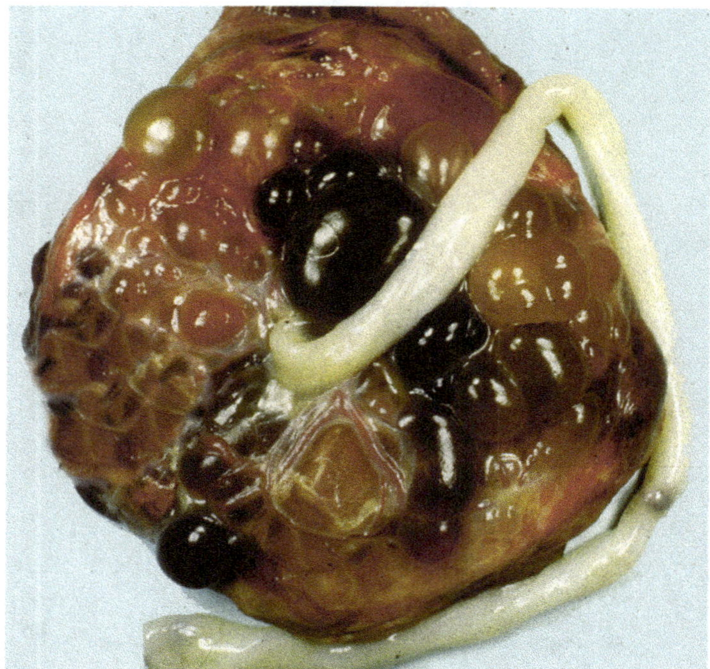

Figure 14.5. Multiple subchorionic cysts, many discolored by previous hemorrhage.

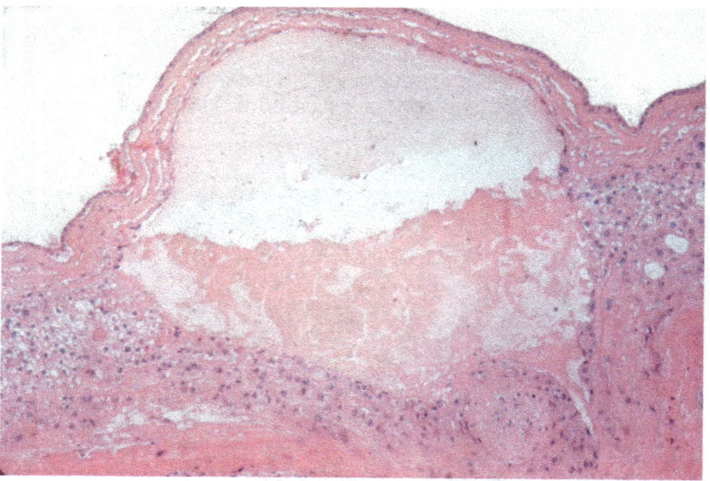

Figure 14.6. Microscopic appearance of a subchorionic cyst under the fetal surface. Note the similarity to the chorionic cyst in Fig. 14.3. H&E ×40.

is a rich source of major basic protein and other proteins. This can be appreciated by the presence of the precipitate found in histological sections (Fig. 14.6). These cysts originate from *collections of extravillous*

trophoblastic cells in which degeneration and central liquefaction has occurred.
Bleeding into such cysts may also occur.

No real tumors have been shown to arise in the fetal membranes,
although **"teratomas"** have been reported. The typical description is of
*a mass in the placenta, often covered with skin, broadly attached to the cho-
rion, which contains a relatively disorganized mass of glia, intestine, cartilage,
fat, and/or other tissues.* These descriptions are reminiscent of **acardiac
twins** (see Chap. 10) despite the lack of umbilical cord, a feature that
is usually held to be a *sine qua non* for acardiac twins. We are of the
opinion that these likely represent a variant of acardiac twinning and
that to invoke their origin from aberrant germ cells seems unwarranted
without supportive evidence. Other teratomas of the placenta fall into
the same category.

Pathogenesis

Amnionic and epidermal cysts have an etiology similar to other types
of epithelial inclusion cysts. **Subchorionic, chorionic, septal,** and
cell island cysts are often found in placentas that show increased
perivillous fibrin, maternal floor infarction (see Chap. 19) or changes
of placental malperfusion (see Chap. 18). They are also more numerous in placentas from high altitudes. These findings support the
view that cyst formation is the result of *degenerative processes due to
malnutrition and hypoxia in the center of large accumulations of extravillous trophoblast.*

Clinical Features and Implications

Amnionic and epidermal cysts are not usually associated with clinical
problems. Large or multiple subchorionic cysts may compress chorionic or umbilical vessels (Fig. 14.5), but there is no evidence that this
actually compromises the fetal circulation. Therefore, other than the
associations noted above, these cysts are thought to have no clinical
significance.

Suggestions for Examination and Report
(Cysts)

Gross Examination: Size, location, character of cysts should be
noted. Sections need only be taken if the true nature of the cyst is in
question and to document large or multiple cysts.

Comment: Not generally necessary.

Embryonic Remnants

Rarely, embryonic **rests** *of cartilage, skin, or bone may be found underneath
the amnionic epithelium* and are of no clinical significance. Some of these
structures may represent the remains of aborted or "vanished" twins
(see Chap. 10). These rests have been interpreted by some as evidence

of the presence of a teratoma within the membranes, but this has not yet been proven.

After regression of the omphalomesenteric duct, remnants of the detached **yolk sac** persist in many placentas. They appear as *3- to 5-mm white-yellow, chalky disks in the chorionic plate* (Fig. 14.7a). The yolk sac remnant is almost invariably located near the margin of the placenta, underneath the amnion. Histologically, it has a lacy appearance, staining deeply purple with hematoxylin, and *appears calcified* (Fig. 14.7b). Minute omphalomesenteric vessels may occasionally

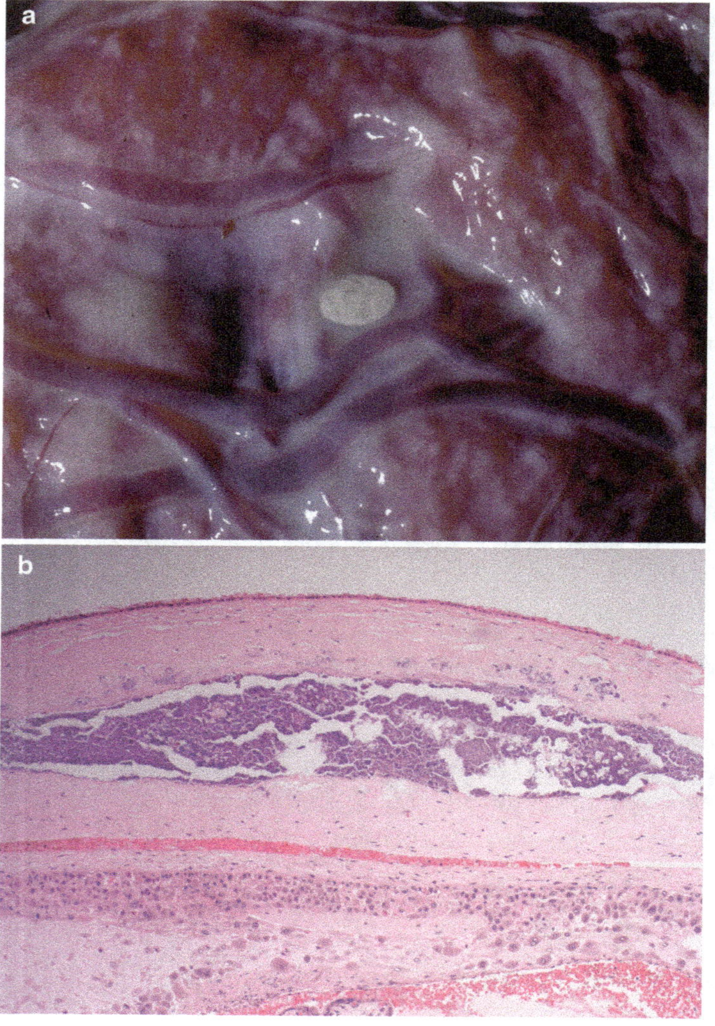

Figure 14.7. (a) Yolk sac remnant on the fetal surface of the placenta. (b) Microscopic appearance of a yolk sac remnant consisting of irregular fragments of calcium phosphate deposits between the amnion and chorion. H&E ×50.

accompany these yolk sac remnants and then can be seen coursing toward the umbilical cord and run along the surface of the cord. These remnants have no associated clinical sequelae.

Vernix Caseosa

Vernix caseosa is *sebum, hair, and other skin secretions from the fetus present in the amniotic fluid.* It is thick, white, and hydrophobic material that may appear as *white flake-like particles or patches of pasty material.* It is sometimes found submitted with the placenta or attached to the membranes (Fig. 14.8). Such accumulations of vernix also occur occasionally in large patches of greasy material that may be mistaken for a fetus papyraceous. After spontaneous rupture of the membranes, it may *dissect underneath the amnion or chorion.* When dissection occurs, fragments *of anucleate squames, fat, hair, and other debris* can be seen under the amnionic epithelium, at times in impressive amounts (Fig. 14.9). Generally, no cellular reaction to this material takes place, but occasionally a histiocytic, giant cell reaction may be identified that is likely due to reaction to the abundant keratin (Fig. 14.10). Vernix has also been identified in the decidua and myometrium of placental bed biopsies and within uterine veins, but has no known clinical significance.

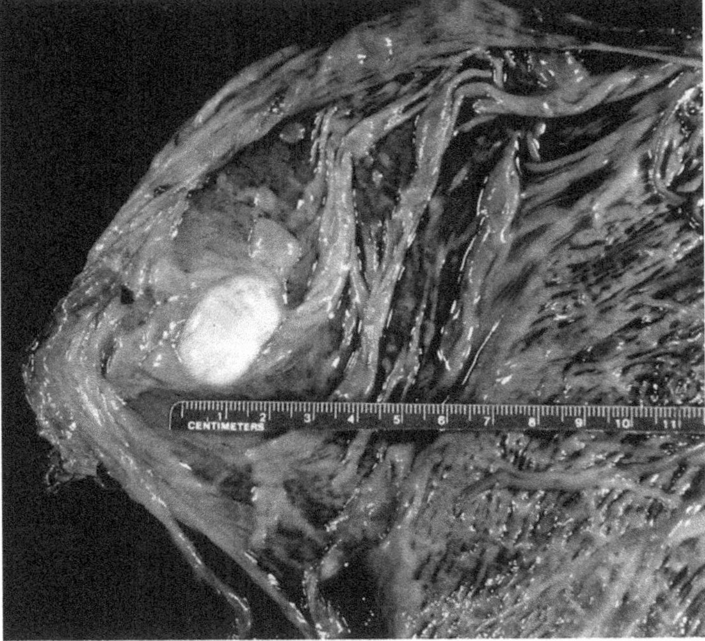

Figure 14.8. Large, white accumulation of pasty vernix caseosa dissected beneath the amnion. It is grossly similar to a yolk sac remnant but is much larger and may be confused with a fetus papyraceous.

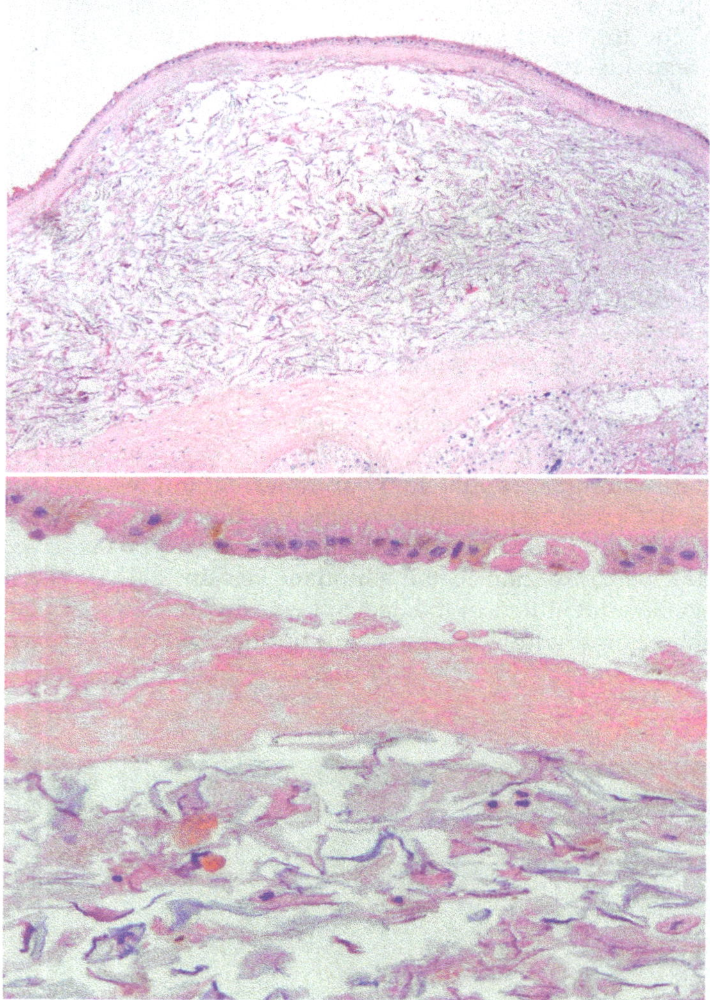

Figure 14.9. Microscopic view of vernix below amnion with readily identifiable squames and occasional hairs and other debris. *Top*: H&E ×20. *Bottom*: H&E ×400.

Hematomas and Breus' Mole

Subamnionic Hematoma

Subamnionic hematomas are seen quite commonly. They usually originate from chorionic plate vessels that have been sampled for tests (pH, blood banking, etc.) or damaged due to excess traction on the umbilical cord during delivery of the placenta. Gross examination reveals a thin layer of recent *blood clot between the amnion and chorion* (Fig. 14.11). Subamnionic hematomas are particularly common in specimens from cesarean section when the placenta is delivered manually. *Rarely is such*

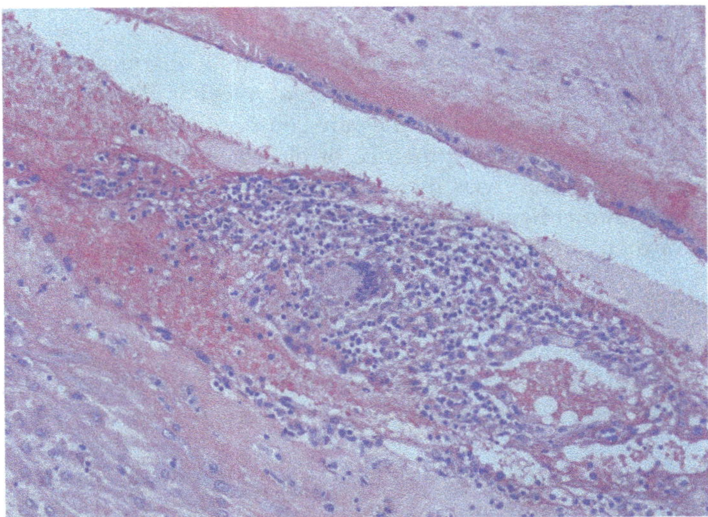

Figure 14.10. Vernix caseosa that has dissected between the amnion and chorion in the fetal membranes. The keratin has resulted in a giant cell reaction (courtesy of Dr. Carmen Stiegman, University of Arkansas for Medical Sciences, Little Rock, Arkansas).

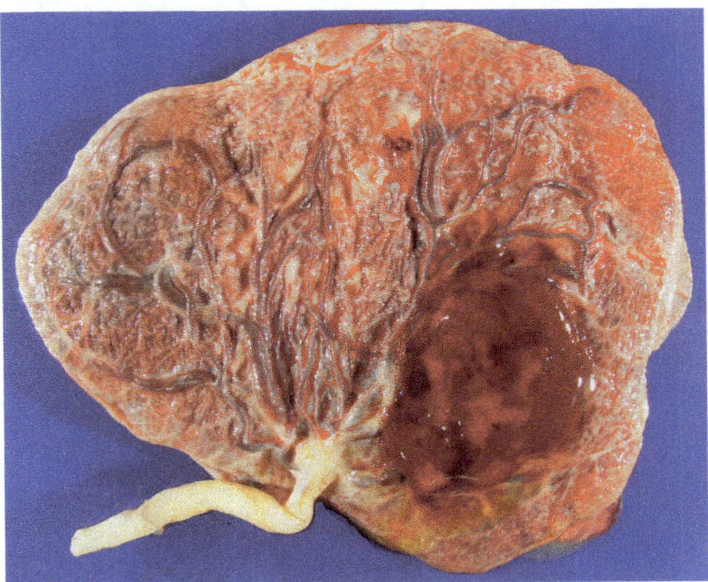

Figure 14.11. Recent subamnionic hemorrhage due to excess traction during delivery. In this case the hematoma forms a plaque. Often the blood dissects under the amnion in a thin layer.

subamnionic blood of prenatal origin. However, since trauma to fetal vessels may occur from invasive antenatal procedures, correlation with clinical history is essential, and if there is a history of anemia or bleeding, evaluation of the extent of the bleeding and disruption of vessels should be documented.

Retromembranous Hematoma

In the delivered placenta, one often finds small plaques beneath the extraplacental membranes, which consist of *recent or old clot* (Fig. 14.12). Older clots may look as though they are composed of fibrotic or necrotic tissue. Microscopically, the presence of old or recent blood is straightforward, and in some cases there may be associated decidual necrosis. **Retromembranous hematomas** are most commonly sequelae of amniocentesis or membrane rupture and are usually of no clinical importance.

Subchorionic Hematoma and Breus' Mole

Pathologic Features

Laminated **subchorionic thrombi or hematomas** form in small quantities almost regularly in the *subchorionic space*. It is at this site where

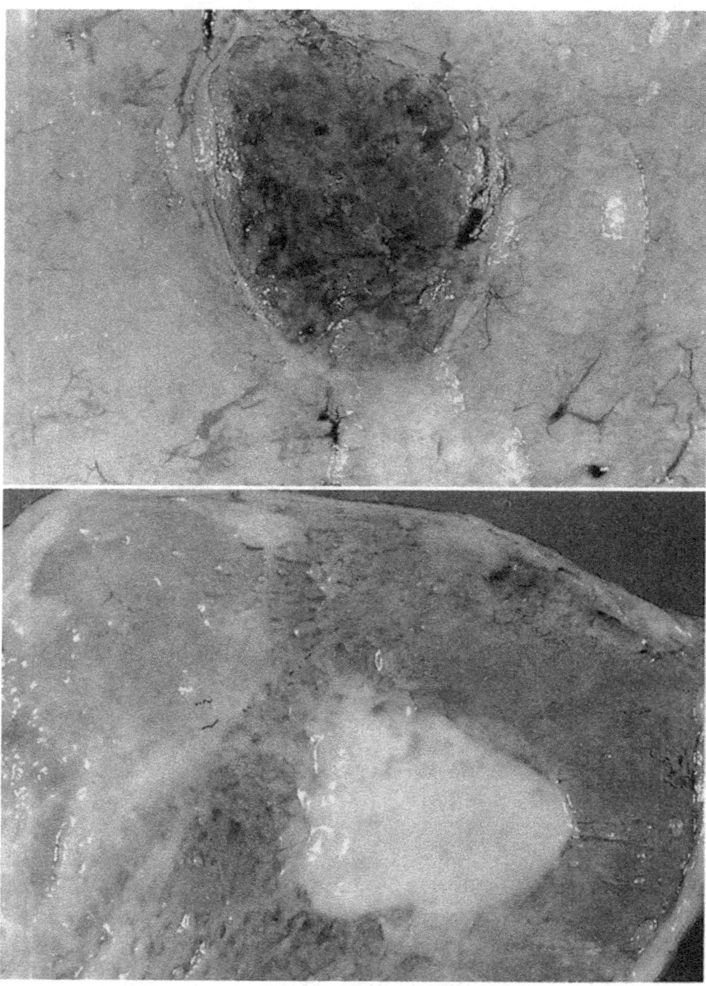

Figure 14.12. Localized retromembranous hematoma. At the *top* there is a dark ovoid blood clot. The *bottom* shows an old, white hematoma. Both are from uncomplicated pregnancies.

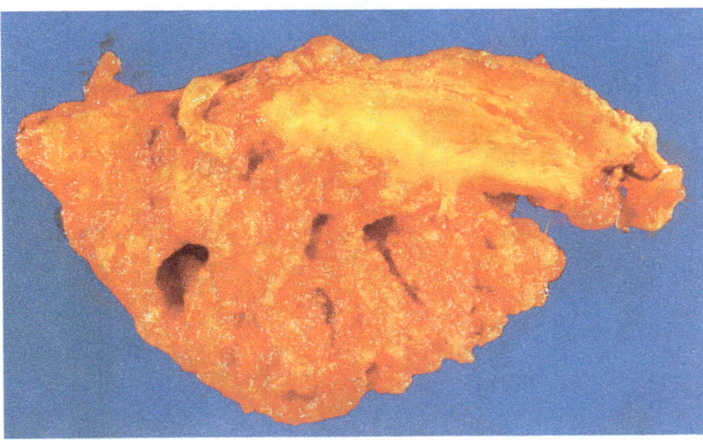

Figure 14.13. Laminated subchorionic hematoma in an uncomplicated term pregnancy.

the intervillous (maternal) blood is deflected backward, and eddying of intervillous blood accounts for the small amounts of fibrin that normally accumulate here. Macroscopically, they appear as *white patches or plaques* of **fibrin** and **laminated clot** under the chorion (Fig. 14.13). They often cause *bosselation of the fetal surface of the placenta.* The fibrin accumulations normally increase with maturation, but material that is much more thrombotic accumulates underneath the chorion in some abnormal placentas, forming distinct **subchorionic hematomas**, which may measure up to 15 cm in diameter (Fig. 14.13).

Clinical Features and Implications

Subchorionic hematomas have been reported in up to 60% of pregnancies evaluated by ultrasonography. They have been associated with *preterm delivery, spontaneous abortion, vaginal bleeding, midtrimester losses, elevated alpha-fetoprotein levels, intrauterine growth restriction,* and *fetal demise.* However, it is estimated that 80% of the subchorionic hematomas recognized before 20 weeks result in a normal term delivery. They are more often found when maternal circulatory disorders exist such as *complex heart disease, and with maternal antinuclear antibodies and thrombophilias.*

Also present and somewhat overlapping with subchorionic hematoma, is the **subchorionic tuberous hematoma**, or **"Breus' mole"** (Fig. 14.14). Breus' mole *differs from subchorionic hematomas in that it is more extensive, is diffusely nodular, and forms "pockets."* Breus' mole was originally described in association with missed abortions and was interpreted as sacculations or diverticula produced by the continued intervillous blood pressure against a decreased amnionic sac pressure, but this mechanism is no longer favored. These lesions have also been associated with *circumvallation, neonatal demise, monosomy X (Turner's syndrome),* and various maternal diseases such as *diabetes, thrombophilias, and hypertension.* The incidence is estimated to be 1:1,200 placentas. At present, there is no consensus as to their etiology.

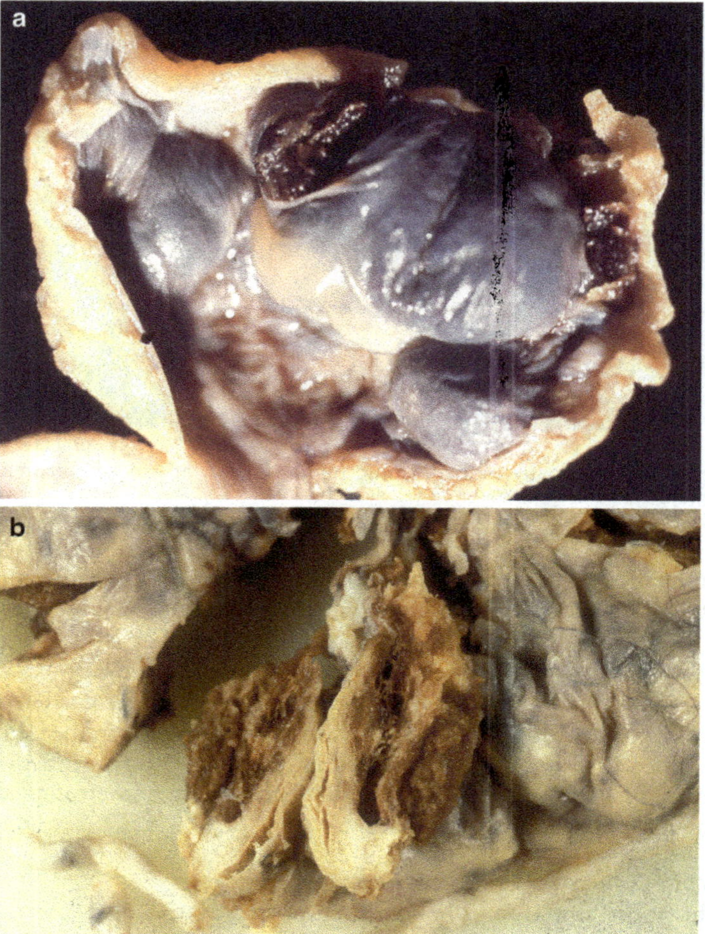

Figure 14.14. Breus' mole in an immature placenta from a missed abortion. Note the numerous blood-filled protrusions on the surface.

Suggestions for Examination and Report
(Subamnionic, retromembranous and subchorionic hematomas)

Gross Examination: Documentation of the size, extent and percentage of the fetal surface involved in a subchorionic hematoma is important, as is estimation of the age of the clot. Subamnionic and retromembranous hematomas should also be measured and described.

Comment: Subchorionic hematomas have been associated with an increased risk of preterm delivery, fetal loss, vaginal bleeding, growth restriction and fetal demise. Correlation with clinical history is suggested. Subamnionic hematomas are usually iatrogenic. Retromembranous hematomas are generally of no clinical significance.

Meconium and Other Pigments

Meconium is the *bile-stained intestinal content of the fetus*. It is present in the fetal intestines long before midgestation but is usually not eliminated until after birth. Its chemical composition is variable and has only been partially determined, but it is known to often contain *mucus, mucopolysaccharides, blood group antigens, enzymes*, and *a small amount of protein*. Meconium discharge in utero is a common event occurring in approximately 17–19% of placentas and is much more common in term and postterm placentas.

Pathologic Features

When meconium is discharged before parturition, *the baby and placenta may be meconium-stained and deeply green* (Fig. 14.15a). An additional feature of meconium is that it causes edema of the membranes, giving them a slimy quality. Microscopically, meconium pigment may be present within macrophages in the fetal membranes, fetal surface, and even the umbilical cord. These **meconium-laden macrophages** are

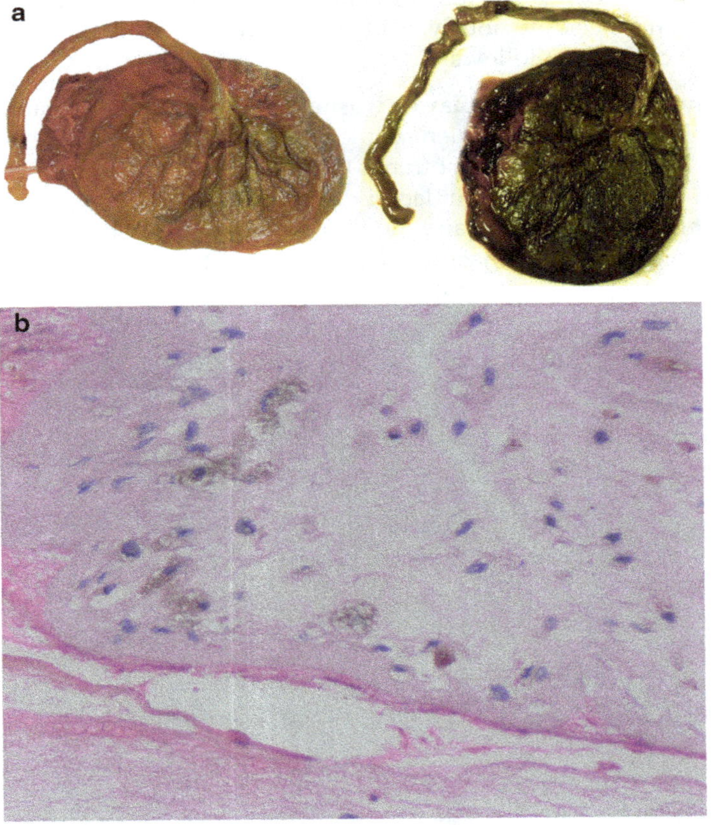

Figure 14.15. (a) Meconium staining of fetal membranes and umbilical cord of term placenta. (b) Many meconium-filled macrophages are present in the amnion of the placenta in part A. H&E ×400.

large, ovoid, or round cells with a slightly translucent, yellow-brown content. They tend to be vacuolated (Fig. 14.15b) but can be inconspicuous in some cases. On electron microscopy, phagolysosomes full of debris are present. The macrophages are normally inactive and thus "lie in waiting" in the membranes until meconium or other substances come by and they spring into functional activity.

When meconium has been present in the amniotic cavity for many hours, the amnionic epithelium begins to show degenerative changes. There is *vacuolization of the cytoplasm, heaping-up of cells, dissociation, loss of cells, and necrosis* (Fig. 14.16). The heaping up of the cells has been called "villous change" or "hyperplasia," but these terms are misnomers since these changes are degenerative in nature. With meconium staining of greater duration, *the smooth muscle cells of the umbilical vessels and their ramifications on the fetal surface may degenerate and show necrosis of individual muscle fibers* (Fig. 14.17). The muscle cells round up, the cytoplasm becomes more eosinophilic, and the nucleus undergoes pyknosis. Eventually, the cells die with complete loss of the nucleus, leaving a degenerated fragment of cytoplasm. How long the vessel must be exposed to meconium to lead to these vascular alterations on histological examination is not known precisely, but it likely to be many hours.

The time from meconium discharge to delivery of the infant and placenta has been previously estimated by in vitro incubation of tissue with meconium, as follows:

- **<1 hours** – meconium may be washed off the placental surface without leaving a stain or microscopic evidence
- **1–3 hours** – the amnion, but not the chorion, will be grossly stained and will contain pigment laden macrophages
- **>3 hours** – the amnion and the chorion will be stained and will contain pigment-laden macrophages

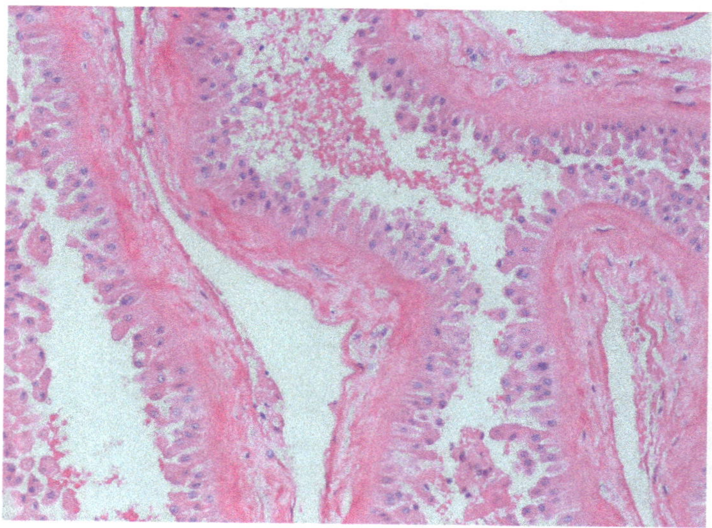

Figure 14.16. Meconium induced degenerative change of the amnion. Note the piling up of the epithelium. H&E ×200.

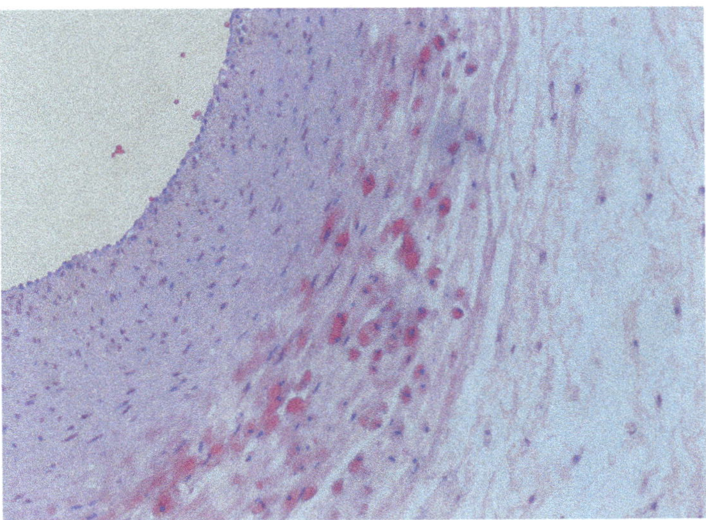

Figure 14.17. Meconium induced muscle damage to the umbilical artery. Note the rounding up of the myofibers, intense eosinophilia, and pyknosis or sometimes loss of the nucleus. H&E ×200.

- **4–6 hours** – the fingernails and toenails of the infant will be stained
- **12–14 hours** – the vernix will be stained.

Recently, a second study of the timing of meconium discharge has been published using similar methods. However, this study shows disparate results in that meconium was not found in the membranes until approximately 24 h. Thus, at present, until these studies can be repeated, the timing of meconium discharge is somewhat in question. After initial staining of the membranes, meconium will stain the decidua capsularis and, after many hours, the umbilical cord. Incubation of umbilical cord has shown uptake of meconium by macrophages in approximately 12–24 h (unpublished data). Staining of the umbilical cord may be seen grossly but is difficult to identify histologically, as there are few macrophages in Wharton's jelly. With very long-standing meconium exposure, meconium-stained macrophages may be identified within the myometrium. When attempting to time meconium discharge before birth, one must keep in mind that meconium is being removed by the macrophages, by fetal swallowing and inhalation, and that in some instances, fetuses discharge meconium repeatedly.

Other pigments, such as **hemosiderin** and **bilirubin**, are very similar to meconium. Bilirubin may cause a yellow discoloration of the fetal surface and fetal membranes and is usually associated with maternal hyperbilirubinemia (Fig. 14.18). Microscopically, pigment-laden macrophages are rare. Hemosiderin derives from hemolyzed red blood cells and is commonly found associated with *circumvallate placentas, erythroblastotic infants, abruptio placentae, thromboses, and other circumstances wherein bleeding has occurred*. Hemosiderin stained placentas have a more **brownish** tint, as opposed to the green of meconium stained

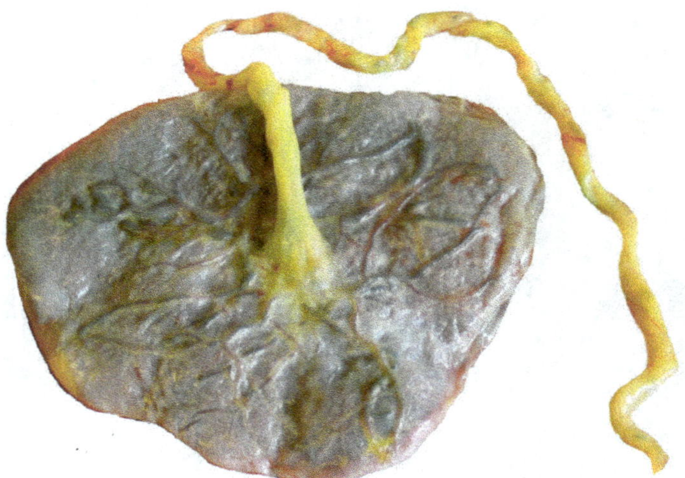

Figure 14.18. Bile staining of placenta. Note the prominent yellow discoloration of the umbilical cord and fetal surface.

placentas (Fig. 14.19). Microscopically, hemosiderin is composed of *brown, granular particles, and it has a characteristic sheen (refringence) when the focus of the light microscope, or its substage, is changed* (Fig. 14.19). In comparison to meconium pigment, hemosiderin is much easier to identify in histologic sections. A **Prussian blue stain** for iron is very helpful for differentiating between these two pigments. While iron stains readily differentiate hemosiderin, the bile in meconium is not readily confirmed. A **Luna-Ishak stain** will stain bile a greenish color. Unfortunately, this stain is technically difficult to perform and difficult to reliably interpret as well. In addition, hemosiderin becomes metabolized to hematoidin in about 7 days, and, regrettably, hematoidin and bilirubin cannot be reliably distinguished from each other, by either light microscopy or special histochemical stains. One should also be aware that the meconium pigment within macrophages bleaches when it is exposed to ambient light.

Pathogenesis
Meconium discharge occurs in approximately 15% of placentas at 39 weeks' gestation, in 27% at 41–42 weeks, and in 32% at over 42 weeks. The reason for the discharge of meconium is complex. It is moved in the intestinal lumen by contractions of the intestinal wall, which is regulated by hormones. One of these is **motilin**. There are lower levels of motilin and other gastrointestinal hormones in immature fetuses than in mature fetuses and higher levels in infants with fetal distress. This is part of the reason why mature fetuses and distressed fetuses often discharge meconium.

Clinical Features and Implications
Meconium discharge is positively correlated with fetal distress *but also occurs without fetal distress.* Many term stillbirths have never discharged meconium despite prolonged periods of distress that may

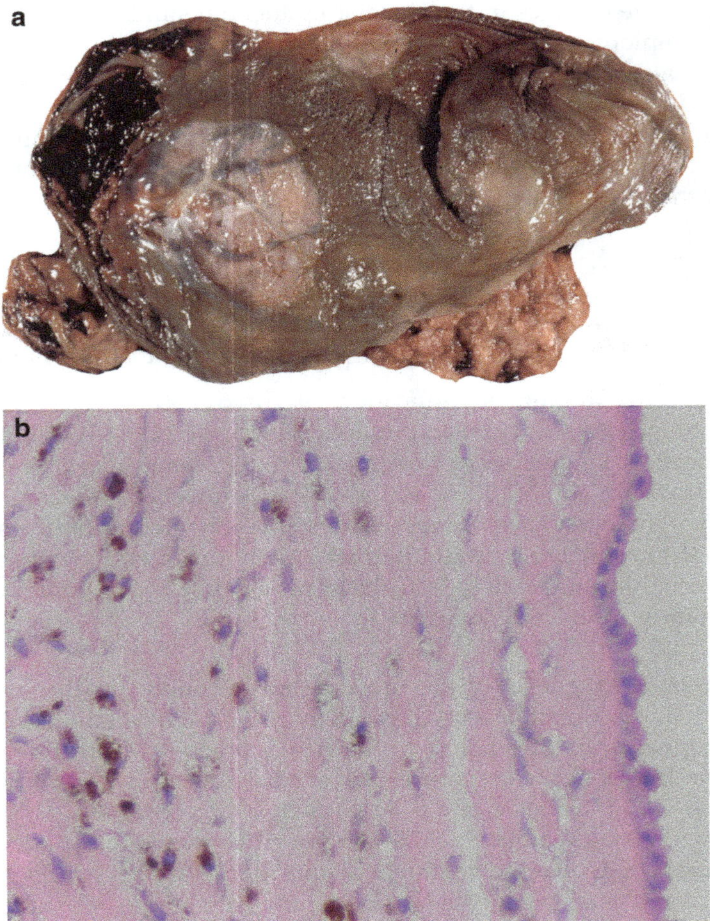

Figure 14.19. (a) Placenta with brown discoloration of the fetal membranes consistent with old bleeding. Some recent hemorrhage is also present on the left. (b) Hemosiderin laden macrophages in the fetal membranes showing yellow-brown particulate material. The nature of this pigment was confirmed with an iron stain. H&E ×200.

eventually lead to their demise. It is equally true that many infants that discharge meconium have **not** experienced fetal distress. Despite this fact, meconium has assumed great importance in medicolegal pursuits (see Chap. 26). Suffice it to say that *meconium discharge may occur in the setting of fetal distress or simply due to fetal maturity.* Thus, discharge of meconium in immature fetuses is more likely to be due to fetal distress, while meconium discharge in term fetuses may be only physiologic.

Despite the controversy over whether meconium discharge occurs secondary to hypoxia, meconium itself has deleterious effects. This includes sequelae due to *aspiration into the lungs as well as direct effects on the amnion and umbilical cord.* One of the major impacts of meconium on fetal morbidity and mortality is related to the meconium aspiration syndrome. Much of the pulmonary damage has been shown to be prenatal in onset, and it is thought that aspirated meconium causes degenerative changes in the alveolar epithelium similar to those seen in the amnionic epithelium and vascular smooth muscle (see above). There is also evidence that damage to the fetal vascular tissue may also have adverse effects. When segments of umbilical veins are exposed in vitro to meconium, the muscular wall contracts markedly and rapidly. Thus, meconium may be a *cause* of hypoperfusion and hypoxia rather than the result.

Suggestions for Examination and Report
(Meconium, hemosiderin or other pigmentation of the membranes)

Gross Examination: Identification of discoloration of the fetal membranes, fetal surface and umbilical cord should each be noted. Meconium staining is most commonly green, hemosiderin is usually brownish and bilirubin is more yellow. However, there is much overlap in appearance. If meconium staining is present on the surface of the cord, this should be particularly noted as the presence of meconium macrophages in the cord are difficult to appreciate. Therefore, discolored areas of the cord should be preferentially sectioned.

Comment: Diagnosis of the presence of meconium in the membranes and/or umbilical cord is usually sufficient (meconium-laden macrophages or meconium histiocytosis) and no comment need be made. Associated myonecrosis should always be mentioned if present. If hemosiderin is identified, a comment on possible sources of bleeding may include retromembranous or retroplacental hematoma, deciduitis, marginal hemorrhage, abruptio, placenta previa and fetal hemorrhage, etc. Yellow discoloration consistent with bilirubin staining should be noted and correlated with the clinical history if possible.

Gastroschisis

Gastroschisis, a fetal anomaly characterized by a defect in the abdominal wall, is associated with a specific abnormality of the amnionic epithelium. The amnionic epithelial cells have a characteristic *fine, uniform, extensive vacuolation* (Fig. 14.20). Although this association was startling when it was first found, it is now known to be regularly present and is virtually diagnostic of gastroschisis. It is not found in fetuses with omphalocele, a similar condition, and appears to have no influence on placental function. The vacuoles contain lipid when examined electron-microscopically, but the origin of the lipid is still obscure. When pregnancies <20 weeks are studied, the vacuolization of the epithelium is not yet present and so it accumulates only later in gestation.

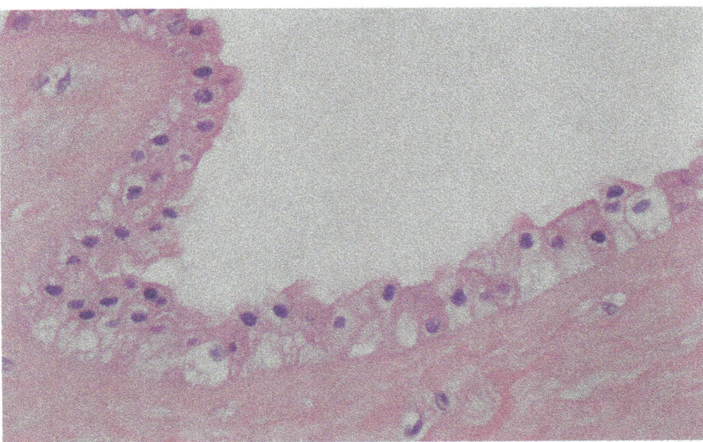

Figure 14.20. Characteristically vacuolated amnionic epithelium in a case of gastroschisis. H&E ×640.

Squamous Metaplasia

Squamous metaplasia is a change of the amnionic epithelium present in up to 60% of term placentas. The term is a misnomer, because the amnion is a type of immature squamous epithelium, being continuous with the fetal surface and the fetal skin. These areas of "metaplasia" do not form in response to some chronic irritation or inflammation, but merely betray maturity. The epithelium becomes *stratified with focal keratinization of the epithelium* (Fig. 14.21), resembling normal epidermis with keratohyaline granules and melanin. Areas of squamous meta-plasia are grossly visible as *whitish, hydrophobic foci of small elevations or irregular plaques* (Fig. 14.21) and are most commonly found near the cord insertion. They are of no clinical consequence.

Amnion Nodosum

Pathogenesis
Amnion nodosum is associated with conditions that lead to *significant, prolonged oligohydramnios*. It is found in the placentas of fetuses with *renal agenesis, following prolonged premature rupture of membranes, in the donor twin of the twin transfusion syndrome, in diamnionic acardiac twins, in sirenomelia,* and in various other disturbances that lead to significant oligohydramnios. Since the amnion lacks blood vessels, it must subsist almost entirely on the amniotic fluid. Lack of fluid leads to degenera-tion and death of the epithelium. Once a defect is present in the epithe-lium, vernix becomes deposited on the denuded basement membrane in a nodular fashion. Amnion nodosum develops only late in fetal life because earlier in gestation there is insufficient vernix. When oligohy-dramnios occurs in the second trimester, amnion nodosum does not develop. Instead, the amnion is either completely normal or shows minute foci of cellular degeneration.

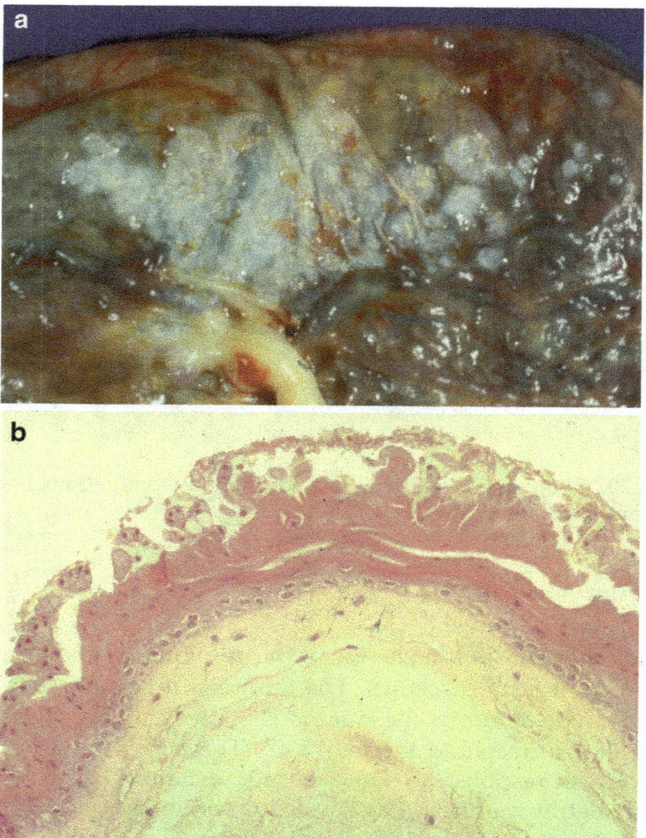

Figure 14.21. (a) Plaques of whitish discoloration on the fetal surface near the umbilical cord characteristic of squamous metaplasia in a mature placenta. (b) Keratinizing squamous metaplasia of the amnion, typical of mature placenta. H&E ×160.

Pathologic Features

Most cases of amnion nodosum show *fine granules on the fetal surface that are best seen in oblique light* (Fig. 14.22). The nodules may be shiny and relatively translucent but also may be more opaque and brown to yellow. The nodules occasionally extend onto the membranes, but are only very rarely found on the surface of the umbilical cord. They are quite different from the lesions seen in squamous metaplasia, which is typically more plaque-like, patchy, and hydrophobic (see above). In addition, amnion nodosum may be scraped off the surface, while plaques of squamous metaplasia may not. Microscopically, nodules of *vernix composed of squames and hair intermixed with sebum are attached to the surface defect* (Fig. 14.23). Generally, there is no associated inflammatory or other tissue reaction.

Clinical Features and Implications

Fetal sequelae of prolonged oligohydramnios primarily consist of **pulmonary hypoplasia** and **various malformations** due to fetal

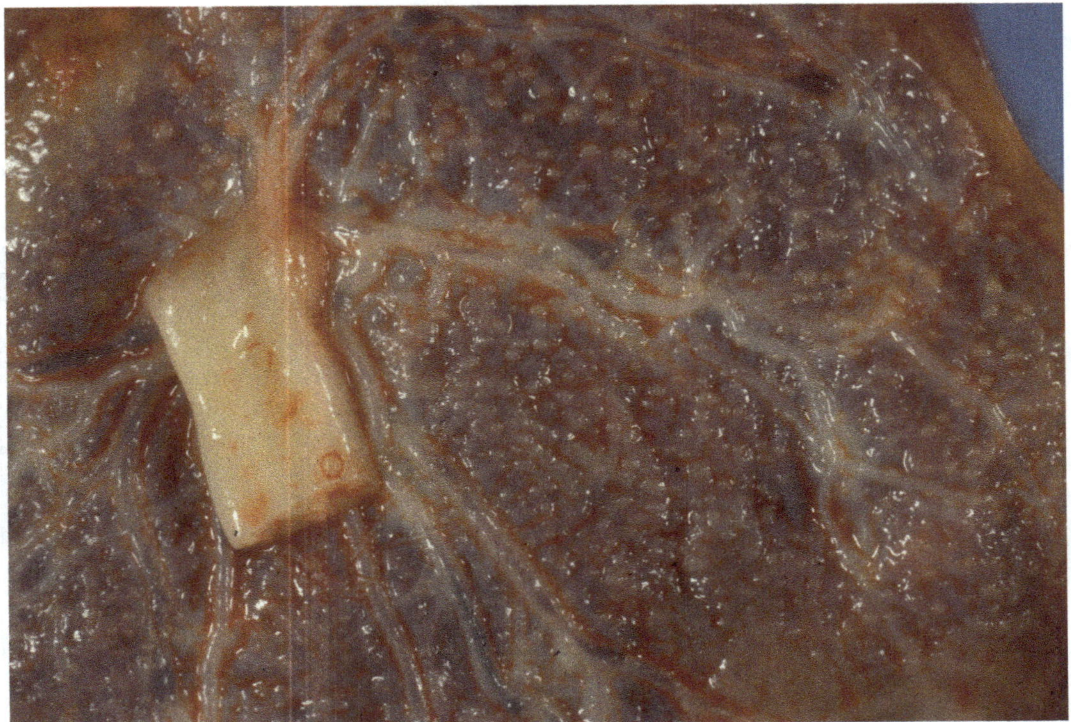

Figure 14.22. Macroscopic appearance of amnion nodosum in a child with renal agenesis. Note the uniform presence of fine pearly, nodules, mostly sparing the vessel surfaces and not present on the cord.

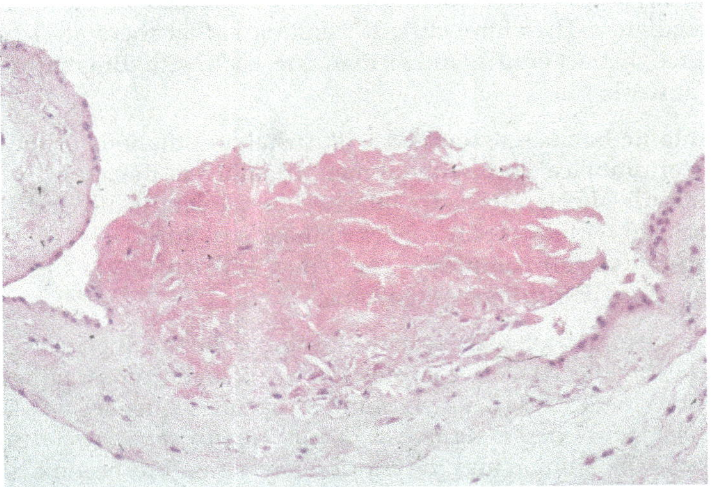

Figure 14.23. Microscopic view of amnion nodosum with absence of amnionic epithelium focally and accumulation of amniotic fluid debris forming an irregular nodule. H&E ×200.

compression from lack of fluid, specifically Potter's sequence with flattened facies and extremities. Amnion nodosum is another complication of the oligohydramnios. *Pulmonary hypoplasia develops due to the inability of the lung to inhale normal amounts of fluid and from compression.* Both breathing motions and the availability of amniotic fluid appear to be necessary for expansion and development of the lung.

Suggestions for Examination and Report
(Amnion Nodosum)

Gross Examination: Lesions should be differentiated from lesions of squamous metaplasia, which are irregular, patchy, and hydrophobic, and cannot be rubbed off. Amnion nodosum consists of smaller, more uniform nodules that can easily be removed. Adequate sampling is important, and in some cases gross photographs may be useful.

Comment: Amnion nodosum is generally associated with oligohydramnios and often with congenital malformations, particularly renal malformations. It occurs when there is a significant reduction in amniotic fluid for a period of time.

Amnionic Bands

Pathogenesis

Amnionic bands are associated with fetal amputations and various major congenital anomalies, and there is no doubt that these bands or sheets are associated with these anomalies. Although the existence of **amnionic bands** as a cause of amputations and other fetal debilities can hardly be disputed, such doubts are expressed in the literature with regularity. Therefore, current thinking is that there are likely at least three distinct entities rather than one, each with different mechanisms at work:

- **Amnionic bands** – associated with distal amputations of the fetus and/or umbilical cord without malformations of the fetus
- **Amnionic sheets** – broadly attached to the fetal skull and facies, associated with major anomalies of those structures
- **Limb-body wall complex** – associated with amnionic sheets and major gross disruptions of the fetus.

Many dysmorphologists refer to these bands and their associated anomalies as the **ADAM complex** (*amnionic deformities, adhesions, mutilation*) or **TEARS** (*the early amnion rupture sequence*).

Amnionic bands most likely develop through rupture of the amnion early in pregnancy. The amnion and the chorion never fuse but become *applied* to each other. Early in gestation, they are separate and do not become applied to each other until the 12th week. If rupture of the amnion occurs prior to this time, the fetus may escape into the chorionic sac. Since growth of the amnion is mediated by stretching of the enlarging sac, rupture will cause the amnion to shrivel and contract producing **amnionic bands**. Parts of the fetus or umbilical cord may become entangled with the bands leading to *fetal amputations or even demise*. The etiology of the early amnion rupture is unknown. There is no apparent hereditary component, increased risk of recurrence, association with amniocentesis, early chorionic villus sampling, or relation to trauma. Suggested etiologies include excessive fetal activity, defective development of the amnion, and vascular disruption. The phenotype is quite variable in that it depends on which part of the umbilical cord or fetus becomes entangled in these contracted bands.

There may be some overlap between categories, particularly the latter two as both seem to be associated *disturbances of early embryogenesis and/or vascular disruption*. Specifically, **amnionic sheets** are frequently associated with specific fetal anomalies such as *exencephaly, meningocele, ectopia cordis, spinal disruptions, clubbed feet, bony defects,* and *single umbilical artery*. Amnionic sheets seem to be associated with amnion rupture as well as abnormalities in development. The last category of amnionic bands is associated with **limb-body wall complex**, and here *the amnion is contiguous with some portion of the abdominal wall*. Associated anomalies also include a *short umbilical cord, single umbilical artery, disruption of the abdominal wall, craniofacial defects, and limb defects*. The limb defects are not the typical isolated amputations seen in amnionic bands. Suffice it to say that the etiology of these entities is still under investigation.

Pathologic Features

Placentas with **amnionic sheets** have broad sheets of amnion tethered to the umbilical cord (Fig. 14.24) that tend to be contiguous with the ectoderm of the fetal face or skull. This leads to typical craniofacial anomalies (Fig. 14.25). These sheets can often be identified by prenatal ultrasonography. Isolated amputations generally are not associated with these sheets, but there are specific anomalies as described above.

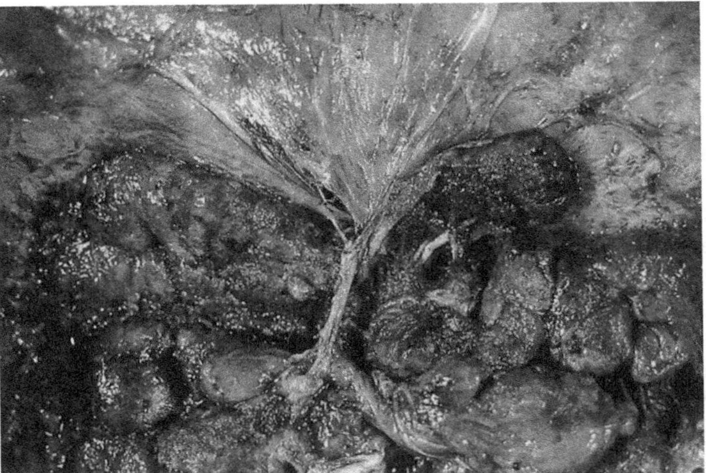

Figure 14.24. Amnionic sheet attached to the fetal surface of the placenta.

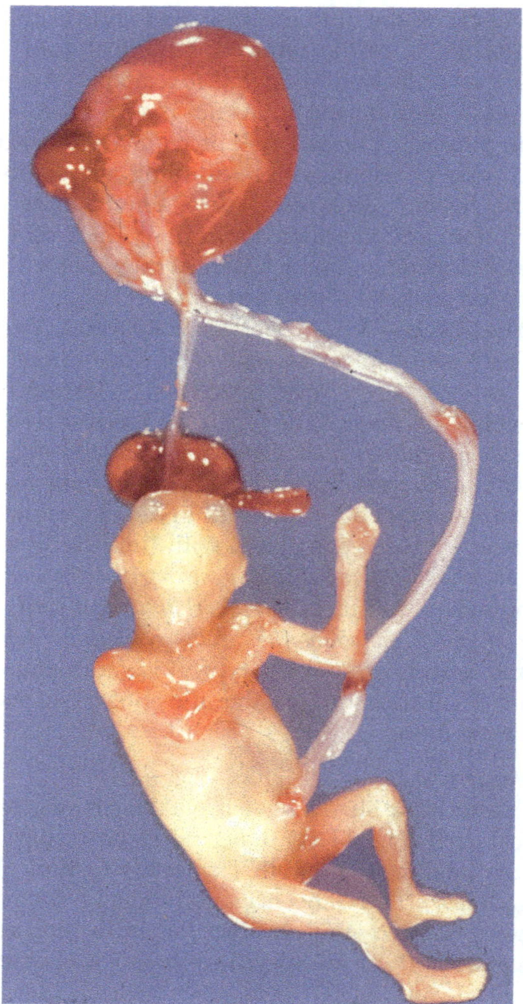

Figure 14.25. Amnionic band/sheet with attached to the fetal head and associated craniofacial anomalies.

The **limb-body wall complex** does not have distinct bands and lacks amputations. They are associated with *single umbilical artery, short umbilical cords, and defects in the abdominal wall.* Characteristic for the limb-body wall complex is an **amnion contiguous with some portion of the body wall, often with the abdomen** (Fig. 14.26). The etiology is still disputed, but incomplete *embryonic folding and neural tube closure* are likely mechanisms rather that early amnion rupture. This is supported by the fact that occasionally unrelated anomalies (e.g., truncus arteriosus) are encountered in such fetuses. They are often associated with fetal growth restriction and hydramnios.

With **amnionic bands,** *the fetal surface of the placenta is usually completely devoid of amnion,* as this has previously ruptured in the formation of bands. As such, the fetal surface is covered only with chorion

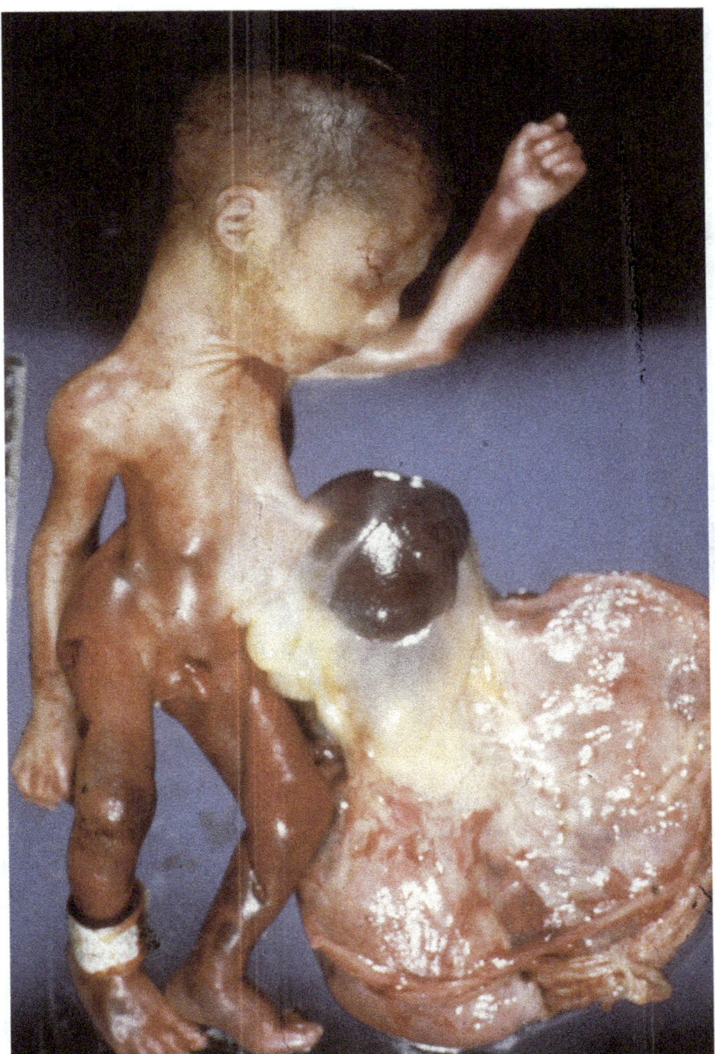

Figure 14.26. Infant with limb body wall complex. Note the short cord tethering the infant to the placenta and the abdominal wall defect.

and is grossly opaque due to increased infiltration of macrophages and fibrin deposition. *Remnants of the amnion can be found attached to the base of the umbilical cord;* this is the only portion that does not detach with rupture. Often a small sac is present at the placental end of the cord where the bands originate (Fig. 14.27). Occasionally, amnionic bands are identified but the placenta shows a somewhat necrotic but relatively intact amnionic surface. In this case, a **focal rupture of the amnion** has occurred with subsequent healing of the amnion over the defect. When histologic sections are made of the bands, they are found to consist of *normal-appearing amnionic epithelium and underlying connective tissue.* There are usually few signs of degeneration, and inflammation is absent.

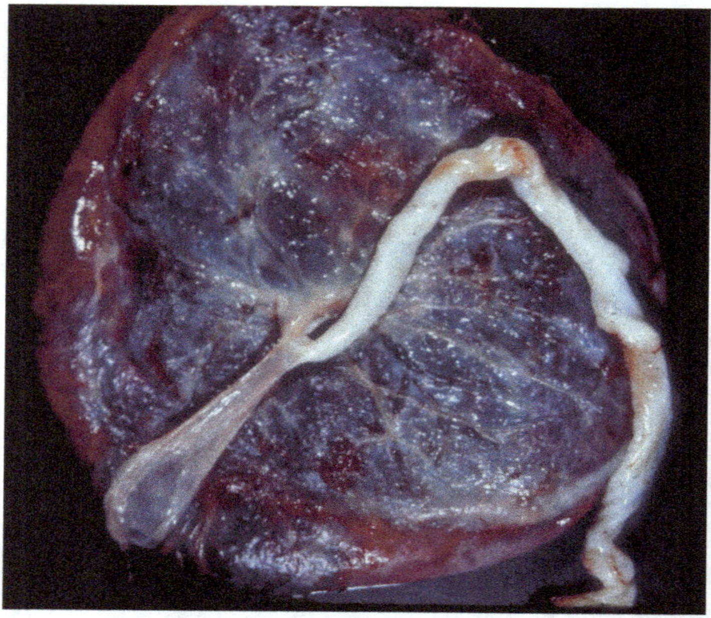

Figure 14.27. Amnionic band attached to the umbilical cord. Note the sac-like configuration of the band. The lack of amnion on the remainder of the fetal surface is not easily appreciated in this case.

Clinical Features and Implications

The *incidence* of amnionic bands is difficult to assess. In previable fetuses, they occur as often as 1 in 53 fetuses. In liveborns, they have been reported to occur in anywhere from 1 per 2,500 to 1 per 10,000 liveborns. The incidence has been reported to be *higher in African-Americans and in younger women.*

The most common and best-known fetal consequence of amnionic bands is *amputation of a portion of an extremity.* One can usually identify the typical constriction of a limb or other body part surrounded by a membranous fragment of amnion. Doubtless, the fetus moves and becomes entangled in these remnants of amnion, and because its fingers move most actively it is this part that is most commonly involved. Rarely, amnionic bands result in amputations with separate delivery of the amputated part. In this case, the amputated foot or other body part is smaller than the infant, as consistent with the gestational age at which the amputation took place. There are also bands that completely encircle the abdomen or an extremity, causing deep furrows and producing sloughing of the skin. Most fetuses with amputations due to amnionic bands are otherwise normal. *Entanglement with the umbilical cord can interrupt its circulation and lead to fetal death* (Figs. 14.28 and 14.29), and mortality is estimated at approximately 30%. At the other extreme, one should consider that *not every case of amnionic rupture necessarily leads to entangling and constrictions.* The phenotypic variations are extremely wide and it is merely a matter of chance which fetal or placental parts become entangled.

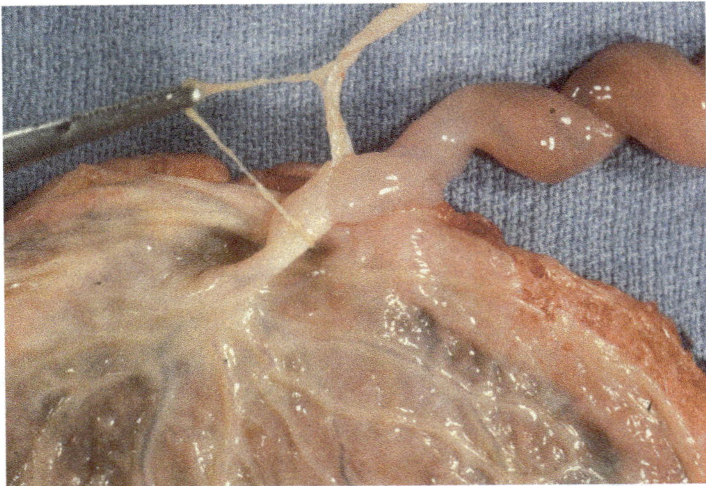

Figure 14.28. Amnionic band encircling the umbilical cord with associated congestion from a stillborn infant.

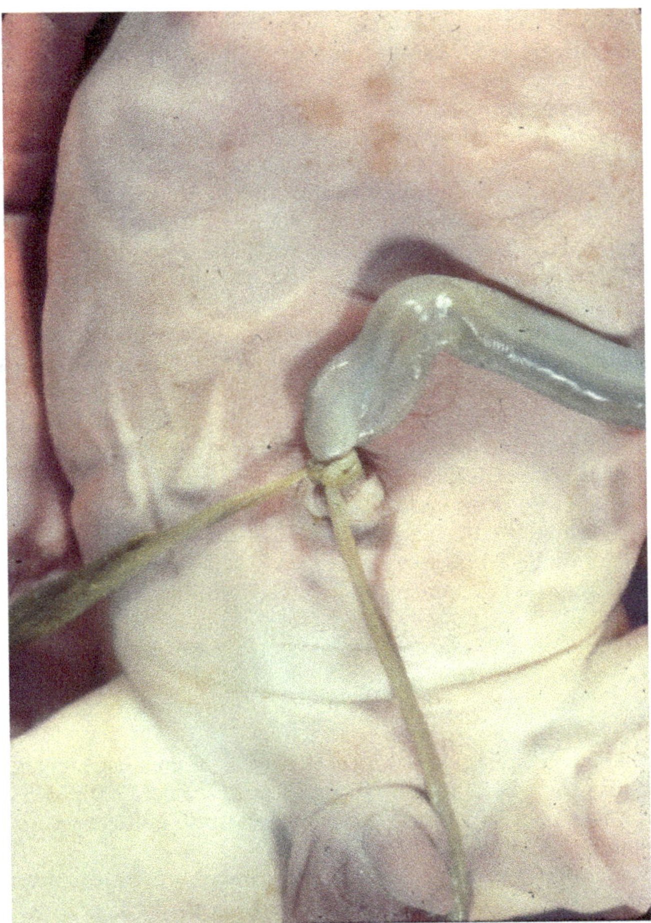

Figure 14.29. Another amnionic band encircling the proximal part of the umbilical cord in a term stillborn infant. Note that the cord and band are stained green secondary to meconium.

Suggestions for Examination and Report
(Amnionic Bands)

Gross Examination: Careful examination of the fetal surface and extraplacental membranes is essential in identification of amnionic bands and is facilitated by a clinical history that is suggestive of that diagnosis, e.g., an isolated amputation or typical anomalies. Usually the band or sheet will be tethered to the umbilical cord and the remaining fetal surface is devoid of amnion, being covered only by chorion. Photographs are very useful. Histologic sections of the bands are unremarkable, revealing only the presence of amnion.

Comment: The sequelae of amnionic bands have an extremely varied phenotype, and correlation with clinical history is essential.

Selected References

PHP5, pages 277–281 (Cysts and Breus' Mole), pages 321–379 (Anatomy and Pathology of the Fetal Membranes).

Altshuler G, Arizawa M, Molnar-Nadasdy G. Meconium-induced umbilical cord vascular necrosis and ulceration: a potential link between the placenta and poor pregnancy outcome. Obstet Gynecol 1992;79:760–766.

Ariel IB, Landing BH. A possible distinctive vacuolar change of the amnionic epithelium associated with gastroschisis. Pediatr Pathol 1985;2:283–289.

Funai EF, Labowsky AT, Drewes Ce, Kliman HJ. Timing of fetal meconium absorption by amnionic macrophages. Am J Perinatol 2009;26:93–97.

Higginbottom MC, Jones KL, Hall BD, et al. The amniotic band disruption complex: timing of amnion rupture and variable spectra of consequent defects. J Pediatr 1979;95:544–549.

Jacques SM, Qureshi F. Subamnionic vernix caseosa. Pediatr Pathol 1994;14:585–593.

Kalousek D, Banforth S. Amniotic rupture sequence in previable fetuses. Am J Med Genet 1988;31:63–73.

Martinez-Frias ML. Epidemiological characteristics of amnionic band sequence (ABS) and body wall complex (BWC): are they two different entities? Am J Med Genet 1997;73:176–179.

Miller PW, Coen RW, Benirschke K. Dating the time interval from meconium passage to birth. Obstet Gynecol 1985;66:459–462.

Morhaime JL, Park K, Benirschke K, Baergen RN. Disappearance of meconium pigment in placental specimens on exposure to light. Arch Pathol Lab Med 2003;127:711–714.

Nickell KA, Stocker JT. Placental teratoma: a case report. Pediatr Pathol 1987;7:645–650.

Pearlstone M, Bax L. Subchorionic hematoma: a review. Obstet Gynecol Surv 1993;48:65–68.

Perlman M, Tennenbaum A, Menash M, et al. Extramembranous pregnancy: maternal, placental, and perinatal implications. Obstet Gynecol 1980;55:34S–37S.

Salazar H, Kanbour AI, Pardo M. Amnion nodosum. Ultrastructure and histopathogenesis. Arch Pathol 1974;98:39–46.

Shanklin DR, Scott JS. Massive subchorial thrombohaematoma (Breus' mole). Br J Obstet Gynaecol 1975;82:476–487.

Stanek J, Weng E. Microscopic chorionic pseudocyts in placental membranes: a histologic lesion of in utero hypoxia. Pediatr Dev Pathol 2007;10:192–198.

Werler MM, Bosco JL, Shapira SK. Maternal vasoactive exposures, amniotic bands and terminal transverse limb defects. Birth Defects Res A Clin Mol Teratol 2009;85:52–57.

Chapter 15
Pathology of the Umbilical Cord

Embryonic Remnants

Allantoic Duct Remnants

Pathogenesis

The **allantoic duct** arises at about the 16th day postconception, as a *rudimentary outpouching of the caudal portion of the yolk sac* (see Fig. 5.4 in Chap. 5). Normally, there is complete obliteration of the allantoic duct at 15 weeks' gestation. A remnant, which connects the umbilicus to the bladder, persists as the **median umbilical ligament**. Occasionally, the duct persists as a minute connection to the fetal bladder. Allantoic duct

R.N. Baergen, *Manual of Pathology of the Human Placenta,*
DOI 10.1007/978-1-4419-7494-5_15, © Springer Science+Business Media, LLC 2011

remnants may be found in estimated 15% of umbilical cords and for unknown reasons; they are more common in males. In most cases they do not have connections with the fetal bladder.

Pathologic Features

Like other umbilical cord remnants, allantoic remnants are most frequently found in the *proximal portions of the umbilical cord closest to the baby*; however, they may exist discontinuously throughout the cord. They are always located centrally *between the two umbilical arteries* and consist of *a collection of cuboidal or flattened epithelial cells, usually without a lumen* (Fig. 15.1). The epithelium is generally of the *transitional type, although mucin-producing epithelium is occasionally found*. Rarely, it is accompanied by muscle. Small vessels or vasa aberrantia may be distributed around vessels, and, rarely, extramedullary hematopoiesis is seen.

Clinical Features and Implications

In most cases, allantoic remnants have no clinical significance. In 1 in 200,000 births, however, the duct is patent, connecting to the fetal bladder. In this situation there may be *urination from the clamped umbilical stump or the presence of cysts* that may persist into adult life. Pyelonephritis and abscess formation are common complications of this rare condition. The cysts may become quite large and give the appearance of a "giant" umbilical cord (Fig. 15.2).

Omphalomesenteric Duct Remnants

Pathogenesis

Early in development, the midgut communicates with the yolk sac via the umbilical stalk. As the embryo grows the umbilical stalk lengthens

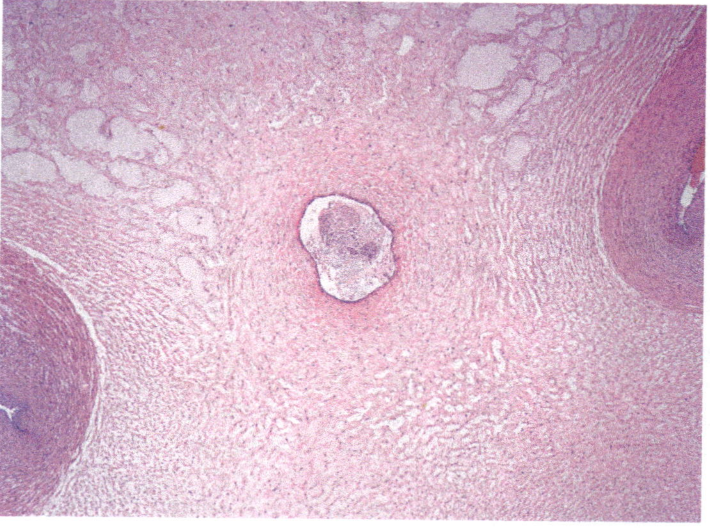

Figure 15.1. Remnants of allantoic duct. Note the absence of the muscular coat. H&E ×40.

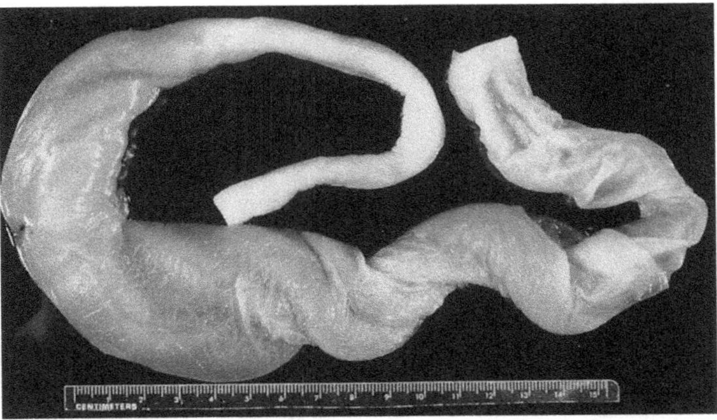

Figure 15.2. Edematous umbilical cord of a 32-week fetus with a large urachal extension into the cord. The cord weighed 180 g (normal weight is 40 g) (courtesy Dr. S. Kassel, Fresno, CA).

and the embryo "prolapses" into the amniotic cavity (see Fig. 5.4). The *connection between the gut and the yolk sac becomes attenuated and forms the* **omphalomesenteric (vitelline) duct**, which is of endodermal origin. When the gut rotates and withdraws to its original cavity between the 7th and 16th weeks, the duct normally atrophies. Persistence of this duct may then be found in an estimated 1.5% of umbilical cords. Remnants of vitelline vessels are found in approximately 7% of cords at term.

Pathologic Features
Like allantoic ducts, remnants of omphalomesenteric ducts are more common at the fetal end of the cord. Again, for unknown reasons, they are more common in males, with a male-to-female ratio of 4:1. Remnants are usually present *near the periphery of the cord and consist of ducts lined by columnar cells similar to intestinal epithelium* (Figs. 15.3 and 15.4). They often have muscular coats and may occur in pairs. Having an endodermal origin, it is not surprising remnants of this duct may contain remnants of *liver, small bowel, pancreatic tissue, adrenal, gastric mucosa, ganglion cells, or other intestinal structures*. Calcific masses have also been reported. The duct remnants are commonly associated with persistent vitelline vessels (Fig. 15.5). These vessels are usually tiny, without a muscular coat, *composed only of endothelium*. The lumen may contain red blood cells. Cysts have been described up to 6.0 cm in diameter and are frequently surrounded by a plexus of small vessels.

Clinical Features and Implications
Clinically, these vestiges are unimportant unless there is direct communication with fetal bowel – an uncommon occurrence. Remnants of omphalomesenteric ducts can be associated with *atresia of the small intestine and Meckel's diverticulum* and are a rare cause of abdominal distention.

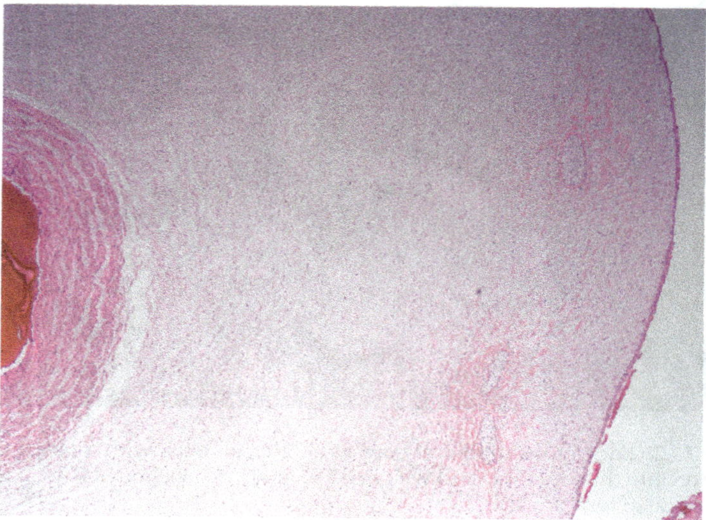

Figure 15.3. Low-power view of a section of a cord with of multiple omphalomesenteric ducts. The marginal position is typical. H&E ×50.

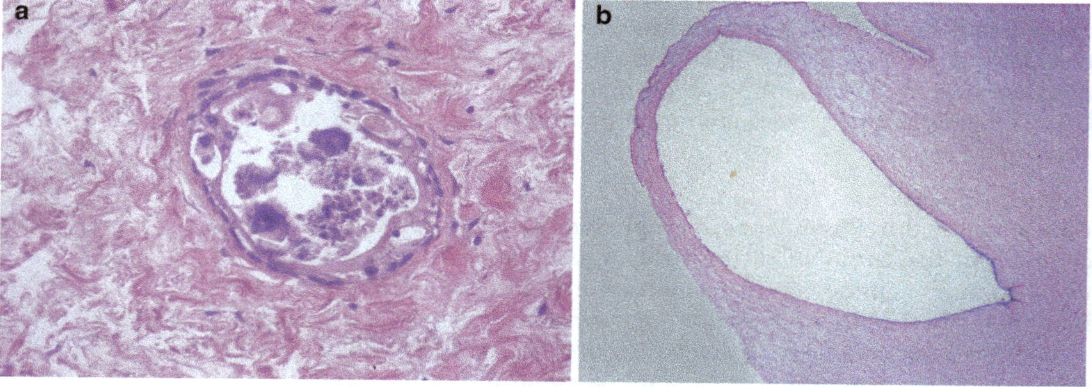

Figure 15.4. The omphalomesenteric duct on the left (**a**) has mucinous epithelium, some calcified luminal content and a small amount of musculature. H&E ×200. On the right (**b**) are the remains of an omphalomesenteric duct at the periphery of the cord. This duct shows moderate cystic dilatation. H&E ×40.

Suggestions for Examination and Report
(Embryonic remnants)

Gross Examination: Unless a cyst is present, remnants are usually not identifiable grossly. Cysts should be measured and additional sections should be taken.

Comment: Embryonic remnants in the cord usually have no clinical significance unless they have persistent connections to the bowel or bladder. This generally requires clinical correlation and a history of bowel or bladder problems in the neonate.

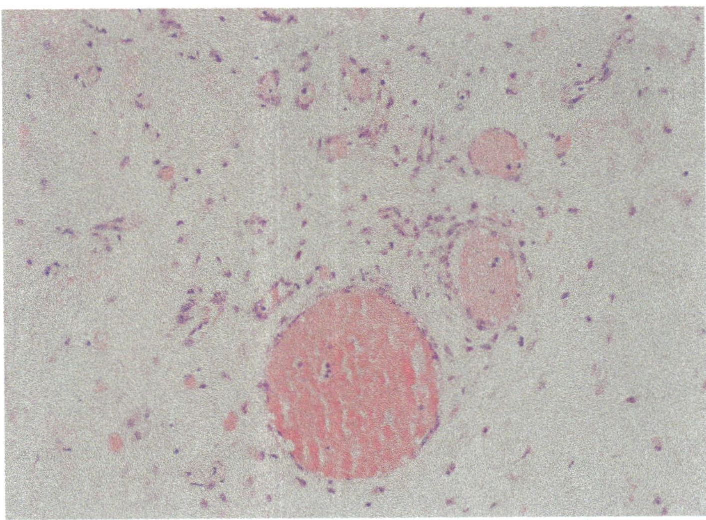

Figure 15.5. A plexus of small vitelline vessels is present in this umbilical cord. H&E ×100.

Umbilical Cord Coiling, Torsion, and Stricture

Pathogenesis

The umbilical cord is usually **coiled, twisted, or spiraled,** more commonly in a counterclockwise direction (a "left" twist) in a ratio of about 4:1 (Fig. 15.6). The helices may be seen by ultrasonographic examination as early as the first trimester of pregnancy but they increase significantly during the third trimester. The coils number up to 40 across the entire length of the cord, but as many as 380 total turns have been described. The **coiling index** has been used to evaluate the degree of twisting, defined as *the number of coils divided by length of cord.* The average coiling index is 0.21/cm or one complete spiral for approximately 5 cm of cord. **Hypocoiled cords** are seen in about 7.5% of cords, **non-coiled cords** are present in 4–5%, and **hypercoiled cords** are reported to be present in anywhere from 10 to 20% (Fig. 15.7). Twisting of the cord is thought to be the result of fetal activity. Lack of coiling may then reflect fetal inactivity, and this concept is supported by the fact that coiling is reduced in cases of restriction of fetal movement due to intrauterine constraint from uterine anomalies or amnionic bands, anomalies that restrict fetal movement such as skeletal dysplasias, and diminished fetal movement resulting from central nervous system (CNS) disturbances.

Pathologic Features

The degree of coiling tends to be rather uniform throughout the length of the umbilical cord. However, focal areas may show excessive or decreased coiling. In addition, excessive coiling may be localized and form a **stricture** (Fig. 15.8). Other terms used for these significant reductions in the diameter of the umbilical cord are **constriction, torsion,** or **coarctation.** They are often seen in fetal demise and most commonly

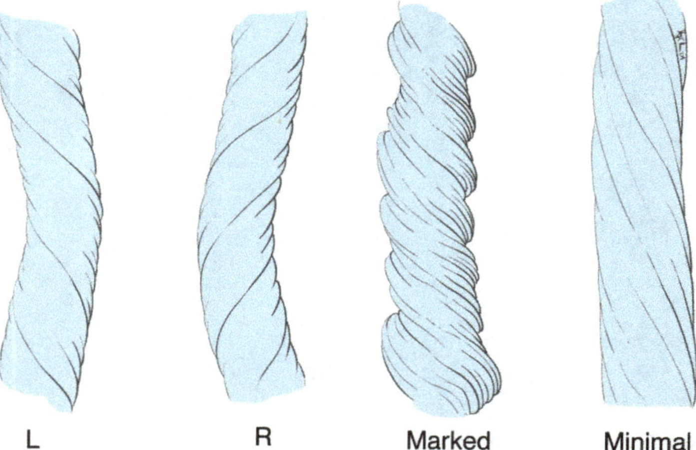

Figure 15.6. Drawing depicting different types of umbilical cord twist including left, right, minimal, and marked twisting.

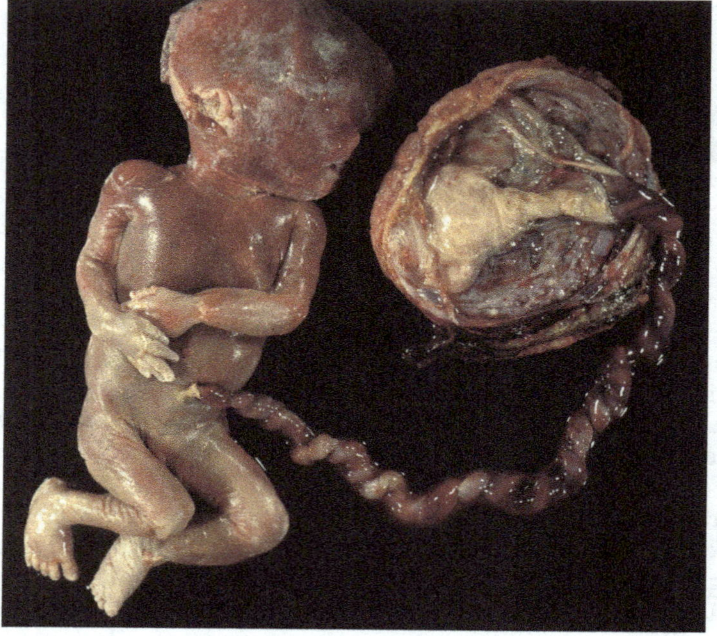

Figure 15.7. Preterm stillborn infant and placenta with a markedly coiled (twisted) umbilical cord. This was the presumed cause of death.

found at the *fetal end of the cord*. This may occur because there is a gradually diminishing amount of Wharton's jelly near the abdominal surface. However, we are convinced that these are **not** artifacts, as some have suggested, and the pathologic changes associated with strictures support this. In addition, not all fetal demises demonstrate this focal decrease in umbilical cord diameter at the fetal surface. Furthermore, cord strictures are most commonly seen in hypercoiled cords and rarely seen in

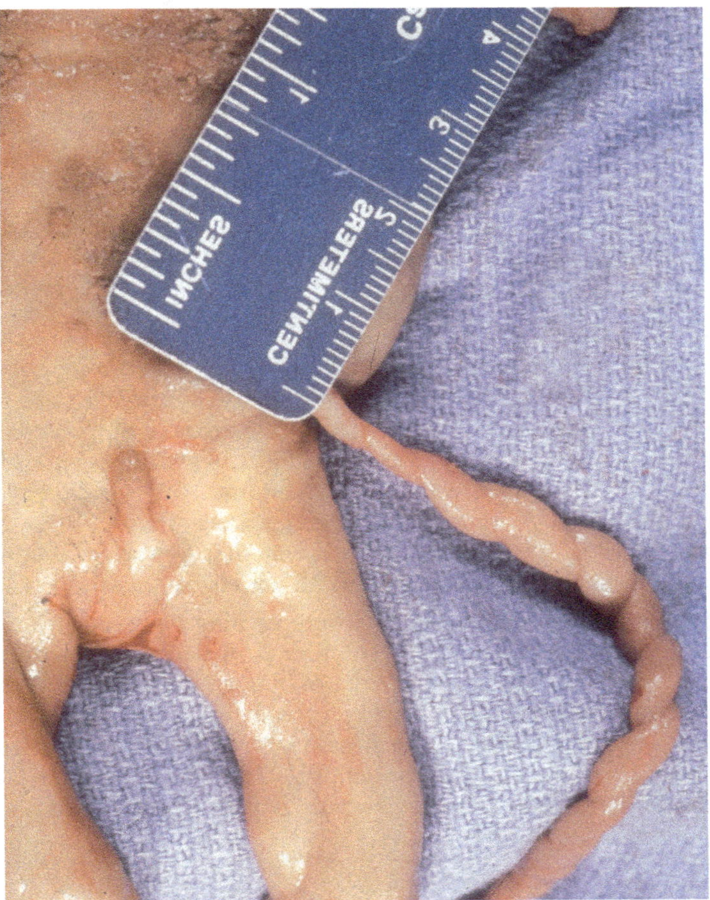

Figure 15.8. Spontaneous abortus at about 14 weeks' gestation with markedly spiraled cord and severe constriction of the cord (torsion) near the fetal surface that led to the death.

hypocoiled or normally coiled cords. Pathologic findings associated with stricture and/or hypercoiling include *congestion of the cord and vessels on one side of the torsion, compression and/or distention of the umbilical vein, long-standing degeneration of the umbilical vessels, and thrombi in the umbilical or placental surface vessels.* Because these fetuses are often macerated and coagulation is inadequately developed in embryos, the demonstration of thrombi is often difficult in early gestation.

Clinical Features and Implications

Hypocoiling and hypercoiling are both associated with adverse perinatal outcome including an increase in *perinatal mortality, intra-uterine growth restriction, and fetal distress* (Fig. 15.7). Hypocoiling, as previously stated, is associated with reduced fetal move-ment in utero and thus has been seen with increased frequency in CNS anomalies and previous intrauterine neurologic injury. Hypercoiling and constrictions are often seen together and have a strong correlation with fetal demise due to mechanical obstruction of blood flow through the cord. If hypercoiling is moderate, a more chronic loss of blood flow may occur leading to growth restriction, although cases of fetal demise may also be associated with growth restriction.

Suggestions for Examination and Report
(Abnormal coiling or stricture)

Gross Examination: Ideally, the direction of the coil or twist and the degree of coiling should be noted (Fig. 15.6). The coiling index described above may be used for this purpose, but may not be necessary if the examiner is experienced. Focal areas with increased or decreased twisting should also be noted. Constrictions should be measured and serially sectioned. In abnormal twisting, attention should always be given to the chorionic plate vessels as these may contain thrombi. It is suggested that additional sections of fetal surface vessels be taken to look for thrombi not visible grossly.

Comment: Abnormal coiling or strictures may be associated with adverse perinatal outcome. If a stricture is present in the setting of a fetal demise and there is evidence of venous obstruction, such as thrombosis, the constriction can be considered the cause of death. If supporting histologic findings are not present, the constriction may be suggested as a cause of demise. Abnormal coiling may also explain other adverse outcome such as growth restriction or neurologic injury if that history is given.

Umbilical Cord Length

Pathologic Features

The normal length of the umbilical cord at term is approximately **55 cm**. Excessively long cords occur in 4–6% of placentas, while abnormally short cords have an incidence of approximately 1–2%. Thus the distribution of cord length is slightly skewed toward longer cords. Short cords are generally considered to be those **less than 35 cm**, as this is the minimum length needed to allow a vaginal delivery with a fundal placental implantation. Long cords are considered to be those **greater than 70–80 cm**, and these numbers are based primarily on normative curves of cord length with long cords being more than two standard deviations from the mean. When evaluating cord length, there are several important points that should be remembered. First, it is important to distinguish between "absolute" and "functional" lengths. A cord that is long but wound about the neck multiple times will be long in the absolute sense but functionally short. This often becomes an issue during fetal descent, either during late pregnancy or during labor, and there is increased traction on the cord. Another point that must be remembered is that the entire cord is almost never submitted to pathology. Four to seven centimeter is always left attached to the infant at delivery and other fragments are discarded, or used for blood gas determinations or other testing. Furthermore, the length of the cord shrinks up to several centimeters in the first few hours following delivery. Thus, the diagnosis of an excessively short cord must be made with caution, if at all, while the diagnosis of a long cord can be made but probably is underestimated. For these reasons, accurate recording at the time of delivery, although difficult to accomplish, is preferable.

Abnormally long cords can be associated with *cord edema, villous congestion, and thrombosis of umbilical or chorionic vessels*. In particular, **fetal thrombotic vasculopathy** is associated with long cords (see Chap. 21). Long cords are also associated with other pathologic changes in the placenta, including *meconium, nucleated red blood cells, and chorangiosis*. The latter two findings are seen in the placenta in the setting of intrauterine hypoxia and imply that long cords are associated with restricted blood flow and resultant fetal hypoxia. The presence of meconium can sometimes be associated with fetal distress.

Pathogenesis

Cord length seems to be determined by several factors – *gestational age, genetics, and fetal movement*. On the 41st day after conception the developing cord has a mean length of about 0.5 cm. By the fourth month it has grown to between 16 and 18 cm and, by the sixth month, to approximately 33–35 cm. Most of the cord's length is achieved by the 28th week of pregnancy. Although growth slows progressively after this time, it never ceases until delivery. Genetics also seems to play a role in that excessively long cords have a tendency to recur, with mothers having a long cord in a previous pregnancy having approximately twice the chance of a long cord in a subsequent pregnancy compared to controls. Males also have longer cords than females and larger babies have a tendency to have longer cords. Finally, movement has been shown to have an affect of the length of cord as well. Short cords are more common in situations in which there is decreased fetal movement due to congenital anomalies such as skeletal dysplasias or trisomy 21, and where there is intrauterine constraint such as uterine anomalies, ectopic pregnancies, amnionic bands, and in twins. This is very similar to the situation for cord coiling. In addition, when pregnant animals are administered drugs that decrease fetal movements, such as curare, alcohol, or beta-blockers, short cords result. The possible relation between long cords and excessive fetal movements is more difficult to assess because of the lack of quantitative data on prenatal movements. However, some authors have indicated that neonates with long cords were noted to be relatively hyperkinetic when compared with those that had shorter cords.

Clinical Features and Implications

Excessively short cords are clearly correlated with neonatal problems. The essential question is whether the length of the cord is determined by prenatal CNS problems or whether the CNS problems result from perinatal problems attending the delivery of a short cord. Many

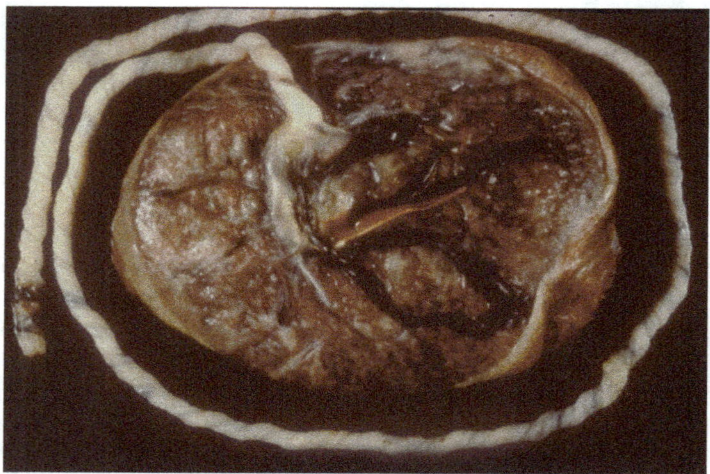

Figure 15.9. An excessively long and twisted umbilical cord. Note the visible thrombus in the fetal surface vasculature seen as a white streak in the vessel.

subsequent neonatal problems associated with short cords are related to excess traction during delivery. These include *premature separation of the placenta (abruptio), cord hemorrhage, cord hematoma, cord rupture, uterine inversion, failure of descent, and prolongation of the second stage of labor.* Short cords have also been associated with *fetal distress, low Apgar scores, depressed intelligence quotient (IQ), and developmental anomalies.* They are also associated with some congenital anomalies, particularly abdominal wall defects as well as amnionic bands. In these latter cases, the defects and the short cord are often the result of some embryonic developmental defect. **Excessively long cords**, on the other hand, are associated with *cord entanglement, cord prolapse, true knots, excessive coiling, constriction, and thrombosis* (Fig. 15.9). Clinical sequelae of long cords include *fetal distress, long-term neurologic impairment, intrauterine growth restriction, and fetal demise.* Cord entanglement, prolapse, and true knots are discussed below.

Cord Diameter

The diameter of the cord is predominantly due to the water content of Wharton's jelly and is usually reflective of the fluid status of the fetus. The diameter increases slowly throughout gestation and then declines slightly in the last few weeks before full maturity. The average cord diameter at term varies from about 1.2 to 1.7 cm. An increased cord diameter is usually due to **edema** (Fig. 15.10). Cord edema is found in 10% of infants and is more common in premature infants. The edema may be *diffusely distributed or occur focally and appear as cysts.* Usually, infants with cord edema have a normal outcome, but cord edema and "thick" cords may be associated with *polyhydramnios, maternal diabetes, and fetal hydrops.*

Excessively thin umbilical cords are often associated with *fetal growth restriction* and can be a potential cause of fetal problems.

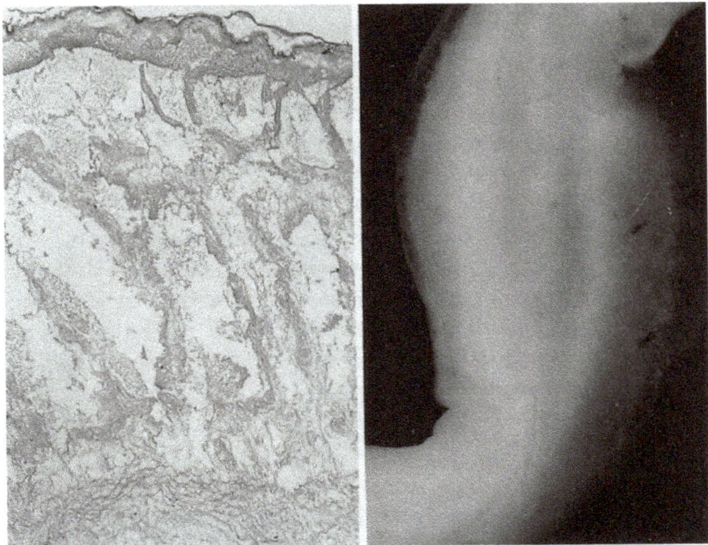

Figure 15.10. Marked edema in the umbilical cord of a normal newborn infant. Note the dissociation of fibrous tissue underneath the surface of the cord. H&E ×160.

The cord may be thin throughout or only portions may be thinned. In the thin areas, there is a decreased amount of Wharton's jelly and thus *compression of vessels is a greater possibility than when they are protected.* The extreme situation of focal thinning of the cord is manifested as the constrictions described above. It is probably incorrect to refer to cases of thin umbilical cord as a "deficiency" of Wharton's jelly as it is not the cellular component of the cord that is diminished but rather the water content. Thus, very thin cords can be thought of as relative "dehydration" and thick cords as a manifestation of increased fluid, which is why the latter is associated with hydramnios and hydrops.

Suggestions for Examination and Report
(Excessively Long or Short Cords, Cord Edema, and Thin Cords)

Gross Examination: Measurement of the total length of all cord fragments submitted is suggested, although the true length cannot be determined without measurement at delivery. Measurement of the cord diameter should be performed as well with particular attention to focal areas of edema or constriction. The chorionic vessels should be evaluated grossly for evidence of thrombi, and in some cases additional sections should be taken of these vessels.

Comment: Abnormalities in cord length and thin cords are associated with adverse perinatal outcome, and these abnormalities should be correlated with clinical history. Fetal vascular thrombosis in the placenta is additional evidence of the clinical significance of abnormal cords. Cord edema is usually not associated with adverse outcome.

Cord Entanglement and Cord Prolapse

Clinical Features and Implications

Cord entanglement is actually quite common, and the incidence of a single **nuchal cord** at term is approximately 20%. The presence of multiple nuchal cords is less common, with two loops around the neck occurring in 2.5% and three nuchal cords in 0.5% of births. Nuchal cords have been identified as early as 20 weeks' gestation, although some of these may resolve before delivery. A nuchal cord that encircles the neck in a locked pattern is of greater significance to outcome than those with an unlocked pattern. The presence of **nuchal cords** or **cord entanglement** is associated with *more admissions to the neonatal intensive case unit, a higher incidence of cesarean section delivery, fetal growth restriction, neonatal anemia, poor long-term neurologic outcome, spastic cerebral palsy, and fetal demise* (Fig. 15.11).

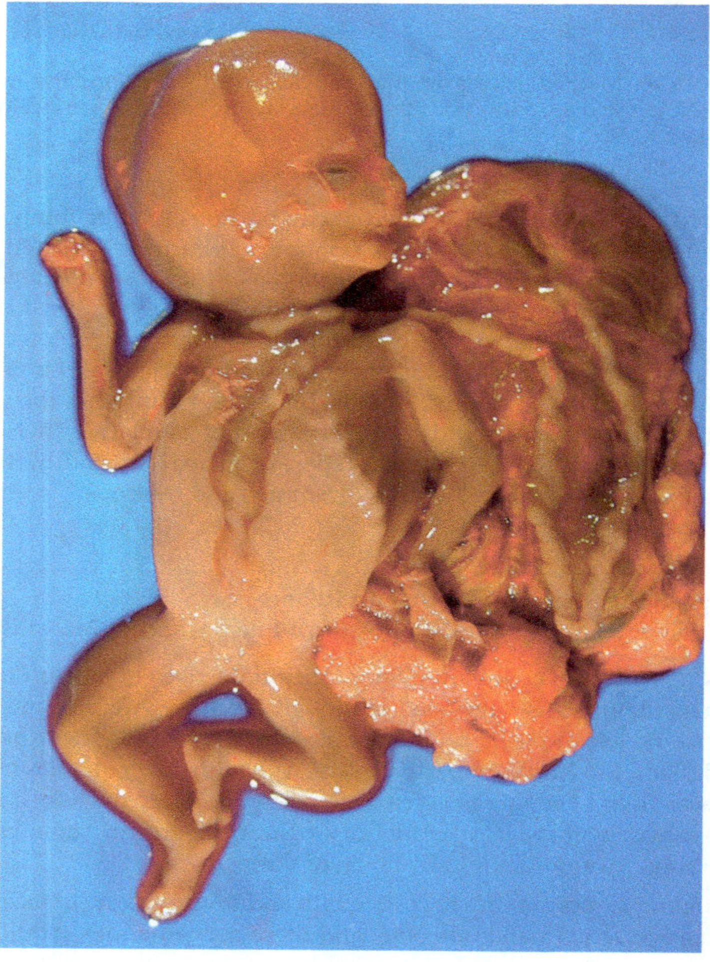

Figure 15.11. Stillborn fetus with a tight nuchal cord. The cord was also long and had obvious hypercoiling. Death presumably came about by obstruction to venous return from the placenta, not by obstruction to vessels of the fetal head.

Cord prolapse *occurs when the umbilical cord precedes the fetal presenting part.* This enables significant compression of cord, particularly against the cervix, during delivery. Prolapse is uncommon and is estimated to occur in 0.41% of deliveries. It is increased in *multiparous patients, premature labor, multiple gestation, fetal malpresentation, and artificial rupture of membranes with high presenting fetal parts and with long cords.* The presence of a prolapsed cord may have grave prognostic significance and is associated with a perinatal mortality of approximately 13%. The manner in which nuchal cords, cord entanglements, or prolapse lead to adverse outcome is by vascular occlusion and decreased venous return from the placenta leading to asphyxia. Cord compression may have serious fetal neurologic consequences, and this is why the "cord compression pattern" of fetal heart monitoring is taken so seriously.

Pathologic Features

The compressed umbilical cord may show profound pathologic changes such as *hemorrhage or even rupture* at the site of compression. However, in many cases, there is no gross evidence of damage in the area of compression. Compression can lead to *thrombosis* of umbilical vessels, but is more commonly associated with thrombosis of the chorionic vessels. These findings are not pathognomonic and so the diagnosis or cord compression or prolapse cannot be made on pathology alone. However, the presence of thrombosis is evidence of decreased flow in the venous system and thus is associated with clinically significant sequelae.

Umbilical Cord Knots

Pathologic Features

True knots of the umbilical cord occur with a *frequency of 0.4–0.5%.* They may be loose (Fig. 15.12) or tight (Fig. 15.13), the latter obviously having greater clinical significance. Tight true knots cause *compression of Wharton's jelly at the site of knotting, congestion on the placental side of the knot (due to decreased venous return to the placenta), and tendency of the unknotted cord to curl* (if the knot has been present for a period of time). In clinically significant knots, the venous stasis that occurs often results in *thrombosis of placental surface veins or even umbilical vein thrombosis.* Mural thrombosis or complete occlusion may be found, and calcifications may occur in long standing thrombosis (Fig. 15.14; see also Chap. 21 for complete discussion on fetal vascular thrombosis).

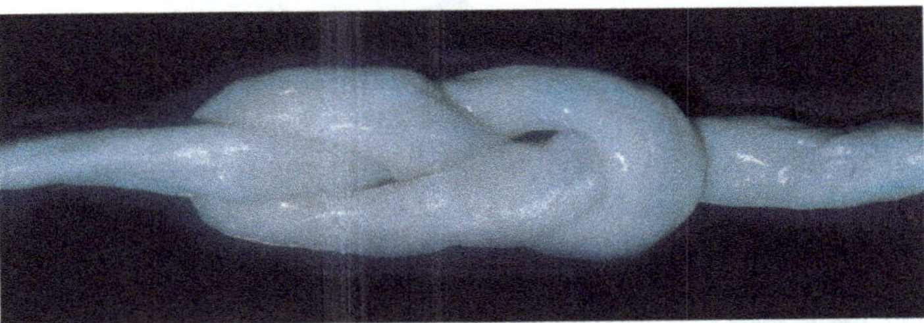

Figure 15.12. Loose true knot in the umbilical cord in infant with no untoward sequelae.

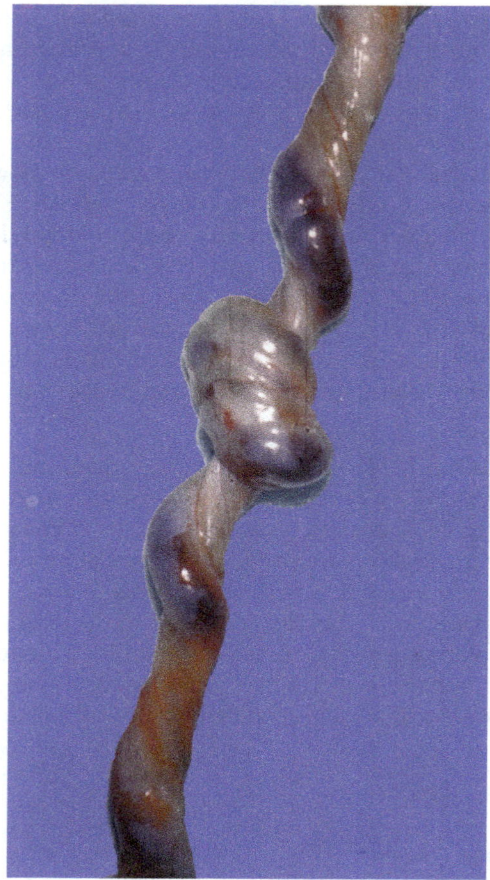

Figure 15.13. Umbilical cord with tight true knot.

False knots should not be called knots at all as they are actually local redundancies of the umbilical vessels, mostly the vein. Some can be quite complex, but the nature of these knots is clear on gross inspection, and confusion with true knots generally does not occur (Fig. 15.15). So far as can be determined, false knots *have absolutely no clinical importance*. Despite their clinical irrelevancy, questions persist just why these redundancies appear at all but answers are elusive at present.

Clinical Features and Implications
True knots are commonly associated with *long cords, multigravidas, male fetuses, and monoamnionic twins*. Knots probably develop early in gestation because the marked fetal movement necessary to cause knotting, or entanglement for that matter, is not possible once the fetus has reached a certain size. The knot often does not become tight until the onset of labor when fetal descent into the birth canal increases traction on the cord. Knots may not only cause *intrauterine or intrapartum fetal death* (Fig. 15.16), but may lead to significant *hypoxia with lasting neurologic damage in the infant*. True knots have an *overall mortality of about 10%*.

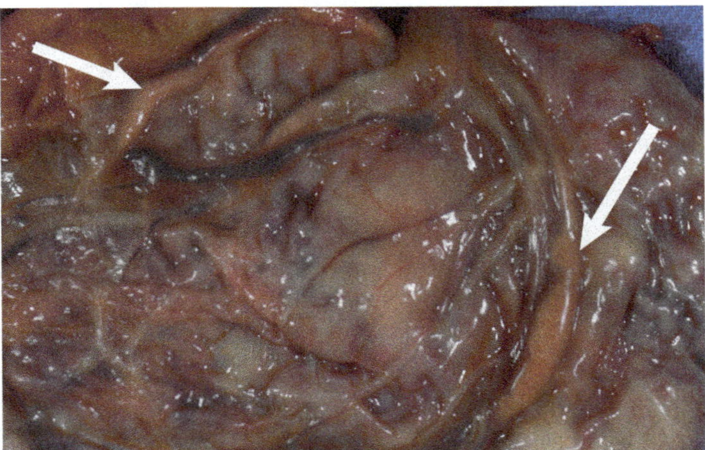

Figure 15.14. Thrombi present in chorionic plate vessels visible as white to yellow streaks within the vessels (*arrows*).

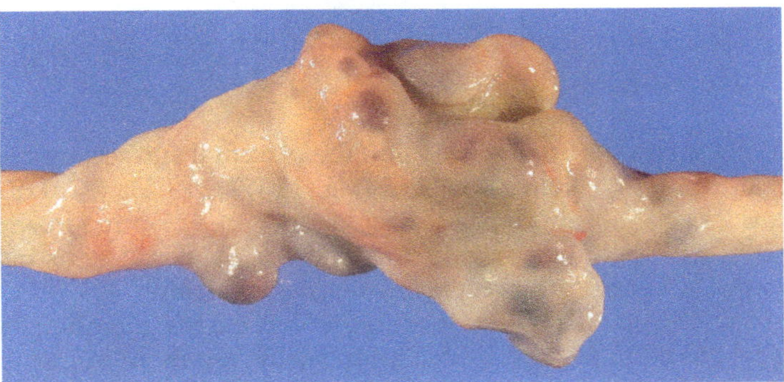

Figure 15.15. "False" knot, representing vascular redundancies.

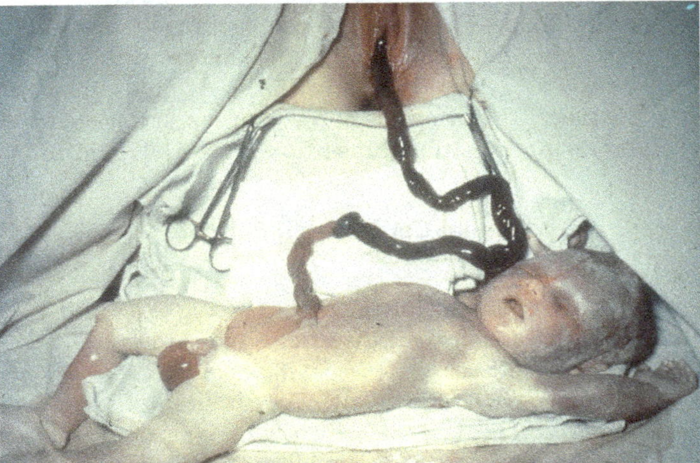

Figure 15.16. Macerated stillborn fetus. Death was due to a true knot is clearly demonstrated here with obstruction of venous return from the placenta. Total cord length was 65 cm. Note the marked congestion of the cord distal to the knot.

> **Suggestions for Examination and Report**
> (Umbilical Cord Knots)
>
> *Gross Examination:* Documentation should be made of the presence
> of the true knot, the tightness of the knot, the presence of congestion
> on either side of the knot, constriction in the area of knot, curling of
> the unknotted cord and gross evidence of thrombosis either in the
> umbilical cord or chorionic vessels. Additional sections should be
> taken through the knot after it has been untied (so cross sections can
> be made). In the case of adverse outcome, a photograph is recom-
> mended. No additional examination is necessary with false knots.
>
> *Comment:* True knots are more clinically significant when tight and
> associated with signs of vascular obstruction such as thrombosis,
> congestion, etc. A comment on the associated findings and an evalu-
> ation of the clinical significance of the knot in each case is recom-
> mended if possible. No comment is necessary when false knots are
> present as they have no clinical consequence.

Cord Insertion

The umbilical cord normally inserts on the placental surface, more often
near or at the center than elsewhere (Fig. 15.17). In nearly 7% of term
placentas it has a **marginal insertion**, a "Battledore" placenta in which it
inserts at the edge of the placenta. In about 1%, the cord inserts into the
membranes, a **velamentous** or **membranous insertion** (Figs. 15.17 and
15.18). Here, the umbilical vessels course within the free membranes and,
having lost their protection by Wharton's jelly, are more vulnerable to
various traumas and disruption. Membranous vessels are not confined to
velamentous cord insertions but also are present in multilobate placentas
(see Fig. 13.2 in Chap. 13) and occasionally in marginal insertions.

Not only are the sites of insertion variable, the insertion itself may
take an abnormal shape. Thus, the vessels may branch of vessels before
the cord inserts onto the surface of the placenta, and this results in a
furcate cord insertion (Figs. 15.17 and 15.19). At times, the cord runs
parallel to the placental surface or in the membranes before its vessels
branch, called an **interpositional insertion** (Figs. 15.17 and 15.20).

Velamentous and Marginal Cord Insertion

Pathologic Features

Velamentous insertion of the umbilical cord occurs in around 1% of singleton term deliveries, **marginal insertion** in approximately 7%. They
are more common with *twins, higher multiples, and in association with a
single umbilical artery (SUA)* (see below). The cord may insert reasonably
close to the edge of the placenta, which is much more common than
the extreme situation, where the cord inserts at the apex of the membranous sac. In the latter configuration, the long membranous course
of the vessels makes them particularly *vulnerable to injury.* It should be

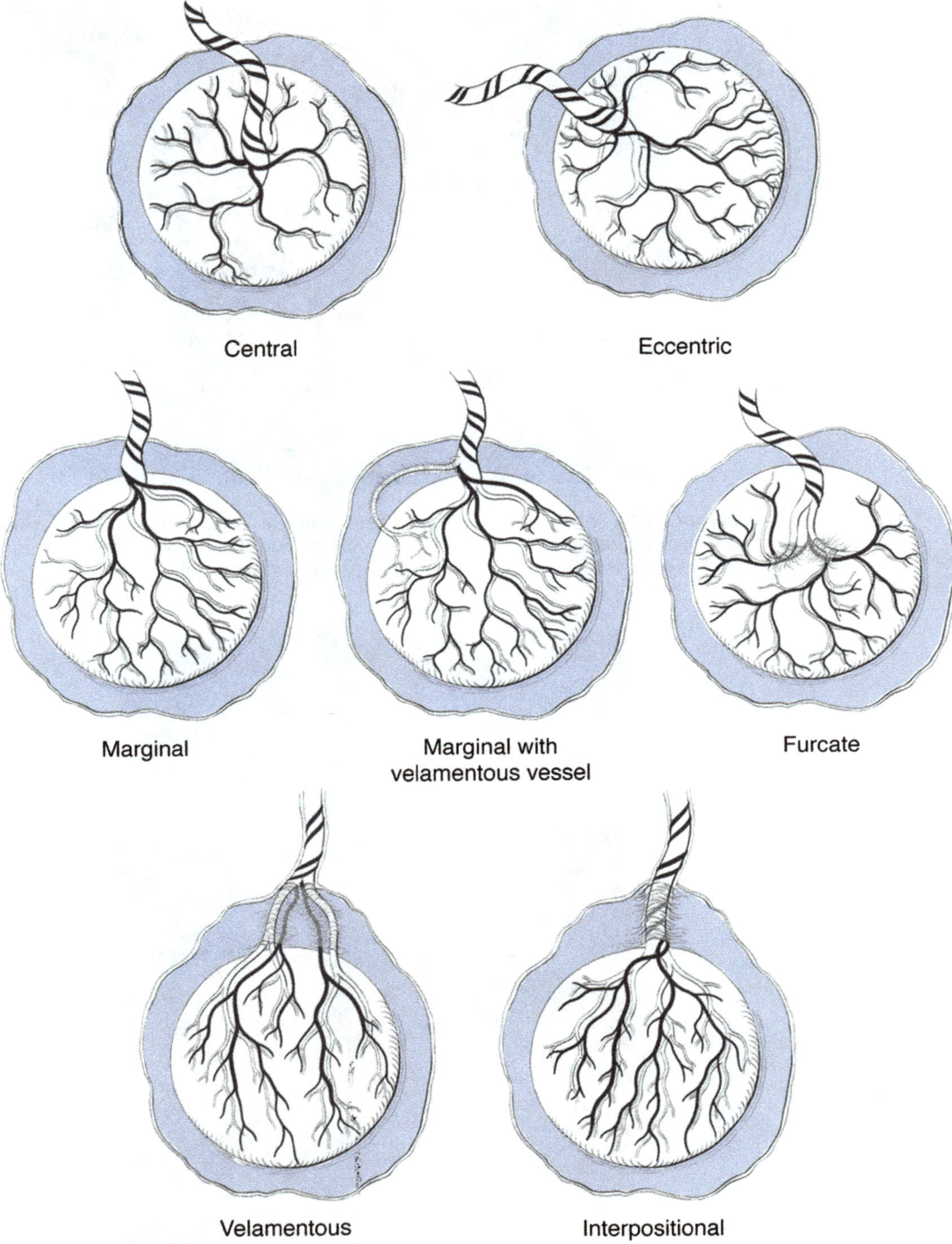

Figure 15.17. Umbilical cord insertion patterns.

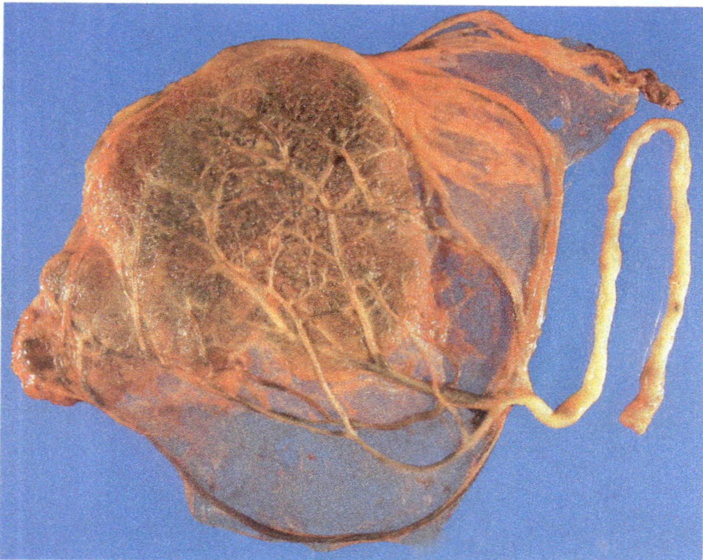

Figure 15.18. Velamentous insertion of umbilical cord. Note that the cord inserts relatively close to the placental margin but the course of the velamentous vessels is long as they branch out around the placental disk.

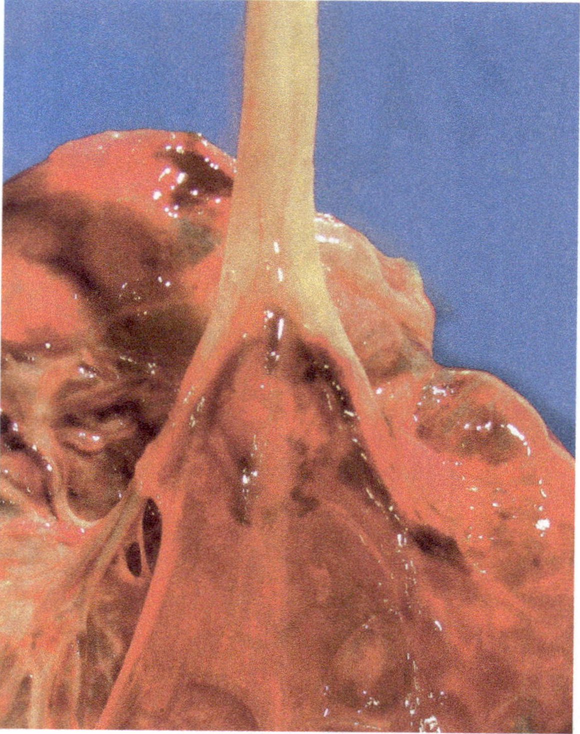

Figure 15.19. Furcate insertion of the umbilical cord. Note that the individual umbilical vessels are visible and have lost some protection of Wharton's jelly as they insert onto the placental surface.

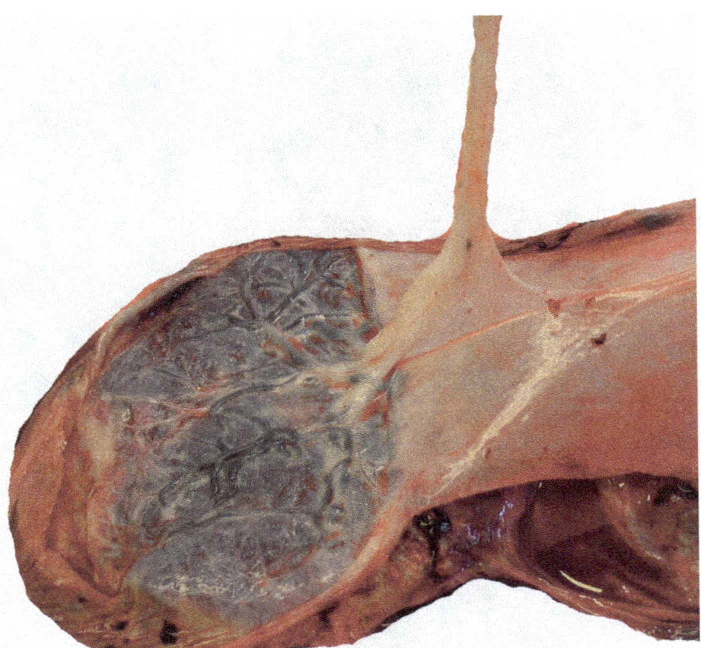

Figure 15.20. Interpositional insertion of umbilical cord. Note that the cord inserts into the membranes, running briefly within the membranes before inserting onto the placental surface. It is clear that the membranous portion of the cord has not lost the protection of Wharton's jelly.

pointed out though, that a membranous course of fetal blood vessels is not reserved to a velamentous insertion of the cord. Quite often there are such membranous vessels issuing from marginally inserted cords or in between multiple placental lobes, and they have the same potential consequences. In multiple gestations, the velamentous cord insertion often arises in the dividing membranes and the membranous vessels are then similarly prone to thrombosis and disruption.

Thrombosis of the velamentous arteries and veins may be seen in this insertional anomaly (Fig. 15.21) and presumably occurs from compression of these easily distensible vessels. Thrombosis may not be limited to the umbilical cord but may also be present in chorionic vessels. *Hemorrhage* can arise due to rupture of the velamentous vessels, most commonly the veins, and is the most frequent complication of membranous vessels (Fig. 15.22). Although hemorrhage may develop during labor and delivery due to increased forces and stress on the vessels during this time, it may commence before labor has even begun. Here, one may find *numerous hemosiderin-laden macrophages derived from the hemolysis of extravasated blood, deposited around the disrupted or thrombosed vessel*. A specific clinical situation occurs when velamentous vessels course over the cervical os, preceding the presenting fetal part, and this is called **vasa previa**. The consequences are quite dire in that the vessels may rupture during a vaginal delivery and lead to exsanguination of the fetus. Recognition of this condition is therefore crucial in preventing this outcome.

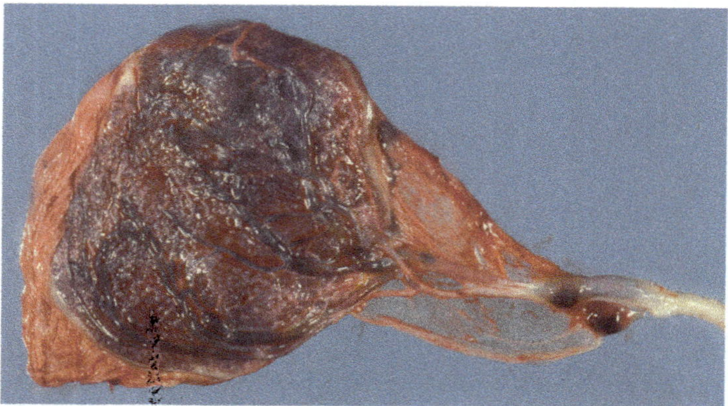

Figure 15.21. Placenta with velamentous cord insertion and thrombosis of velamentous vessels seen at the *right*.

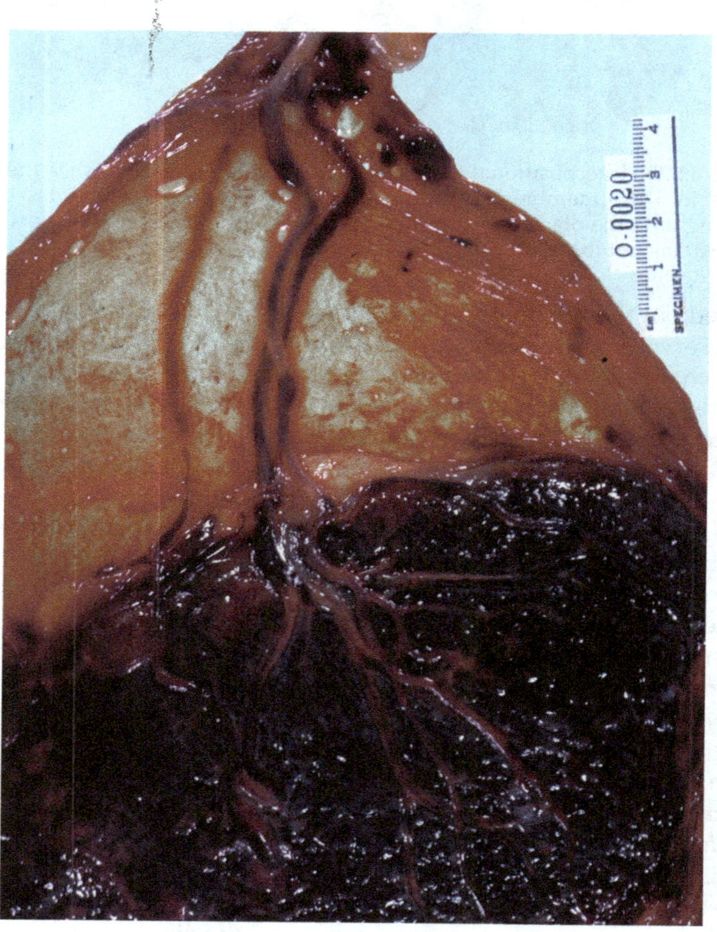

Figure 15.22. Recent hemorrhage in the membranes from rupture of a velamentous vessel. Note discoloration of membranes in area of hemorrhage.

Pathogenesis

Two mutually contradictory theories have been put forward to explain marginal and velamentous cord insertions as well as abnormal placental shapes. These are the **abnormal primary implantation** ("polarity theory"), and **trophotropism**. The abnormal implantation theory postulates that, at the nidation of the blastocyst, the embryo does not face the endometrium; rather, it is located at the opposite side, or obliquely oriented. Thus, when the early umbilical cord develops, it has to seek its connection with the future area of placentation by extending its vessels from the embryo to the base of implantation. Eventually, the vessels must become membranous in location. However, virtually all early embryos studied that have been described with this problem have had a "normal" endometrial position. The second theory of **trophotropism** postulates that the placenta grows in areas in which there is good blood supply and nutrition and atrophies in areas where there is not. This theory is favored for the following reasons. Serial ultrasonograms during early pregnancy show that the placenta actually changes location during gestation. This placental "movement" is accomplished through *marginal atrophy on one side and growth and expansion on the other*. In abnormal cord insertions, atrophy near the cord insertion with growth and expansion of the opposite site results in the cord insertion *being left behind in the membranes*. Lesser degrees would result in a marginal insertion. Trophotropism also plays a role in the development of abnormal placental shapes (see Chap. 13). In both abnormal cord insertions and abnormal placental shapes, areas of infarction and/or atrophy are quite common, lending additional support for this theory.

Clinical Features and Implications

Velamentous and marginal cord insertions are found relatively frequently in early abortions and are highly correlated with *congenital anomalies*. One of most serious complications of velamentous vessels is **vasa previa** in which membranous vessels are present over the internal cervical os. In this situation, membranous vessels may be disrupted by the exiting fetal head or by the obstetrical attendant who ruptures the membranes (Fig. 15.22). *Exsanguination* from ruptured membranous vessels can proceed within minutes. The frequency of hemorrhage is difficult to assess but has been estimated to be 1 in 50 cases of velamentous insertions. However, the mortality rate from intrapartum rupture and hemorrhage is high and estimated to be around 58% overall and 73% when the hemorrhage occurs before delivery. Velamentous vessels are also more susceptible to compression by fetal parts, resulting in obstruction of blood flow. Clinical associations of velamentous insertion therefore include *fetal distress, low Apgar scores, neonatal thrombocytopenia, fetal growth restriction, prematurity, growth restriction, cerebral palsy, and death*. Marginal insertions do not have the same sequelae as velamentous insertion, unless membranous vessels are present.

Furcate Cord Insertion

Furcate cord insertion is a rare abnormality in which the *umbilical vessels split and separate from the cord substance prior to reaching the surface* *of the placenta* (Figs. 15.17 and 15.19). They may lose the protection afforded by Wharton's jelly and are thus *prone to thrombosis and injury,* but in many cases Wharton's jelly is still present. There is much confusion between furcate and velamentous insertions, which have many features in common. *Stillbirth, fatal hemorrhage, varices, thrombosis of fetal vessels, and intrauterine growth restriction* have all been described in association with furcate cord insertion but less commonly than with velamentous insertion and most infants are normal.

Interpositional Cord Insertion

Interpositional insertion is also a type of membranous insertion. Here, the cord inserts in the membranes but unlike velamentous insertion, *the vessels do not lose the protection of Wharton's jelly* (Figs. 15.17 and 15.20). The cord does not divide but actually runs within the membranes. Interpositional insertion therefore does not have the same clinical consequences as velamentous insertion.

Suggestions for Examination and Report
(Abnormal Cord Insertion)

Gross Examination: In velamentous insertion, the distance from insertion to the placental margin should be measured and the membranous vessels evaluated for rupture, hemorrhage, or thrombosis. It is recommended that membranous vessels be rolled with the fetal membranes and submitted as a separate section. Photographs of the intact specimen should be considered, particularly in cases of poor outcome. If there is a history of vasa previa, particular care should be taken in evaluating the presence of blood within the membranes, as rupture of a velamentous vessel may be difficult to identify on gross examination.

Comment: If there is rupture or thrombosis of velamentous vessels, the possibility of fetal hemorrhage should be mentioned and correlated with the clinical history.

Single Umbilical Artery

Pathologic Features
Single umbilical artery (SUA) is the commonest congenital anomaly of humans (Fig. 15.23a). It has an incidence of 0.5–1% in singletons and 8.8% in twins. It can now be detected prenatally by ultrasonography and should always be ascertained at birth. A remnant of the second umbilical artery can sometimes be identified on microscopic examination (Fig. 15.23b). *It must be cautioned that SUA may be found at one end of the cord and not the other.* At times, the arteries fuse far above the cord insertion on the placenta in a manner that is similar to their normal communication near the placenta. These are called Hyrtl's anastomoses, and occasionally this communication is many centimeters from the cord insertion onto the placenta. Therefore, documentation of a SUA should include sections from the fetal end of the cord.

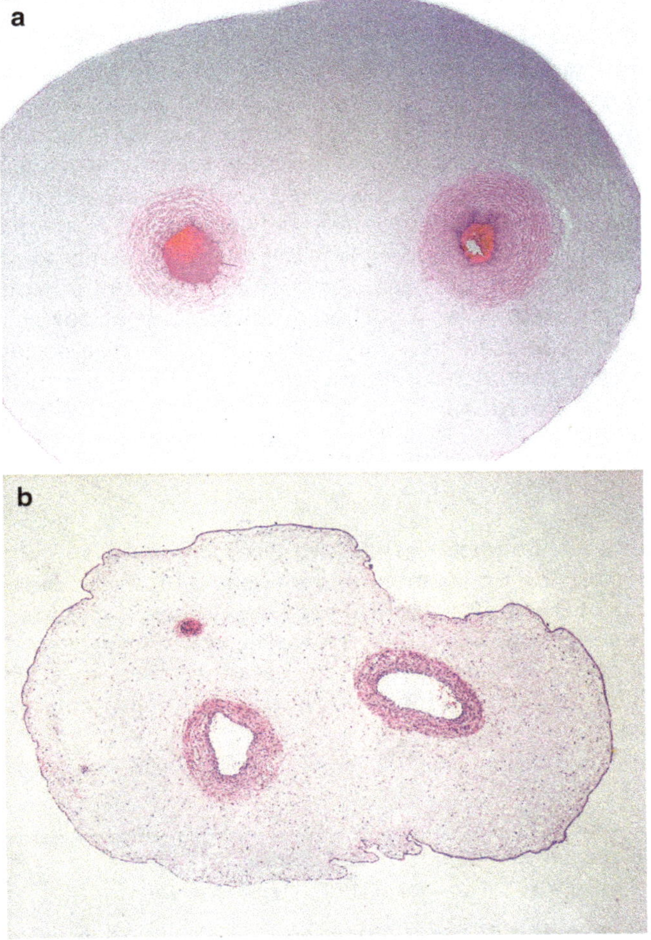

Figure 15.23. (a) Umbilical cord with SUA. There is no evidence of the second umbilical artery. H&E ×10. (b) Umbilical cord with SUA in which the muscular remnant of a "vanished" second umbilical artery can be seen on the *upper left*. H&E ×10.

Clinical Features and Implications

SUA has been associated with *growth restriction, maternal diabetes, antepartum hemorrhage, polyhydramnios, and oligohydramnios.* Cord accidents are also more common in these cords. Congenital anomalies are present in 30–44.7% of infants in autopsy studies, and other placental abnormalities are found in 16.4%. Since *renal anomalies* are relatively frequent with an incidence of 18.5%, neonatal renal sonography is often recommended when SUA is found. Hollow organ anomalies, such as *intestinal atresia,* are also relatively frequent in these infants. An isolated SUA (without other sonographic anomalies) overall does not usually affect outcome and is often found in perfectly health infants. To be sure, the pediatrician should be notified of its existence in order to perform a more detailed physical examination to ensure that the infant has no hidden anomalies.

Pathogenesis

In 73% of cases, the defect locates to the left artery. Cytogenetic and complex anomalies are associated nearly exclusively with the left-sided absence. *Absence of one umbilical artery may occur as aplasia or as the consequence of atrophy of one artery.* The latter mechanism is probably more frequent and can be seen to have occurred in many specimens when histologic examination is undertaken and incomplete atrophy is present (Fig. 15.23b). Atrophy occasionally occurs late in pregnancy but when it takes place long before birth, the arterial lumen gradually vanishes, and only a tiny muscular remnant may remain. In some cases, atrophy of an artery when a portion of the placenta atrophies and one umbilical artery loses its "territory." Thus, SUA may be associated with trophotropism and therefore with placental shape aberrations and abnormal cord insertions.

Supernumerary Vessels

More than three umbilical vessels are normal for many species, but are *rare in humans.* The right umbilical vein usually does not develop, but **persistence of the right umbilical vein** has been reported to be associated with congenital anomalies. However, considering its rarity, one must take care, when assessing an increased number of vessels, not to be misled by the frequent looping that occurs in many cord vessels or by false knots.

Suggestions for Examination and Report
(Single Umbilical Artery and Persistence of the Right Umbilical Vein)

Gross Examination: Several cross sections of the cord must be examined to ensure that the correct number of vessels is documented. Sections away from the insertion site are recommended, as these may show only one artery due to anastomoses or may show more vessels due to false knots.

Comment: Single umbilical artery and persistence of the right umbilical vein are both associated with an increased risk of congenital anomalies. Therefore, although the majority of these infants are normal, evaluation for anomalies may be suggested.

Thrombosis of Umbilical Vessels

Pathologic Features

The incidence of **umbilical vessel thrombosis** is 1 in 1,300 deliveries, 1 in 1,000 perinatal autopsies, and 1 in 250 high-risk gestations. *Venous thromboses are more common than arterial thromboses, but the latter are more often lethal.* Thrombi in the branches of the umbilical vessels in the chorionic plate are much more common than thrombi in the umbilical cord, but are often associated with these same underlying etiologies (see Chap. 21). Grossly identifiable thrombi may show slight swelling and discoloration of the entire cord and may be directly visible on cut section (Fig. 15.24a). Microscopically, they show a typical configuration with organizing fibrin and clot within the lumen (Fig. 15.24b). Old thrombi in umbilical vessels, primarily the vein, may calcify, and occasionally massive calcification has made it difficult to ligate the cord at delivery.

Pathogenesis

Thrombosis in umbilical vessels most frequently occur near term. They may develop due to velamentous insertion, inflammation (funisitis), varices, entanglement, knotting, torsion, abnormal coiling, amnionic bands, maternal diabetes, and funipuncture. Coagulation problems caused by thrombophilias of mother or infant are sometimes the cause. The formation of thrombi with velamentous insertion

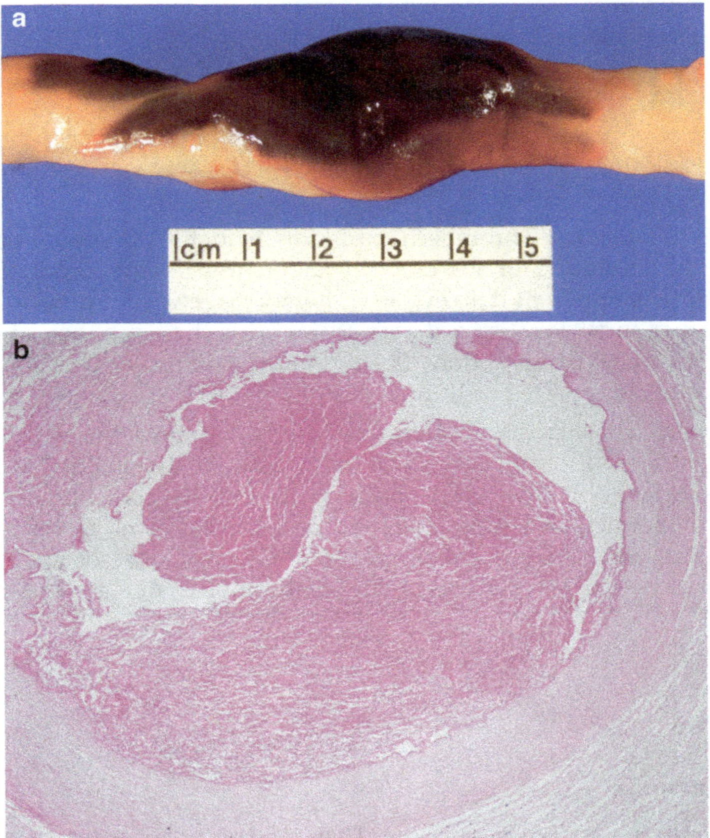

Figure 15.24. (a) Gross photograph of a thrombus in an umbilical vessel. Note that the discoloration and fusiform shape is similar to that seen in a hematoma (see Fig. 15.26), but on cross section a dilated thrombosed vessel was identified. (b) Microscopic view of the umbilical cord in (a). There is a nearly occlusive thrombus present within the umbilical vein. H&E ×20.

of the cord is readily understandable as is thrombosis that may occur in varices, from knotting as well as the entangling of cords in monoamnionic twins (see Chap. 10). Physical compression of umbilical vessels and/or damage to vessel walls is usually the primary cause, but it is a hypercoagulable state in thrombophilias and maternal diabetes.

Clinical Features and Implications

Thrombosis can compromise the circulation and lead to *growth restriction, fetal death, or neurologic injury*. This is particularly true of thrombosis in umbilical vessels as these are the main supply conduits of blood for the fetus. Thrombi may also break off and potentially *embolize to the fetus* or to the placenta, where they may cause infarction of various tissues or systemic thrombosis. More remarkable are the thrombi that occur in the absence of all of these more readily understood complications, and they are perhaps the most common. Very frequently thromboses of vessels in the cord are associated with similar events in the villous ramifications (see Chap. 21). Thrombosis due to coagulation defects has been associated with extensive CNS lesions in the infants as well as stroke and neonatal thrombosis.

Suggestions for Examination and Report
(Thrombosis of Umbilical Vessels)

Gross Examination: Thrombi that are grossly identified should obviously be submitted for microscopic examination. As the cord is often multiply clamped at delivery, local hemorrhage is common, so the examiner must take special care to look for the serrations of the clamp when taking sections from hemorrhagic areas. This should not be misinterpreted as thrombosis.

Comment: Thrombosis of umbilical vessels may be associated with compression of umbilical vessels from cord entanglements, knots, hypercoiling, or other cord problems as well as from underlying coagulopathies, and some maternal or fetal disorders. If there are cord abnormalities present or a clinical history of an associated disorder, these can be correlated with the thrombosis in a comment.

Tumors

Hemangiomas

Angiomas are benign neoplasms. They tend to occur at the placental end of the cord and arise from one or more umbilical vessels. Unlike chorangiomas that occur in the villous tissue (see Chap. 22), they are not usually associated with hydramnios. The neoplasms may attain a large size, up to 18 cm in length and 14 cm in diameter, with weights up to 900 g. They have a fairly uniform histologic appearance (Fig. 15.25),

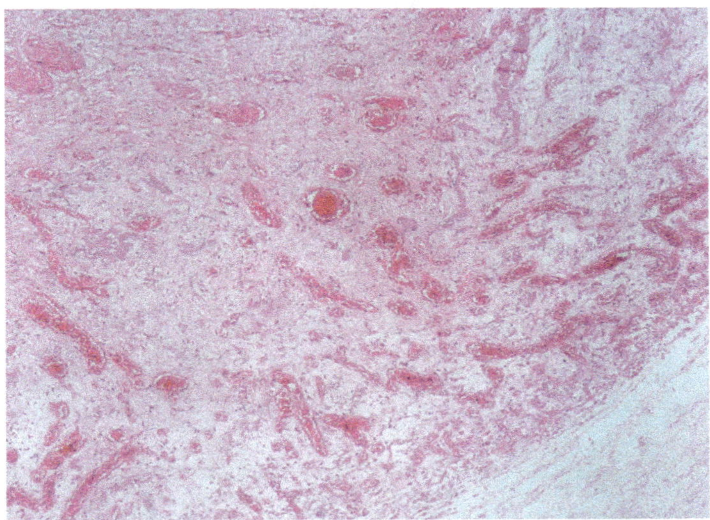

Figure 15.25. Histologic appearance of a hemangioma of the umbilical cord. H&E ×40.

consisting of a *proliferation of small capillaries in a loose connective tissue stroma. Some have myxoma-like stroma and are then called angiomyoxomas;* however, some have referred to these as hamartomas. Hemangiomas may be associated with *fetal hemorrhage, high output cardiac failure, elevated maternal α-fetoprotein (AFP) levels, disseminated intravascular coagulation, fetal hemangiomas, fetal anomalies, and fetal death.*

Teratomas

Teratomas are much less common than angiomas and in fact are very rare. There is some controversy about the diagnosis of these lesions and their differentiation from acardiac twins (see Chap. 10). If the lesion does not contain axial skeleton or umbilical cord, it likely represents a true tumor. As with other teratomas *skin, connective tissue, and various other tissues* such as colonic or respiratory epithelium are often present.

Miscellaneous Cord Lesions

Hemorrhages and **hematomas** of the umbilical cord are relatively rare. They have serious consequences as the fetus may *exsanguinate or sustain significant neurologic injury from compression of umbilical vessels.* A 50% fetal mortality has been reported (Fig. 15.26). Cord hematomas occur due to rupture of one or more umbilical vessels and underlying etiologies include with *short cords, trauma (amniocentesis, cordocentesis), aneurysms, hemangiomas, and cord entanglement.* At times there are associated thrombi. Grossly they appear as fusiform swelling of the cord with marked discoloration due to the extravasated blood. Cord rupture may also occur with dire consequences (Fig. 15.27).

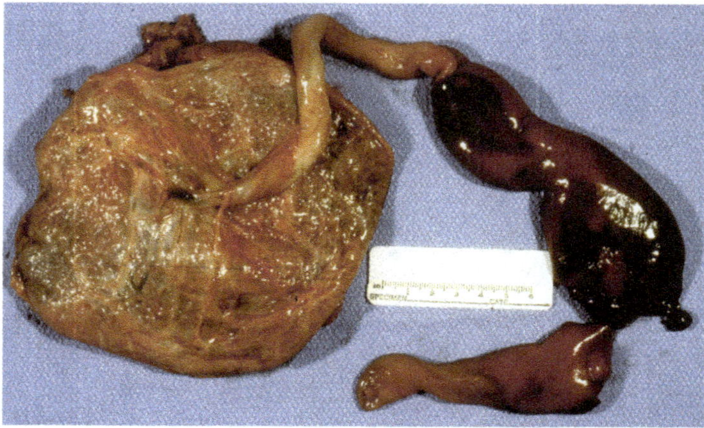

Figure 15.26. Umbilical cord with hematoma and rupture resulting in an intrapartum fetal death. The cord shows marked discoloration and hemorrhage with a somewhat fusiform shape due to accumulation of blood in Wharton's jelly.

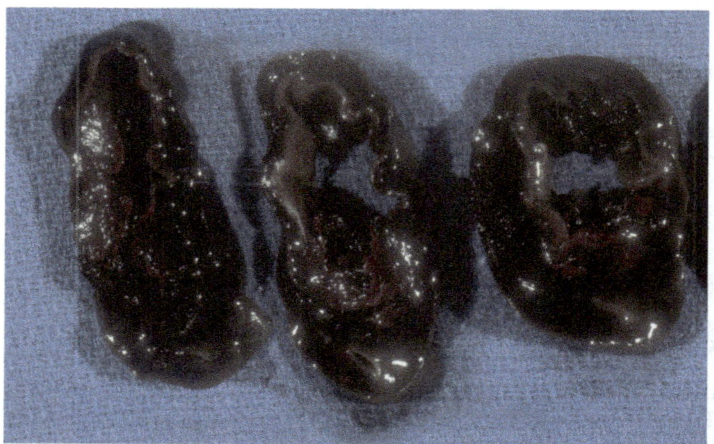

Figure 15.27. Cut sections of the umbilical cord seen in Fig. 15.26. Note that there is extensive hemorrhage throughout Wharton's jelly and the umbilical vein is thin and ruptured (*lower left* and *upper right*).

False knots, or vascular redundancies, previously discussed, may sometimes be confused with varicosities in the umbilical cord. Real **varix** formations are rare (Fig. 15.28) and show *marked, focal thinning of the wall of the umbilical vein that may be associated with muscle necrosis.* Fetal death may occur from *fetal hemorrhage or compression of the aneurysmally dilated veins* (Fig. 15.29). When elastic stains are done on such cords, it has been repeatedly found that the elastic fibers of the vein are focally deficient.

The umbilical cord may **rupture**, either completely or partially (Figs. 15.26 and 15.27). This will inevitably lead to bleeding and often results in cord *hematomas.* Excessively *short cords* may rupture during descent, but *velamentous cord insertion* is the most frequent antecedent

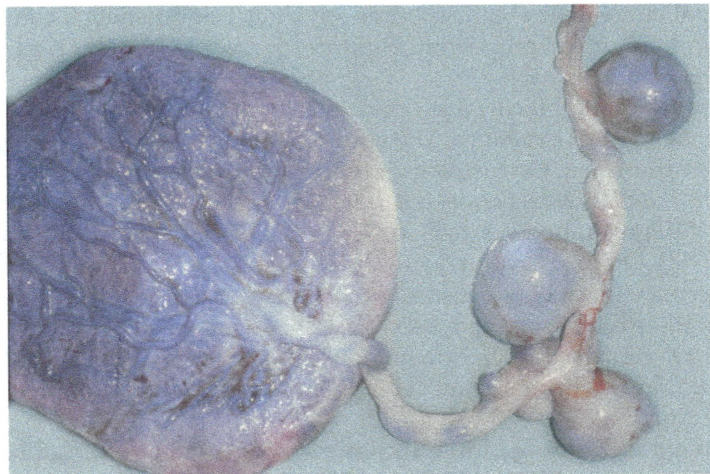

Figure 15.28. Unusual placenta with multiple varices of the umbilical vein.

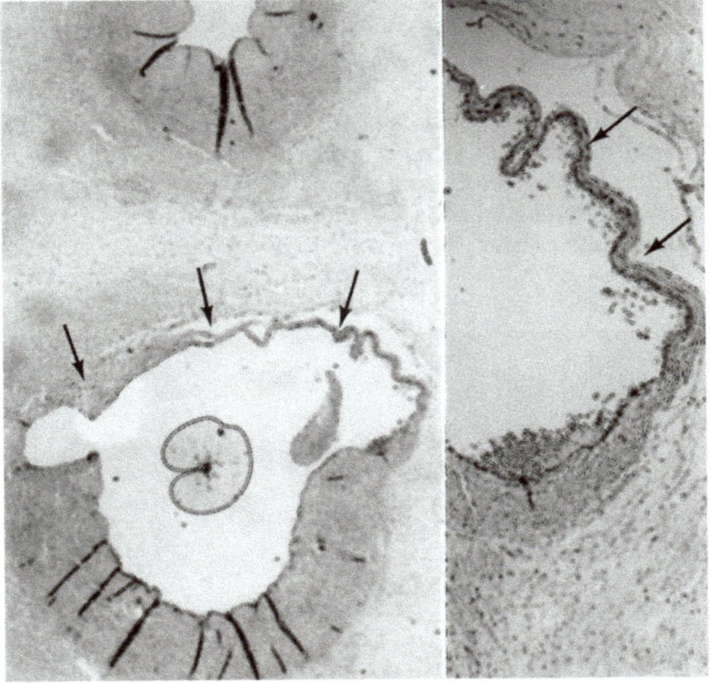

Figure 15.29. Aneurysmal dilatation of the umbilical vein with fatal compression of arteries. No cause was identified for this lesion.

of this complication. Rupture is associated with the some of same underlying causes as hematoma, and includes *varices, cord entanglement, trauma from amniocentesis or therapeutic intrauterine transfusion, and severe acute funisitis.* If rupture occurs, it is most often at the site of its placental attachment, but can occur anywhere. Spontaneous complete rupture is an uncommon event; *most ruptures are partial and cause local hematomas or hemorrhage.*

Necrosis of umbilical vessel walls may result from chronic and severe **meconium exposure**. The cord will usually be discolored green or greenish-brown. On histologic section one sees *rounded, degenerating myocytes with loss of nuclei and cell death* (see Fig. 14.17 in Chap. 14). Such areas of degeneration not only occur in the vein but may affect arteries as well. On occasion, they are the sequelae of thrombosis, but they may occur without it. Necrosis of umbilical arteries and a linear **ulceration** of Wharton's jelly have been described associated with intestinal atresia. Obviously, this leads to hemorrhage into the umbilical cord and amniotic fluid with resultant fetal anemia and the potential for fetal exsanguination.

Segmental thinning of umbilical vessels has also been described as a focal thinning of the vessel wall with virtual absence of the vascular media. It is seen predominantly in the umbilical vein (Fig. 15.30) and has been associated with congenital malformations and fetal distress.

Squamous metaplasia of the amnionic epithelium covering the umbilical cord may occur as it does in the fetal membranes. These may grossly visible as *irregular, white, hydrophobic patches on the surface of cord.* Microscopically, *keratinizing squamous epithelium* partially replaces the more usual cuboidal epithelium. These plaques may be confused with the surface nodules present in *Candida* infection. In the latter situation, the nodules tend to be *slightly elevated, more circumscribed, round, and may be white to yellow in color* (see Chap. 16). Finally, the cord may show various **discolorations** similar to those seen in the fetal membranes (see Chap. 14). Green discoloration may be present in meconium exposure, brown

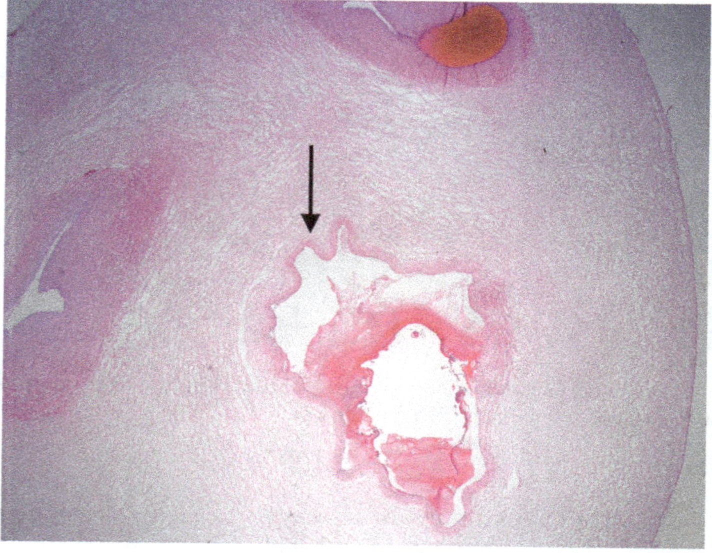

Figure 15.30. Segmental thinning of the umbilical vein (*arrows*). No cause was apparent. H&E ×40.

discoloration is usually due to hemosiderin from old hemorrhage, yellow discoloration from maternal bilirubinemia, and red-brown discoloration is usually secondary to **hemolysis** after fetal death.

Suggestions for Examination and Report
(Hemangioma, Hematoma, Hemorrhage, Varices, and Rupture)

Gross Examination: Any time a hemorrhagic lesion of the cord is identified, multiple serial sections should be cut to determine the underlying cause. If this is not readily apparent, serial sections of the entire lesion should be submitted. Care must be taken in avoiding areas of cord clamping.

Comment: If there is extensive hemorrhage in the cord, compression of umbilical vessels may occur, leading to significant embarrassment of blood flow to the fetus, with potentially dire consequences. Correlation with outcome, fetal hematocrit, etc. is suggested if this information is available.

Selected References

PHP5, pages 380–451 (Anatomy and Pathology of the Umbilical Cord).

Baergen RN, Malicki D, Behling CA, Benirschke K. Morbidity, mortality and placental pathology in excessively long umbilical cords. Pediatr Dev Pathol 2001;4:144–153.

Bendon RW, Tyson RW, Baldwin VJ, et al. Umbilical cord ulceration and intestinal atresia: a new association? Am J Obstet Gynecol 1991;164:582–586.

Benirschke K. Obstetrically important lesions of the umbilical cord. J Reprod Med 1994;39:262–272.

Benirschke K, Bourne GL. The incidence and prognostic implication of congenital absence of one umbilical artery. Am J Obstet Gynecol 1960;79:251–254.

deLaat MW, Franx A, van Alderen ED, Nikkels PG, Visser GH. The umbilical coiling index, a review of the literature. J Matern Fetal Neonatal Med 2005;17:93–100.

Heifetz SA. Single umbilical artery: a statistical analysis of 237 autopsy cases and review of the literature. Perspect Pediatr Pathol 1984;8:345–378.

Heifetz SA. Thrombosis of the umbilical cord: analysis of 52 cases and literature review. Pediatr Pathol 1988;8:37–54.

Heifetz SA, Rueda-Pedraza ME. Hemangiomas of the umbilical cord. Pediatr Pathol 1983;1:385–398.

Jauniaux E, De Munter C, Vanesse M, et al. Embryonic remnants of the umbilical cord: morphologic and clinical aspects. Hum Pathol 1989;20:458–462.

Lacro RV, Jones KL, Benirschke K. The umbilical cord twist: origin, direction, and relevance. Am J Obstet Gynecol 1987;157:833–838.

Naeye RL. Umbilical cord length: clinical significance. J Pediatr 1985;107:278–281.

Qureshi F, Jacques SM. Marked segmental thinning of the umbilical cord vessels. Arch Pathol Lab Med 1994;118:826–830.

Sun Y, Arbuckle S, Hocking G, et al. Umbilical cord stricture and intrauterine fetal death. Pediatr Pathol Lab Med 1995;15:723–732.

Tantbirojn P, Saleemuddin A, Sirois K, Crum CP, Boyd TK, Tworoger S, Parast MM. Gross abnormalities of the umbilical cord: related placental histology and clinical significance. Placenta 2009;30:1083–1088.

Section V

Disease Processes and the Placenta

This section is concerned with diseases or disease processes that affect the placenta and includes both maternal and fetal conditions. Chapter 16 discusses infections, such as acute chorioamnionitis, ascending infection, chronic villitis, and chronic intervillositis, and also discusses causative organisms. Chapter 17 covers maternal diseases and the various drugs and physical agents that may affect the placenta. There are numerous maternal diseases that complicate pregnancy, but only the most important or prevalent of those that affect placental function are covered here. Because of their particular importance, preeclampsia, systemic lupus erythematosus, and thrombophilia are discussed separately in Chap. 18. Chapter 19 presents a miscellaneous group of placental lesions, some of which are associated with maternal or fetal disease. However, these lesions either do not have one specific etiology, or the etiology is unknown and so they do not fit easily in other chapters. Therefore, they are placed in this chapter for convenience. The final two chapters discuss fetal conditions. Placental changes in hydrops, fetomaternal hemorrhage, and metabolic disorders are covered in Chap. 20, while fetal thrombotic lesions and fetal thrombotic vasculopathy are discussed in Chap. 21.

Chapter 16

Infectious Diseases

General Considerations

The pathogenesis of prenatal infections and related circumstances must be understood if the associated pathological lesions are to be interpreted correctly. Infections may reach the placenta and fetus in several ways (Fig. 16.1):

- By **ascension** from through endocervical canal
- By **hematogenous transmission** from maternal blood

R.N. Baergen, *Manual of Pathology of the Human Placenta,*
DOI 10.1007/978-1-4419-7494-5_16, © Springer Science+Business Media, LLC 2011

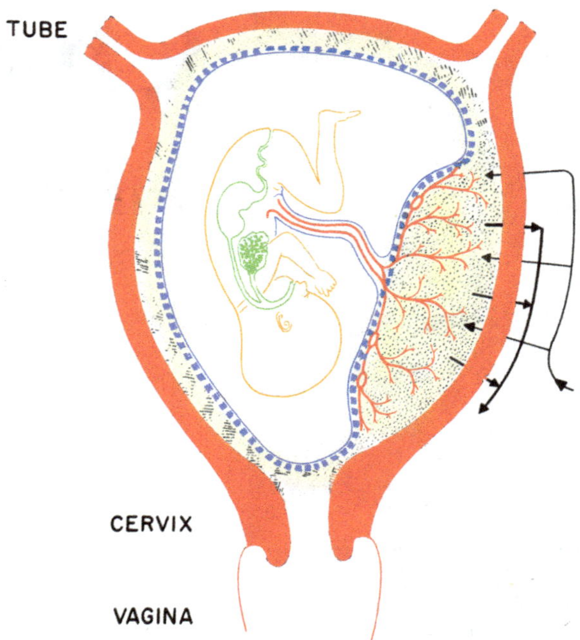

Figure 16.1. Intrauterine position of fetus and placenta. Infectious organisms ascend through the endocervical canal. They first infect the membranes covering the internal os and then penetrate the amniotic cavity.

- By **direct introduction** via amniocentesis, chorionic villus sampling, amnioscopy, percutaneous umbilical blood sampling, or intrauterine fetal transfusion
- By **direct extension** from infection in the endometrium

The majority of infections arise by one of the first two methods, and they will be the focus of this chapter. Ascending infections in particular are the most common type of infections involving the placenta.

Ascending Infection and Acute Chorioamnionitis

Acute chorioamnionitis is common, with an incidence of 20–24% of live births and up to 67% of preterm deliveries. It is an important cause of *preterm labor* and *preterm deliveries*, which in turn are significant causes of perinatal morbidity and mortality. Acute chorioamnionitis has also recently been implicated in the development of *lung disease, poor long-term neurologic outcome, and cerebral palsy.*

Pathogenesis
Ascending infection, also called "amniotic sac infection syndrome," develops from *an infection that commences in the vagina and endocervix and then ascends to the uterine cavity* (Fig. 16.1). Acute chorioamnionitis, when properly defined, is *always* due to infection, and the

ascending nature of this infection is supported by three pathological findings:

- It is usually associated with severe acute deciduitis.
- In twin gestations, it is invariably the lower twin that has chorioamnionitis or whose membranes are more severely inflamed.
- The point of spontaneous membrane rupture, which is in proximity to the cervical os, has the most severe inflammation.

It is often stated that infection occurs secondary to membrane rupture but in actuality, *it is the loss of membrane integrity resulting from inflammation that makes rupture a probability.* In fact, ascending infection occurs most often in the **presence of intact fetal membranes.** Furthermore, it is now the predominant opinion that *amniotic sac infection is the primary cause of premature labor and delivery,* at least in those pregnancies that terminate spontaneously before 30 weeks' gestation. In approximately 72% of patients with preterm labor, bacteria can be cultured from the amniotic fluid. It is interesting to note that antimicrobial therapy usually fails to prolong pregnancy when chorioamnionitis is already extant.

Acute Chorioamnionitis and Preterm Delivery

Causes or associations of preterm labor include *intrauterine infection (acute chorioamnionitis), maternal smoking, poor maternal nutrition, maternal drug use such as alcohol or cocaine, young maternal age, prior cervical surgery, and cervical incompetence.* Maternal disorders such as preeclampsia and hypertensive disease may also lead to preterm birth iatrogenically, as delivery must be accomplished prematurely due to maternal indications. It has also been suggested that *intercourse during late pregnancy* may initiate premature delivery, but this is still controversial. There is now a very large body of investigation *incriminating inflammatory mediators in the initiation of labor during the process of ascending infection.* Interleukin-1 (IL-1), IL-6, and IL-8 are elevated in the amniotic fluid and cord blood in the presence of an ascending infection. Tumor necrosis factor (TNF) activates the cytokine machinery and may well be at the starting point of labor initiation by stimulating prostaglandin production from the decidua. Deciduitis, decidual macrophage activation, and neutrophils exudation, in particular, play an important role in the initiation of premature labor. However, the precise chemical cascade that ultimately leads to myometrial contractions is not yet elucidated. Suffice it to say that the cytokine system is intimately involved in premature labor when it is caused by infection.

Incompetent Cervix

It has been suggested that 1% of pregnancies and up to 20% of midtrimester abortions result from an **"incompetent cervix."** It is clinically defined as painless cervical dilatation occurring preterm and is thought to most commonly develop secondary to previous surgery or abnormal cervical development. Thus, a truly incompetent cervix is an *anatomical defect* that develops due to *congenital anomalies or trauma.* Trauma, specifically a history of previous surgery, is the most common antecedent. In a study of cervical laser conizations, the frequency of premature births increased from 6 to 38%. However, in the majority of cases of preterm labor, the cervix is anatomically normal and is *affected by severe chronic cervicitis, causing the cervix to be patulous and prone to premature dilatation.* Often, an incompetent cervix is diagnosed, the pregnancy delivers prematurely and the histology shows a significant acute chorioamnionitis. In these cases, the painless cervical dilatation is most likely *not* due to an "incompetence" of the cervix but rather due to underlying ascending infection. This underlying inflammation may be associated, if not due to, deficient endocervical mucus production.

"Clinical" Acute Chorioamnionitis

Making the diagnosis of **"clinical" chorioamnionitis** is problematic as only some gravidas with amniotic sac infection show clinical evidence of infection. Histologic chorioamnionitis must be considered the gold standard for the diagnosis of chorioamnionitis and ascending infection. Clinical chorioamnionitis is usually based on manifestations of local or systemic inflammation including *fever, leukocytosis, uterine tenderness, foul-smelling vaginal discharge, and maternal or fetal tachycardia.* Indeed, close to 75% of women with histologic acute chorioamnionitis do not fulfill the criteria for clinical chorioamnionitis, and many have no symptoms at all; many women with some symptoms of "clinical chorioamnionitis" ultimately do not have an ascending infection. On the other hand, only a minority of patients with a diagnosis of clinical chorioamnionitis ultimately show histologic chorioamnionitis. Other tests such as culture and Gram stain of the amniotic fluid, assays of the amniotic fluid for cytokines, esterase or endotoxin, and fetal fibronectin have provided better correlation with histologic chorioamnionitis than clinical evaluation. Despite these statistics, there is a significant correlation between histologic and clinical chorioamnionitis.

Pathologic Features

The pathologic features of an **ascending infection** are those of **acute chorioamnionitis**, that is, a neutrophilic inflammatory infiltrate in the amnion and chorion. Inflammatory lesions are present **only** when microbacterial contamination exists in the amniotic cavity. Typically, the fetal surface of the placenta lacks the blue sheen of the normal organ, and both *the membranes and fetal surface are white and opaque,* being obscured by the inflammatory exudate of polymorphonuclear leukocytes (PMNs) (Fig. 16.2). The surface may become *yellow or green when much leukocytic exudate has accumulated or the process has been of long duration.* The placenta is frequently malodorous, and the very astute observer may sometimes identify the prevailing organism by the odor. The fecal odor of *Fusobacterium* and *Bacteroides* infections and the sweet odor of *Clostridium* and *Listeria* infections are useful identifiers for the adept examiner. *The membranes are typically more friable, and the decidua capsularis is frequently detached and hemorrhagic.* In many cases, the membranes are incomplete and consist of mere fragments of amnion without chorion or decidua capsularis. Particularly in preterm placentas, the inflammation is often accompanied by an *acute marginal hemorrhage* that undermines the edge of the placenta. Although this mimics abruptio placentae clinically, this process (Fig. 16.3) markedly

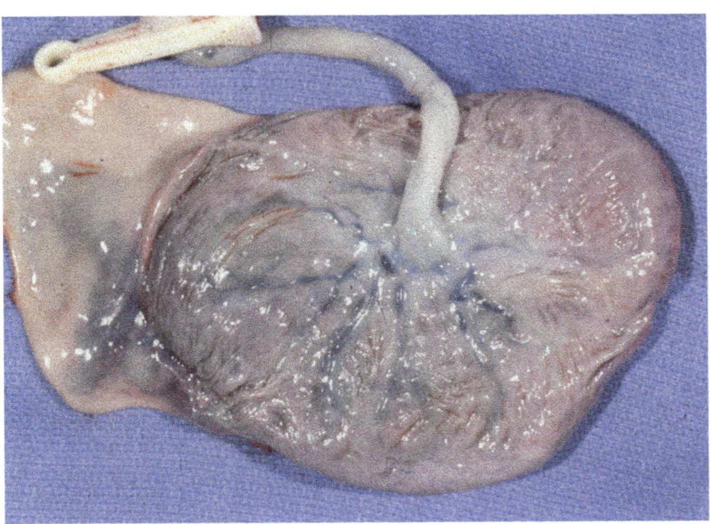

Figure 16.2. Term placenta with severe chorioamnionitis. The surface of the placenta is obscured by a whitish exudate; the vasculature is also indistinct.

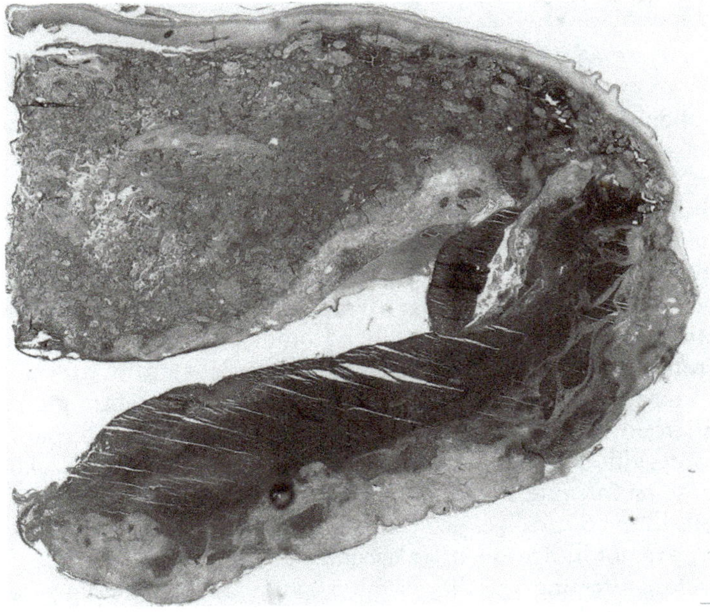

Figure 16.3. Placenta at 23 weeks' gestation with massive chorioamnionitis and marked marginal hemorrhage that undermines the placenta and originates from deciduitis and disrupted vessels. H&E ×3.5.

differs from the typical abruptio placentae as it originates from the associated acute deciduitis.

Acute chorioamnionitis, by definition, is *the presence of acute inflammatory cells, PMNs in particular, within the fetal membranes* (Fig. 16.4). Eosinophils are found at times but usually only in protracted infections.

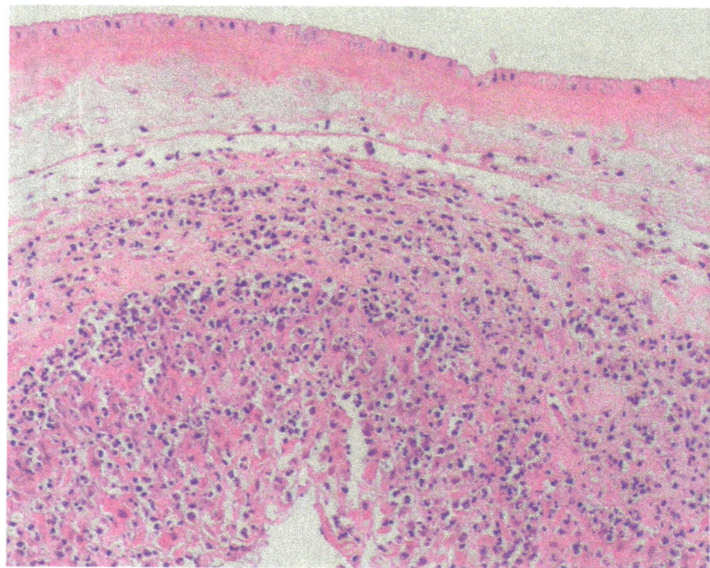

Figure 16.4. Massive chorioamnionitis in immature placenta. Exudate is present in the amnion and chorion. The placenta had a purulent surface and marked funisitis. H&E ×200.

Macrophages may participate to a variable extent. Chronic inflammatory cells, such as lymphocytes and plasma cells, are generally **not** present in acute chorioamnionitis. When present and admixed with acute inflammatory cells, the diagnosis of **subacute chorioamnionitis** is made (see below). It is important to note that initially, when bacteria enter the uterine cavity, a localized inflammation/infection occurs in the decidua capsularis and extraplacental membranes at the internal cervical os, which ultimately will become the rupture point of the membranes. The infection ascends and expands laterally up the walls of the uterine cavity as the bacteria spread into the amniotic cavity. Once there, inflammatory cells are recruited from the maternal blood in the intervillous space and migrate through the chorionic plate. At this point, an intrauterine infection is established. Similarly, inflammatory cells in the decidua capsularis, which only focally extends into the chorion, are not indicative of an ascending infection but may be due to local factors affecting viability of the decidua and is sometimes seen in cases of ruptured membranes without ascending infection.

There is a grading system for acute chorioamnionitis, the idea being that grade correlates with neonatal outcome. However, grading is not always reliable for this purpose. We believe that *the most important features of ascending infection are the infectious agent and whether there is a fetal response.* For example, *Trichomonas* can be enormously leukotactic, yet have little effect on neonatal morbidity and mortality. Conversely, *group B Streptococcus* may be associated with minimal leukocyte infiltration but have a devastating effect upon fetal and neonatal life.

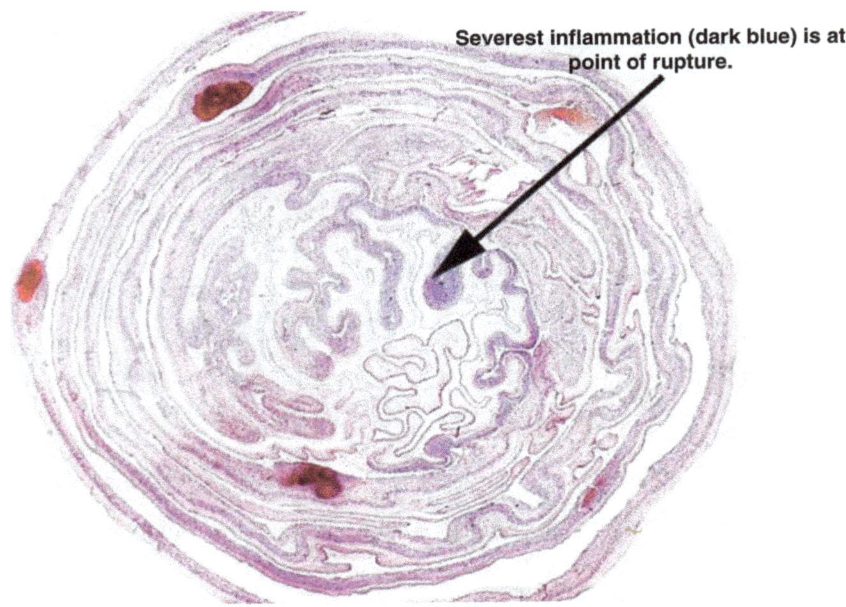

Figure 16.5. Membrane roll of placenta with chorioamnionitis. The edge of the membrane rupture is in the center and shows a dark exudate. H&E ×2.

Maternal Response, Fetal Response, and Fetal Infection
In acute chorioamnionitis, the inflammatory infiltrate may be **maternal** or **fetal** in origin. The **maternal component** of the leukocytic reaction originates in the intervillous space and in the maternal vessels of the decidua in the free membranes. The *emigration of leukocytes is always directional, toward the amniotic cavity*, presumably toward an antigenic source in the amniotic fluid. Initially, when organisms first gain access to the uterine cavity, the fetal membranes covering the internal cervical os may show an inflammatory infiltrate (Fig. 16.5). This is often accompanied by acute deciduitis (Fig. 16.6). This local phenomenon does not indicate an intra-amniotic infection is present. *The first evidence that true intra-amniotic infection has occurred is the presence of leukocytes that marginate from beneath the fibrin under the chorionic plate.* As the infection progresses, the leukocytes then infiltrate the chorion and eventually the amnion of the chorionic plate. Abscess formation underneath the chorionic plate and dissemination of exudate between villous trunks are rare events.

As the fetus normally swallows and breathes in amniotic fluid, exposure to organisms present in the amniotic fluid can occur and result in a fetal response to the infection. Fetal inflammatory *cells migrate from the umbilical vessels and the superficial fetal vessels in the chorionic plate* constituting a **fetal inflammatory response.** Fetal response, however, is rare prior to the 20th week of gestation due to immaturity of the fetal immune system. In general, **acute funisitis** occurs first, with the vein becoming involved before the arteries. The inflammatory cells migrate toward the amnionic surface, marginate first at the vascular intima, *and*

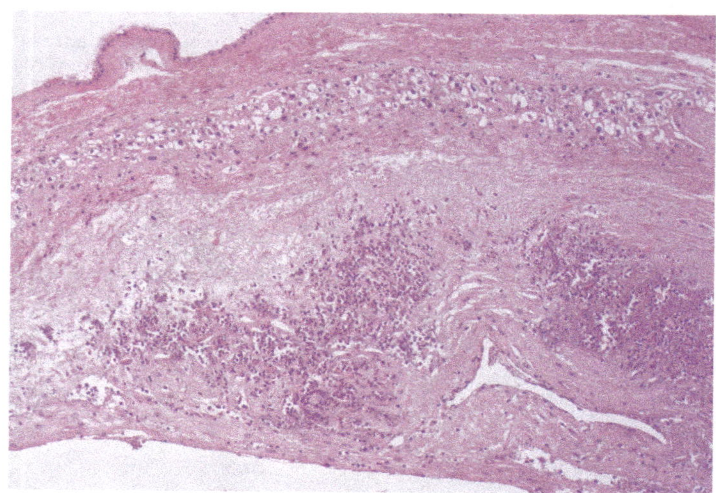

Figure 16.6. Acute deciduitis in an immature placenta. H&E ×160.

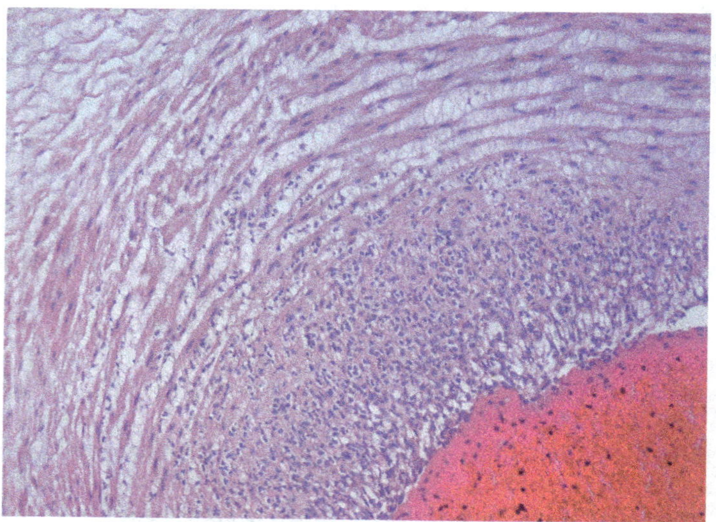

Figure 16.7. Acute funisitis involving umbilical vein. Leukocytes have penetrated between muscle fibers toward the cord surface. H&E ×100.

then begin to dissect among the muscle bundles of the umbilical vein and arteries, finally infiltrating Wharton's jelly (Figs. 16.7 and 16.8). They also reach the cord's surface and may accumulate there in substantial numbers. Funisitis does *not* signify the existence of fetal sepsis or even fetal infection. Fetal sepsis is a relatively late event in the course of an ascending bacterial infection and often results from invasion of organisms into the fetal lung, intestinal tract, and even the middle ear. *If fetal infection occurs, PMNs can be found in the lung and stomach of the neonate intermixed with squames.* Initially, this pus is likely aspirated from the amniotic fluid and not produced in the fetal lung, as only later in the infectious process can one find an inflammatory accumulation within the alveolar tissue.

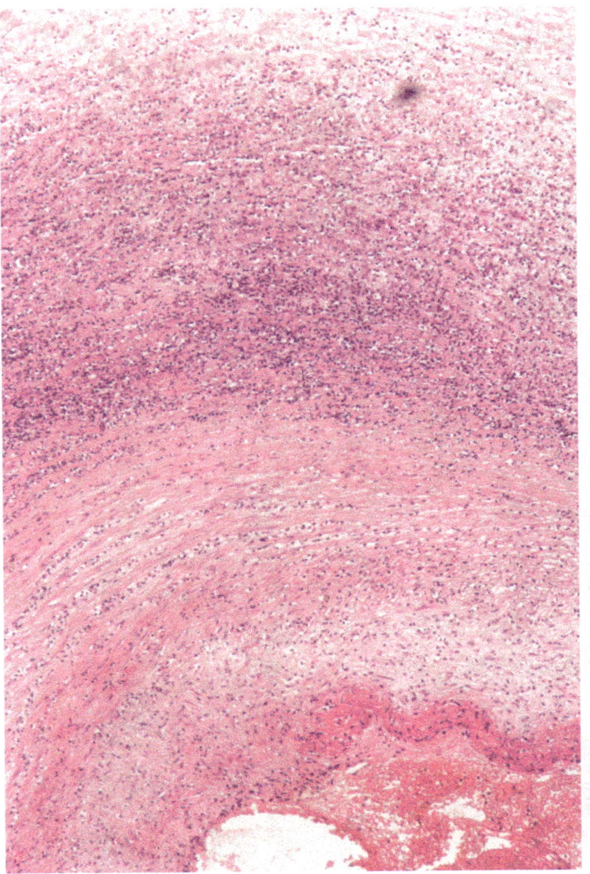

Figure 16.8. Necrotizing funisitis with rings of exudates, some of which are degenerated. H&E ×40.

In longer-standing infections, **necrotizing funisitis** may occur. Compared to the fetal membranes, the umbilical cord is not able to efficiently remove the chronic accumulation of inflammatory debris. The connective tissue cells of the umbilical cord often then degenerate completely. This results in *exudate being deposited in successive waves, which accumulate in concentric perivascular rings* (see below). This exudate is more prone to develop mineralization than the exudate of the fetal membranes and thus may become *calcified*. The calcification may reach extraordinary proportions at times, so that the cord cannot be readily clamped at delivery. *Mural thrombosis* may also be present. Necrotizing funisitis is classically associated with congenital syphilis infection (see below) but is not specific, as other organisms, such as *Candida*, *Streptococci*, and other bacteria have been isolated from these cases. **Mural thrombosis in chorionic veins** is also frequently present when the infection has been of longer duration and there is some destruction of the vessel walls through which the neutrophils migrate. The thrombi may be grossly apparent as yellow-white streaks and are usually attached to the intima of the veins, toward the amnionic surface (Fig. 16.9).

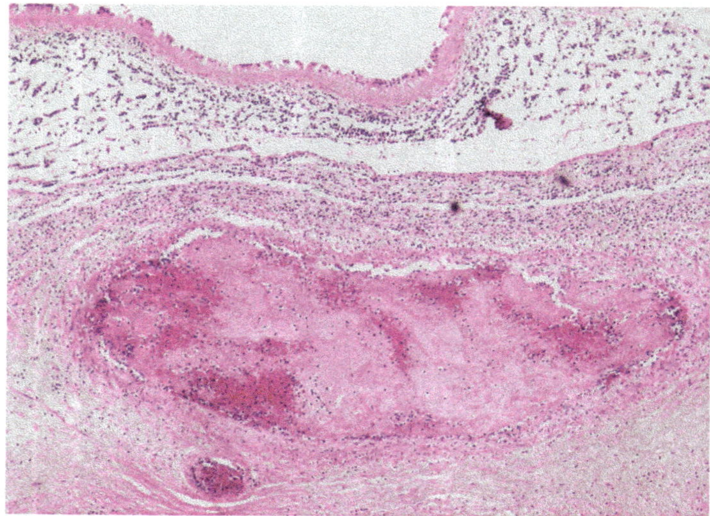

Figure 16.9. Chorioamnionitis with involvement of chorionic vessels. Early mural thrombosis is present at the surface of the vein. H&E ×20.

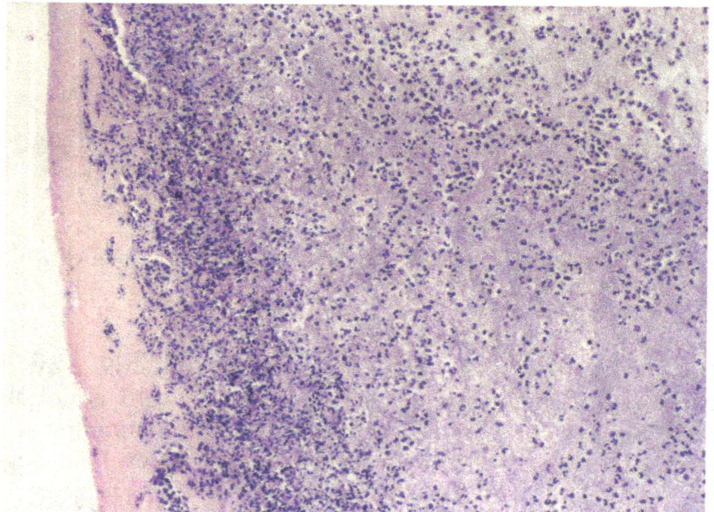

Figure 16.10. Subacute chorioamnionitis with massive infiltration of acute and chronic inflammatory cells and necrosis. H&E ×40.

Subacute Chorioamnionitis
In the amniotic infection syndrome, the amnionic epithelium may be *degenerated or necrotic*, especially in areas of severe inflammation. If the infection progresses, the PMNs die and the *dead inflammatory cells* may accumulate in large quantities underneath the amnion in the potential space that exists between amnion and chorion. There may be accumulation of *mononuclear cells* as well. This has been referred to as **subacute chorioamnionitis** (Fig. 16.10). It occurs in situations

where the causative organism is of *low pathogenicity* and does not result in immediate delivery or when there are *repetitive bouts of infection*. Like necrotizing funisitis and thrombosis, this is indicative of a longer-standing infection. Ultimately, some of the necrotic exudate underneath the amnion may calcify, forming linear depositions of calcium underneath the amnion. However, the fetus usually delivers before this happens. Subacute chorioamnionitis should be distinguished from chronic chorioamnionitis (see below) in which the infiltrate is predominantly mononuclear.

Suggestions for Examination and Report
(Acute chorioamnionitis)

Gross Examination: The discoloration and opacity of the fetal surface and membranes should be described. Sections of the membrane roll should include the rupture point of the membranes (furthest from the margin of the placental disc) as this gives the highest yield. If desired, bacterial cultures may be done prior to examination by lifting the amnion and swabbing between the amnion and chorion. Visible calcifications or thrombi in the umbilical cord should also be noted.

Comment: The diagnosis should include descriptions of the *severity, location and characterization* of the inflammatory infiltrate. For example – mild, moderate or severe infiltrate involving chorionic plate and chorionic plate vessels. Additional findings of necrosis indicative of *subacute chorioamnionitis*, inflammation associated *thrombosis of chorionic vessels, acute villitis, intervillous abscesses*, and *funisitis* should always be specifically mentioned.

Specific Microorganisms

The organisms most frequently associated with **preterm infants** are *group B Streptococcus, Fusobacterium*, and *Peptostreptococcus*, while the organisms associated with **term infants** are *group B Streptococcus, Fusobacterium, Escherichia coli, Bacteroides*, and *Ureaplasma*. Microorganisms are difficult to identify on histologic sections of infected placentas, and Gram stains or other special stains are rarely helpful. However, some organisms such as *Listeria, Candida, Fusobacterium*, and some cocci may be visible on careful microscopic examination and in some cases may be visible with the use of additional special stains (see below). The *pattern of inflammation* is often the most important clue to diagnosis of a specific organism. The most common organisms causing acute chorioamnionitis will be discussed in some detail, while a summary of the less common infections are summarized in Table 16.1.

Group B *Streptococcus*

Clinical Features and Implications
Group B streptococci are *gram-positive cocci*, which are often, but not always, beta-hemolytic. Infections with this organism are frequent and it is considered one *of the most virulent perinatal infections.* Prematurity and premature rupture of membranes are strongly correlated with group B streptococcal infections. *Sepsis, pneumonia, and meningitis* are common sequelae and infection is an important cause of *fetal asphyxia, stillbirth, and neonatal death.* A significant number of women will have a positive screen for this organism. Antibiotic treatment does not ensure eradication of the organism throughout pregnancy. Although rapid detection and screening are possible currently using DNA probes, there is no agreement on when to screen for the colonization, or how to respond when positive results are obtained. Recent studies show rapid neonatal or intrapartum administration of antibiotics does not prevent neonatal sepsis, nor does it reduce mortality. There is still a great deal of controversy on how and when to treat mothers and infants in this setting.

Pathologic Features
Intra-amniotic infection with group B *Streptococcus* and even neonatal sepsis may occur *without chorioamnionitis being present.* In fact, there is little to no inflammation in the placentas of 75% of newborns in which the organism has been cultured. This is one of the peculiarities of this organism and is primarily due to host-related factors and the toxins produced by the bacteria that enable its proliferation. This lack of inflammatory response is one of the factors responsible for the virulence of the organism. With careful search, it is often possible to identify the cocci, particularly on the amnion (Fig. 16.11). In fact, *the presence of minimal inflammation and readily identifiable cocci in the membranes*

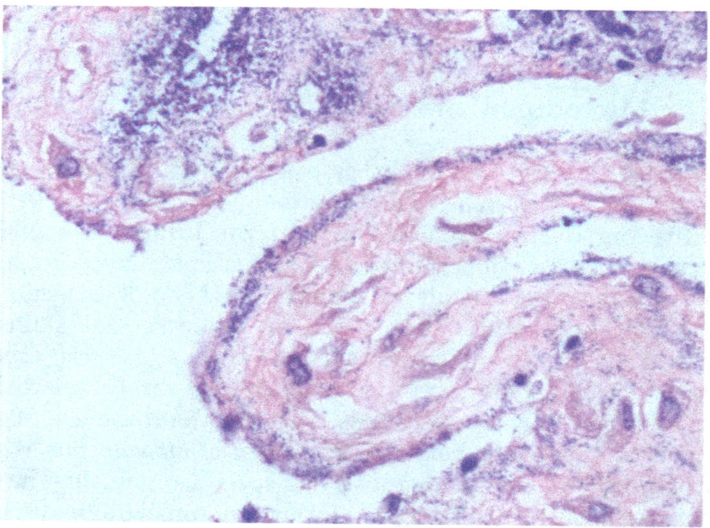

Figure 16.11. Group B *Streptococcus* infection. Note the abundance of bacterial organisms (cocci) and the minimal associated inflammation. H&E ×250.

is almost pathognomonic for group B Streptococcus. In some cases, focal abscesses may form underneath the amnion associated with epithelial necrosis and accumulation of bacterial colonies.

Listeriosis

Clinical Features and Implications
Listeriosis is caused by a *gram-positive bacillus*, **Listeria monocytogenes**. The organism is a danger principally to *pregnant women, newborns, and immunocompromised individuals*. In infants, listeriosis is known as **granulomatosis infantiseptica** and is characterized by visible abscesses and a 60% perinatal mortality. *Neonatal meningitis* is another serious complication of fetal infection with this organism. A rash is often present in the neonate, and Gram stains of the skin or gastric aspirates are helpful in identification. The diagnosis is also easily established from cultures. Anti-listeriolysin O titers quickly develop after infection, and so may be useful in diagnosis.

Pathogenesis
Listeriosis occurs in a wide variety of mammals and birds, as well as in humans. There is transmission to neonates from mother's milk or as a nosocomial infection in nurseries. Direct contact with infected animals and consumption of certain foods such *as pasteurized milk, certain fresh cheeses, cabbage, poorly cooked sausage, and chicken and pâté.* The organism survives moderate heat and thrives at low temperature so that it grows well even in food kept refrigerated. The presence of organisms in the vagina and in stool and the *typically severe chorioamnionitis* suggest that the mode of infection is ascending.

Pathologic Features
Aside from the usual *opacity of the fetal surface and membranes* of the placenta, which is occasionally described as greenish, the typical **intervillous abscesses** may be visible in cross sections of the placenta (Fig. 16.12). If smears are done on these lesions, a Gram stain will

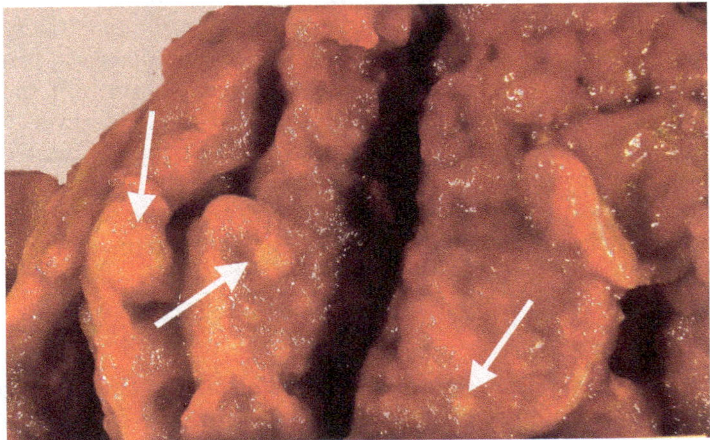

Figure 16.12. Numerous placental abscesses (*arrows*) due to *Listeria* infection.

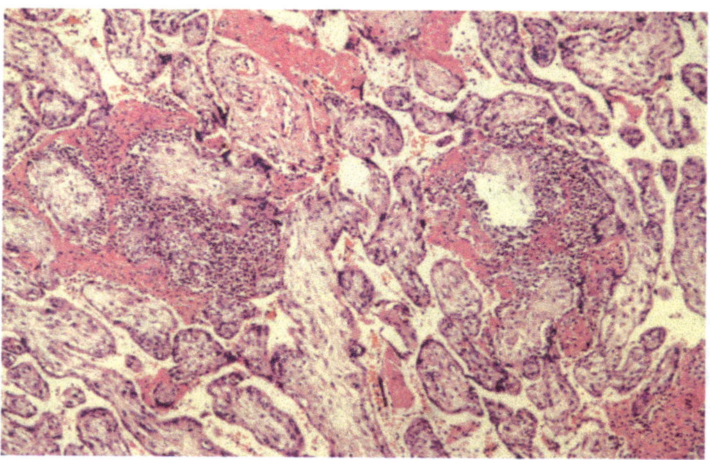

Figure 16.13. *Listeria* abscess in the intervillous space. There is much necrosis of villi, fibrinoid deposition, and infiltration with PMNs. Numerous organisms were found on Gram stain. H&E ×200.

often reveal the organism. On microscopic examination, one sees *villous abscesses, villous necrosis, and acute villitis.* The abscesses frequently have a central area of necrosis and are usually composed of massive numbers of neutrophils, which surround and infiltrate the villi (Fig. 16.13). The villitis may be necrotizing and associated with villous destruction. This pattern may also occur occasionally in maternal septicemias due to *Staphylococcus* and *E. coli,* and uncommonly with other organisms such as *Campylobacter* and *Chlamydia.* Generally, in maternal sepsis the mothers are usually so ill that labor and delivery occur before abscesses develop. The villi are otherwise almost never involved in common cases of chorioamnionitis, however severe that process may be. In the case of *Listeria,* the presence of *placental abscesses* may be due to fetal septicemia, corresponding to similar abscesses in the fetus.

The amnion commonly contains abundant bacterial growth and the *acute chorioamnionitis is usually severe. Acute funisitis* may also be present. Since the *bacteria thrive under low temperature conditions,* they will often proliferate during cold storage of the placenta prior to examination. Rapid diagnosis is important because prompt therapy with ampicillin rapidly cures the maternal and fetal infection. When listeriosis is recognized during pregnancy and adequately treated, the *placental abscesses may undergo "scarring."* They are then sometimes still recognizable histologically as a former abscess, as true scar formation does not occur in the placenta. The abscesses in the fetus in a resolved infection probably have a similar fate.

Escherichia coli

Gram-negative bacilli, in particular **Escherichia coli,** are a frequent cause of acute chorioamnionitis. They normally colonize the gastrointestinal tract and commonly cause urinary tract infections. There is a strong association with maternal rectal colonization of the organism and subsequent vertical transmission. Infection of the infant may result in *pneumonia, intestinal infection, sepsis, or meningitis*. Neonatal meningitis may occur through the aspiration of amniotic fluid via the middle ear. Uncommonly, acute chorioamnionitis *may be associated with intervillous abscesses and acute villitis*.

Fusobacterium

Fusobacterium necrophorum and ***Fusobacterium nucleatum*** are *pleomorphic, filamentous, gram-negative, anaerobic organisms*, which are common causes of acute chorioamnionitis. They normally colonize the mucous membranes or the mouth, intestines, and urogenital tract. It is estimated that as many as 30% of patients with "occult" chorioamnionitis may be infected with *Fusobacterium* species. They are considered an important cause of premature labor. *Acute chorioamnionitis may be severe*, but the organisms are often invisible on routine stains and difficult to identify on tissue Gram stains. Bouin's fixative makes their demonstration particularly difficult. *Giemsa* and *Warthin–Starry stains* may be used for identification of these organisms (Fig. 16.14).

Clostridia

Infection with ***Clostridium perfringens***, *a gram-positive rod*, occasionally complicates pregnancy. Among anaerobic infections it is particularly feared because it causes postabortal sepsis and uterine gas gangrene, which may be life threatening for the mother. The infection is often quite severe and associated with frequent *abortion and fetal loss*. The placenta may have a *greenish amnionic surface and a putrefactive odor*.

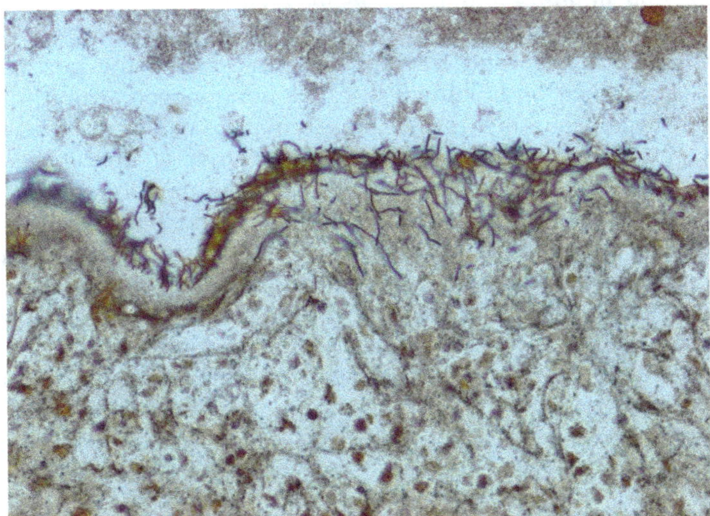

Figure 16.14. Chorioamnionitis due to fusobacteria in the placenta at 23 weeks' gestation. The placental surface was opaque. Silver stain showing massive bacterial growth. The dark filaments radiating from the amnionic basement membrane are easily identified as the filamentous organisms. ×240.

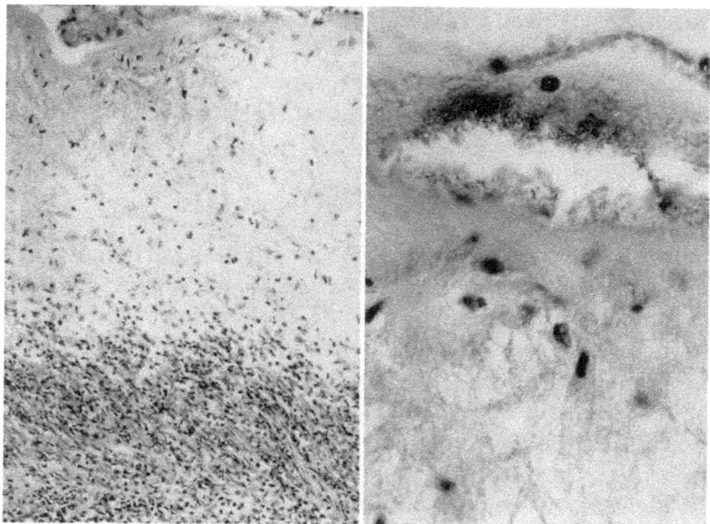

Figure 16.15. Clostridial chorioamnionitis at term. There was intensive deciduitis and chorionitis. Note the pocket of gram-positive rods underneath the amnion. H&E ×640.

Purulent exudate will be present within the membranes and fetal surface and it may contain *gram-positive rods* (Fig. 16.15). Inflammation and necrosis of villous tissue may be found in septic cases. Fetal infection may also occur.

Mycoplasma

Mycoplasma hominis and ***Ureaplasma urealyticum*** are known urogenital pathogens for humans. *M. hominis* is a known cause of pelvic inflammatory disease and febrile conditions during the postpartum period. *U. urealyticum* is known to cause nongonococcal urethritis in men. The organism attaches itself to spermatozoa and may thus more readily penetrate the endocervical mucous barrier. *U. urealyticum* may be the cause of *repetitive abortions, sterility, and premature birth*. Both organisms are a cause of *neonatal meningitis* and have been associated with *chronic neonatal lung disease*. The organisms may cause *acute chorioamnionitis* similar to that caused by other bacteria. Some villous alterations such as *villous sclerosis, degenerative changes of villous vessels, thrombosis, and villous edema* have been reported. Study of these organisms is hampered by our current inability to demonstrate the organism in tissue sections and their specific culture requirements.

Chlamydia

Chlamydia trachomatis is responsible for the most common sexually transmitted disease in the United States. *C. trachomatis* also causes *trachoma, lymphogranuloma venereum, nongonococcal urethritis in men,* and *mucopurulent cervicitis, chronic salpingitis,* and *sterility in women.* It is estimated that between 10 and 20% of sexually active men and women are infected with this organism. Approximately one-half of infants born to infected mothers develop *ophthalmia neonatorum ("inclusion body blennorrhea")* and others develop *pneumonitis*. Approximately 3–4% of all neonates have ophthalmia, and 1–2% have pneumonitis from infection with this organism. This organism has not been isolated from the placenta and thus has not been conclusively demonstrated to be a direct cause of acute chorioamnionitis, but it *has* been found in the amniotic fluid, and in the eye and nasopharynx of neonates. The *bacterium-like intracellular microbe* can be visualized in the cytoplasm of infected cells by *direct immunofluorescence*. The infection can also be diagnosed by culture, by immunoperoxidase and by polymerase chain reaction (PCR) amplification.

Chlamydia psittaci infection is rarely recognized as a cause of human abortion, although it commonly causes abortions in sheep and other domestic species. Sheep farmers and their wives have a high exposure to this pathogen, and abortion has been described in this population. When abortion ensures, it is then associated with *acute intervillositis, villous necrosis,* and *inclusions in syncytiotrophoblast*. Electron microscopy and immunofluorescence have confirmed the presence of the organism.

Bacterial Vaginosis

Bacterial vaginosis has been defined as the *"replacement of the lactobacilli of the vagina by characteristic groups of bacteria accompanied by changed properties of the vaginal fluid."* The bacterial species include *Bacteroides, Gardnerella vaginalis, Mycoplasma hominis, Ureaplasma urealyticum,* and perhaps others. A relation to premature rupture of membranes, preterm birth, and amniotic sac infection has been reported to exist.

Candida Species

Clinical Features and Implications

Vaginal infection with **Candida albicans** is common during pregnancy, and it is estimated that 26% of women harbor these organisms. Neonatal candidiasis can be traced to maternal vaginal infection in most cases and may manifest as *skin rash, dark red skin discoloration, pneumonia, meningitis, sepsis, and intestinal contamination*. Although infection may cause neonatal demise, successful treatment has been reported. *Candida* infection has also been associated with abortions. Although C. *albicans* is the most common candidal organism, infection with C. *parapsilosis*, a common skin inhabitant, has also been reported, as has infection with C. *tropicalis*.

Pathologic Features

Prenatal infection of the placenta, cord, and fetus may be associated with severe acute chorioamnionitis but *typically involves only the umbilical cord*. Grossly, *the umbilical cord shows numerous tiny, round, white or yellow plaques* (Fig. 16.16). Histologically, the nodules consist of *focal infiltrates of acute inflammatory cells underneath areas of*

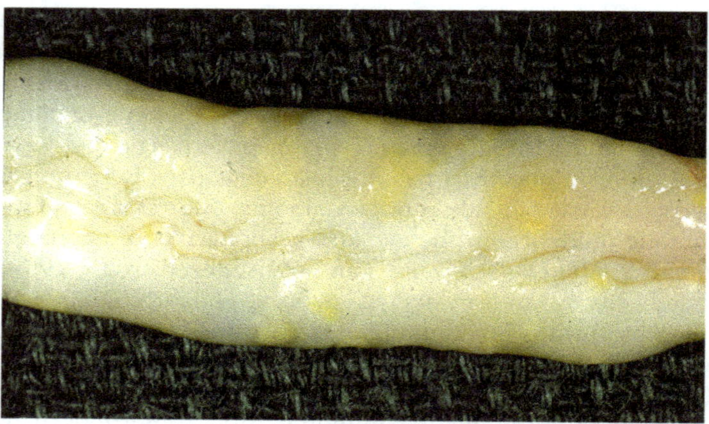

Figure 16.16. Congenital candidiasis showing numerous small, yellow-white plaques, representing abscesses.

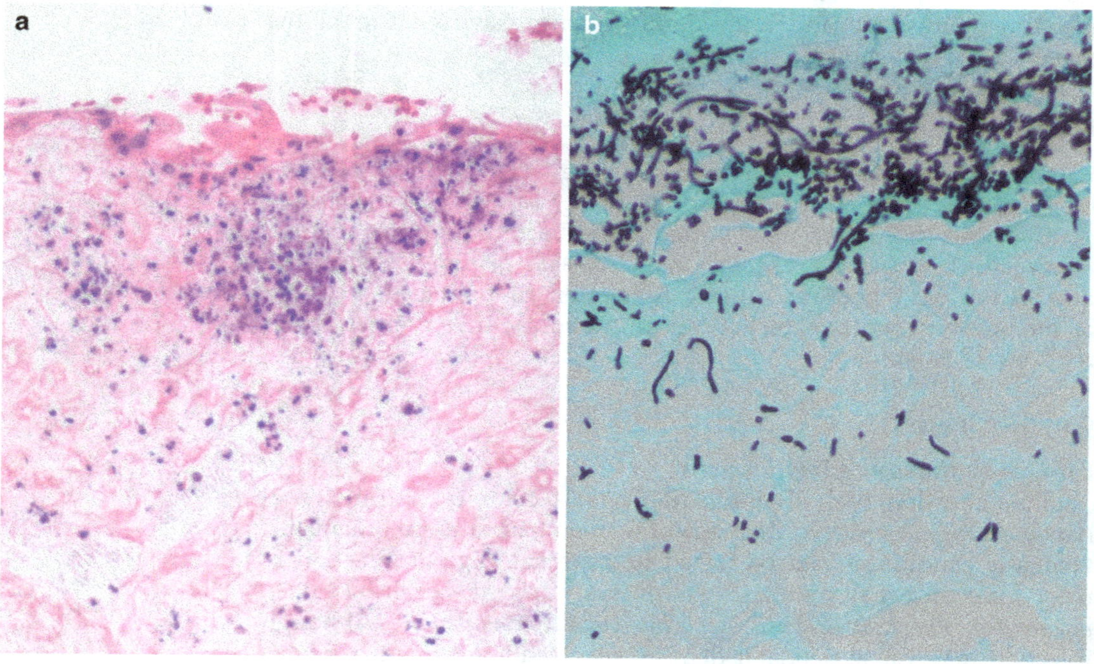

Figure 16.17. (a) Candidiasis of umbilical cord. There are accumulations of inflammatory cells, debris, and organisms associated with epithelial necrosis. H&E ×200. (b) GMS stain showing pseudohyphae and yeast forms. GMS ×200.

epithelial necrosis in the periphery of the umbilical cord (Fig. 16.17a). *Fungal pseudohyphae and yeast forms* are readily demonstrated with silver stains but are quite difficult to identify in routine preparations (Fig. 16.17b). Villous lesions are rarely identified, but when they occur consist of *focal necrosis, chronic villitis, and intervillous abscesses.*

> **Suggestions for Examination and Report**
> (Specific infections causing acute chorioamnionitis)
>
> *Gross Examination:* There are no gross techniques or sections to submit to identify specific organisms except in the case of *Candida*. Extra sections of cord are suggested if lesions are identified grossly. Culture remains the gold standard for identification of specific organisms and this should be undertaken if there is a request for identification.
>
> *Comment:* Use of special stains for microorganisms is helpful only in looking for certain organisms such as *Fusobacterium*. However, if the pattern of inflammation is suggestive of a particular organism, such as group B *Streptococcus*, *Candida*, *Fusobacterium*, or *Listeria*, special stains are sometimes useful for confirmation.

Chronic Villitis

Chronic villitis is defined by a *chronic inflammatory infiltrate in the chorionic villi*. Chronic villitides are divided into two general groups, those of *infectious* etiology and those of *unknown* etiology [**villitis of unknown etiology** (VUE)]. In infectious villitides, maternal infections are transmitted *hematogenously* and *transplacentally* from the mother to fetus. Causative organisms include *Toxoplasma gondii,* rubella virus, cytomegalovirus, herpes simplex virus, hepatitis, and HIV. However, many other organisms such as spirochetes, parasites, and other viruses are implicated. Close to 90% of infectious villitides are due to cytomegalovirus and syphilis. Selected infections will be covered in some detail, while features of the remaining organisms are summarized in Table 16.2.

Syphilis

Pathogenesis
Infection with **Treponema pallidum** may occur at any time during pregnancy. The organism may pass to the fetus via the placenta during all stages of maternal syphilis infection. Most frequently, disseminated infection in the neonate arises from *hematogenous spread of the spirochetes between the first and second stages of infection of the mother*. Spirochetes can be demonstrated by immunofluorescence and electron microscopy in fetuses as early as 9–10 weeks' gestation. Expression of the disease's pathologic features depends on the fetus's ability to produce antibody to spirochetal antigen. Therefore, since young fetuses cannot mount a proper antibody response, the histopathological changes cannot be seen in early infection.

Pathologic Features
The more severely the fetus is affected, the greater are the pathological changes in the placenta. The placenta usually shows an *increase in weight*, which may be quite impressive. Placentas up to 2,500 g have been reported. Microscopically, *the villi tend to be "bulky" and enlarged.* Classically there is *endothelial and fibroblastic proliferation and chronic villitis with prominent plasma cells* (Figs. 16.18 and 16.19). The decidua also may

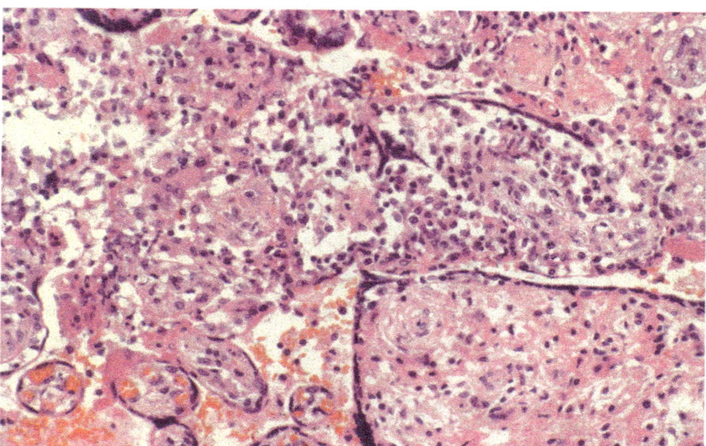

Figure 16.18. Villi of placenta in congenital syphilis. Villi are hypercellular, infiltrated with mononuclear cells. Note the focal necrosis and vascular obliteration. H&E ×240.

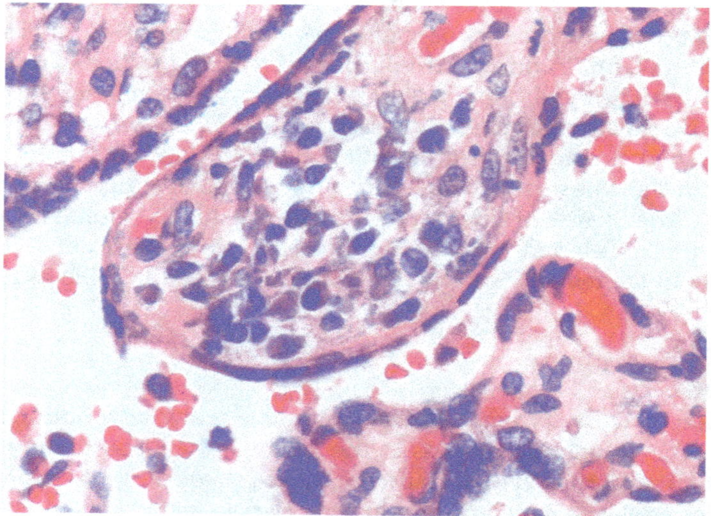

Figure 16.19. Plasma cell infiltration of chorionic villi in congenital syphilis. H&E ×240.

show plasma cell infiltration with necrosis, although this is obviously not specific for infection with this organism (Fig. 16.20). Chronic chorioamnionitis is uncommonly present (see below). Abscesses or villous necrosis is seen in severe infections, but gummas or granulomas have never been reported in the placenta. *Necrotizing funisitis* may also be present (Figs. 16.21 and 16.22), which is a classic finding in syphilitic infection, but is not considered pathognomonic as was previously thought. Here, numerous inflammatory cells form incomplete rings around the umbilical vessels and over time may calcify.

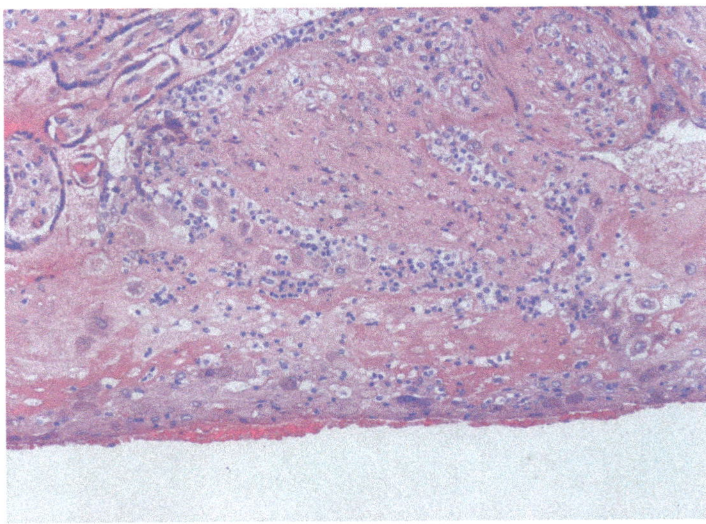

Figure 16.20. Chronic deciduitis of decidua basalis in an infant afflicted with typical congenital syphilis. The placenta was large (580 g). H&E ×160.

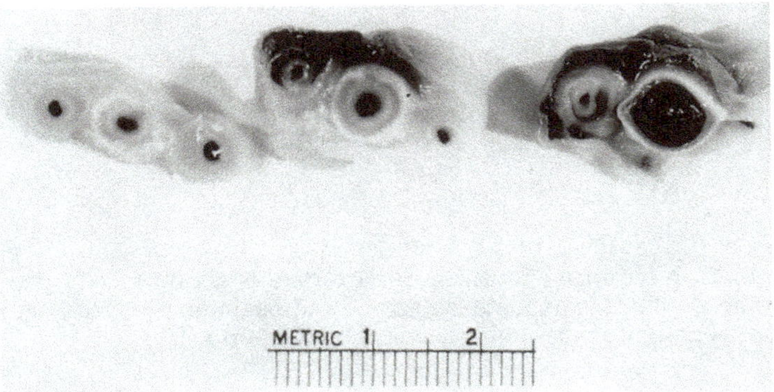

Figure 16.21. Concentric rings of perivascular exudate in necrotizing funisitis.

Cytomegalovirus

Clinical Features and Implications

Congenital **cytomegalovirus (CMV)** infection is a common disease, with 3,000–4,000 infected infants born in the United States each year. From 1.6 to 3.7% of seronegative women convert to seropositivity for CMV during pregnancy. The rate of transmission to the fetus after recent maternal infection is between 20 and 50%. Fetal infection is more serious when it occurs during a primary maternal infection than when it follows recurrent maternal disease and when it occurs during the first half of pregnancy. Fetal and neonatal infection has many manifestations, including *hearing loss, blindness, hydrops fetalis, obstructive uropathy, meconium peritonitis, growth restriction, hydrocephaly, stillbirth, and cerebral palsy*. The *hallmark of fetal infection is intracranial calcifications* and *perivascular echogenic signals in the basal ganglia*, both of which may

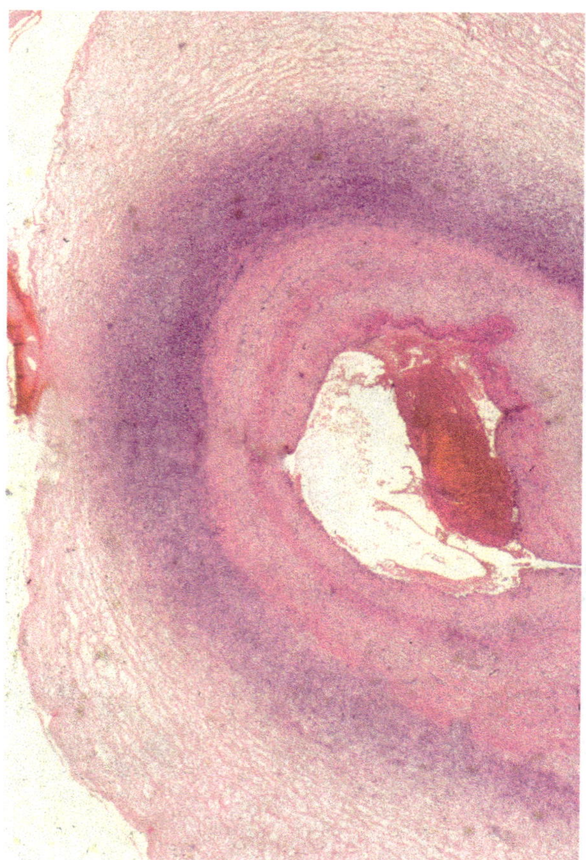

Figure 16.22. Necrotizing funisitis. The exudate is concentrically deposited around the vessels; the exudate is necrotic and beginning to calcify. A mural thrombus is present in the umbilical vein. von Gieson ×12.

be identified on ultrasound examination. Some of these manifestations may be ascertained only years later. Neonates with this infection may excrete virus for years and may become a major source for infection of pregnant mothers and toddlers in day-care centers.

Pathogenesis

The virus is *often acquired by sexual contact.* Fetal infection is undoubtedly most often acquired during primary maternal infection from *maternal viremia and by the passage of virions through the trophoblast, which it infects and destroys.* Congenital infection is also *occasionally acquired from infected endometrium,* and CMV inclusions in endometrial glands have been demonstrated in abortion specimens.

Pathologic Features

Cytomegalovirus infection in the placenta is characterized by *chronic lymphoplasmacytic villitis* (Fig. 16.23) and deposition of hemosiderin in the villous stroma. The chronic villitis typically causes bulky enlargement of the chorionic villi. Diagnosis of this infection in this placenta may be made, as it is in other organs, by identification of *inclusion-*

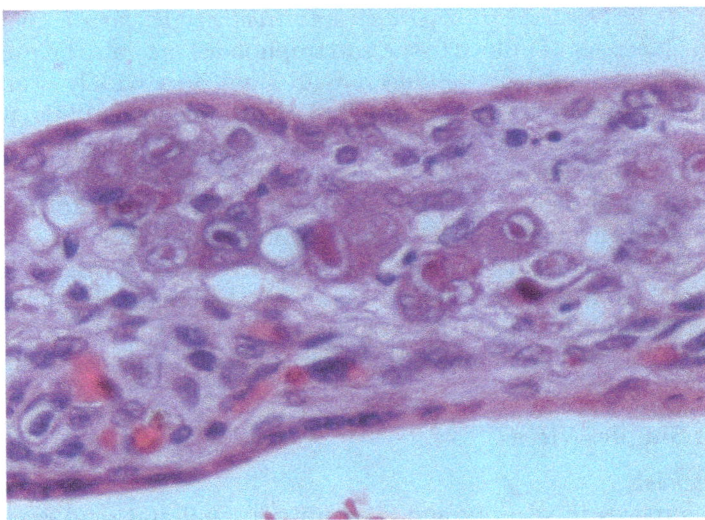

Figure 16.23. Congenital cytomegalovirus infection. Marked chronic villitis, composed almost entirely of plasma cells, is evident, as is focal necrosis of the trophoblast and capillary walls. H&E ×650.

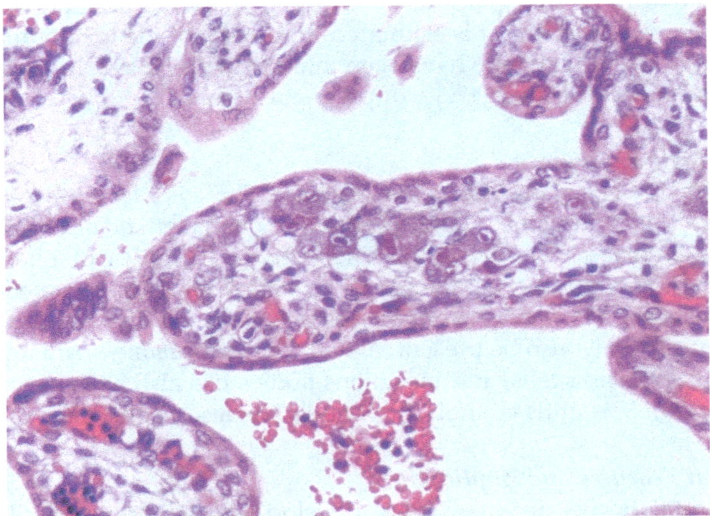

Figure 16.24. Owl-eye nuclear inclusion of a cytomegalic cell in the villus of a patient with CMV infection. This cell also contains many cytoplasmic inclusions as well. H&E ×200.

bearing cytomegalic cells. The inclusion bodies may be the typical nuclear "owl-eye cells," but cytoplasmic inclusions are also commonly seen (Fig. 16.24). *Inclusions may be seen in villous capillary endothelium, villous stromal cells, the amnion, and even the decidua.* Vasculitis of chorionic vessels may occur leading to thrombosis and calcification in long-standing cases and is the source of the *hemosiderin deposits* seen in the adjacent stroma. Even without typical inclusions, the presence of *plasma cells and hemosiderin deposition are virtually pathognomonic of CMV infection.* Necrosis of villous tissue and trophoblast may also be present. The villitis is commonly *multifocal* with small foci widely scattered through the villous tissue in contrast to other infectious villitis, which tends to be more confluent. Thus, extreme scrutiny of many sections may be necessary to make the diagnosis from tissue sections.

When typical inclusions are not present, CMV can be detected by immunohistochemistry, in situ hybridization, and PCR, which are more sensitive than routine histology. Positivity in these cases is found to be mostly in the *villous stroma,* but may also be present in *syncytiotrophoblast* and *endothelial cells.* Serological studies, virus isolation, or PCR may be performed on amniotic fluid or neonatal samples as well.

Herpes Simplex Virus

Pathogenesis

The differences in severity and types of placental and fetal reactions in prenatal herpes infection suggest that *both transplacental and ascending infection* occur. *Herpetic endometritis* has been demonstrated, which is suggestive of direct spread as well. Infection with **herpes simplex virus (HSV)** occurs only occasionally, and this is likely due to the protective nature of transplacentally acquired maternal antibodies. The latter are common, and it is estimated that 16.4% of the US population from 15 to 74 years of age have been infected with HSV-2. In addition, HSV is "silently" shed by 2.3% of pregnant women.

Pathologic Features

The placenta is usually *grossly unremarkable.* There is a *lymphoplasmacellular infiltrate* within the villous stroma. The characteristic *inclusion bodies and "ground-glass nuclei,"* when present, are diagnostic of a herpetic infection. The chronic villitis can be extensive or may be associated with necrosis. *Necrotizing deciduitis, amnion necrosis, chorionic vasculitis,* and *funisitis* may also be present. *Necrotizing chorioamnionitis* with true "blisters," plasma cells, and inclusions bodies has also been described (Fig. 16.25). Vasculitis of chorionic vessels can also result in *thrombosis.*

Clinical Features and Implications

Congenital herpes infection may develop without maternal illness or the presence of herpetic lesions. When infection occurs during the first 4 months of pregnancy, abortion is common as is *stillbirth* in later gestation. At autopsy *ocular, renal,* and *cerebral anomalies* may be found including *massive destructive of the brain, resembling hydranencephaly.* Calcifications in fetal organs have also been described.

Parvovirus B19

Clinical Features and Implications

Infection with this highly contagious virus is an important cause of *second trimester abortion and hydrops fetalis.* Approximately 40–60% of adults have immunoglobulin G (IgG) antibodies from previous

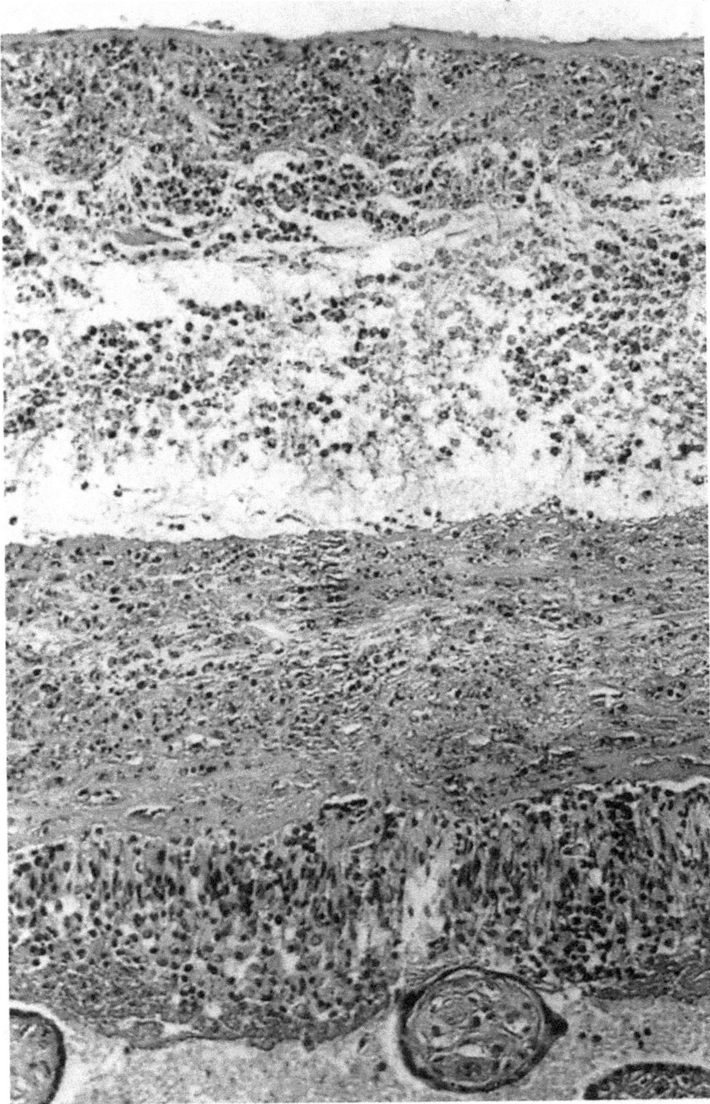

Figure 16.25. Congenital HSV-2 infection resulting in stillbirth. Note the sub-amnionic blister filled with plasma cells. The amnion and chorion are necrotic. H&E ×160.

infection. Maternal infection is asymptomatic in up to 75% of cases, but transmission of the virus to the fetus still occurs. Women with acute infection during pregnancy show viral transmission from mother to fetus in approximately 25–33% of cases; serious fetal disease occurs in 9% of these cases. Fetal infection is typically associated with *anemia* and in some cases *hydrops* due to the predilection of the virus for erythrocyte precursors. It is estimated that 16–18% of fetal hydrops may be caused by infection with this organism. Thus, it is an important cause of stillbirth. While intrauterine transfusion therapy in documented cases has been shown to be beneficial, recovery from this infection has also been witnessed without therapy. *Myocarditis and ocular anomalies have also been described.*

Pathologic Features

Macroscopically, the placenta is enlarged and when fetal hydrops is present, the placenta is *pale, friable, enlarged, and edematous.* Infection can usually be diagnosed by the *typical ground-glass inclusion bodies of nucleated red blood cells* it produces. The intranuclear inclusions are lightly stained and eosinophilic and are composed of crystals of the small, 20-nm virus particles. The infected cells are called "**lantern cells**" since they resemble Chinese lanterns (Fig. 16.26). The inclusions are present in circulating normoblasts, nucleated red blood cells, and in their precursors in fetal organs and the placenta. These are usually very numerous in cases in which anemia and hydrops are present. Chronic villitis may be present, and in this situation the villi may be large and bulky. Additional findings include hemosiderin in chorionic macrophages, *villous destruction, necrosis, endothelial damage, and perivascular lymphocytic infiltrate.*

Many methods are available to identify the organism. Immunohistochemistry, DNA hybridization studies, and electron microscopy can demonstrate parvovirus in the placenta, and a rapid and sensitive PCR test for detection of the antigen has been developed

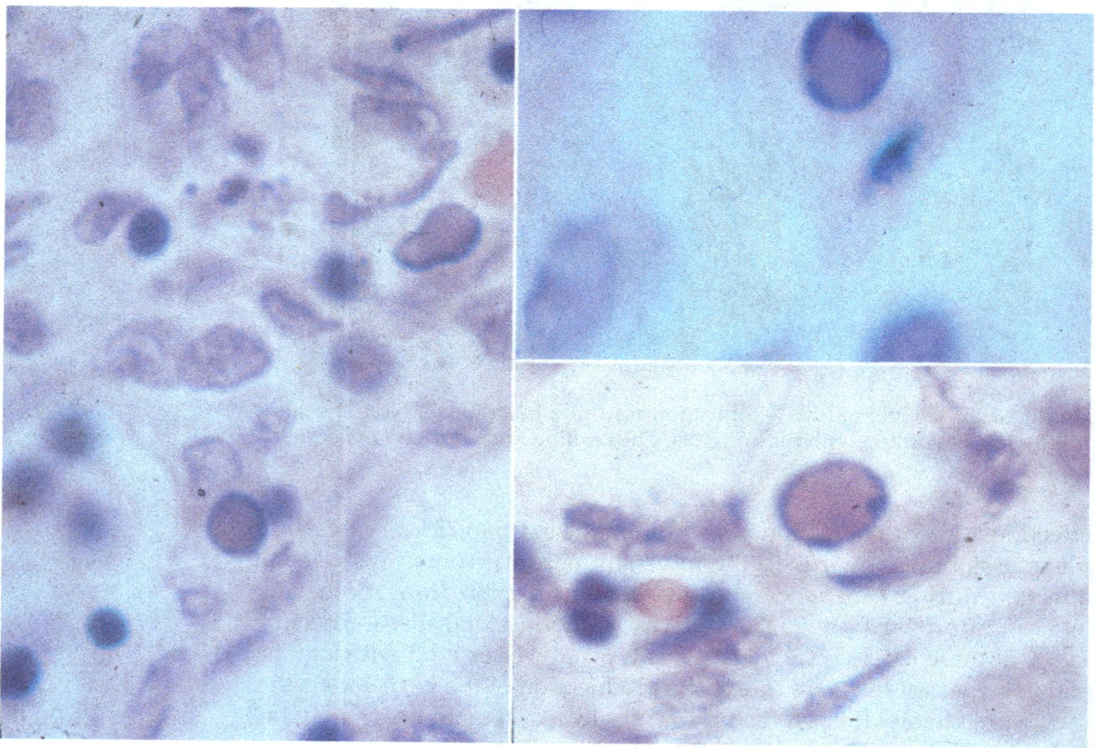

Figure 16.26. Infection with parvovirus B19. Normoblastic nuclei have smudged intranuclear inclusion bodies (*arrow*). H&E ×240.

for use on fetal blood and amniotic fluid. Serologic detection of the B19 antigen is also now widely available. As is true in many infections, elevated IgG titers in maternal blood denote former infection, while an elevated IgM titer diagnoses recent or active disease.

Mycobacteria

Leprosy, due to *Mycobacterium leprae,* is now an uncommon disease in the United States. Vertical transmission from mother to infant is either uncommon or does not occur. However, abortion has been associated with isolation of the organisms from the placenta and cord blood. Documented cases show *granulomatous lepromatous lesions* in the chorionic villi and *a few acid-fast bacilli.* The placentas tend to be relatively small. *Acid-fast organisms have been found in decidua, trophoblast,* and *villous stroma.*

In contrast to leprosy, congenital infection with **Mycobacterium tuberculosis** has been repeatedly demonstrated to occur. In fetal infection, *caseating granulomas in the lungs and acid-fast bacilli in the liver, spleen, and kidneys* are found. There may be difficulty in distinguishing transplacentally acquired tuberculosis from infection transmitted by inhalation of infected amniotic fluid and from neonatal disease acquired nosocomially. The placenta may be *grossly normal* or may *contain firm, white plaques.* Microscopically, typical but rare *granulomas with giant cells* in the chorionic villi or intervillous space may be seen. *The bacilli may be found in fetal vessels, intervillous fibrin, septa, or villous stroma.* Special stains for acid-fast bacilli will assist in identification of the rare organism. In some cases, congenital infection is present but the placenta is unaffected. *The decidua may also contain areas of extensive necrosis and the placental floor may also contain granulomas.* These findings suggest direct transmission from decidua to placenta. Occasionally, acute granulomas occur, consisting of neutrophils in the intervillous space causing local villous destruction. In other cases, one may find isolated giant cells in the stem villi but no inflammation.

Toxoplasma

Pathogenesis

The *coccidian,* **Toxoplasma gondii,** is a pan-global parasite of cats, other felids, and many domestic animals. In infected cats, oocysts are shed in the stools. Rodents and other animals then ingest the oocysts and acquire the disease. Cats, preying on infected rodents, complete the life cycle. In humans, infection is acquired by two means: contamination with oocysts from feces of infected cats; and ingestion of oocysts and tachyzoites in raw, infected meat, mostly pork and mutton. Pregnant women are advised not to eat undercooked or raw meat, and should avoid having contact with "wild" cats. Cats raised solely on commercial diets are very rarely infected. Emptying the litter box daily to prevent drying and dust-producing feces is recommended, but best done by another member of the household.

It is generally assumed that almost all congenital *Toxoplasma* infections develop from a *primary infection* during pregnancy. Large prospective studies of toxoplasmosis in pregnancy have shown that in women with primary infection during pregnancy, 45% of the infants develop congenital toxoplasmosis. The rate of infection increases with gestation, and is 17, 25, and 65% in the first, second, and third trimesters, respectively. Although infection is less likely in early gestation, fetal sequelae are the most severe when infection develops during this period.

Clinical Features and Implications

Transplacental toxoplasmosis can cause severe disease in the offspring. *Hydrops* and *hepatosplenomegaly* are common in infected neonates and *chorioretinitis, encephalitis, hydrocephaly,* or other organ involvement may cause crippling disease. Late onset of symptomatology is seen in children with congenital toxoplasmosis, and new lesions continue to appear well after the age of 5 years.

Pathologic Features

Placental infection with *Toxoplasma* is presumably produced by organisms circulating in the maternal blood, although the isolation of cysts from endometrium in chronic aborters makes direct infection from the endometrium possible. *Cysts are often present in the subamnionic/chorionic tissues and under the surface of the umbilical cord* (Fig. 16.27) unaccompanied by inflammation. They also may be identified in chorionic villi and trophoblast. The villi show an *increase in Hofbauer cells and vascular proliferation in the villi and an increase in circulating fetal normoblasts. Lymphocytic-plasmacellular villitis* is seen only when cysts rupture, and then may be associated with *villous necrosis of granulomatous villitis.* As with CMV infection, *thrombosis of chorionic or umbilical vessels* may occur and the thrombi may become calcified. Identification is difficult in histological sections, and positive identification may require PCR, immunohistochemistry, fluorescence antibody technique, or electron microscopy. Although cysts can be identified with diligence on histologic section, without ancillary techniques, tachyzoites

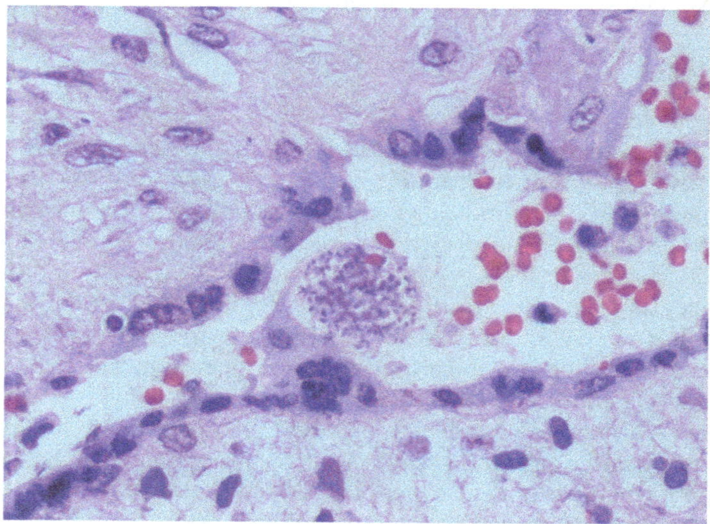

Figure 16.27. *Toxoplasma* cysts in syncytium in a child with congenital infection. H&E ×240.

cannot be recognized with certainty. Handling and culturing this organism is often avoided because of the hazards of infection.

Malaria

Pathogenesis

Malaria, which is an infection with one of the four species of **Plasmodia**, is the commonest infectious disease in the world. True congenital infection has been described only rarely, and the mechanism of fetal/neonatal infection is still uncertain. It is thought that transplacental infection most likely occurs during delivery; however, some severely infected patients have died undelivered with an infected fetus still in utero. There is no agreement as to whether the organisms cross the placenta into the fetal circulation. It seems likely that the plasmodium does not cross by itself, and when transplacental infection occurs, the parasites are probably transferred within red blood cells. Maternal to fetal transfer of red blood cells occurs, but is rare.

Clinical Features and Implications

Pregnancy substantially increases the severity of malaria in the mother and is associated with *premature births, low birth weight, and decreased placental weight.* Perhaps because of transferred immunity, symptomatic disease in the neonate is virtually never recognized at birth. It becomes evident only after several weeks.

Pathologic Features

On occasion the placenta has been described as *"diagnostically black at parturition"* owing to malarial pigment. In most cases, however, there is no macroscopic abnormality. Some cases show diffuse placental enlargement. Histological studies of the placenta reveal *malaria-infected erythrocytes in the intervillous space* in 40% of cases, and an additional 35% of cases show evidence of malarial pigment without the presence

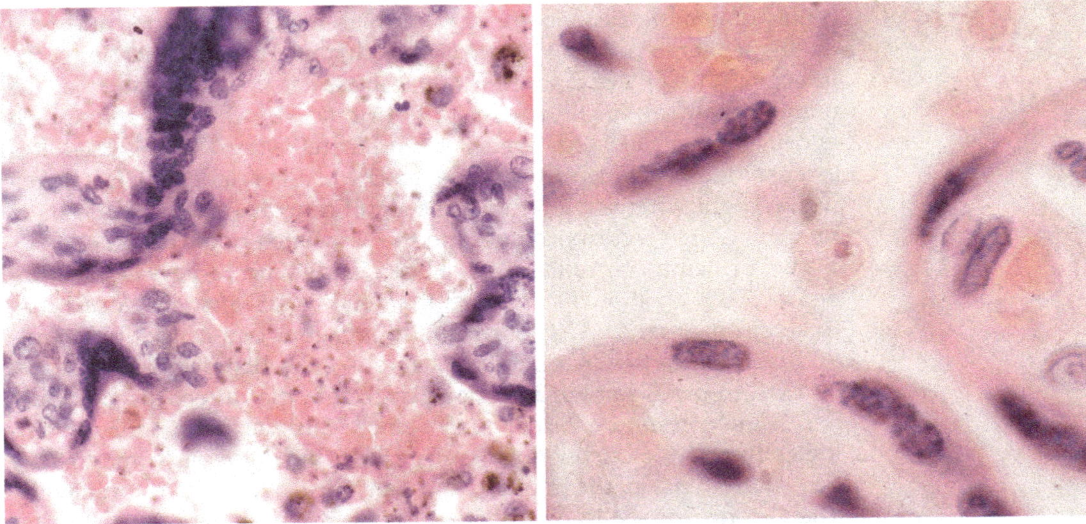

Figure 16.28. Malaria infection with presence of pigment and malarial organisms within the intervillous space. An intracellular organism is present in the right figure. *Left*: H&E ×200. *Right*: H&E ×400.

of organisms (Fig. 16.28). The *pigment*, which is a breakdown product of hemoglobin, may be present in *fibrinoid, macrophages or free in the intervillous space*. Chronic intervillositis with accumulation of macrophages in the intervillous space is present to at least some degree in the majority of cases, and *massive chronic intervillositis* (see below) is seen in about 6% of cases. There may be a necrotizing villitis as well. An increased *amount of intervillous fibrinoid* and *thickening of the trophoblastic basement membrane* is often seen. Placentas may rarely have infarcts, abruptions, or fetal vascular thrombosis.

Suggestions for Examination and Report
(Specific infections causing chronic villitis)

Gross Examination: If abnormalities in villous tissue are noted, or infection is suspected, additional sections of grossly normal villous tissue should be submitted.

Comment: If the pattern of the villitis is consistent with a particular organism, based on the clinical history, one may do additional studies. With some organisms, such as CMV, definitive diagnosis of the organism can be made on histology alone or with the aid of immunohistochemistry. Specific infections in the differential diagnosis can generally not be ruled out on the basis of lack of pathologic findings.

Villitis of Unknown Etiology

Pathogenesis

Chronic villitis is frequent, occurring in 5–15% of all placentas. When placentas of complicated pregnancies, growth-restricted infants, and fetal deaths are studied, the incidence is much higher, up to 34%. At times, the infectious etiology of chronic villitis is apparent from the history or the pathological features. In the majority of cases, however, despite much effort, no specific etiology is elicited, and then the term **VUE** is used. It is estimated that VUE represents close to 95% of all villitides. VUE is now a well-recognized entity but remains a significant challenge because of its frequency, high recurrence rate, and the associated poor outcome.

Two principal suggestions have been made with respect to the etiology of VUE. First, it is suggested that VUE is an *infectious disease* due to a yet unrecognized agent or due to an agent that cannot be identified from placental examination. There is great histological similarity of VUE to other known infectious disorders that affect the placenta, and some common viruses are extremely difficult to recognize histologically or by electron microscopy (EM). Infections also may cause few symptoms in the mother and may not be detected prenatally. The second theory is that VUE is an immune reaction akin to placental *"rejection" or graft-versus-host disease*. This is supported by the histiocytic and T-cell lymphocyte predominance of the inflammatory reaction, its frequent location in an area of maternal–fetal tissue interaction, its frequent recurrence, and its tendency to recur in families. Furthermore, 60% of the infiltrating immunocytes of VUE are maternal CD3 positive T-cells from the intervillous space. An immunological pathogenesis of VUE with maternal cells infiltrating the villi has long been championed. Whether this is tantamount to immune "rejection" mounted by the mother against the placenta needs further investigation. Furthermore, recurrent VUE has often been associated with various autoimmune diseases in the mother. In addition, VUE is more common in pregnancies with assisted reproductive technology when donor eggs are used compared with nondonor eggs. At this time, the only certain conclusion is that VUE is **not** the result of infection with common, known pathogens since no virus or other agent has been consistently identified.

Pathologic Features

Macroscopically the placentas of VUE have been described as *stiff*. The placentas are occasionally *smaller*, particularly in growth-restricted fetuses. If areas of villitis are large and associated with necrosis, the *villous tissue may appear mottled* (Fig. 16.29). The mottling is a subtle finding and is only present when villitis is extensive. There are no specific changes that allow definitive macroscopic identification.

Microscopically, lesions have a wide spectrum, from focal to extensive involvement wherein virtually all villi have some pathological reaction. The villitis is characterized by *infiltration primarily by histiocytes* with lesser numbers of *lymphocytes*. The chronic villitis may be *necrotizing* with *villous destruction* and secondary changes of *ischemia*,

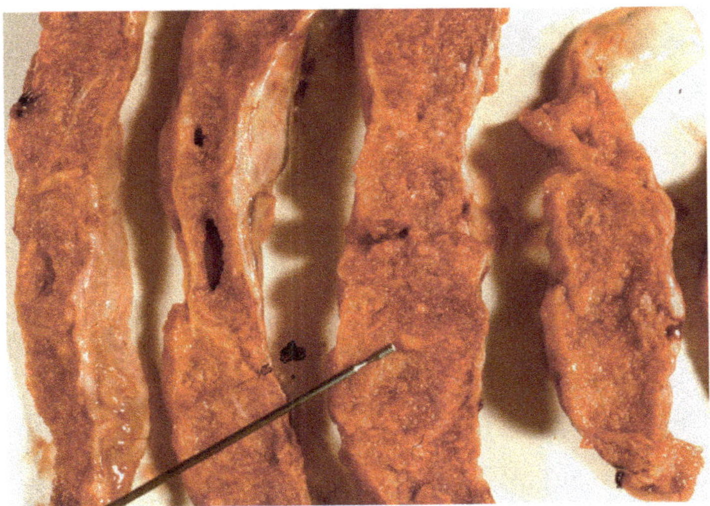

Figure 16.29. Placenta with diffuse VUE. Note the mottling of the villous tissue. The probe indicates one area of subtle whitish discoloration which represents villitis.

infarction, fetal vascular thrombosis, and *avascular villi* (Figs. 16.30 and 16.31). VUE is especially *frequent in the basal villi* in the maternal floor of the placenta. Associated findings in VUE include *villous dysmaturity, an increase in nucleated red blood cells, hemosiderin deposition,* and *chorangiosis.* All or none of these abnormalities may be found. If villitis affects

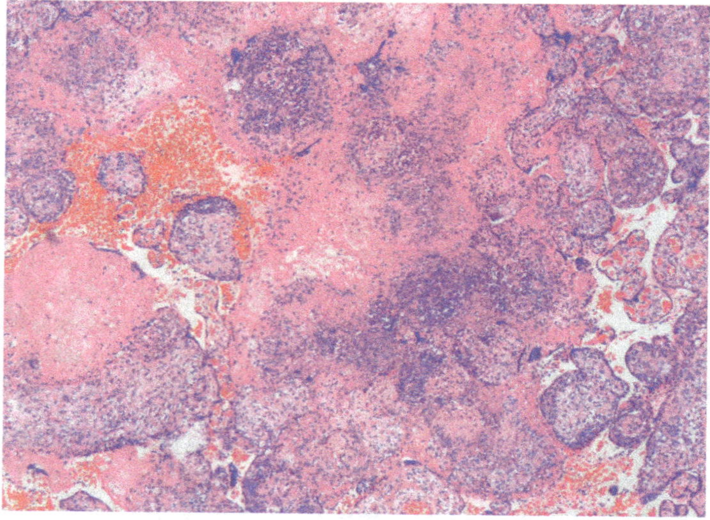

Figure 16.30. Low-power view of diffuse chronic villitis of unknown etiology. H&E ×40.

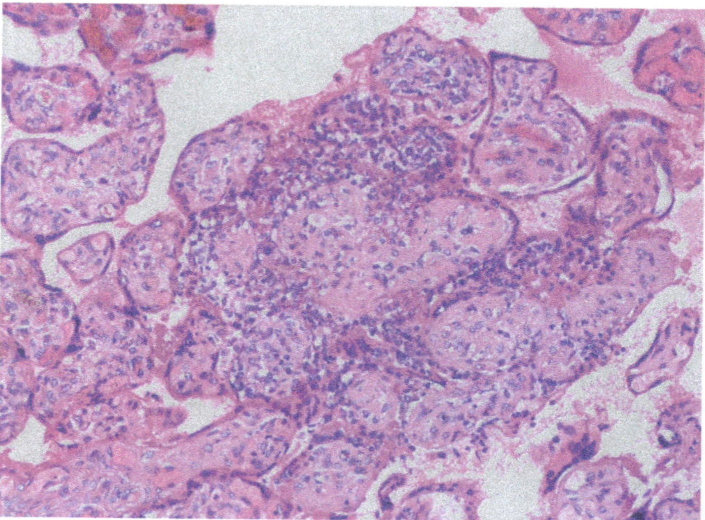

Figure 16.31. VUE with intense infiltration with lymphocytes and histiocytes. The vessels are obliterated. H&E ×240.

larger vessels leading to destruction, there may be extensive fetal vascular thrombosis.

The similarity to known infectious causes of villitis, such as seen with CMV and rubella, is striking and based on inflammatory infiltrate alone, differentiation is not generally possible. However, in general VUE tends to be *more multifocal, is much less commonly associated with plasma cell infiltration, and tends to be concentrated in the basal plate.* In infectious villitis there may be involvement of the umbilical cord, chorionic plate, and membranes. There is, however, much overlap. One should also note that degenerative lesions simulating VUE can be present peripheral to infarcts, and these should not be confused with typical VUE as discussed here.

Clinical Features and Implications

There is little doubt that VUE is able to eliminate a considerable amount of placental parenchyma from nutrient transfer. Therefore, the presence of *fetal growth restriction* in as many as 33% of cases is not surprising. One must emphasize, however, that there is no absolute relation between the severity of VUE and the severity of fetal growth restriction. VUE is also associated with *recurrent abortions, prematurity, abnormal neurologic development, cerebral palsy, encephalopathy,* and *intrauterine fetal demise.* Of great interest is the frequently recurrent nature of this lesion with recurrence rates of 10–25%. Furthermore, the reproductive loss is 60% in patients with recurrent villitis in contrast to a 37% loss in nonrecurrent villitis.

Suggestions for Examination and Report
(Villitis of unknown etiology)

Gross Examination: If mottling of the villous tissue is identified, or there is a history of infection, growth restriction, or fetal demise, at least several additional sections of villous parenchyma should be submitted.

Comment: The diagnosis is consistent with VUE if the pattern is typical and there is no evidence of infectious etiology. Infectious etiologies cannot be ruled out. Extensive VUE can explain and be correlated with stillbirth, intrauterine growth restriction (IUGR), and other adverse outcomes if this history is provided.

Chronic Chorioamnionitis

Chronic chorioamnionitis is a recently described lesion in which the *inflammatory infiltrate in the fetal membranes consists predominantly of a mononuclear cells, lymphocytes,* and *histiocytes* rather than acute inflammatory cells (Fig. 16.32). The diagnosis should not be made if scattered chronic inflammatory cells in the membranes or if the infiltrate

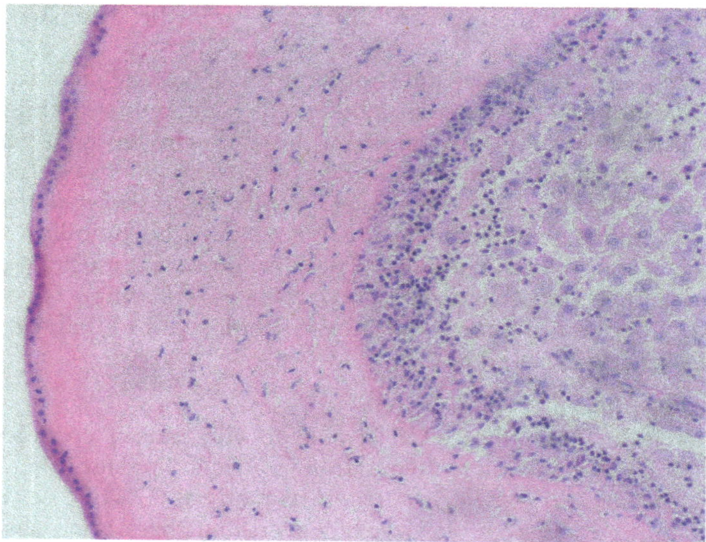

Figure 16.32. Chronic chorioamnionitis involving the fetal surface. H&E ×60.

is primarily in the decidua. Chronic chorioamnionitis is found in association with VUE in approximately 79% of cases. Thus, its identification should alert the examiner to search for foci of chronic villitis. Clinically, chronic chorioamnionitis has been associated with *maternal hypertension, diabetes, fetal hydrops, growth restriction,* and *oligohydramnios.* If a mixed acute and chronic inflammatory infiltrate is present, subacute chorioamnionitis is present (see above).

Suggestions for Examination and Report
(Chronic chorioamnionitis)

Gross Examination: Chronic chorioamnionitis cannot be appreciated on gross examination.

Comment: Chronic chorioamnionitis may be associated with chronic villitis and adverse perinatal outcome.

Chronic Intervillositis

Chronic intervillositis is an infiltrate of *mononuclear cells in the intervillous space* (Fig. 16.33). This entity has also been called massive chronic intervillositis, chronic intervillositis of unknown etiology, and chronic histiocytic intervillositis. The inflammatory cells are

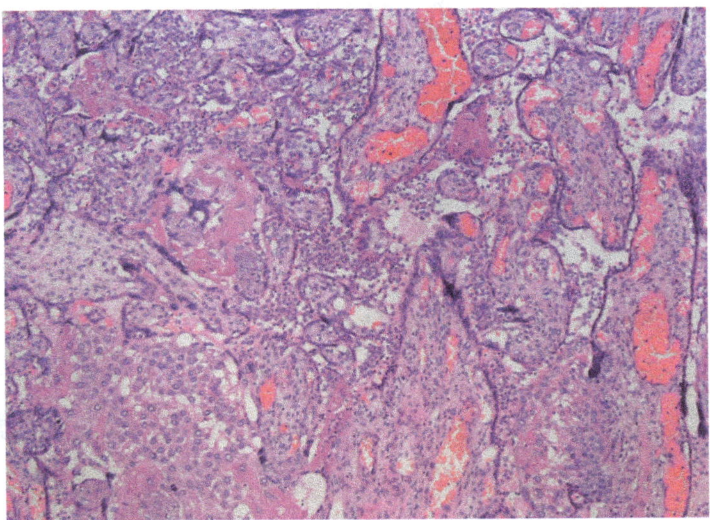

Figure 16.33. Severe chronic intervillositis associated with chronic villitis consisting of infiltrates of lymphocytes and histiocytes. H&E ×250.

predominantly CD68-positive macrophages but lesser numbers of lymphocytes are also present. There is a *variable amount of intervillous fibrinoid deposition* as well, sometimes containing extravillous trophoblastic cells. Thus, at times it is confused with massive perivillous fibrin deposition or maternal floor infarction (see Chap. 19). This entity has most commonly been described in *recurrent abortion* specimens but also occurs in the second and third trimester where it is associated with *fetal growth restriction* and *intrauterine demise*. *Chronic villitis* is often also seen in association with chronic intervillositis. Since the macrophages are of maternal origin, it has been suggested that the etiology of the associated reproductive problems is of immunologic origin. Like VUE, chronic intervillositis has been associated with a high recurrence rate (67%) and autoimmune disease has been described in 52%.

Suggestions for Examination and Report
(Chronic intervillositis)

Gross Examination: Chronic intervillositis is generally not recognized grossly.

Comment: Chronic intervillositis may be associated with recurrent abortion, fetal loss, or fetal growth restriction.

Table 16.1. Miscellaneous bacteria in ascending infection.

Bacteria	Morphology	Pathologic features	Potential clinical sequelae	Comment
Actinomyces	GP filamentous anaerobe	Foul smelling placenta Severe ACA may be necrotizing Identifiable organisms	Preterm labor	May show massive invasion by organism
Bacteroides fragilis	GN anaerobe	ACA	Meningitis	Other neonatal infections described
Brucella		No characteristic lesion	Abortion Fetal infection may be fatal or self-limited	Acquired from animal and animal products
Campylobacter	GN aerobe	ACA Villous necrosis Acute villitis	Recurrent abortions Fetal death	Common enteric pathogen
Corynebacteria	GP diphtheroids	ACA Gray-brown plaques on placental surface with invading organisms	Sepsis not described	Normal vaginal flora Occasional infection
Coxiella burnetii (Q fever)	GN obligate intracellular	Severe necrotizing villitis	Congenital infection Fetal death	Rare zoonosis Organisms may be identified in placenta
Ehrlichiosis	GN obligate intracellular	No lesions	Neonatal infection (of granulocytes)	Probable transplacental infection
Francisella tularensis		Granulomatous lesions	Granulomatous lesions	
Gardnerella	G variable	Occasionally mild ACA	Preterm delivery Fetal demise (rare)	Common vaginal organism
Group A *Streptococcus* (*S. pneumoniae*, *Enterococcus*)	GPC	ACA	Pneumonia	Common
Haemophilus influenzae	GNR	ACA	Preterm delivery Pneumonia Sepsis	Uncommon May mimic group B *Streptococcus* infection
Neisseria gonorrhoeae	GN diplococcus	ACA associated with cervical infection	Sepsis Ophthalmia neonatorum	Uncommon
Rickettsia	GN obligate intracellular	No lesions	Full recovery	Very rare
Salmonella	GNR	ACA	Meningitis Pneumonia Fetal demise	Mothers are symptomatic or carriers
Shigella	GNR	ACA	Sepsis Enterocolitis	Uncommon
Staphylococcus	GPC	ACA	Neonatal sepsis	Common pathogen
Streptobacillus	GNR	ACA	Rare	Causes "rat bite fever" or Haverhill fever

G gram, *P* positive, *N* negative, *C* cocci, *R* rods, *ACA* acute chorioamnionitis, *AF* acute funisitis

Table 16.2. Miscellaneous organisms causing villitis.

Organism	Category	Pathologic features	Potential clinical sequelae	Comment
Borrelia (relapsing fever)	Spirochete	No lesions	Found in neonatal and placental blood	Follows bite of infected tick Geographically widespread
*Borrelia burgdorferi*Lyme disease (erythema migrans)	Spirochete	Rare plasma cells Increased nucleated red blood cells	Stillbirth Congenital anomalies	
Leptospira	Spirochete	No lesions	Abortion	Rare
Blastomyces	Fungus	Granulomas Chronic villitis	No neonatal infection reported	
Coccidioides immitis	Fungus	Fungal spherules Acute inflammatory response Fibrinoid deposition and necrosis Infarction and necrosis	Fetal death reported Disseminated infection	
Cryptococcus	Fungus	Colonies of organisms in intervillous space Scant inflammation No villous invasion	Cryptococcosis or meningitis in mother Infants not affected	Associated with lupus and immunodeficiency
Coxsackie B	Virus	Villous necrosis Severe intervillositis	Fetal hydrops Myocarditis Meningitis	Rare fetal infection May not show placental lesions
ECHO	Virus	Chronic villitisChronic intervillositis Mural thrombosis	Congenital infection	Rare
Epstein–Barr virus	Virus	Deciduitis Lymphoplasmacytic villitis Trophoblastic necrosis Endothelial damage	Early abortion Congenital anomalies (rare)	Uncommon
Hepatitis	Virus	Yellow green discoloration of placenta Bilirubin in Hofbauer cells and chorionic macrophages Relative villous immaturity Focal syncytial necrosis	Abortion Fetal ascites Meconium peritonitis	Usually hepatitis B
Human immunodeficiency virus	Virus	No lesions	Prematurity Endometritis	Transmission rate to fetus 24%
Influenza	Virus	No lesions		Transplacental infection occurs
Mumps	Virus	Severe villous necrosis Small cytoplasmic inclusion bodies in decidua	Possible congenital anomalies	Virus isolated from placenta

(continued)

Table 16.2. (continued)

Organism	Category	Pathologic features	Potential clinical sequelae	Comment
Poliomyelitis	Virus	No lesions		Virus isolated from the placenta
Rubella	Virus	Endothelial damage in villi Obliteration of stem vessels Focal trophoblastic necrosis Villous inflammation and sclerosis Swollen Hofbauer cells (in early infection)	Congenital anomalies in early infection	
Rubeola	Virus	Not described	Not teratogenic Fetal mortality	Rare
Smallpox	Virus	Villous, membrane and trophoblastic necrosis Intervillous fibrinoid deposits Calcification	Fetal demise Early abortion	May occur with primary vaccination
Varicella	Virus	Chronic villitis Occasional multinucleated giant cells Rare granulomas Remote infection: occluded stem vessels	Cutaneous scars Limb hypoplasia Chorioretinitis Cataracts Hydrops Visceral calcifications	
Babesia microti	Protozoa	No lesions	Infection of neonatal red blood cells	Very rare
Leishmania major (Kala-Azar)	Protozoa	Thrombosis of villous vessels Amastigotes within and outside macrophages Trophoblastic degeneration No inflammation		Occasional congenital infection
Trichomonas vaginalis	Protozoa	No specific lesions	Preterm delivery Low birth weight Neonatal infection Pneumonia	Rare
Trypanosoma cruzi (Chagas disease)	Protozoa	Enlarged, pale placenta Chronic destructive villitis Chronic intervillositis Amnionic epithelium, Hofbauer cells, or syncytium may contain amastigotes	Stillbirth Maternal myocarditis, esophagitis, and encephalitis	Transmitted by triatomid the "kissing" bug
Enterobius vermicularis	Nematode	Embryo with worm in abdomen and no inflammation	One case reported	
Schistosomes	Trematode	Eggs with granulomas Occasional worms		

Selected References

PHP5, pages 535–540 (Parvovirus Anemia), pages 657–761 (Infectious Diseases).

Altshuler G, Hyde SR. Fusobacteria. An important cause of chorioamnionitis. Arch Pathol Lab Med 1985;109:739–743.

Benirschke K, Mendoza GR, Bazeley PL. Placental and fetal manifestations of cytomegalovirus infection. Virchows Arch B Cell Pathol 1974;16:121–139.

Doss BJ, Greene MF, et al. Massive chronic intervillositis associated with recurrent abortions. Hum Pathol 1995;26:1245–1251.

Driscoll SG, Gorbach A, Feldman D. Congenital listeriosis: diagnosis from placental studies. Obstet Gynecol 1962;20:216–220.

Fojaco RM, Hensley GT, Moskowitz L. Congenital syphilis and necrotizing funisitis. JAMA 1989;261:1788–1790.

Heller DS, Rimpel LH, Skurnick JH. Does histologic chorioamnionitis correspond to clinical chorioamnionitis? J Reprod Med 2008;53:25–28.

Hillier SL, Witkin SS, Krohn MA, et al. The relationship of amniotic fluid cytokines and preterm delivery, amniotic fluid infection, histologic chorioamnionitis, and chorioamnion infection. Obstet Gynecol 1993;81:941–948.

Jacques S, Qureshi F. Chronic chorioamnionitis: a clinicopathologic and immunohistochemical study. Hum Pathol 1998;29;1457–1461.

Kaplan C, Benirschke K, Tarzy B. Placental tuberculosis in early and late pregnancy. Am J Obstet Gynecol 1980;137:858–860.

Kapur P, Rakheja D, Gomez AM, Sheffield J, Sanchez P, Rogers BB. Characterization of inflammation in syphilitic villitis and in villitis of unknown etiology. Pediatr Dev Pathol 2004;7:453–458.

Menon R, Taylor RN, Fortunato SJ. Chorioamnionitis – A complex pathophysiologic syndrome. Placenta 2010;31:113–120.

Ohyama M, Itani Y, Yamanaka M, et al. Re-evaluation of chorioamnionitis and funisitis with a special reference to subacute chorioamnionitis. Hum Pathol 2002;33:183–190.

Parant O, Capdet J, Kessler S, Aziza J, Berrebi A. Chronic intervillositis of unknown etiology (CIUE): Relation between placental lesions and perinatal outcome. Eur J Obstet Gynecol Reprod Biol 2009;143:9–13.

Popek EJ. Granulomatous villitis due to *Toxoplasma gondii*. Pediatr Pathol 1992;12:281–288.

Qureshi F, Jacques SM, Bendon RW, et al. *Candida* funisitis: A clinicopathologic study of 32 cases. Pediatr Dev Pathol 1998;1:118–124.

Redline RW. Inflammatory responses in the placenta and umbilical cord. Semin Fetal Neonatal Med 2006;11:296–301.

Redline RW. Villitis of unknown etiology: noninfectious chronic villitis in the placenta. Hum Pathol 2007;38:1439–1446.

Redline RW, Patterson P. Villitis of unknown etiology is associated with major infiltration of fetal tissues by maternal inflammatory cells. Am J Pathol 1993;143:473–479.

Samra JS, Obhrai MS, Constantine G. Parvovirus infection in pregnancy. Obstet Gynecol 1989;73:832–834.

Walter PR, Garin Y, Blot P. Placental pathologic changes in malaria: a histologic and ultrastructural study. Am J Pathol 1982;109:330–342.

Chapter 17
Maternal Diseases Complicating Pregnancy

General Considerations

In certain maternal diseases, placental findings may be confirmatory of the disease, while in others, placental pathology may be the first indication of an abnormality. In many of the diseases complicating pregnancy, the associated placentas are often not examined, or examination is not reported. This is unfortunate because those placentas could aid in diagnosis and knowledge of the pathogenesis of these conditions and the mechanisms by which these conditions affect the fetus.

R.N. Baergen, *Manual of Pathology of the Human Placenta,*
DOI 10.1007/978-1-4419-7494-5_17, © Springer Science+Business Media, LLC 2011

For convenience, the diseases covered in this chapter are summarized in Table 17.1, which also includes those disorders in which little information is known or has been reported. Some more common conditions are discussed below. Maternal neoplasms are discussed in Chap. 22.

Connective Tissue Disorders

Systemic lupus erythematosus is a relatively common connective tissue disorder that has a significant affect on pregnancy and the placenta. This disease as well as the associated lupus anticoagulant and antiphospholipid antibody syndrome is discussed in greater detail in the next chapter on placental malperfusion (Chap. 18).

Scleroderma, also called **systemic sclerosis**, is a disease of unknown etiology characterized by the production of autoimmune antibodies and the deposition of fibrous tissue in many organs. It has been reported on many occasions to occur in pregnancy, although the usually late onset of scleroderma makes it an uncommon association. *Stillbirths, abortions, and premature births* are common in women with this disorder and *maternal deaths* have also occurred. Pathologic features of the placenta include *infarcts, decidual vasculopathy, abruptio placentae, extensive fibrinoid deposits, X-cell (extravillous trophoblast) proliferation, and cysts.* These are findings often associated with disorders of placental malperfusion and are seen in other autoimmune disorders (see Chap. 18).

Dermatomyositis, which is an autoimmune disease with primarily cutaneous expression, has been reported during pregnancy uncommonly. Pathologic findings of reported cases include *subamnionic necrosis and hemorrhage, infarcts, and fibrinoid deposition* similar to maternal floor infarction (see Chap. 19).

Ehlers–Danlos syndrome is a heterogeneous disease. It rarely occurs during pregnancy, with an estimated incidence of one in 150,000 pregnancies. *Premature delivery and premature rupture of membranes* have been reported, suggesting that the membranes are exceptionally fragile in these patients. The placentas have otherwise been reported to be normal.

Renal Disease

In general, renal disease, when associated with hypertensive disease in pregnancy, will be associated with decidual vascular lesions and lesions of malperfusion that are seen with preeclampsia (see Chap. 18). Renal disease not associated with hypertension is usually associated with histologically normal placentas, although fetal and placental weights are often diminished.

Specifically patients in **acute renal failure** from any cause usually have normal infants when appropriately managed and in those cases, the placentas are found to be normal. Pregnant women with **chronic renal failure** have a high perinatal mortality rate, and their placentas often are quite abnormal with numerous placental lesions. Most notable among them is *diminished growth of the placenta*, presumably secondary to maternal decidual vascular disease and hypertension. The histologic findings may be similar to preeclampsia, but tend to be less pronounced. In particular, the *decidual vessels may show nonspecific thickening of the walls* (see Fig. 18.6 in Chap. 18) without overt decidual vasculopathy or atherosis.

Patients with successful **renal transplantation** have a 30% incidence of preeclampsia during pregnancy and suffer occasional rejection of the transplant. Intercurrent infection is a serious hazard, but cyclosporine immunosuppression apparently does not interfere with placentation. The placenta, however, is rarely described.

Liver Disease

Acute fatty liver of pregnancy does not usually affect the placenta directly. It has a dismal prognosis, with a survival rate between 18 and 23%. *Hemolysis, coagulation, and other disturbances occur clinically, and preeclampsia* may result with its complications. It has recently been suggested that this disorder has a similar pathogenesis to preeclampsia and HELLP syndrome (see Chap. 18). When maternal bilirubin is high, *gross examination of the placenta can identify the pigment, particularly in the perivascular connective tissue of the fetal surface* (Fig. 17.1). Microscopically, however, no abnormalities are detected, and visible pigment-laden macrophages are rare. **Cholestasis of pregnancy** has been associated with a high rate of *stillbirth* and other perinatal complications. *Meconium staining, preterm labor, and fetal distress* are common. Other than frequent meconium staining, no specific placental findings have been recorded.

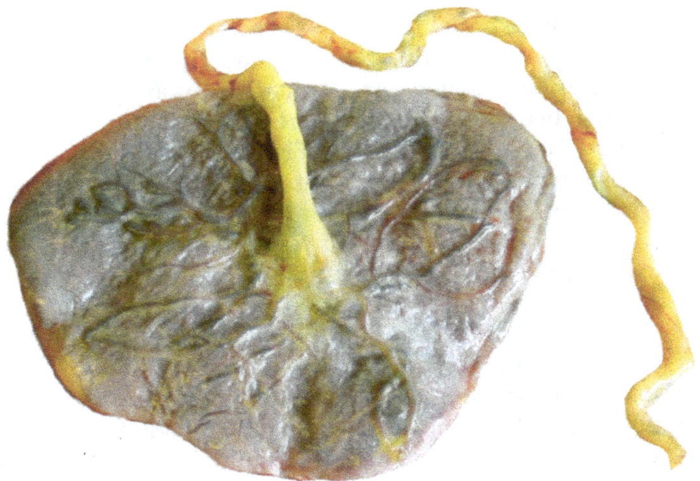

Figure 17.1. "Yellow"-stained placenta due to hyperbilirubinemia in the mother.

Cardiac Disease

The effect maternal **heart disease** has on pregnancy, fetal outcome, and placental development is variable. Patients with valvular disease such as **aortic stenosis**, severe **rheumatic heart disease**, or **cardiomyopathies** may have placentas with *infarcts* and *intervillous thromboses. The villous surface may be reduced,* and fetal growth restriction has also been described. Patients with less severe disease often have normal placentas. If there is associated maternal hypoxia, increased villous capillaries may be identified.

Hematologic Disorders

Sickle Cell Anemia

Clinical Features and Implications
Sickle cell anemia occurs predominantly in the African-American population. The heterozygous condition, **sickle cell trait**, occurs with a frequency of 9% in the United States African-American population and is as high as 45% in central Africa. The homozygous condition, **sickle cell anemia** is characterized by the presence of *sickling of red blood cells,* which result from crystallization of the abnormal hemoglobin S into "tactoids," which occurs particularly under conditions of reduced oxygen tension. Pregnant patients with sickle cell disease have many serious problems. *Urinary tract infection (45%), preeclampsia (25%), and puerperal sepsis (20%)* are the main complications. *Increased perinatal mortality, lower birth weights, and fetal growth restriction* have also been reported. In heterozygotes, these complications are significantly less frequent and less severe. Prophylactic transfusion reduces the frequency of painful crises but does not secure a beneficial pregnancy outcome, presumably because the significant placental lesions are present prior to this therapy.

Pathologic Features
Macroscopically, placentas may be *small* and the associated fetuses have *growth restriction.* They may contain grossly visible *infarcts.* Formalin fixation usually allows the microscopic identification of *sickle cells in the intervillous space* in sections (Fig. 17.2). It is thought that the hypoxia of postpartum placental separation induces the sickling of red blood cells in the intervillous space. Of note, Bouin's fixation results in red blood cell lysis and thus may compromise identification of sickle cells, while Zenker's solution causes reversal of the sickling phenomenon. Often, *nucleated red blood cells* can be found as well. *Increased syncytial knots, accelerated villous maturity, infarcts, increased fibrin, abruptios, and villous edema* have also been identified (see Figs. 18.12 and 18.17). Maternal sickle cells traverse the placenta to the fetal side, and in about one-half of placentas, and sickle cells are then found in aspirated cord blood. Doubtless, this is a traumatic feature of delivery of the placenta.

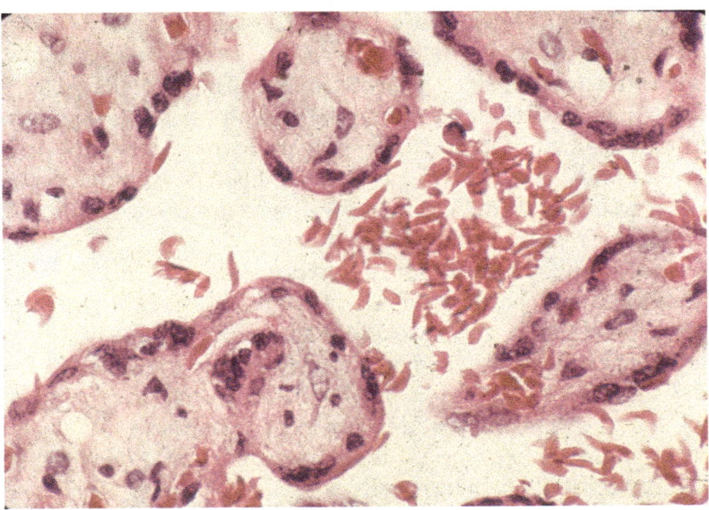

Figure 17.2. Sickled red blood cells in the intervillous space in a case of maternal sickle cell disease. H&E ×400.

Other Hematologic Disorders

Mothers with **β-thalassemia** often have normal infants, but may have *growth restricted infants or spontaneous abortions*. Placentas have not been found to have any associated abnormalities; however, in *infants* with sickle cell thalassemia (**hemoglobin SC disease**), placental infarcts may be found. Maternal **anemia** may cause *significant placental enlargement and in some cases an increase in villous capillaries (see below)*. It seems logical that the anemia leads to inadequate oxygenation of the fetoplacental unit, which, in turn, evokes a physiologic, compensatory placental hypertrophy. However, in severely anemic patients, the placentas are *small with pronounced morphologic changes of decreased uteroplacental perfusion* (see Chap. 18). In **thalassemia trait**, only mild placental enlargement with an increased placental-to-fetal ratio is seen. Simultaneously existing malnutrition is often associated with severe anemia, and this may explain differences in findings in the various studies.

The finding of placental hypertrophy with anemia has raised the question as to what changes may be observed in placentas of chronic oxygen deficiency at **high altitude**. Some studies have shown that the placenta at high altitude is considerably *larger than normal*, while other studies have found the placenta to be of normal size but the infants were smaller. Placentas at high altitude have shown histologic abnormalities such as *an increase in the villous capillaries and a larger capillary volume*. This effect (presumably due to chronic hypoxia), leads to an altered capillary/villous ratio at high altitude. The capillaries are also more closely applied to the trophoblastic surface than is the case at sea level. At times, the increased capillaries are sufficient for a diagnosis of chorangiosis (see Chap. 19).

Idiopathic thrombocytopenia (ITP) is a rare complication of pregnancy. It carries with it the risk of *postpartum hemorrhage and, less commonly, neonatal hemorrhagic complications.* The latter is particularly an issue when obstetricians obtain fetal scalp samples for fetal pH determination or when cordocentesis is performed. On rare occasion, the placenta may have *intervillous thrombi, infarcts,* or *decidual vascular lesions.* It is not clear, however, whether these are caused by the ITP or are perhaps the result of preeclampsia.

Thrombotic thrombocytopenic purpura during pregnancy is a serious disease and carries a high mortality rate. *Stillbirth* has also been described. Often the disease is mistaken clinically for severe preeclampsia, perhaps because of the similarity of the vascular lesions. *The decidual arterioles may show hyaline thrombi or fibrin deposition that resembles atherosis.* This has been called the "snowman sign," as it often presents as a sort of segmented thrombus or hyaline deposit looking like several circles connected together.

Neonatal thrombocytopenia has many causes, including the *transfer of maternal human leukocyte antigen (HLA) antibodies, maternal thiazide administration,* and *alloimmunization.* The latter condition has special dangers of fetal intracranial hemorrhage, and is now being treated with prenatal platelet transfusions. Unfortunately, the placenta in these cases has not been well studied, and in the cases that have been described, the placenta was normal.

Thyroid Disease

Thyroid disease has *no known direct impact on placental structure and function,* but many thyroid disorders enhance the probability of preeclampsia. Thus, *placental infarcts, decidual vasculopathy, and abruptio* are more common. Hyperthyroidism during pregnancy may be complicated by *polyhydramnios,* and *hydrops fetalis* has been reported in a number of patients with treated Graves' disease. Infants of hyperthyroid patients may be *growth-restricted or hyperthyroid* and more frequently have *prenatal distress, meconium staining, and fetal demise.* Diabetes is also more frequent in hyperthyroid patients during pregnancy.

Untreated **hypothyroidism** renders most patients anovulatory. It is therefore not often encountered as a complication of pregnancy. *Abortions, congenital anomalies, anemia, preeclampsia, abruptio, and postpartum hemorrhage* are more common in those patients who do become pregnant. *Fetal death* occurs 12% and *growth restriction* in 31%.

Diabetes Mellitus

Clinical Features and Implications

Abnormalities of glucose metabolism, including **gestational diabetes** and **insulin-dependent diabetes**, are among the most common medical complications of pregnancy. These conditions cause *increased fetal wastage, abortion, prematurity, macrosomia, and certain congenital anomalies.* Glucose passes the placenta readily, and the fetus responds to hyperglycemia with hyperplasia of the islets of Langerhans and increased insulin secretion; the primary reason for macrosomia in maternal diabetes. Periodic hyperglycemia is thought to cause fetal polyuria and resultant polyhydramnios. More severe disease, with vascular complications, may be associated with *fetal growth restriction.*

Pathologic Features

The placentas of diabetic women are often severely abnormal. Placental abnormalities are subject to many variations, mostly due to the degree of diabetic control during gestation. In addition, because of the high fetal mortality during the last 2 weeks of pregnancy, many pregnant diabetic patients are now delivered before term. The placenta of most poorly controlled diabetics is *enlarged, thick, and plethoric* (Fig. 17.3), which is generally thought to be a manifestation of *fetal hypervolemia and maternal hyperglycemia.* There is a decrease in collagen content and mucopolysaccharide in diabetic placentas and they are therefore remarkably *friable.* They may also be edematous. Microscopically, the villous structure of the placenta in maternal diabetes may be focally *dysmature or immature* (Fig. 17.4) with *"persistence" of the cytotrophoblastic layer, increased cytotrophoblastic mitoses, thickening of the trophoblastic basement membrane, and increased perivillous fibrin.* There is frequently some degree of *villous enlargement and hypervascularity, sometimes meeting the criteria for chorangiosis* (see Fig. 19.8), and *nucleated red blood cells* are often present in villous capillaries. In contrast, when diabetes is well controlled during pregnancy, the placental weight does not usually deviate from that of normal organs and the villous tissue is usually microscopically normal.

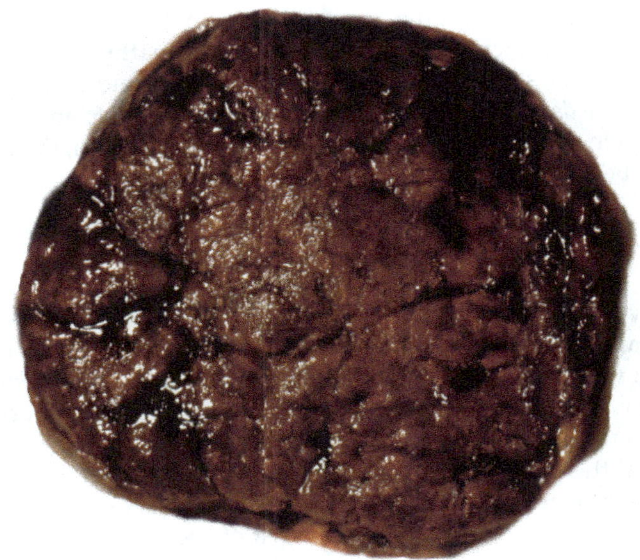

Figure 17.3. Placenta from a diabetic. The maternal surface shows congestion. Friability of the placental tissue leads to tears and depressions in the surface, as seen here, even with careful handling. The placental disk was also markedly thick.

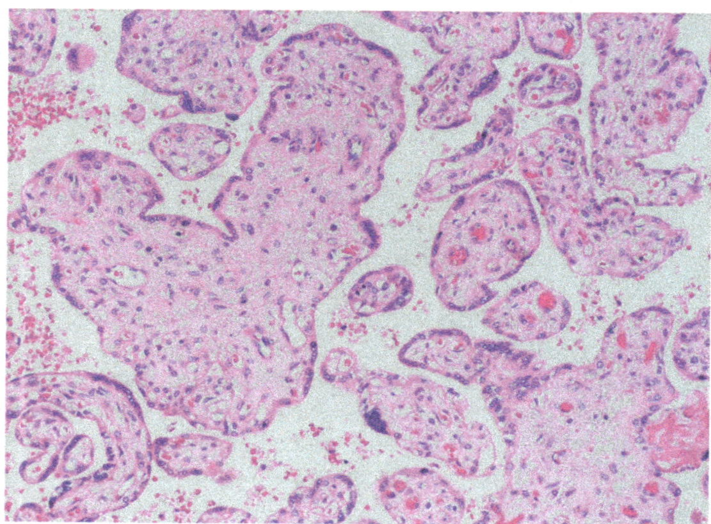

Figure 17.4. Villous dysmaturity in a diabetic placenta showing enlarged and immature appearing villi and increased villous vascularity. H&E ×100.

Fetal and placental vascular thrombosis is more common in the infants of diabetic mothers. This problem is occasionally reflected in *fetal renal and adrenal vein thrombosis*. There is a slight increase in the frequency of *single umbilical artery* (3–5% in diabetic progeny compared to a <1% average incidence). The umbilical cord is usually more "edematous" or, more accurately, it contains more Wharton's jelly. **Sacral agenesis** (caudal regression syndrome) is a highly characteristic fetal anomaly associated with maternal diabetes, but no specific placental lesions have been associated with this congenital anomaly.

When the pregnancy is complicated by **nephropathy (class F diabetes)**, fetal *growth restriction and placental infarcts* are found with increased frequency. *The decidua is also often unusually thick.* Infarcts are otherwise uncommon in diabetic mothers' placentas. In this situation, the placenta may even be smaller than expected for that gestational age.

Miscellaneous Conditions

Pregnancy complicated by **hypercholesterolemia** or **hypobetalipoproteinemia** has resulted in entirely normal placentas but may be associated with fetal growth restriction. In one reported case, *numerous lipid-laden macrophages were present in the intervillous space*, concentrated in the maternal floor, but not within the placental villi. The infant was normal and the placenta had a normal gross appearance.

Pheochromocytoma complicating pregnancy has serious implications for the fetus and mother. It is estimated that pheochromocytoma is associated with fetal death in 45% of cases, abortions in 12%, and maternal mortality in 25%. *Thrombosis of the umbilical cord* has been found in one case and *abruptio placentae* in four cases. The disease is often mistaken for preeclampsia because of the hypertension and albuminuria.

Maternal Drug Use

Tobacco

Clinical Features and Implications
Smoking during pregnancy has been the topic of numerous studies, which unfortunately have yielded contradictory results. Smoking is often considered the cause of an increased frequency of *low birth weight infants*. It has also been associated with *abortions, premature rupture of membranes, preterm delivery, placenta previa, perinatal death, and abruptions. Passive smoking* may also have a similar deleterious effect on fetal development.

Pathogenesis
The adverse effects of smoking may be mediated through reduced blood flow to placenta and fetus. When umbilical and uterine blood flow velocities have been studied, the effect on fetal growth appears to result from a significant rise in fetal placental vascular resistance. The relative hypoxia has been incriminated as the cause of the significant elevation of fetal erythropoietin levels with maternal smoking.

Pathologic Features
There is an increase in the placental to fetal weight ratio in smokers, which is due to the lower fetal weights, rather than to larger placentas. An increased frequency of *single umbilical artery* (SUA) and *abnormal cord insertions* is seen in smokers. Smokers' placentas have *more calcifications, increased perivillous fibrin,* and an increased incidence of *abruptions,* although the latter association is often overstated. *Chorangiosis* has also been seen with increased frequency in the placentas of smokers. **Electron microscopy** of the placenta has also yielded significant changes induced by smoking. Alterations and damage to the endothelium of the umbilical arteries and vein have been identified as well as a reduction in the microvillous surface of the syncytial cells and other changes, which adversely affect oxygen exchange from mother to fetus.

Alcohol

A direct effect of **alcohol** on the placenta is disputed, although fetal growth restriction and other consequences of the fetal alcohol syndrome are well delineated in the offspring of patients with alcohol abuse during pregnancy. Several studies have shown that the placenta is smaller than that of controls, and there is an *increased incidence of chorioamnionitis, chronic villitis, meconium staining, chorangiomas, abruptio placentae, and embryologic remnants in the umbilical cords.* The significance of the increase in these lesions is unknown.

Cocaine

The use of **cocaine** (benzoylmethylecgonine) and **"crack"** (the free-base smokable form of cocaine) during pregnancy has increased appreciably. Consuming cocaine in pregnancy has been linked to *abruptio placentae, prematurity, preeclampsia, fetal growth restriction, transient* *hypertension, and severe placental vasoconstriction.* Much of the effect of cocaine, at least during pregnancy, seems to be mediated through its known hypertensive and vasoconstrictive activity. Following cocaine exposure, there is a rise of maternal arterial pressure combined with a reduction of uterine blood flow. The frequency of abruptio placentae is, in our experience, not as excessive as given in the many reports. It must be admitted that cocaine abuse is often combined with alcohol and other drug abuse and with maternal cigarette smoking, which may confound the issue. The vasoconstriction caused by these agents may be transmitted to the fetus, in which *cerebral infarction* has occasionally been observed.

Miscellaneous Therapeutic Medications

Few other drugs have shown well-recorded effects on placental structure, the notable exception being **methotrexate** in which there is *severe trophoblast toxicity.* This is apparently the reason it is used successfully in the eradication of early ectopic pregnancies and in gestational trophoblastic disease. A number of other chemotherapeutic agents have been used on pregnant women in the treatment of malignancies, generally with little ill effect on the fetus or placenta. Severe fetal growth restriction occurred with a patient who attempted to cause abortion by taking **aminopterin**; the placenta was not described. **Cyclophosphamide** is considered teratogenic and therefore is generally not used in the first trimester. The data on **6-mercaptopurine** and **azathioprine** suggest that the risk for congenital anomalies early in pregnancy is low. **Alkylating agents** have been used successfully and have been attended without ill effect. Neither fetal toxicity nor placental abnormalities have been described with use of a variety of cytotoxic drugs. In general, malignancy and the need for administration of chemotherapy are not considered an indication for termination of pregnancy.

Irradiation during pregnancy is usually avoided because of the known deleterious effects it has on the fetus. Occasional reports of the effect of therapeutic irradiation on fetuses have shown variable findings including *fetal anomalies (such as hydronephrosis)* and placental abnormalities, including *decidual inflammation and necrosis, necrosis of the fetal membranes, and nonspecific degenerative changes.*

Suggestions for Examination and Report
(Maternal diseases and conditions)

Gross Examination: In the setting of maternal disease, gross examination is relatively routine. Specific attention should be given to any gross lesions that are associated with the specific maternal condition present. As usual, any gross lesions identified should be sampled.

Comment: Correlation of findings with those typical for the specific maternal disease should be attempted, however, diagnosis of maternal disease from placental pathology can only be suggested.

Table 17.1. Reported features of maternal disorders.

Disorder	Clinical prenatal features	Pathology
Connective tissue disorders		
Dermatomyositis	–	Subamnionic necrosis, infarcts, ↑fibrinoid
Ehlers–Danlos	PM, PROM	?Fragile membranes
Myositis ossificans	PROM	–
Periarteritis nodosa	–	NL
Rheumatoid arthritis	IUGR	Small infarcts, calcification
Scleroderma	IUFD, Ab, PM, abruptio, maternal death	Infarcts, DV, ↑fibrinoid
Takayasu's arteritis	–	–
Renal and liver disease		
Chronic renal disease	–	Small, abnormal decidual vessels
Acute fatty liver of pregnancy	PEC, coagulation abnormalities	Gross bilirubin staining
Cholestasis of pregnancy	IUFD, PM	Meconium macrophages
Hyperlipidemia	IUGR	Rare foam cells in intervillous space
Miscellaneous inherited disorders		
Cystic fibrosis	–	–
Cystinosis	–	Vacuolization of decidual cells
Cystinuria	IUGR	–
Gaucher's disease	Thrombocytopenia	NL
Gordon's syndrome	–	NL
Impetigo herpetiformis	IUFD	"Placental insufficiency"
Niemann–Pick disease	–	NL
Phenylketonuria	–	NL
Pruritus gravidarum	Cholestasis, PM, IUFD	Meconium macrophages
Sarcoidosis	–	Granulomas
Smith–Lemli–Opitz	–	NL
Wilson's disease	–	NL
Hematologic disorders		
Heart disease	fetal/placental weight ratio, IUGR	Infarcts, intervillous thrombi
β-Thalassemia	Ab, IUFD	Occasional infarcts
Factor VII deficiency	–	–
Folate deficiency	Ab, abruption	Retroplacental hematoma

(continued)

Table 17.1. (continued)

Disorder	Clinical prenatal features	Pathology
Hematologic disorders		
Hemorrhagic hereditary telangiectasia	–	–
High altitude	–	Placentomegaly, increased syncytial knots, chorangiosis
ITP	Postpartum hemorrhage	Intervillous thrombus, infarcts, decidual vasculopathy
Leukoagglutinins	–	–
Maternal anemia	–	Placentomegaly or small placenta with increased syncytial knots
SC disease (sickle thalassemia)	Ab, IUFD	Infarcts
Sickle cell disease	PEC, sepsis, perinatal mortality, IUGR, abruptio	Small placenta, sickle cells in intervillous space, increased syncytial knots, infarcts, increased fibrin, villous edema, retroplacental hematoma
Sickle cell trait	Similar to disease but less severe	Similar to sickle cell disease but less severe
TTP	IUFD, high mortality	Hyaline thrombi in decidual vessels
Von Willebrand's disease	–	–
Endocrine disorders		
Cushing's disease	Ab, IUFD, PM	NL
Diabetes insipidus	Severe oligohydramnios	–
Diabetes mellitus	Macrosomia, PM, Ab, IUGR, congenital anomalies, fetal vascular thrombopathy	Placentomegaly, dysmature villi, hypervascular villi, NRBCs, thrombosis
Thyroid disease (general)	PEC, abruptio, IUGR, IUFD	Infarcts
Thyroid-hyperthyroidism	Polyhydramnios, fetal distress	Meconium macrophages
Thyroid-hypothyroidism	Ab, congenital anomalies, postpartum hemorrhage	–
Zollinger–Ellison	–	NL

(continued)

Table 17.1. (continued)

Disorder	Clinical prenatal features	Pathology
Maternal drug use		
Alcohol	IUGR, fetal alcohol syndrome, abruptio	Acute chorioamnionitis, meconium macrophages, chorangioma, umbilical cord remnants
Cocaine	Abruptio, IUGR, maternal hypertension, PM, PEC	Retroplacental hematoma
Heroin	IUGR	Acute chorioamnionitis, meconium macrophages
LSD	Ab, chromosome breakage	NL
Tobacco	IUGR, Ab, PROM, IUFD, abruptio	Single umbilical artery, abnormal cord insertions, calcifications
Marijuana	–	–

"–" Not been reported; *Ab* abortion; *IUFD* intrauterine fetal demise; *IUGR* intrauterine growth restriction; *NL* normal; *NRBC* nucleated red blood cell; *PEC* preeclampsia; *PM* prematurity; *PROM* premature rupture of membranes

Selected References

PHP5, pages 584–599 (Maternal Diseases Complicating Pregnancy: Diabetes, Hematologic Disorders, Endocrine Disorders).

Akbulut M, Sorkun HC, Bir F, Eralp A, Duzcan E. Chorangiosis: The potential role of smoking and air pollution. Pathol Res Pract 2009;205:75–81.

Baldwin VJ, MacLeod PM, Benirschke K. Placental findings in alcohol abuse in pregnancy. Birth Defects Orig Artic Ser 1982;18:89–94.

Davis LE, Leveno KJ, Cunningham FG. Hypothyroidism complicating pregnancy. Obstet Gynecol 1988;72:108–112.

Davis LE, Lucas MJ, Hankins GDV, et al. Thyrotoxicosis complicating pregnancy. Am J Obstet Gynecol 1989;160:63–70.

Dombrowski MP, Wolfe HM, Welch RA, et al. Cocaine abuse is associated with abruptio placentae and decreased birth weight, but not shorter labor. Obstet Gynecol 1991;77:139–141.

Evers IM, Nikkels PG, Sikkems JM, Visser GH. Placental pathology in women with type I diabetes and in a control group with normal and large-for-gestational age infants. Placenta 2003;24:819–825.

Haust MD. Maternal diabetes mellitus: effects on the fetus and newborn. In: Naeye RL, Kissane JM, Kaufman N (eds) Perinatal diseases. Baltimore: Williams & Wilkins, 1981:201–285.

Meyer MB, Tonascia JA. Maternal smoking, pregnancy complications and perinatal mortality. Am J Obstet Gynecol 1977;128:494–502.

Naeye RL. Relationship of cigarette smoking to congenital anomalies and perinatal death: a prospective study. Am J Pathol 1978;90:289–294.

Saad J, Kouides P, Shan R, Cramer S. Pathology of thrombotic thrombocytopenia purpura in the placenta, with emphasis on the "snowman sign." Pediatr Dev Pathol 2007;10:455–462.

Shanklin DR. Clinicopathologic correlates in placentas from women with sickle cell disease. Am J Pathol 1976;82:5a.

Singer DB. The placenta in pregnancies complicated by diabetes mellitus. Perspect Pediatr Pathol 1984;8:199–212.

Chapter 18
Placental Malperfusion

General Considerations

Placental insufficiency is a term often used in connection with **placental malperfusion** and is sometimes defined as a critical reduction of the placental exchange membrane. It is a most difficult term to define precisely. Ratios of placental to fetal weight have been used to correlate with placental function, but alterations of this ratio are so frequent that one cannot deduce placental dysfunction from an abnormal ratio (see Table 3.7 in Chap. 3). "Placental insufficiency" may be due to a variety of factors including *abnormal fetal genome, chronic infection, maternal disease, localization of the placenta in the uterus, cord insertion, preeclamptic changes, chorangiosis, tumors, fetal thrombotic vasculopathy, excessive fibrinoid deposits, and so on.* We prefer to specify the lesions that are present rather than to embrace them all in the imprecise terminology of "placental insufficiency." Placental malperfusion, on the other hand, also has many synonyms, including placental underperfusion, uteroplacental malperfusion, uteroplacental underperfusion, and placental bed underperfusion. These all describe the same thing and have in common a number of features, with the primary defect being an abnormality in uteroplacental vessels. These abnormalities and their sequelae are described below.

R.N. Baergen, *Manual of Pathology of the Human Placenta,*
DOI 10.1007/978-1-4419-7494-5_18, © Springer Science+Business Media, LLC 2011

The classic disorder of placental malperfusion and "placental insufficiency" is **preeclampsia**. The constellation of placental findings, however, is also seen in the syndrome of **lupus anticoagulant, systemic lupus**, occasionally in **coagulation disorders**, and even without underlying maternal disease. The fact that the same pattern of placental lesions occurs in different disorders suggests that there is a common thread in the underlying pathophysiology of these disorders. However, the pathophysiology of these disorders is still not fully understood.

Preeclampsia and Gestational Hypertension

Clinical Features and Implications
The diagnosis of preeclampsia (PEC) is made based on clinical criteria:

- **Hypertension** associated with pregnancy after 20 weeks gestation, and
- **Proteinuria.**

Previously, edema was also included in the definition, but currently the above criteria are sufficient. The diagnosis of hypertension and the amount of proteinuria are specifically defined, as are the criteria for severe preeclampsia, but the specifics are beyond the scope of this text. Hypertension associated with pregnancy and not associated with proteinuria is frequently referred to as **pregnancy-induced hypertension**, and more recently as **gestational hypertension. Eclampsia** is merely preeclampsia with seizures; however, in 38% of pregnant women who develop eclampsia, hypertension or proteinuria was not previously present. It is important to note that preeclampsia is a pregnancy-induced disease and that, typically, after delivery, the disease ceases, although in rare cases sequelae persist into the early postpartum period. Inasmuch as preeclampsia occurs in the absence of a fetus, as it occurs with increased frequency in hydatidiform moles, it is clearly dependent on the presence of placental tissue, a fact that has provided some clues to the study of its pathogenesis. Recent work has shown that abnormal placentation and resultant placental damage, inflammation, and oxidative stress are implicated in the development of the clinical syndrome of preeclampsia.

Preeclampsia is a common complication of pregnancy, occurring in 2–7% of all pregnancies and in 7–10% of primigravidas. It is most often mild and occurs near term (75% of cases), in which case there is a minimal risk of adverse pregnancy outcome. *The disease is much more frequent in primigravidas, and in very young gravidas.* The frequency and severity of the disease is significantly higher in women with *multiple gestation, chronic hypertension, previous preeclampsia, pregestational diabetes, and thrombophilia.* Paternal risk factors also exist, some having to do with family history and some relating to sperm exposure.

Preeclampsia is responsible for substantial maternal and perinatal morbidity and mortality. Outcome is poorer in early-onset preeclampsia and in women with other underlying diseases. Maternal or obstetric complications include *abruption, disseminated intravascular coagulation, pulmonary edema, acute renal failure, liver failure, stroke, and death.* Perinatal complications include *preterm delivery, fetal growth-restriction, hypoxia and/or neurologic injury, and death.* Fetal complications generally result from the characteristic placental alterations (see below). Preeclampsia is also thought to be associated with the **HELLP syndrome** *(hemolysis, elevated liver enzymes, low platelets).* Indeed, approximately 80% of patients who develop HELLP syndrome were previously diagnosed with preeclampsia.

Pathologic Features
The principal pathologic changes of the placenta in preeclampsia are:

- **Decidual vasculopathy,**
- **Infarcts,**
- **Abruptio placentae,**
- **Villous maldevelopment,** and
- **Diminished growth**

These pathologic features do not necessarily correlate with the clinical disease. Even in severe clinical disease, they are not always present. Severe placental changes may also occur when no maternal symptoms are present and placental lesions may occur long before clinical manifestations. Finally, these lesions are not pathognomonic for preeclampsia as they may be found in other disorders such as lupus anticoagulant and thrombophilias (see below). They are, however, indicative of abnormal uteroplacental perfusion.

Decidual Vascular Changes
Various changes occur in the decidual (spiral) arterioles, which are collectively referred to as **decidual vasculopathy, decidual arteriopathy, or decidual arteriolopathy.** These lesions are the underlying cause of the other placental changes such as infarcts and abruptios. Vascular changes include:

- **Lack of physiologic conversion,**
  - **Focal or complete,**
  - **Persistence of arteriolar smooth muscle,**
  - **Decreased luminal diameter,**
- **Thrombosis,**
- **Vasculitis,**
- **Atherosis,** and
- **Fibrinoid necrosis.**

Under physiologic conditions, trophoblast of the placental shell infiltrates the arterial beds of the decidua and superficial myometrium, destroys the muscular walls of the arterioles, and replaces them with fibrinoid. This infiltration of the implantation site ultimately opens the lumens and renders the vessels incapable of a vasoconstrictive response to the various vasoactive mediators. Therefore, in normal *physiologic conversion,* the arteries are transformed into *enlarged, tortuous but rigid channels.* In preeclampsia and other disorders of malperfusion, on the other hand, the invasion of trophoblast is more superficial, and there is *failure of trophoblastic invasion of the proximal, myometrial branches. Invasion of decidual vessels is also impeded* to some degree. The smooth muscle persists either partially or completely. These changes are designated as **lack of physiologic conversion** (Fig. 18.1).

Fatty infiltration in the walls of the endothelial cells can be observed and later the presence of *macrophages containing phagocytosed fat from degenerating lipid-laden myogenic foam cells.* This change is called **atherosis** or sometimes acute atherosis (Figs. 18.2 and 18.3) and is very characteristic of preeclamptic changes. Proliferative activity of intimal and muscle cells along with damage to the vascular endothelium leads to **decidual vascular thrombosis** (Fig. 18.3). Eventually, **fibrinoid necrosis** of the media occurs (Fig. 18.4). Inflammatory changes such

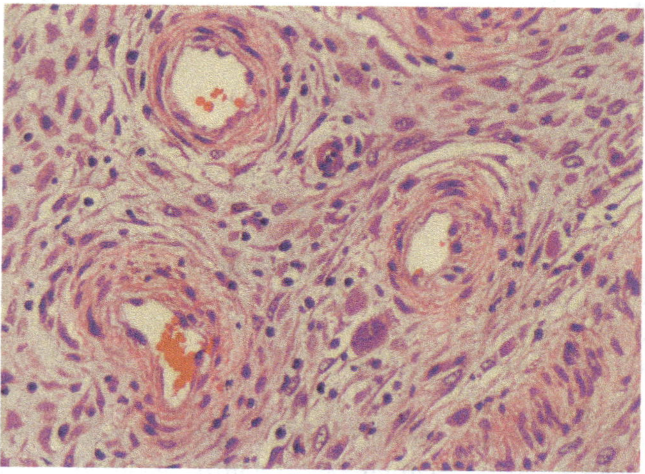

Figure 18.1. Lack of physiologic conversion of decidual vessels. The arterioles retain their thick muscular coat in spite of abundant extravillous trophoblast in the implantation site. H&E ×200.

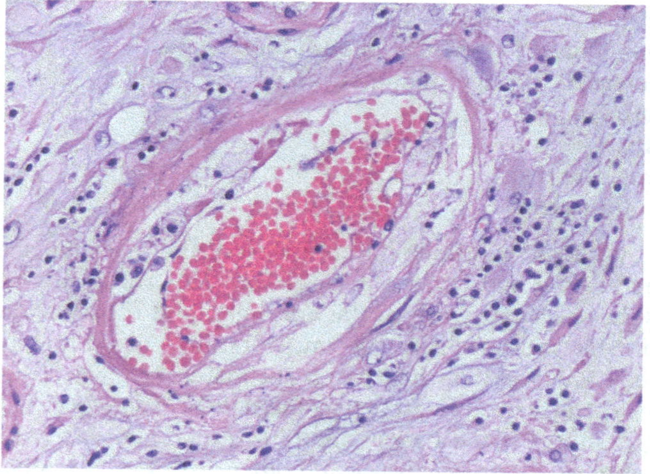

Figure 18.2. Acute atherosis and fibrinoid degeneration. H&E ×400.

as *chronic inflammation of the decidual tissue and decidual vessels* are also found in association with the vascular lesions, sometimes referred to as **decidual vasculitis** (Fig. 18.5). Although lymphoid cells may be present, plasma cells are conspicuously absent. There is often secondary necrosis of the decidual tissue as well (Fig. 18.4). *Vascular thickening or "spasm" has also been described, but is more common in chronic hypertension without pregnancy-induced hypertension or preeclampsia* (Fig. 18.6).

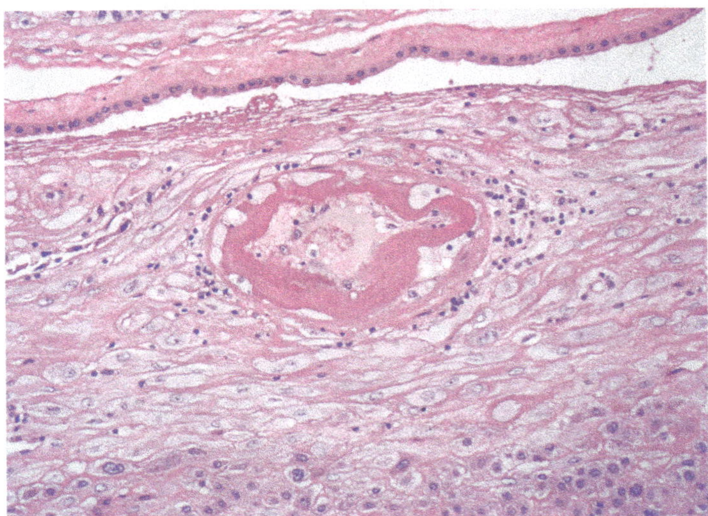

Figure 18.3. Atherosis in decidual arterioles of patient with preeclampsia. The vessel wall has been replaced by fibrin, the intima replaced by cholesterol-laden macrophages, and there is early mural thrombosis. H&E ×400.

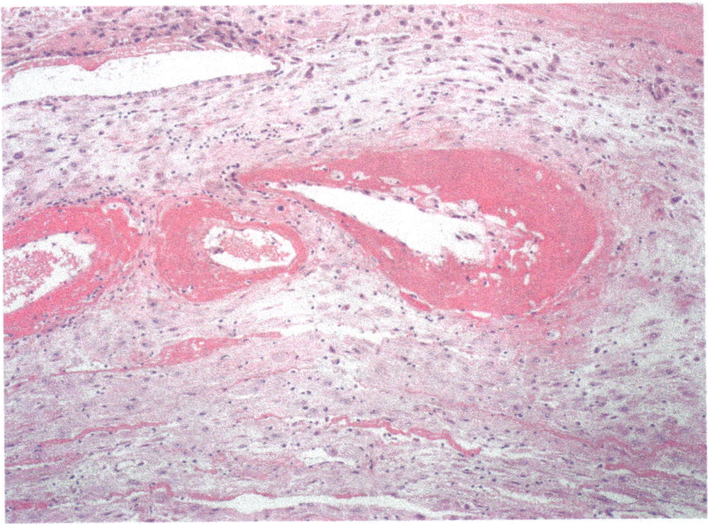

Figure 18.4. Hyalinized decidual vessels with thrombosis and marked fibrinoid necrosis. H&E ×200.

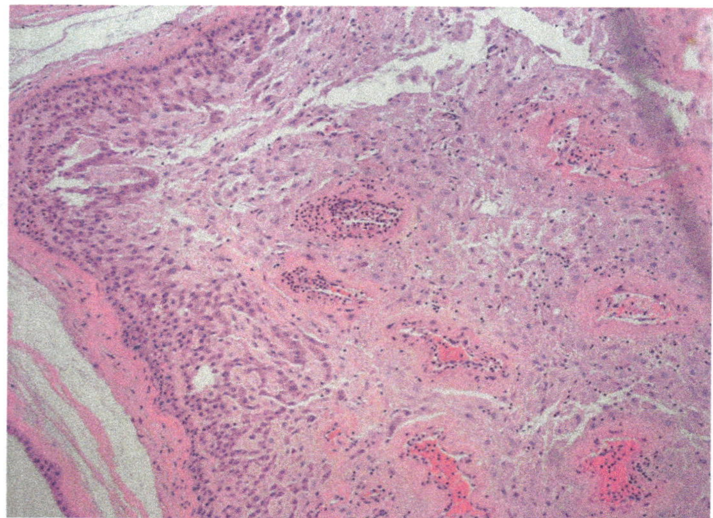

Figure 18.5. Decidual vessels show lymphocyte and macrophage infiltration (decidual vasculitis). H&E ×200.

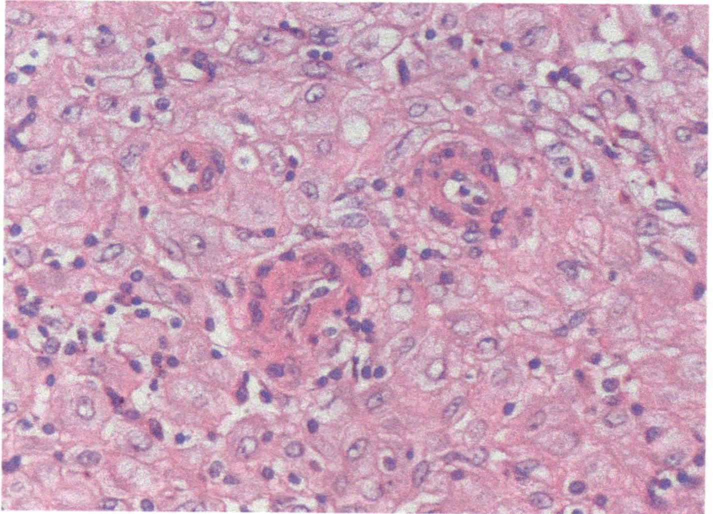

Figure 18.6. Vessel from the implantation site of a patient with hypertensive disease. Note the thickened vascular wall, which may be secondary to spasm. H&E ×220.

The vascular changes are not easily found in the delivered placenta. For that reason, it has been suggested that *en face* sections of the maternal floor be prepared in order to obtain more cross sections of maternal arterioles. While this makes intuitive sense, we have not found that it enhances our ability to diagnose atherosis or other lesions. Depending on the skill of the histotechnologist preparing the section, variable success is achieved. However, the vessels in the decidua capsularis that accompany the membranes are often pathologically altered and

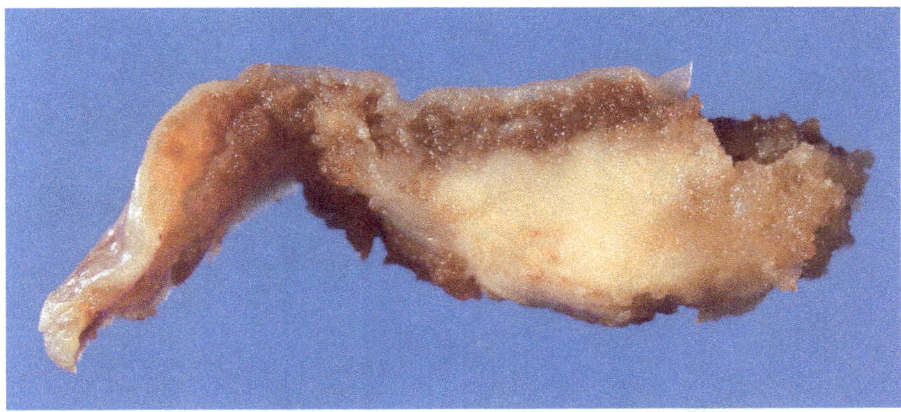

Figure 18.7. Placental sections from a patient with severe preeclampsia and stillbirth. A large, old infarct is present; it is white and firm on cut section.

so in some respects may be superior for diagnosis. Sections of the membranes from the placenta margin are particularly good in showing these changes.

Infarcts

Placental infarcts are the most common and conspicuous lesions observed by the pathologist. They represent *villous tissue that has died because of deficient intervillous (maternal) circulation.* Infarcts are firm, condensed dead areas of villous tissue that often encompass the entire thickness of the placenta (Figs. 18.7 and 18.8). Frequently, they involve the base of the placenta and are particularly common at the placental edge. Generally, marginal infarcts at term actually represent a somewhat different process in that they represent atrophy of placental tissue due to local factors rather than true infarcts, although they are histologically indistinguishable. *When infarcts are found away from the placental margins, and particularly when they are randomly distributed, conditions of malperfusion almost invariably exist.* Infarcts in any location in first- and second-trimester placentas are always abnormal.

Macroscopically, infarcts are *firmer than the surrounding villous tissue and have a granular surface.* Early infarcts are initially dark red and congested and can be distinguished from normal tissue by their firmness and by their lack of a spongy texture (Fig. 18.8). *As they age, infarcts become progressively yellow, then tan-gray, and finally white and firm* (Fig. 18.9). Microscopically, the earliest change is congestion of villous capillaries and intravillous hemorrhage followed by *villous agglutination,* or collapse of the intervillous space (Fig. 18.10). Shortly thereafter, there is *loss of distinct nuclear basophilia of the syncytium with "smudging" of nuclei* (Fig. 18.11). *Pyknosis and karyorrhexis then follow.* The endothelium and intravascular erythrocytes then lose staining and become pale and ghost-like. Occasionally, acute inflammatory cells are seen at the edge of the infarct, and this should not be interpreted as villitis. With time, the trophoblast and villous stromal cells completely lose their staining characteristics. The resultant *pale-staining ghost villi*

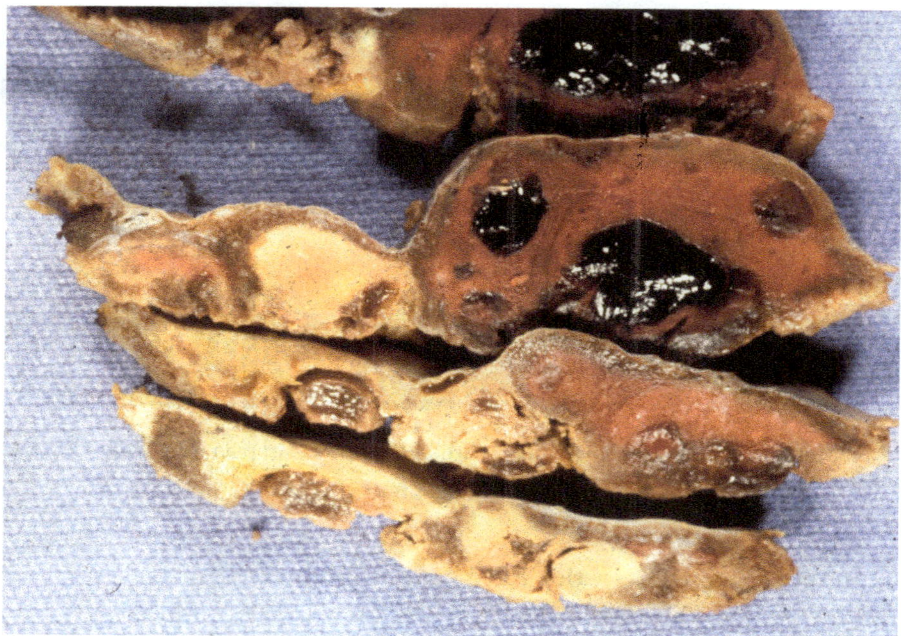

Figure 18.8. Placental sections from a patient with preeclampsia and infarcts of varying age. Recent infarcts show *dark* discoloration, which gradually changes to *pink*, *tan*, and then *white* in the oldest infarcts.

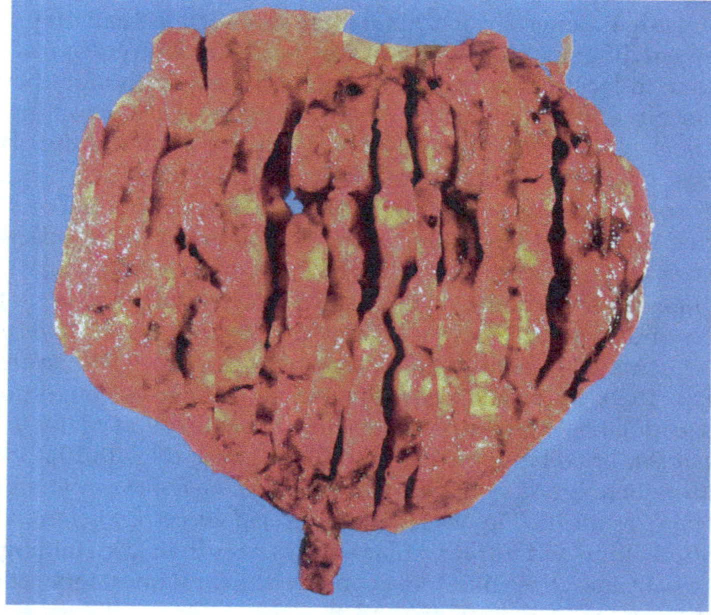

Figure 18.9. Multiple old infarcts involving primarily the placental floor seen as *yellowish* discolorations of the placental parenchyma.

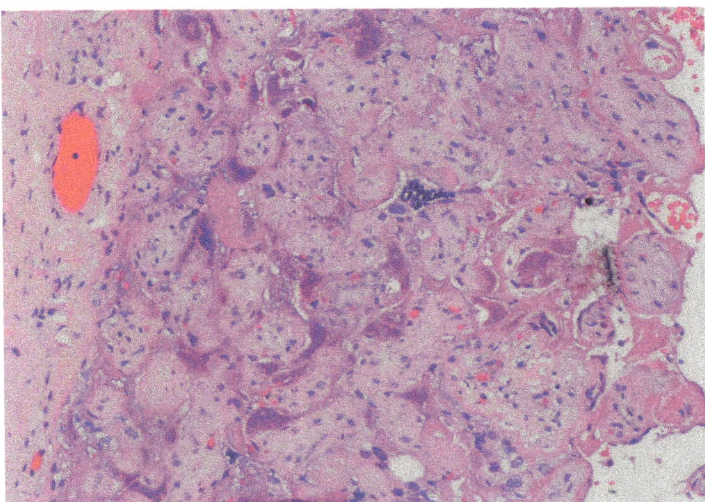

Figure 18.10. Early infarct with ischemic change, collapse of villi, and loss of the intervillous space and smudging of the trophoblastic nuclei. H&E ×250.

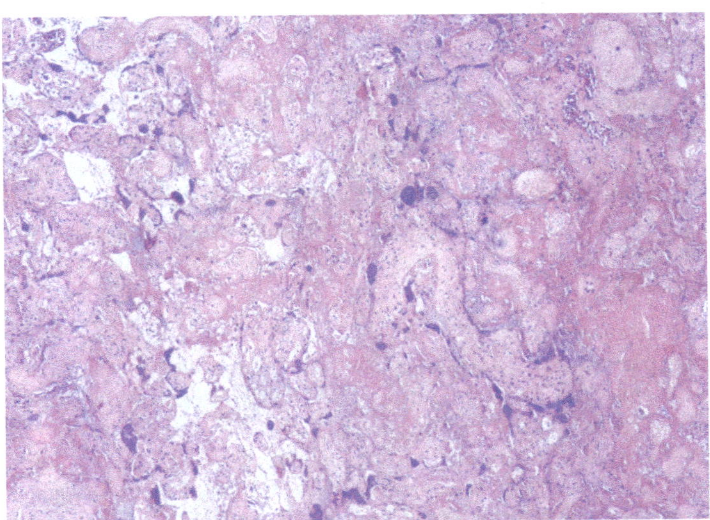

Figure 18.11. Intermediate age infarct with smudging and karyorrhexis of trophoblastic nuclei. Focally there is loss of the basophilic staining of the nuclei. H&E ×100.

are completely collapsed, interspersed only with a thin layer of fibrinoid material (Fig. 18.12). The periphery of the infarct often shows less well-developed changes. Unlike infarcts of other organs, such as the spleen or kidney, placental infarcts do not "organize" and are never invaded by organizing fibrous tissue or blood vessels; in their subsequent evolution, they only become atrophic. The number of infarcts, and more importantly, *the percentage of the placental mass involved*, has important clinical significance for the fetus. It has been stated that a minimum

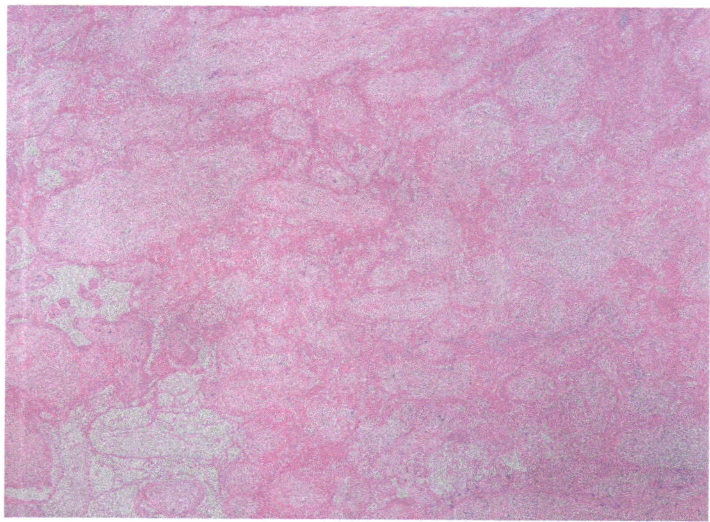

Figure 18.12. Old infarct with ghost-like villi showing virtually no basophilic staining. The villous are collapsed on one another with a thin layer of fibrinoid interposed. H&E ×100.

of 190 g placental tissue is needed for fetal survival. Thus, large infarcts, or multiple small infarcts involving a substantial portion of the placenta may be fatal. Usually, infarcts involving less than 10% of the placental parenchyma do not affect oxygenation per se. However, the higher percentage of involvement of villous tissue, the less placental reserves exist, which can ultimately affect fetal outcome if additional problems arise.

Abruptio Placentae

Abruptio placentae is defined as detachment of the placenta from its decidual seat. The most common predisposing cause is preeclampsia. Here, the hemorrhage begins with the decidual vascular lesions described above, specifically, *thrombosis of the decidual arterioles leads to necrosis and subsequent venous hemorrhage.* Pathologically, this results in a **retroplacental hematoma** (Figs. 18.13 and 18.14). The hematoma pulls the placenta away from the uterus, and, ultimately, the villous tissue underlying the hematoma will become infarcted, as it has lost its blood supply. Abruptios are discussed in more detail in Chap. 19.

Villous Maldevelopment and Syncytial Knotting

Reconstructions of serial paraffin sections show that most "syncytial knots" seen in term placentas are in fact tangential sections of irregularly shaped villous surfaces. Although they are due to tangential sectioning, they are representative of a characteristic deformation or contour of the surface of the terminal villi and so are not technically an artifact. Correct interpretation of syncytial knots is of considerable importance, as increased syncytial knotting is widely accepted as a diagnostic indicator of placental ischemia and malperfusion.

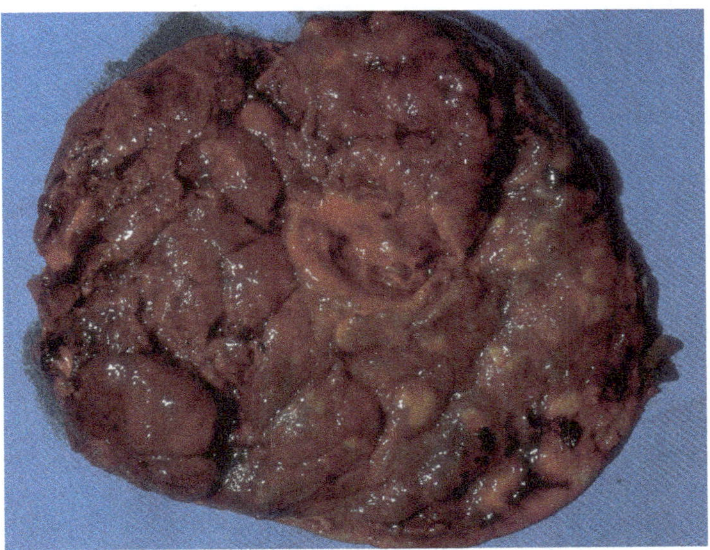

Figure 18.13. Abruptio with a layered retroplacental clot (*center*) and adjacent old infarct.

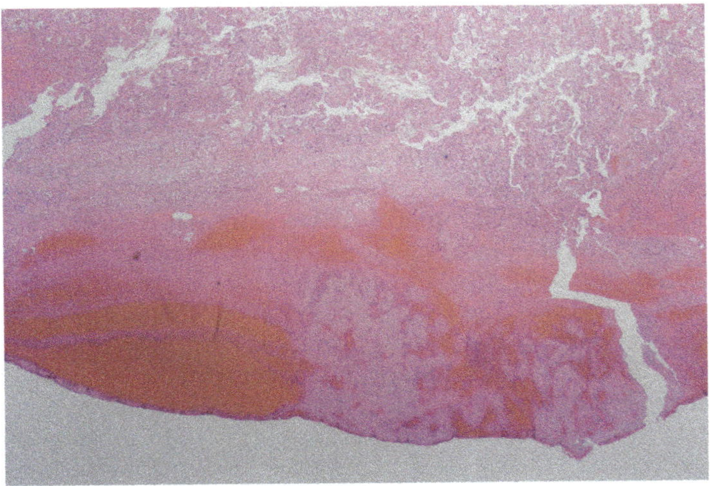

Figure 18.14. Fresh abruptio with minimal infarction of villous tissue. The clot below is elevating the decidua basalis. H&E ×60.

Furthermore, the percentage of villi with syncytial knots increases with gestational age to a maximum of about 28% at term. Thus, when *more than 28–30% of terminal villi possess syncytial knots*, especially in the premature placenta, *it is diagnostic of some level of perfusional compromise.* Even so, diagnosis is particularly difficult for inexperienced observers, as recognition of this finding is dependent on precise knowledge of what is normal for a specific gestational age.

Villous Maldevelopment and Hypoxia:
Several different patterns of villous maldevelopment emerge that are associated with preplacental, uteroplacental, or postplacental hypoxia. **Preplacental hypoxia** *may be associated with maternal anemia, pregnancy at high altitude, maternal cyanosis, or other conditions in which the mother experiences hypoxia*, and the blood flowing to the placenta has reduced oxygen levels. Mother, placenta, and fetus all experience hypoxia. The classic example of **uteroplacental hypoxia** *is pregnancy-induced hypertension* and *preeclampsia* in which the placenta experiences hypoxia by virtue of diminished blood flow via the uteroplacental vessels. In this case, the mother is normally oxygenated but the placenta and fetus are hypoxic. **Postplacental hypoxia** is strongly linked to *intrauterine growth restriction associated with absent or reversed end-diastolic umbilical flow*. It may or may not be associated with preeclampsia, and the mother and placenta have normal oxygen levels, while only the fetus is hypoxic. The resulting histologic appearance in each case is due to several aspects of villous development. First is the degree **of maturation**. Accelerated maturation results in a developmental shift from immature intermediate villi towards mature intermediate and then terminal villi. This results in smaller and smaller villi with more increased syncytial knots. Second, is the **degree and type of fetoplacental angiogenesis.** This is controlled by intraplacental oxygen levels, which in turn influences the numbers and shapes of terminal villi (Fig. 18.15).

In postplacental hypoxia, there are high oxygen levels that induce nonbranching angiogenesis, resulting in *poorly developed, long, slender, or filiform terminal villi with minimal branching, minimal syncytial knots, and long, largely unbranched capillary loops* (Fig. 18.15). In the past, this has been referred to as **terminal villus deficiency** (Fig. 18.16) but is also called **villous hypoplasia**. In preplacental hypoxia, the low oxygen levels induce branching angiogenesis, resulting in clusters of *richly capillarized, short, highly branched, and notched terminal villi, showing increased syncytial knots* or **Tenney–Parker changes** (Fig. 18.17). The highly branched, net-like capillary beds are easy to perfuse, as their structure provides less flow resistance than comparably large capillary beds composed of longer, less branched capillaries. Placentas from cases of uteroplacental hypoxia are similar to those with preplacental hypoxia irrespective of whether they are complicated by preeclampsia.

Terminal Villus Deficiency: Villous Hypoplasia:
Terminal villus deficiency is associated with *postplacental hypoxia and intrauterine growth restriction (IUGR) with absent or reversed end-diastolic flow*. Terminal villus side branches of the mature intermediate villi are largely missing. *The terminal capillary loops, resulting from nonbranching angiogenesis, are long, slender, and usually unbranched*, thus explaining the high Doppler resistance index. The straight course of the largely unbranched, filiform terminal villi results in *predominance of small, round villous cross sections of minimum diameters (30–60 μm) with admixture of some longitudinal sections* (Fig. 18.16). The prevalence of the smallest villous diameters, in combination with occasional unbranched, filiform,

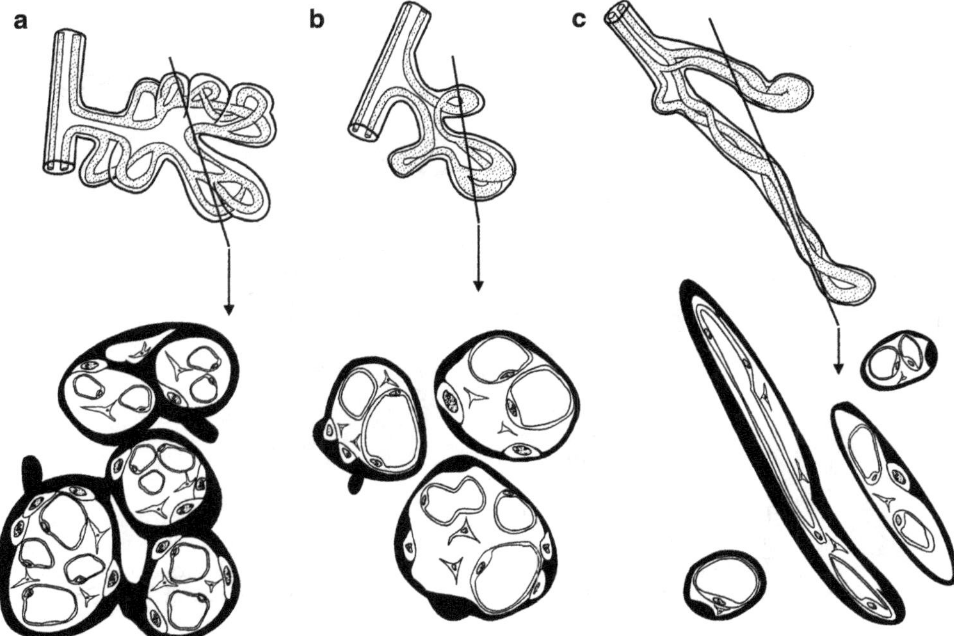

Figure 18.15. Capillary branching patterns and their effect on shapes of terminal villi in histologic section. (**a**) Predominance of branching angiogenesis, resulting in highly branching capillaries and short, knob-like, multiply indented terminal villi, which on section show increased syncytial knotting. This is seen in both preplacental and uteroplacental hypoxia. (**b**) Groups of grape-like terminal villi with smooth surfaces are the result of a balanced mixture of branching and nonbranching angiogenesis. The resulting histologic sections reveal less trophoblastic knotting than in (**a**) and the terminal villi contain sinusoidally dilated capillaries. This is the pattern in normal pregnancy. (**c**) Prevalence of nonbranching angiogenesis causes long, poorly branched, and minimally coiled capillaries in long, filiform terminal villi. Due to the absence of parallel capillary loops within the villi, they have unusually small diameters ranging between 30 and 40 μm. Histologically, these features result in small-caliber villous cross sections and a few longitudinal sections. This is terminal villus deficiency and is seen in postplacental hypoxia associated with absent or reduced end diastolic umbilical flow.

low-caliber villous sections, absence of syncytial knotting, and an unusually wide intervillous space, makes this an easily identifiable condition. The abnormalities in end-diastolic flow in the umbilical arteries by Doppler measurement provide evidence that the resulting blood flow impedance is considerably increased. Clinically the Doppler findings are considered evidence of fetal compromise, often with the need for immediate delivery.

Other Placental Changes in Preeclampsia
Aside from the liability of infarcts, abruptio, villous maldevelopment, and the nearly invariable decidual vascular alterations, the placenta in PEC undergoes some additional and mostly minor structural changes. More often than not, the placenta is *smaller and "drier"* than expected for that gestational age. When sectioned, the placenta is much *darker than normal organs*, reflecting the hemoconcentration of the fetus. The umbilical cord is often thin as well. In preeclampsia, and particularly

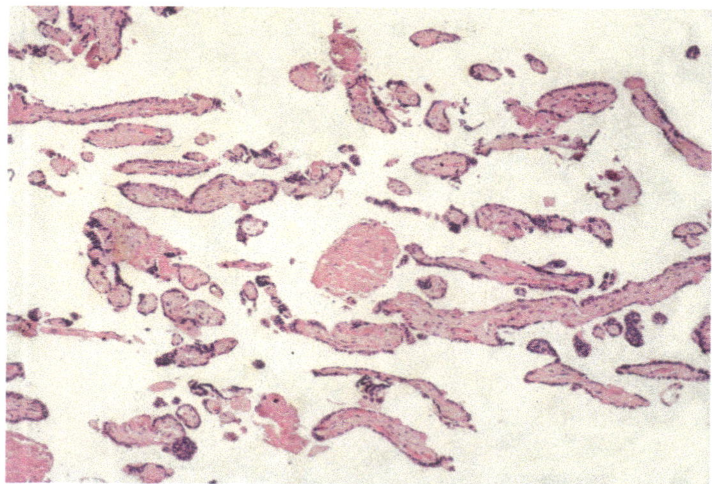

Figure 18.16. Placenta from a patient with intrauterine growth restriction and absent end-diastolic flow (postplacental hypoxia) at the 40th week of gestation. There is a striking predominance of small villous calibers and filiform longitudinal profiles and an unusually wide intervillous space. H&E ×55.

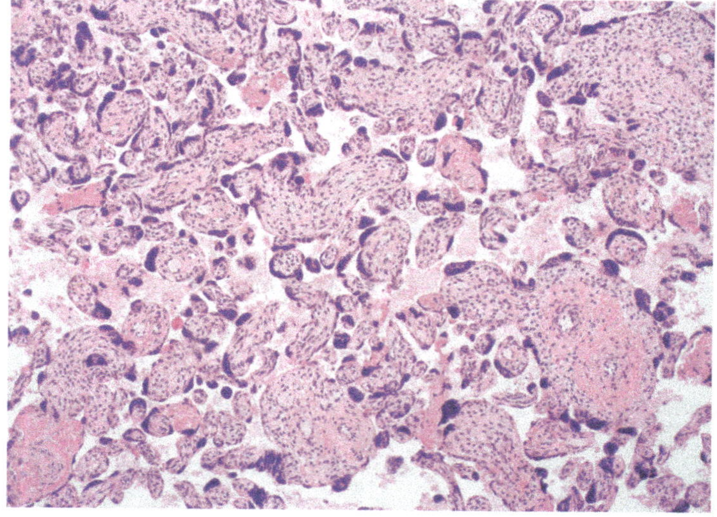

Figure 18.17. "Tenney–Parker" changes in a placenta at 25 weeks' gestation. There is obvious acceleration of villous maturation and increased syncytial knots, which appear *enlarged* and *bulbous* in shape compared to syncytial knots seen in cross sections of a mature placenta. H&E ×64.

in eclampsia, there is enhanced pulmonary embolization of syncytial cells. Occasional authors have even suggested that excessive pulmonary embolization with syncytial buds may cause maternal death. It is probably fortunate that these cells are swiftly disposed of in the lung. Interestingly, women who have increased numbers of syncytial remnants in their circulation early in pregnancy have a statistically higher risk of the development of preeclampsia and may provide an early screening tool in the future.

Pathogenesis

The principal cause of preeclampsia is still unknown. Preeclampsia is more likely to develop in *primigravidas, in women with increased placental tissue (moles and multiple gestation), and in women with preexisting vascular disease or with a predisposition to vascular disease*. While it is certain that the disease relates to the presence of placental tissue, the proximate cause is obscure. Theories involving immunologic mechanisms, genetic predisposition, environmental and dietary factors, vasoactive mediators, and endothelial dysfunction have all been suggested. The pathophysiology of preeclampsia is complex, but **vasospasm** and **diffuse endothelial injury** are key events. Small vessels in affected organs undergo *vasoconstriction, which causes increased resistance to flow and subsequent arterial hypertension*. The associated endothelial damage has serious sequelae, including vascular thrombosis and end-organ ischemia and damage. Placental injury and ischemia also appear to play a role in pathophysiology of preeclampsia, and investigation in this area has shown much promise in understanding this complex disorder.

Lupus Erythematosus

Clinical Features and Implications

Systemic lupus erythematosus (SLE) occurs primarily in young women (M/F ratio 10:1), and it often complicates pregnancy. Fetal survival is reduced due to *an increased number of abortions, maternal renal insufficiency*, and *preeclampsia*. Pregnancy itself does not constitute a risk to patients with SLE, and some patients with SLE have essentially normal placentas and normal infants.

The disease is accompanied by a variety of **circulating antibodies,** of which the best known is the **antinuclear antibody** (ANA). It must be remembered, however, that up to 50% clinically normal pregnant women have antinuclear antibodies at least once during the course of their pregnancy. **Lymphocytotoxic antibodies** possessing antitrophoblastic activity have been found in about 80% of patients with SLE. Fluorescent antibodies (fibrinogen, IgG, IgM, IgA, and C3) have been found localized to the trophoblastic basement membranes, which show thickening on electron microscopy. **Anticoagulant antibodies** also occur in SLE patients, and patients with these antibodies have more spontaneous abortions (58.7%) than those who do not (24.7%).

Some antibodies of patients with SLE are transferred to the fetus. These antibodies may cause *thrombocytopenia, leukopenia, hemolytic anemia, skin lesions, discoid lupus, fetal growth restriction*, and a variety of other conditions, including the LE phenomenon. LE cells may be observed in the neonates of mothers with SLE, but these usually disappear within 7 weeks after delivery and there is subsequent normal development of the infant. In infants of mothers with discoid lupus, neonatal skin lesions develop but disappear within 5 months leaving only small scars. *Congenital heart block* has recently been described to occur in an estimated one of 60 SLE pregnancies. The constellation of congenital heart block with fetal hydrops and skin lesions is now considered part of the **neonatal lupus syndrome.**

Pathologic Features

Although the placentas of patients with SLE may be normal, more often they show changes that are frequently impossible to differentiate from the lesions of preeclampsia. Preeclampsia is also more frequently seen in patients with SLE. When both are present, it is difficult to know whether the placental pathology is due to PEC or to SLE. Histologic study of placentas with SLE reveals *decidual vasculopathy* and/or *atherosis (17%), villitis of unknown etiology (28%),* and *infarcts (18%),* which are principally associated with the simultaneous presence of antiphospholipid antibodies. *Thrombosis of decidual vessels and ischemic/hypoxic changes are also prominent* (Fig. 18.3). One may see intensive chronic deciduitis with infiltration of the decidual vascular walls by abundant chronic inflammatory cells in which, unlike preeclampsia, *plasma cells predominate.* The decidual vascular lesions result in *placental* infarcts and abruptios, which in turn result in retarded placental and fetal growth (Figs. 18.10–18.14). The villous tissue displays *Tenney–Parker changes,* the increased syncytial knotting, which is best known in preeclampsia and is due to reduced maternal perfusion (Fig. 18.17). While Tenney–Parker change, infarcts and other lesions are usually not seen until the third trimester in preeclampsia, in SLE they are seen in the second trimester as well. Thus the presence of decidual vasculopathy and infarcts in the second trimester, whether in association with preeclampsia or not, suggests the possibility of undiagnosed SLE.

Lupus Anticoagulant and Antiphospholipid Antibodies

Clinical Features and Implications

Lupus anticoagulant is the most commonly observed of several **antiphospholipid antibodies.** Others include **anticardiolipin** and **antiphosphatidylserine.** Lupus anticoagulant was first described in patients with SLE who had thrombotic complications. Since then it has been recognized that women with histories of *repeated abortion and premature births* often possess circulating lupus anticoagulants that may indirectly be responsible for this excessive fetal wastage. The term *anticoagulant* is clearly a misnomer because lupus anticoagulant is more frequently encountered in patients **without** lupus, and it is **not** associated with abnormal bleeding in most patients. In some patients, however, thrombotic sequelae may occur, especially in the arterial circulation.

Antiphospholipid antibodies correlate with *early spontaneous abortions, fetal demise, IUGR, and rarely with neonatal stroke.* It is strongly associated with recurrent fetal loss. *Vascular occlusions, aortic thrombosis, carotid artery thrombosis, and central nervous system (CNS) lesions* have also been observed in the neonate. Prednisone and aspirin administration has been advocated for treatment, but studies of the efficacy of various modes of treatment have shown that heparin plus low-dose aspirin is preferable resulting in improved outcome.

The antibodies that characterize this group are heterogeneous but generally prolong phospholipid-dependent coagulation tests by binding to epitopes on the phospholipid portion of prothrombinase (factors Xa and Va, calcium, and phospholipid). Laboratory test results may be discordant, necessitating measurements of specific coagulation factors in order to establish the diagnosis. The antibodies are usually IgG molecules, but may be also be IgM and IgA, or combinations. When abnormal immunologic findings are present in pregnant patients, such as an unexpectedly positive Venereal Disease Research Laboratory (VDRL) test, further investigation is required, particularly a search for the presence of lupus anticoagulant and anticardiolipins.

Pathologic Features

The placenta is often morphologically indistinguishable from that of patients with severe preeclampsia or SLE. Anticoagulants have a coagulative ability in the placenta, leading to the *thrombosis in the intervillous space. Abruptios are also seen.* There is often *extensive placental infarction* and *decidual vascular lesions,* which are found at much younger gestational ages than in preeclampsia. Frequently, the lesions occur before the 20th week of pregnancy. The decidua often shows a marked degree of *acute and chronic inflammation and necrosis.* Similar to hypertensive disease, *infarcts, increased syncytial knots, and increased intervillous fibrin deposition* are frequent findings. When these lesions are present in the early second trimester in patients with no history of preeclampsia or pregnancy-induced hypertension, the likelihood of the presence of an antibody or other procoagulant condition is great. The degree of *infarction* and compromise of the intervillous circulation adequately explain resultant stillbirth and growth restrictions.

Thrombophilias

Clinical Features and Implications

Inherited thrombophilias include **activated protein C resistance, prothrombin mutation, deficiency of antithrombin III, protein C deficiency, protein S deficiency**, and **hyperhomocysteinemia** (homozygous deficiency of methylene tetrahydrofolate reductase [MTHFR]). The most common defect is "activated protein C resistance," which is usually due to a point mutation in the factor V gene (**factor V Leiden mutation**). The allele frequency is highest in Europeans, while it is absent from many non-European populations. *Increased spontaneous abortions, fetal loss, IUGR, and preeclampsia* have all been reported to be increased in maternal thrombophilias. The association with fetal loss is strongest in activated protein C resistance and prothrombin mutations and with protein S deficiency. Maternal deep vein thrombosis is uncommonly reported, but often women with these defects have no history of thrombotic events and present with an unexplained pregnancy loss. Peripartum thrombosis in the fetus has been reported in protein C deficiency and neonatal stroke has also been described.

Pathologic Features

The placentas of such pregnancies have been reported to show an increased incidence of thrombosis, including *intervillous thrombi, intervillous fibrinoid deposition, abruptio, and fetal thrombotic vasculopathy.* Placentas have occasionally shown changes similar to that seen in preeclampsia, including *atherosis, infarcts, and increased syncytial knots,* but placental lesions are not found in all women with these disorders. There is also some controversy about the etiology of the placental lesions and the reproductive losses in these women. Although the assumption has been that abnormal coagulation was responsible, other factors such as the activation of complement may be implicated.

Suggestions for Examination and Report
(Conditions of placental malperfusion)

Gross Examination: The presence of infarcts and abruptios should be noted, and, importantly, the percentage of placental tissue involved. Location of the infarcts (central versus peripheral) and age of the lesions should also be recorded. It is not necessary to record the location, size and age of each infarct but an overall comment in the report should be made, e.g., "multiple central infarcts, recent and remote, comprising 20% of the villous tissue." This is also true for abruptios. It is most important that the percentage of viable (or nonviable) placental tissue be estimated grossly as this cannot be done microscopically. Representative sections of the infarcts and abruptio should be taken along with routine sections. Extra sections to evaluate decidual vessels are also advised. These may be additional sections of maternal surface, membranes or enface sections. Additional sections of "grossly normal" tissue should also be taken as gross assessment usually underestimates the percentage of involved tissue.

Comment: A comment on the extent of the infarcts and/or abruptio is helpful with an estimation of percentage of placental tissue involved. Morphologic changes such as increased syncytial knots and so on should all be listed individually. Decidual lesions may be all listed individually or included under the category of "decidual vasculopathy." If there is no history of hypertensive disease, preeclampsia or other systemic disease associated with these findings, workup for the disorders noted above may be suggested.

Selected References

PHP5, pages 155–165 (Oxygen and Oxygen-Controlled Growth Factors as Regulators of Villous and Vascular development), 249–261 (Uteroplacental Vessels), 473–490 (Histopathologic Approach to Villous Alterations), 491–518 (Classification of Villous Maldevelopment), 604–656 (Maternal Diseases Complicating Pregnancy: Preeclampsia, Lupus Erythematosus and Lupus Anticoagulant).

Baergen RN, Chacko SA, Edersheim T, et al. The placenta in thrombophilias: a clinicopathologic study. Mod Pathol 2001;14:213A.

Infante-Rivard C, David M, Gauthier R, et al. Lupus anticoagulants, anticardiolipin antibodies and fetal loss. A case-control study. N Engl J Med 1991;325:1063–1066.

Khong TY, Pearce JM, Robertson WB. Acute atherosis in preeclampsia: Maternal determinants and fetal outcome in the presence of the lesion. Am J Obstetr Gynecol 1987;157:360–363.

Kingdom JCP, Kaufmann P. Oxygen and placental villous development: origins of fetal hypoxia. Placenta 1997;18:613–621.

Kupferminc MJ, Eldor A, Steinman N, et al. Increased frequency of genetic thrombophilia in women with complications of pregnancy. N Engl J Med 1999;340:9–13.

Levine JS, Branch DW, Rauch J. The antiphospholipid syndrome. N Engl J Med 2002;346(10):752–763.

Magid MS, Kaplan C, Sammaritano LR, et al. Placental pathology in systemic lupus erythematosus: A prospective study. Am J Obstet Gynecol 1998;179:226–234.

Rand JH, Wu XX, Andree HAM, et al. Pregnancy loss in the antiphospholipid-antibody syndrome – a possible thrombogenic mechanism. N Engl J Med 1997;337:154–160.

Rey E, Kahn SR, David M, Shrier I. Thrombophilic disorders and fetal loss: a meta-analysis. Lancet 2003;361:901–908.

Robertson WB, Brosens I, Dixon HG. The pathological response of the vessels of the placental bed to hypertensive pregnancy. J Pathol Bacteriol 1967;93:581–592.

Tenney B, Parker F. The placenta in toxemia of pregnancy. Am J Obstetr Gynecol 1940;39:1000–1005.

Van Horn JT, Craven C, Ward K, Branch DW, Silver RM. Histologic features of placentas and abortion specimens from women with anti-phospholipid and antiphospholipid-like syndrome. Placenta 2004;25:642–648.

Yoon BH, Lee CM, Kim SW. An abnormal umbilical artery waveform: A strong and independent predictor of adverse perinatal outcome in patients with preeclampsia. Am J Obstet Gynecol 1994;171:713–721.

Chapter 19
Miscellaneous Placental Lesions

Intervillous Thrombi

Pathogenesis

Intervillous thrombi are common lesions, occurring in approximately one fifth of term placentas. They are defined as localized clots in the intervillous space and were previously known as Kline's hemorrhages. Intervillous thrombi may occur secondary to *leakage from the fetal capillaries* and thus may be a manifestation of **fetomaternal hemorrhage**. If they are large or numerous, they may be an indication of significant hemorrhage (see Chap. 20). Immunohistochemistry for fetal hemoglobin has identified fetal red blood cells in intervillous thrombi, and in fact, a good correlation exists between the presence of fetal red blood cells in the maternal circulation and intervillous thrombi. It should also be mentioned that when the maternal and fetal bloods are compatible, clotting might not take place even in a significant fetal

R.N. Baergen, *Manual of Pathology of the Human Placenta*,
DOI 10.1007/978-1-4419-7494-5_19, © Springer Science+Business Media, LLC 2011

hemorrhage. However, in many cases, intervillous thrombi have no clinical impact on mother or infant.

On the other hand, intervillous thrombi may develop due to *increased thrombosis in the maternal circulation* in the setting of **maternal thrombophilias** or **preeclampsia**. When associated with the latter, they are often found in the maternal floor in relation to decidual vasculopathy. Intervillous thrombi are also seen in cases of **erythroblastosis fetalis** and in **hydatidiform moles**. In these situations, the edema so alters the intervillous blood flow as to cause local eddying and stasis, with thrombosis the end result. Fresh intervillous thrombi may also simply be the result of **local stasis of blood flow during labor**. Finally, small breaks may occur, perhaps from fetal movement, injuring the villi in some way. This may explain the frequency of fetal bleeding in otherwise normal placentas. It is not possible to differentiate the different etiologies on routine microscopic examination alone.

Pathologic Features

The maternal "jet" of blood enters in the center of the cotyledon. In this region, the villous tissue is usually composed of larger, more immature villi, which are separated by wide intervillous clefts. This is the most common site of intervillous thrombi. Gross examination of fresh intervillous thrombi reveals *red, shiny lesions with sharp, angular outlines* (Fig. 19.1). At times one can see that their triangular shape originates from vessels in the placental floor. They are *often laminated with light tan-gray and red alternating lines*. Older intervillous thrombi tend to be more white-tan (Fig. 19.2). They are sometimes confused with infarcts but can be differentiated from them grossly by the granular consistency and round contour in the latter.

Microscopically, intervillous thrombi *displace adjacent villous tissue* and form a clot in the intervillous space (Fig. 19.3). Older clots may contain macrophages that have engulfed red blood cells. *If intervillous thrombi become large, or if they are of longer duration, the compressed*

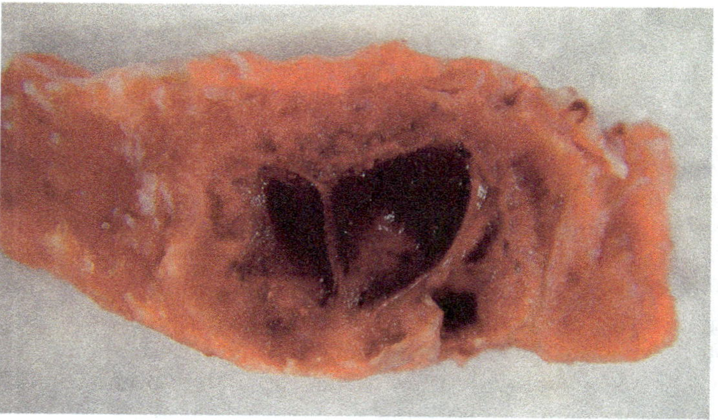

Figure 19.1. Intervillous thrombus in a term placenta shows recent clot with laminated fibrin.

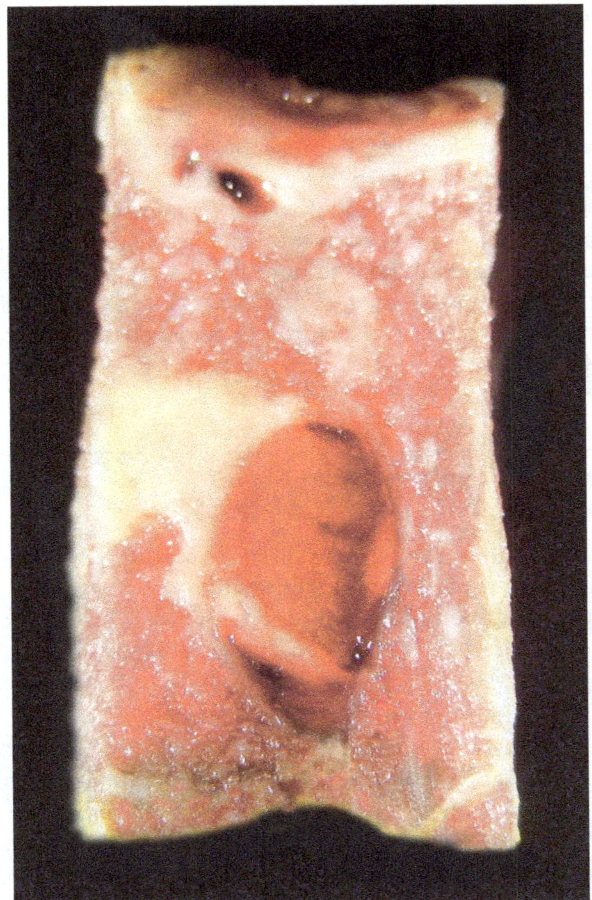

Figure 19.2. Layered fibrin is present in this older intervillous thrombus.

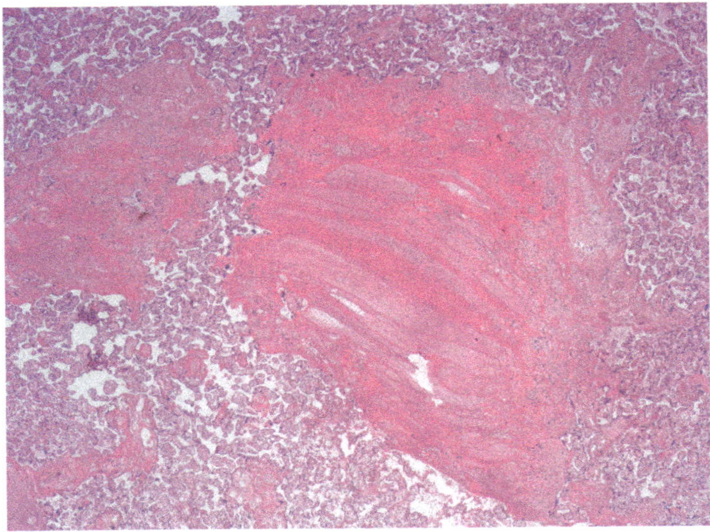

Figure 19.3. Layered fibrin with "lines of Zahn" in an intervillous thrombus H&E ×10.

adjacent villous tissue will become infarcted. Thus, older lesions may be difficult to differentiate from infarcts. They may also be found in the subchorionic region, forming because of eddying of the intervillous blood as it is reflected beneath the chorion and in this case would be better described as subchorionic thrombi or hematomas. This type of intervillous thrombus is common and increases with gestational age. It is of parenthetic interest here to note that intervillous thrombi *never undergo the repair process known to pathologists as "organization"* and so do not show the fibrous tissue ingrowth and neovascularization that occurs in other organs.

Suggestions for Examination and Report
(Intervillous thrombi)

Gross Examination: Description of the number and size of the intervillous thrombi is important in evaluating the clinical significance. Representative sections are recommended but in the case of multiple lesions, not all lesions need to be sampled.

Comment: If intervillous thrombi are large or numerous, the possibility of a fetomaternal hemorrhage should be raised and a Kleihauer–Betke test recommended (see Chap. 20). This is particularly important in the case of a fetal demise or if there is evidence of fetal anemia. The latter may be given in the clinical history or indirect evidence of fetal anemia may be concluded from the presence of pale villous tissue (see Chap. 20).

Intravillous Hemorrhage

Intravillous hemorrhage is most commonly due to sudden placental ischemia with disruption of the capillaries and therefore by nature is an acute process. Trauma to the placenta, particularly abruptios resulting from motor vehicle accidents, leads to this type of "bruising" of the villous tissue. Histologically, it consists simply of extravasation of red blood cells from the villous capillaries into the stroma without associated alternation of the villous structure (Fig. 19.4). As this is an acute change, it precedes evidence of the early ischemic change of the villi following an abruption or an infarction, e.g., collapse of the intervillous space.

Suggestions for Examination and Report
(Intravillous hemorrhage)

Gross Examination: This lesion is not usually visible grossly.

Comment: Intravillous hemorrhage is seen in conditions of early ischemia, trauma or acute hypoxia.

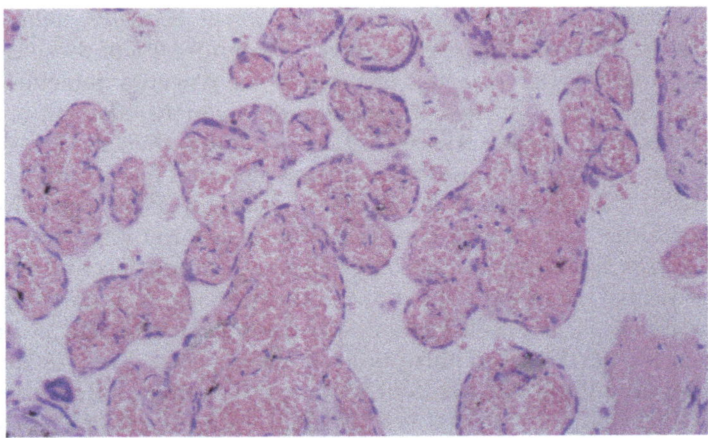

Figure 19.4. Intravillous hemorrhage in an immature placenta 14 h after an automobile accident. H&E, *left* ×40, *right* ×160.

Retroplacental Hematoma and Abruptio Placentae

Pathogenesis

An **abruptio placentae** is defined as the *detachment of the placenta from its decidual seat*. There are many causes of abruptio, including *maternal vascular disease, trauma from accidents, amniocentesis, uterine anomalies, placenta previa, folic acid deficiency, grand multiparity, and rarely pheochromocytoma*. Most abruptios are the result of either *maternal vascular disease or trauma*, with preeclampsia being the cause in 13% and eclampsia in 35%. Thus, hypertensive disease in pregnancy is the most common cause of abruptios. Automobile accidents are the commonest cause of *traumatic* placental hemorrhages and abruptios.

Clinical Features and Implications

The frequency of abruptio placentae is estimated to be between 0.96 and 3.75% of all deliveries. With a total abruptio, or with a large acute abruptio, there may be pain due to sudden stretching of the uterine peritoneal covering, sometimes accompanied by vaginal bleeding or backache. More often, abruptio is partial and is often painless. If the separation and thus the bleeding are not in close proximity to the cervical os, no vaginal bleeding may be present, and this is referred to as a "concealed abruption." Since not all abruptios bleed externally or produce the classical clinical signs of a painful, rigid abdomen, the diagnosis is bound to be missed clinically in some cases. Clinical "abruptio" may also mimicked by *active peripheral bleeding that ultimately leads to circumvallation and by marginal hemorrhage associated with severe ascending infection*. Therefore, placental examination is essential in these cases to determine the cause of the symptomatology.

When pregnant women are involved *in car accidents with blunt trauma to the abdomen, fetal loss occurs in 25%,* with 50% of these due to maternal death. When one-half or more of the placenta detaches suddenly, the fetus usually dies. If placental detachment takes place over a long period, in stages and with infarcts ensuing, then the fetus may survive but will suffer from deficient transplacental oxygen and nutrient supply. This may result in *hypoxia, growth restriction, or neurologic injury.* In some cases, if the placenta itself is also torn by trauma, *severe fetal hemorrhage and anemia* may develop, and transplacental hemorrhage may also accompany the trauma. *Vaginal bleeding, uterine rupture, fetal brain damage, and skull fractures* also have been reported in motor vehicle accidents. Delayed abruptio has been reported to occur up to 5 days after an automobile accident, but careful examination of the placenta will reveal damage that is coincident with the trauma. If extension of the abruption occurs over time, fetal death may be the result, but this usually occurs within 48 h.

Pathologic Features

Premature placental separation, or abruptio, is diagnosed pathologically by the presence of a **retroplacental hematoma**. Abruptio placentae and retroplacental hematoma are very similar, but not equivalent diagnoses. A retroplacental hematoma is the pathologic lesion that results from the clinical condition of abruptio. Alternatively, retroplacental hematomas by their nature will lead to separation of the placenta from the uterus or an abruption. Grossly, fresh retroplacental hematomas, those less than an hour or so old, may not be distinguishable from the normally present postpartum maternal blood clot that is loosely adherent. *After several hours, however, the retroplacental clot will become adherent to the maternal surface* and identifiable on gross examination. These clots are most commonly present at the margin of the placenta. *Compression of the underlying villous tissue then follows* (Fig. 19.5; see also Fig. 18.13 in Chap. 18) in a few hours. With time, the blood dries, becomes firmer and stringy, and then changes color to brown and eventually may become greenish. The placental tissue underneath the clot becomes compressed and will ultimately become infarcted (Figs. 19.6 and 19.7). Over time, *the blood cells begin to degenerate and there is laminated fibrin present. Hemosiderin-laden macrophages will be present after approximately 4–5 days.* The decidua basalis becomes degenerated and necrotic and is often replaced by the hematoma. Depression of the villous tissue disappears as the overlying placenta becomes infarcted and then atrophies.

Since most abruptios are the result of maternal vascular disease or trauma, assessment of the decidual spiral arterioles is desirable. In the locale of the abruption, this may be impossible as the vessels here are often destroyed by the process or have remained behind during the delivery of the placenta. One must therefore look in adjacent portions of decidua and, especially, in the decidua capsularis. *Atherosis and thrombosis are* often well displayed in these vessels. In some cases, it may be impossible to rule out vascular changes as the cause of abruption, and thus the etiology remains obscure.

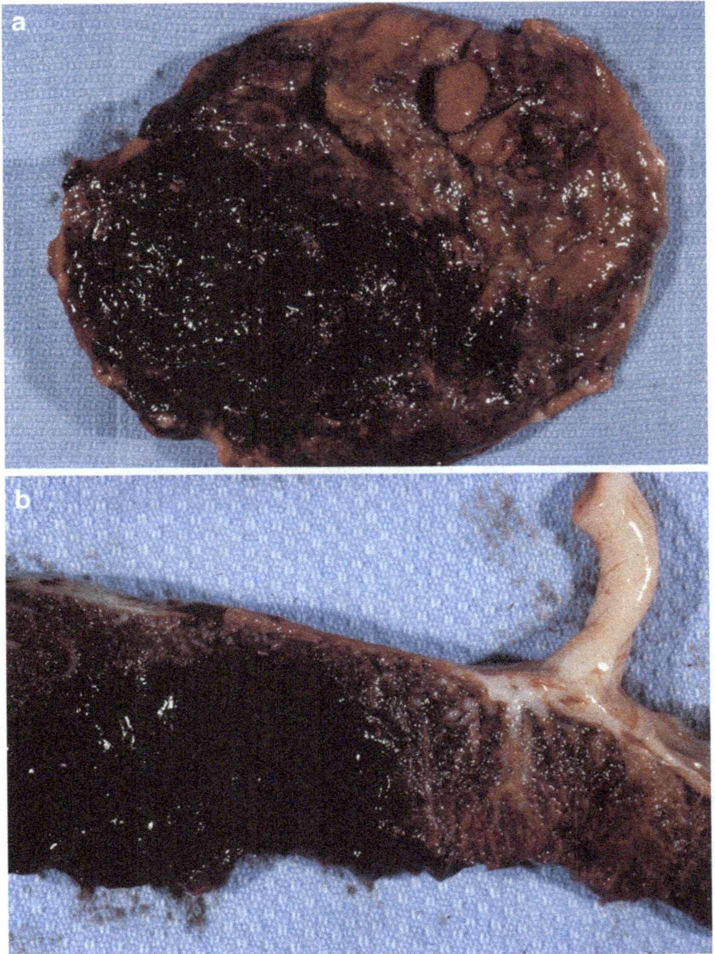

Figure 19.5. (a) Maternal surface of the placenta with a retroplacental hematoma showing recent adherent blood clot. (b) Cross section of the placenta shows that the recent blood clot compresses the underlying villous tissue, which shows no alteration.

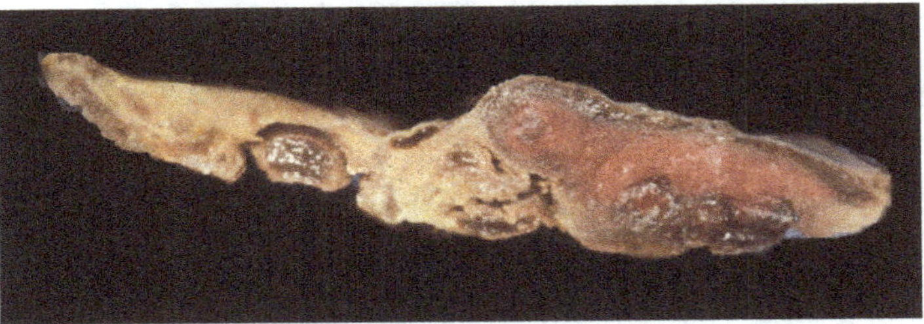

Figure 19.6. Several retroplacental hematomas are seen in this cut section of a placenta from a woman with severe preeclampsia. The fetal surface is at the *top* of the figure and maternal surface at the *bottom*. The hematoma on the *left* is old with infarction of the underlying villous tissue presenting as white, firm tissue. A more recent hematoma is seen on the *right* with mild discoloration of the underlying villous tissue consistent with a more recent infarct.

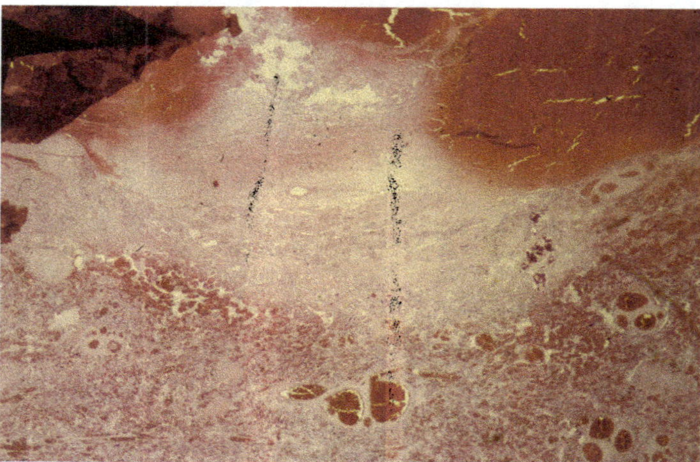

Figure 19.7. Histologic picture of a retroplacental hematoma from a recent abruption. The maternal surface is at the *top* and shows a recent clot with some compression of the villous tissue but no obvious infarction. H&E ×20.

Suggestions for Examination and Report
(Retroplacental hematoma)

Gross Examination: Identification of the retroplacental hematoma, the percentage of the placenta involved and the age of the hematoma is essential. Representative sections of the clot and underlying villous tissue should be taken. If parts of the hematoma appear grossly older, it recommended that the oldest and most recent clot both be submitted.

Comment: The presence of the retroplacental hematoma, percentage of the surface involved and the findings of maternal vascular disease or other associated lesions should be included in the report as well as the acuteness of the lesion.

Chorangiosis and Chorangiomatosis

Chorangiosis, chorangiomas, and chorangiomatosis are related lesions and can be generally defined as follows:

- **Chorangiosis** – a diffuse increase in the number of villous capillaries
- **Chorangioma** – a benign neoplastic proliferation of capillaries and stroma within a villus forming an expansile nodular lesion
- **Chorangiomatosis** – a multifocal lesion characterized by an increase in villous capillaries that tends to permeate the normal villous structures and commonly involves stem villi

Chorangiosis and chorangiomatosis are discussed in the following sections while chorangiomas are discussed with other neoplasms in Chap. 22.

Chorangiosis

Pathologic Features

Chorangiosis is diagnosed principally by low-power lens inspection of histological sections. It has been specifically defined as *ten or more capillaries in each of ten villi in ten fields inspected with a 10× objective in three different, noninfarcted areas of the placenta* (Fig. 19.8). Three or more areas are best interpreted in separate sections from three different areas of the placenta. A grading system has been developed but is seldom used. Meeting the full criteria requires counting a total of 3,000 capillaries and thus may not be practical or even necessary in every case. With experience, counting a number of fields in different areas and confirming that the process is diffuse throughout the placenta is often sufficient for the diagnosis. Furthermore, if the criteria is not completely met but a significant number of villi contain 15 or 20 or more vessels, this is also evidence of increased capillary proliferation and therefore may be diagnosed as chorangiosis with a comment for the basis of the diagnosis. At times "focal chorangiosis" is sometimes diagnoses based on the focality of the changes. Normally three to five capillaries are present in normal terminal villi and when there are more than five but less than 10, the term "borderline chorangiosis" has been used. Neither of these terms has been well studied, and so their clinical significance is not known precisely.

The increase in capillary lumen cross sections seen in this lesion comes about through endothelial proliferation. It thus takes *weeks to develop full-blown chorangiosis*. Villous congestion should not be misinterpreted as chorangiosis (Fig. 19.9). Congestion of the terminal villi may occur when the cord has been clamped soon after delivery of the neonate, from cord compression, knots, torsion, cord entanglements, and the like.

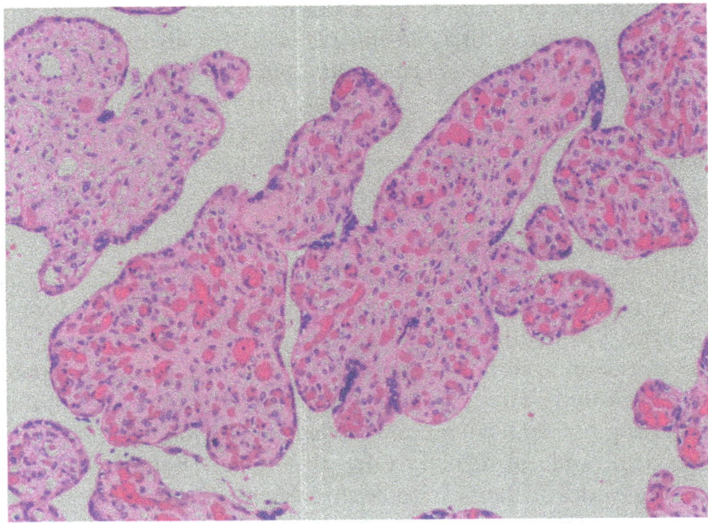

Figure 19.8. Chorangiosis showing a marked increased in the number of villous capillaries. H&E ×200.

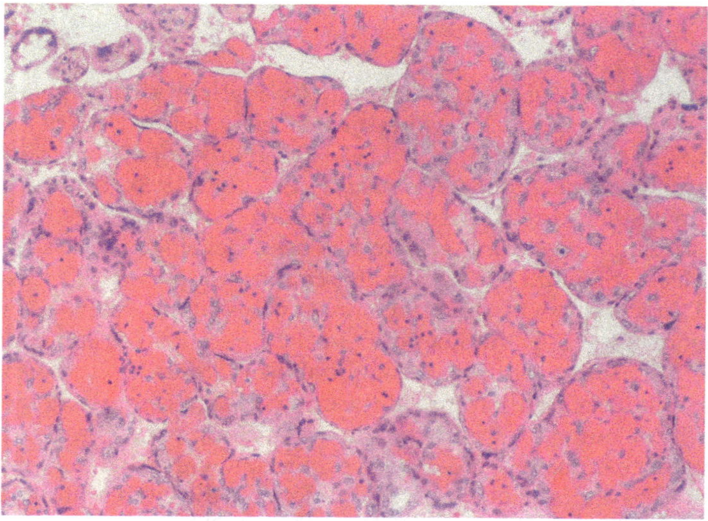

Figure 19.9. Villous congestion. Contrast this appearance with that of chorangiosis in Fig. 19.8. Here the capillaries are enlarged and distended with blood but their number is not increased. H&E ×200.

Pathogenesis

At term, the terminal villi comprise nearly 40% of the villous volume and about 60% of villous cross sections. These figures explain why a remarkable reduction of terminal villi, as in terminal villus deficiency (see Chap. 18), may lead to fetal hypoxia. *There is a clear-cut inverse relation between the area of villous vasculosyncytial membranes and fetal hypoxia.* Conversely, the proliferation of villous capillaries seen in chorangiosis is an adaptation to chronic oxygen deficiency. This is supported by the fact that chorangiosis occurs in placentas of women *at very high altitude, in preeclampsia,* and in *severely anemic mothers.* It is also seen in mothers who *smoke, are exposed to heavy pollutants, and in mothers who have chronic hypoxia to heart disease or other conditions.* Further support comes from experiments in guinea pigs in which an increase in capillaries can be demonstrated when they are chronically (45 days) deprived of oxygen. Thus, *an altered capillary/villus ratio is characteristic of hypoxic placentas.*

Clinical Features and Implications

Chorangiosis is presently underrated as an indicator of *chronic prenatal hypoxia.* In an unselected population, chorangiosis is relatively rare but it is found with increasing frequency in the placentas of infants admitted to neonatal intensive care units. It is strongly correlated with *perinatal mortality,* and a wide variety of pregnancy and placental disorders, including *perinatal circumstances that suggest long-standing hypoxia.* It is more commonly observed in the placentas of babies who develop *cerebral palsy* and in infants with *cord problems* of one kind or another. Its presence betrays a deleterious intrauterine environment for the fetus and a manifestation of an attempt (teleologically speaking) of the placenta to enlarge its diffusional surface.

> **Suggestions for Examination and Report**
> (Chorangiosis)
>
> **Gross Examination**: Chorangiosis is not diagnosed grossly.
>
> **Comment**: Chorangiosis is associated with conditions of chronic hypoxia and is strongly correlated with perinatal morbidity and mortality.

Chorangiomatosis

Like chorangiosis, **chorangiomatosis** is characterized by an increase the villous capillaries. However, chorangiosis involves terminal villi, while in chorangiomatosis, the process involves immature intermediate or stem villi and the terminal villi are generally spared. In chorangiosis, the capillaries are surrounded by basement membranes only, while in chorangiomatosis the vessels are surrounded by loose bundles of reticular fibers that blend into the surrounding stroma. Chorangiomatosis also has many features in common with chorangiomas, namely the presence of *perivascular cells around vessels, increased cellularity, and stromal collagen.* Chorangiomas are also thought to arise from immature intermediate or stem villi.

Chorangiomatosis may be divided histologically into two main patterns, **localized (focal or segmental)** and **diffuse multifocal. Focal** and **segmental chorangiomatosis** involve focal areas of contiguous villi, with segmental chorangiomatosis involving greater than five villi and focal chorangiomatosis involving five or less. Microscopically, small-clustered groups of *stem villi or immature stem villi show increased cellularity of the stroma as well as increased vessels.* Perivascular cells are present but are not easily identified on routine tissue stains. **Diffuse, multifocal chorangiomatosis** involves multiple independent areas of the placenta. Although it is not considered a gross lesion, occasionally it may be identified as multiple nodules within the villous parenchyma (Fig. 19.10). In this pattern, *there are multiple nodules of expanded chorionic villi, which contain numerous small capillaries* (Fig. 19.11). While localized chorangiomatosis is associated with prematurity, preeclampsia, and multiple gestation, diffuse multifocal chorangiomatosis is associated

> **Suggestions for Examination and Report**
> (Chorangiomatosis)
>
> **Gross Examination**: If nodules are identified grossly, generous sampling of the villous tissue is recommended. Lesions may be difficult to identify on gross examination if small.
>
> **Comment**: A comment on the clinical associations may be made, i.e., preeclampsia, prematurity and multiple births for localized chorangiomatosis and IUGR, extreme prematurity, preeclampsia, placentomegaly and congenital anomalies for diffuse multifocal chorangiomatosis.

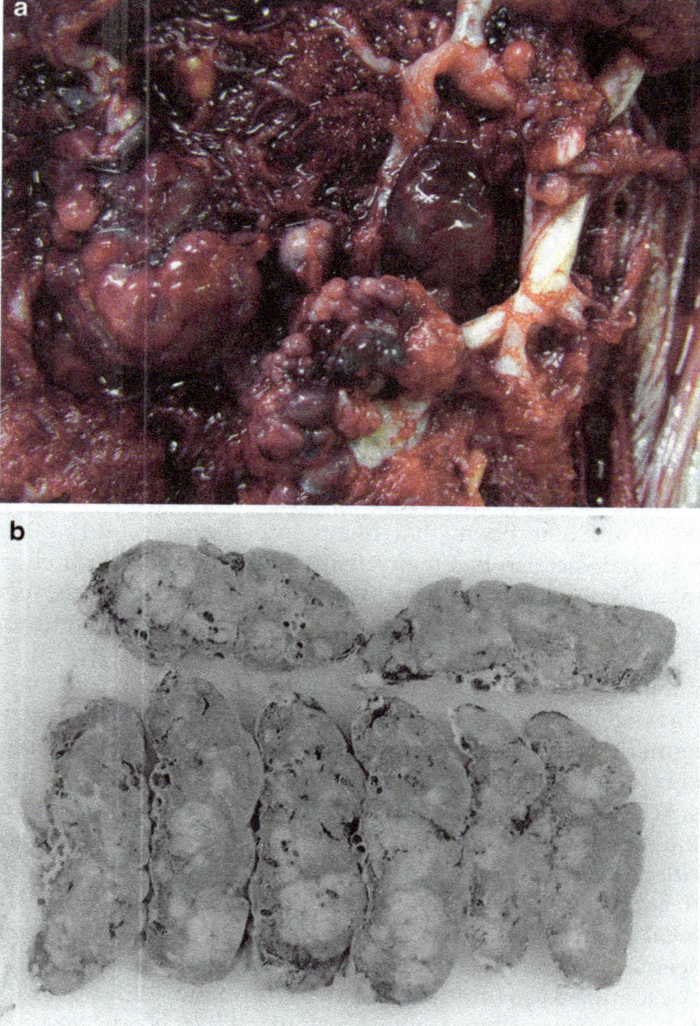

Figure 19.10. (a) Multifocal chorangiomatosis may be visible grossly as nodular areas in the placenta. (b) Cross sections of villous tissue may show nodular pale lesions as well.

with extreme prematurity, preeclampsia, intrauterine growth restriction (IUGR), placentomegaly, and congenital anomalies. It has been suggested that the diffuse multifocal form of chorangiomatosis may be a developmental abnormality of the villi.

Fibrinoid Deposition

Normal Perivillous Fibrinoid

Perivillous fibrin or fibrinoid deposition is a normal feature of term placentas. It likely develops secondary to damage of the syncytiotrophoblast with subsequent clotting in the intervillous space and closure

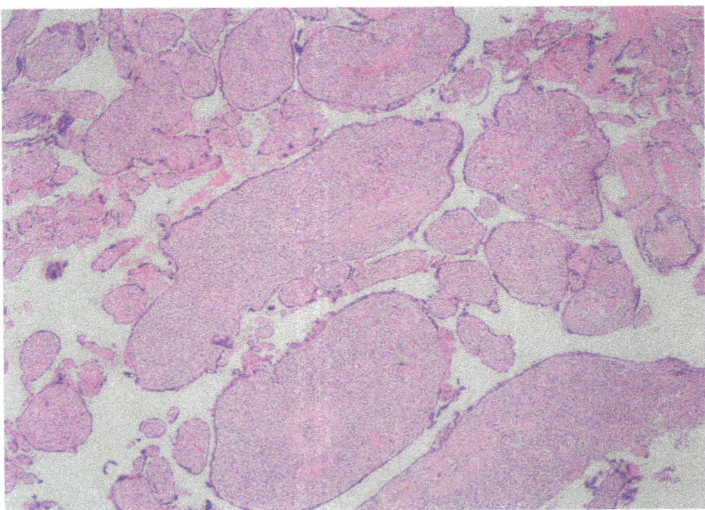

Figure 19.11.   Diffuse, multifocal chorangiomatosis. Note the multiple, nodular foci of villi with increased capillaries. H&E ×100.

of the trophoblastic defect by a fibrinoid plug. It is particularly prominent in stem villi, whose trophoblastic surface is largely replaced by fibrinoid at term. One normally finds some increase in fibrinoid encasing larger groups of villi below the chorionic plate (*subchorionic laminated fibrin or fibrinoid*), and in the *marginal zone*. The amount of fibrinoid increases with advancing pregnancy. Although modest amounts are considered normal, a diffuse increase may be interpreted as reflecting *chronic intervillous perfusional problems* as it is seen in *preeclampsia and abnormal maternal coagulation*. If the perivillous fibrinoid is excessive, it is referred to as **maternal floor infarction** or **massive perivillous fibrin deposition** (see below). In foci of more significant fibrinoid deposition, *shiny, white irregular deposits* may be grossly visible in the villous tissue. Microscopically fibrinoid is *pink and lamellar in structure*. Perivillous fibrinoid either *fills gaps in the syncytiotrophoblastic cover of villi, or encases villi or small groups of villi* (Fig. 19.12). The syncytiotrophoblast of these villi is often degenerated and may be absent.

Maternal Floor Infarction and Massive Perivillous Fibrin Deposition

Pathogenesis
Maternal floor infarction (MFI) is a placental lesion with specific pathologic features and clinical associations. The incidence has been reported to be as high as one in 200 placentas, but that figure is much higher than is our experience. The cause is unknown but suggested etiologies have included *congenital infection, immune mediated rejection, and abnormal extravillous trophoblastic proliferation*. It appears to be a specific entity, in part because of its frequently recurrent nature. It may be related to an *abnormal host/placental interaction*, but the interaction may not necessarily be an immunological one. Some investigators have differentiated cases in which the maternal floor was primarily involved from those

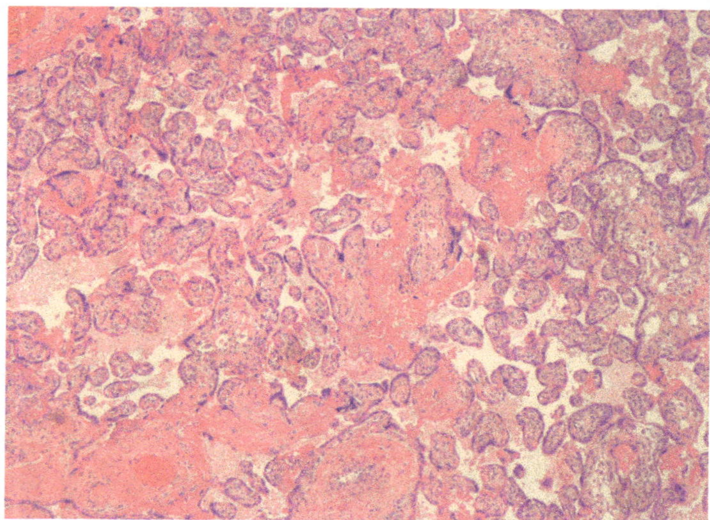

Figure 19.12. Mature placenta with typical amount of perivillous fibrinoid. H&E ×40.

with diffuse fibrinoid deposition; hence the designation of "**massive perivillous fibrin deposition**." At this time, there is no convincing evidence that these are two different entities. However, since in many cases, the fibrin deposition is not primarily in the maternal floor and the infarction of villous tissue that occurs is not primary but secondary, massive perivillous fibrin deposition may be a more appropriate term.

Pathologic Features

Excessive fibrinoid deposition is the main diagnostic feature of **MFI**. In this condition, the decidual floor is heavily infiltrated by fibrinoid, which also disseminates throughout the villous tissue. This infiltration is visible and even palpable on gross examination. The maternal surface loses its normal cotyledonary development and shows a corrugated appearance. The *floor of the placenta is thick, stiffened, and often yellow* (Fig. 19.13). On cut section, the villous tissue is diffusely penetrated with gray fibrinoid (Figs. 19.14 and 19.15), even though the process is not always completely expressed. Thus, in some placentas, the characteristic fibrinoid deposition does not involve the entire floor or portions of the villous tissue are inexplicably spared.

Microscopically, *fibrinoid encases villi in a net-like pattern* while intervening villi are normal. Initially the encased villi appear viable (Fig. 19.16). Over time, the syncytiotrophoblast degenerates and eventually disappears completely. A thickened trophoblastic basal lamina then surrounds the fibrotic villous stroma. In some cases, chronic villitis may be associated with the lesion. The fetal vessels sometimes remain intact, but ultimately become obliterated. The villi are literally strangled by the fibrinoid. Therefore, older lesions appear quite similar to true villous infarcts. However, the *diffuse pattern of fibrinoid infiltration, the lack of confluence of infarcted villi, and the fact that the process is*

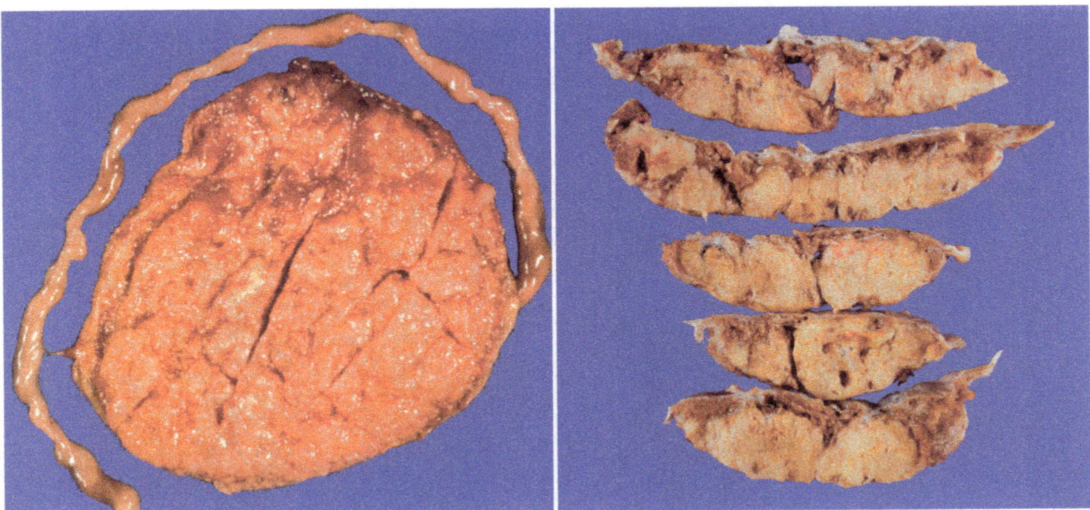

Figure 19.13. Maternal floor infarction. On the *left*, the maternal surface of the placenta shows loss of normal cotyledonary structure with yellow discoloration of the surface. On the *right*, cross sections of the placenta demonstrate the typical "net-like" deposition of fibrinoid material throughout the parenchyma.

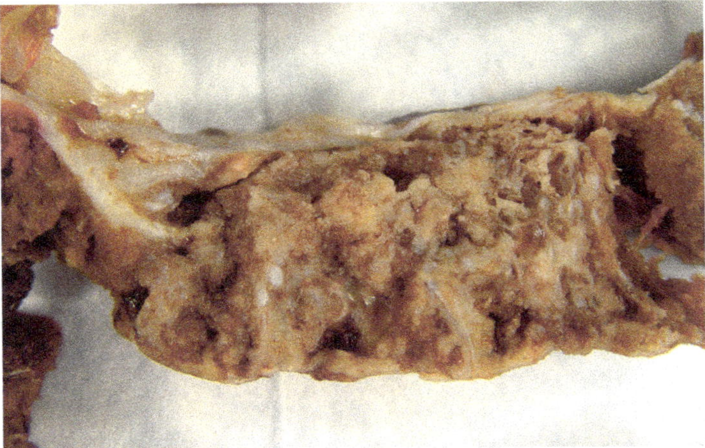

Figure 19.14. Another placenta showing grossly identifiable fibrinoid deposition consistent with a maternal floor infarction.

often confined to the placental floor favors the diagnosis of maternal floor infarction (Fig. 19.17). In addition, in true infarcts, the villi are collapsed and only a thin layer of fibrinoid encases the villi. *Proliferation of extravillous trophoblast* is occasionally associated with this lesion, and in some cases the proliferation may be quite striking (Fig. 19.18). In most cases, extravillous trophoblastic cells are present in *strings or as single cells deep within the fibrinoid.*

Clinical Features and Implications

In maternal floor infarction, the excessive fibrinoid deposits reduce blood flow in the intervillous space, obstructing maternofetal exchange.

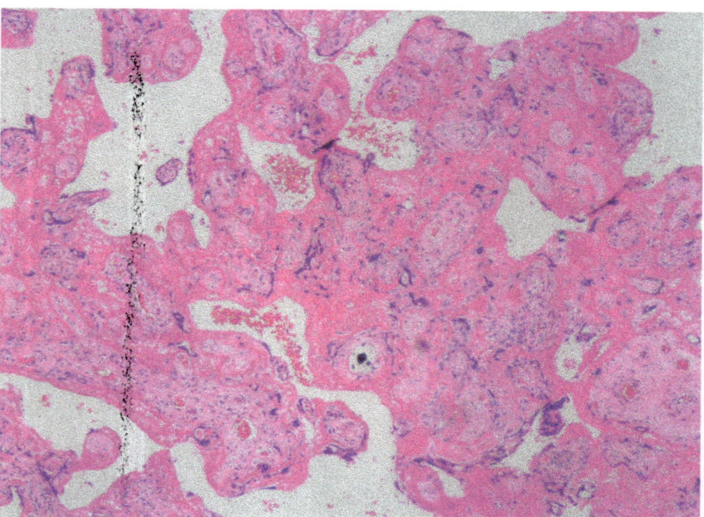

Figure 19.15. Maternal floor infarction with villi encased in fibrinoid material. Here, the villi are still viable and have begun to show only minimal degenerative change. H&E ×100.

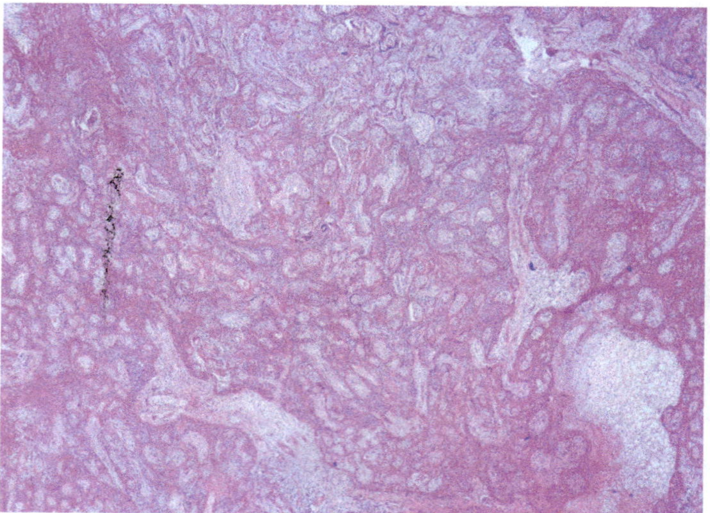

Figure 19.16. More advanced maternal floor infarction with almost complete infarction of villous tissue. The vague net-like pattern can still be appreciated and strands of fibrinoid are still present. H&E ×20.

If a large enough area is involved, fetal growth and survival may be endangered. Typically, the pregnant patient who develops maternal floor infarction is clinically normal and drop-off of fetal growth or decreased fetal movements in the late second or third trimesters is the only indication of problems. Some reports have shown an association with MFI and *maternal thrombophilias*. Oligohydramnios may be associated with the

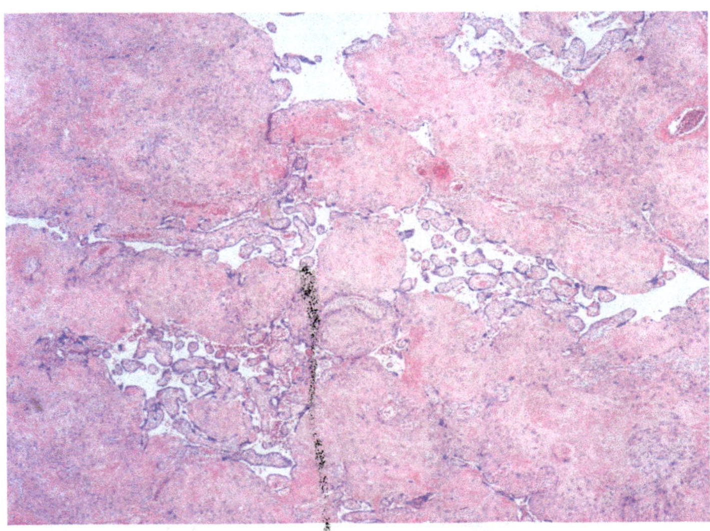

Figure 19.17. Maternal floor infarction with excessive fibrinoid associated with a more prominent proliferation of extravillous trophoblast. H&E ×20.

lesion, particularly when growth restriction is present. MFI *strongly correlates with IUGR, intrauterine fetal demise (IUFD), and neurologic impairment. Microcephaly* has also been described. Importantly, the condition recurs frequently in subsequent pregnancies at rates of 30% or more. One patient had nine consecutive losses due to maternal floor infarction. With other patients in whom the lesion had previously occurred, the anticipation of its recurrence has led to intense fetal monitoring and improvement outcome. *Elevations in maternal serum alpha-fetoprotein*, likely due to disruption of the maternal–fetal interface, may be detected from the second trimester on. Major basic protein (MBP) levels in maternal serum are also significantly elevated in some patients with maternal floor infarction. Ultrasonographic criteria for the diagnosis of maternal floor infarction have been established and are useful in anticipating the disease.

Suggestions for Examination and Report
(Maternal floor infarction)

Gross Examination: Recognition and description of the gross pathologic features is essential. These include firmness and discoloration of the maternal surface and deposition of fibrinoid in the placental parenchyma. An estimate of the percentage of involvement of the placental tissue by fibrinoid is also important. Sections should be taken of any grossly "normal" tissue as well as additional section of abnormal tissue.

Comment: Maternal floor infarction has been associated with IUGR, IUFD and poor neurologic outcome as well as recurrence in subsequent pregnancies.

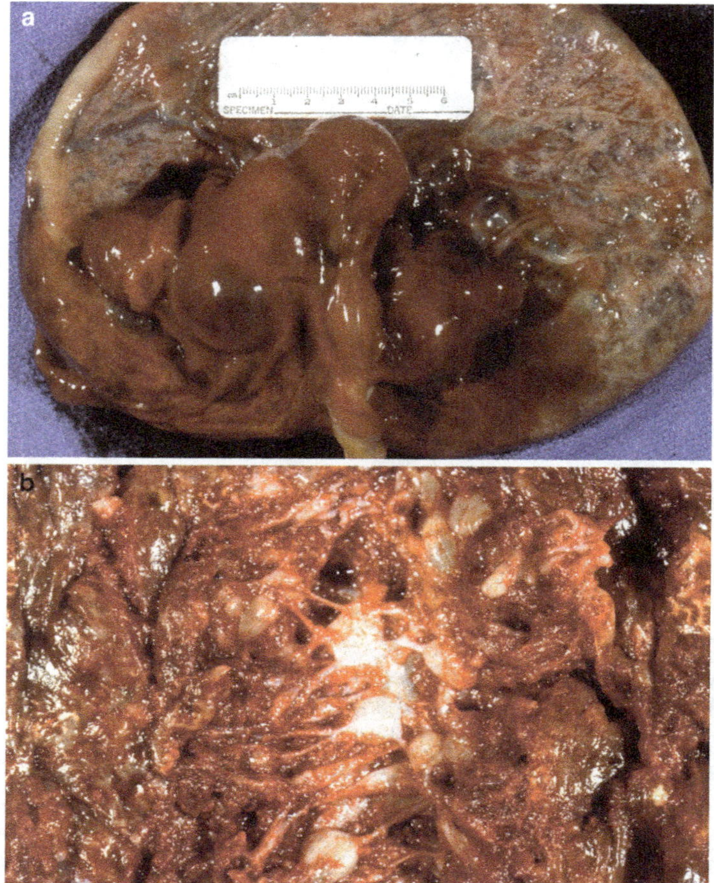

Figure 19.18. (a) Fetal surface of a placenta with mesenchymal dysplasia demonstrating large, dilated and tortuous vessels surrounded by gelatinous material and blood. (b) Maternal surface of the same placenta with dilated chorionic villi similar to those seen in a partial mole. The remaining villous tissue appears grossly normal.

Placental Mesenchymal Dysplasia

Clinical Features and Implications

Mesenchymal dysplasia is a rare condition of unknown etiology with specific gross and microscopic placental abnormalities. Over 80 cases have been reported at present, and 20% of these have been associated with Beckwith–Wiedemann syndrome. Approximately half of the remaining cases have been associated with IUGR. Fetal or neonatal demise occurs in 43%. Mesenchymal dysplasia has also been associated with *preeclampsia, maternal hypertension, polyhydramnios, macrosomia, omphalocele, and kidney abnormalities.* In addition, some cases have reported *congenital hemangiomas, vascular hamartomas, and hepatic mesenchymal hamartomas* in the fetus in these cases. Most commonly, the fetus has a 46, XX karyotype, and 82% of the cases that have been reported are in female fetuses. Clinically, mesenchymal dysplasia may be misdiagnosed as a partial hydatidiform mole since it has a similar appearance on prenatal ultrasound examination. Imaging may also reveal large vascular areas with features consistent with both arterial and venous signals under the chorionic plate. There are also gross and microscopic features that may be confused with a partial mole as well (see below).

Pathogenesis

The pathogenesis of this disorder is unknown; however, there is much recent work on the possible etiology or etiologies. The thrombosis noted in many fetal vessels has led some authors to suggest the possibility of maternal thrombophilia as an etiologic factor, but this has not been well studied. Another theory is that chronic hypoxia develops due to fetal thrombotic vasculopathy and decreased gas exchange in the dysplastic villi. This is supported by the often-associated finding of chorangiosis and the association with IUGR. A few cases have shown genetic mosaicism in the placenta with a mixture of androgenetic cells and biparental cells in amnion, chorion, and mesenchyme but not in the trophoblast, and it is suggested that this leads to the abnormal develop of the mesenchymal tissue in the placenta. This is supported by the congenital hamartomas reported in some fetuses. These findings, the association with Beckwith–Wiedemann, and the female preponderance all suggest that imprinting may have an important role in the etiology.

Pathologic Features

Grossly, there is significant *placentomegaly* with an increase in both placental size and weight. This is usually true even in cases that are not associated with Beckwith–Wiedemann syndrome. Abnormalities of the umbilical cord have been seen in a number of cases including excessively long or twisted cords, single umbilical artery, and abnormal insertions. The *surface chorionic vessels are markedly dilated and somewhat tortuous, and gelatinous material may be visible around the vessels* (Fig. 19.19a). Thrombosis in these vessels is common, which can be visible on gross inspection. *Grossly enlarged and cystic villi* may also be visible (Fig. 19.19b). These changes are usually focal, with more grossly normal areas intervening, but may involve up to 80% of the placental parenchyma.

Histologically, the *stem villi are enlarged and contain loose connective tissue and cistern-like formations* (Fig. 19.20). Some stem villi may measure up to 1.5 cm in diameter. The enlargement and hydropic change of the villi is the basis for confusion with partial moles. However, there is no trophoblastic proliferation, and *the hydropic villi are well vascularized.* They may contain *cisterns,* but, unlike moles, there is often a concentration of vessels under the trophoblastic cover. *These smaller vessels tend to be abnormally small and thick walled* but may show *thrombosis or aneurysmal dilatation.* Occasionally, *some villi have a more fibromatous stroma with a myxoid core.* Overall, there appears to be an increase in the amount of villous stromal tissue leading some authors to suggest the term "placental mesenchymal hyperplasia" rather than dysplasia for this entity. The grossly normal areas usually show immature appearing

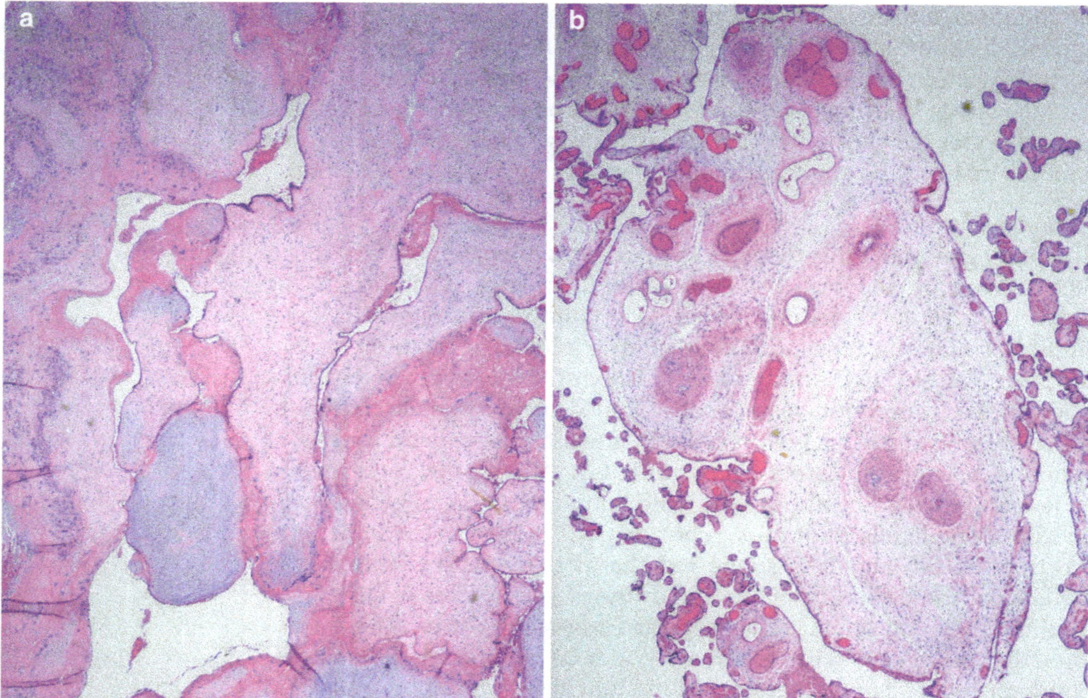

Figure 19.19. (**a**) Mesenchymal dysplasia showing dilated and hydropic villi underneath the chorionic plate. In contrast to moles, there is no trophoblastic proliferation. Myxoid stroma is present in some villi. H&E ×20. (**b**) Mesenchymal dysplasia showing an enlarged villus with persistence of fetal vessels which appear thick walled and abnormal. Normal villi are seen in the vicinity. H&E ×20.

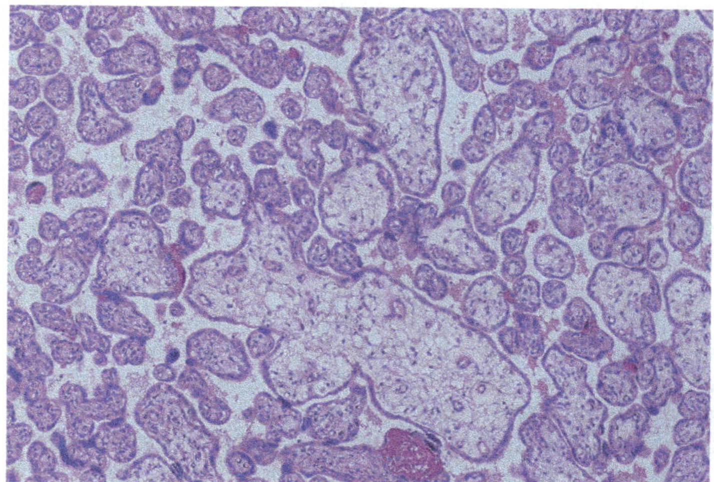

Figure 19.20. Villous immaturity or dysmaturity in a term placenta. The villi are larger than would be expected in a term placenta, with well-defined trophoblastic cover rather than the rarified trophoblast seen normally. In addition, the vessels are more centrally located and thus there are decreased vasculosyncytial membranes with a resultant decrease in diffusional capacity. H&E ×100.

villi, which are occasionally hydropic. *Villous chorangiosis* is also a relatively common finding in the remaining "normal" villi. These changes are less prominent in earlier gestations.

Suggestions for Examination and Report
(Mesenchymal dysplasia)

Gross Examination: Additional sections of the abnormal vessels and cystically dilated villi should be submitted with a full description of all the changes.

Comment: Mesenchymal dysplasia is a disorder of unknown etiology, which may be associated with fetal anomalies and adverse perinatal outcome. Correlation with clinical history, if given, is suggested.

Villous Edema and Villous Immaturity

Villous edema, when severe and diffuse, is associated with **fetal hydrops** and is often referred to as **placental hydrops**. The placenta is usually markedly enlarged and pale on gross examination, corresponding to severe, widespread edema of terminal villi. (Fetal hydrops is discussed in further detail in Chap. 20.) On occasion, focal severe villous edema is seen in term or near-term placentas not associated with fetal hydrops or severe fetal anemia. This is a relatively nonspecific finding and of unclear etiology. However, it has been seen with increased frequency in infants who develop neurologic impairment and cerebral palsy.

Villous immaturity, also called **distal villous immaturity** or **villous dysmaturity**, is an interesting maturation defect of the terminal villi. Microscopically, the terminal villi are *enlarged with increased numbers of capillaries, macrophages, and fluid within the villi*. They are often considered to have *increased vasculosyncytial membranes* and thus there is often a greater distance between the villous capillaries and the syncytiotrophoblastic basement membrane. This in turn is thought to decrease the efficiency or maternal–fetal exchange. This finding is most often associated with *maternal diabetes* (see Chap. 17) and has also been seen in infants with *Beckwith–Wiedemann syndrome*. Infants with this finding are at an increased risk of *IUFD*, but at this time this finding requires further study and characterization (Fig. 19.21).

Suggestions for Examination and Report
(Villous edema and villous immaturity)

Gross Examination: These lesions are not visible on gross examination.

Comment: Severe villous edema, when focal and not associated with hydrops, should be diagnosed but no comment is recommended. If villous immaturity is present in the setting of a fetal demise, then a comment about the association with this outcome can be made with the proviso that the etiology of this change is still unclear.

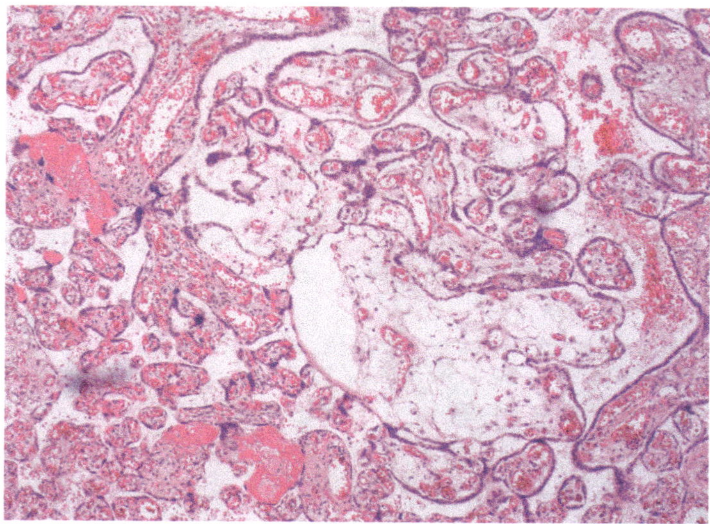

Figure 19.21. Focal villous edema. In contrast to Fig. 19.20, the changes are focal. A few villi in the central portion of the figure are larger and swollen with identifiable edema of the stroma. Fluid spaces are easily identifiable but peripherally located capillaries are still present.

Selected References

PHP5, pages 565–567 (Intervillous Thrombus), 480, 615–620 (Retroplacental Hematoma/Abruptio Placentae), 871–873 (Chorangiosis and Chorangiomatosis), 226–233 (Fibrinoid), 281–284 (Maternal Floor Infarction), 873 (Placental Mesenchymal Dysplasia).

Adams-Chapman I, Vaucher YE, Bejar RF, et al. Maternal floor infarction of the placenta. Association with central nervous system injury and adverse neurodevelopmental outcome. J Perinatol 2002;22:236–241.

Altshuler G. Chorangiosis: an important placental sign of neonatal morbidity and mortality. Arch Pathol Lab Med 1984;108:71–74.

Benirschke K, Gille J. Placental pathology and asphyxia. In: L Gluck (ed) Intrauterine asphyxia and the developing fetal brain. Chicago: Year Book Medical Publishers, 1977.

Fox H. Perivillous fibrin deposition in the human placenta. Am J Obstet Gynecol 1967;98:245–251.

Khong TY. Chorangioma with trophoblastic proliferation. Virchows Arch 2000;436:167–171.

Ogino S, Redline RW. Villous capillary lesions of the placenta: distinctions between chorangioma, chorangiomatosis and chorangiosis. Hum Pathol 2000;31:945–954.

Parveen Z, Tongson-Ignacio JE, Fraser CR, Killeen JL, Thompson KS. Placental mesenchymal dysplasia. Arch Pathol Lab Med 2007;131:131–137.

Pham T, Steele J, Stayboldt C, Chan L, Benirschke K. Placental mesenchymal dysplasia is associated with high rates of intrauterine growth restriction and fetal demise. Am J Clin Pathol 2006;126:67–78.

Reshetnikova OS, Burton GJ, Milovanov AP. Effects of hypobaric hypoxia on the fetoplacental unit: The morphometric diffusing capacity of the villous membrane at high altitude. Am J Obstet Gynecol 1994;171:1560–1565.

Vernof KK, Benirschke K, Kephart GM, et al. Maternal floor infarction: Relationship to X cells, major basic protein, and adverse perinatal outcome. Am J Obstet Gynecol 1992;167:1355–1963.

Chapter 20

Placental Abnormalities in Fetal Conditions

Hydrops Fetalis

Hydrops fetalis is defined as severe, diffuse edema of the fetus. It has an overall incidence of 0.02–0.07% and is usually divided into immune and nonimmune hydrops. The majority of cases are nonimmune hydrops, the etiology of which is extremely varied. Nonimmune hydrops may be separated into the general categories of *congenital anomalies, infections, genetic disorders, hematologic disorders, fetomaternal hemorrhage, trauma, and miscellaneous.* Cardiac abnormalities are the most common, comprising approximately 40% of cases of nonimmune hydrops. About 35% of cases can be ascribed to genetic diseases; chromosomal anomalies make up 10–15%, hematologic disorders about 10%, and miscellaneous causes make up the remaining cases (Table 20.1).

R.N. Baergen, *Manual of Pathology of the Human Placenta,*
DOI 10.1007/978-1-4419-7494-5_20, © Springer Science+Business Media, LLC 2011

Immune Hydrops

Pathogenesis

Erythroblastosis fetalis, hemolytic disease of the newborn, or **immune hydrops** is a condition caused by *maternal antibodies directed against fetal red blood cell antigens*. The antibodies form due to "sensitization" from previous exposure to the antigen, usually from a previous pregnancy. These antibodies cause destruction of fetal red blood cells with resultant severe fetal anemia. In the majority of cases, the antibodies are directed against Rh-(D) antigens, but cases directed against other Rh antigens occur and unusual cases of sensitization against other antigens such as Kell or ABO have been described. Since immunoglobulin G (IgG) antibodies and not IgM antibodies are able to cross into the placenta, antigens that result in IgG antibodies are the most likely to result in disease. Hemolytic disease due to other antibodies does not differ *histopathologically* from anti-D-caused erythroblastosis, but clinical disease due to ABO-incompatibility and many other blood groups tends to be mild compared to Rh disease. Fetal hemolysis may rarely result from *glucose-6-phosphate dehydrogenase (G-6-PD) deficiency or virus infections* and it is important to differentiate these causes for the purposes of prognosis and treatment. As Rhogam prophylaxis has become more widespread, Rh incompatibility disease has become relatively uncommon in the United States, except in immigrant patients.

In typical erythroblastosis, there is transplacental transfer of maternal Rh antibodies leading to hemolysis in the fetus. The fetus attempts to replace this loss of red blood cells by overproduction and premature dissemination of immature red cell precursors [nucleated red blood cells (NRBCs)]. Fetal hematopoiesis becomes increasingly activated, and the peripheral blood thus contains a markedly increased number of **NRBCs** and **erythroblasts**. Over time, the severe anemia leads to *cardiomegaly and high-output congestive heart failure*. With extensive hemolysis, the fetus becomes *progressively anemic, and large iron stores may be present in the liver and spleen*. When the fetal hematocrit falls much below 15%, severe edema, ascites, and anasarca develop – the condition known as **hydrops fetalis**.

Pathologic Features

The pathologic features of the placenta in erythroblastosis fetalis are not specific. They develop largely because of the fetal anemia and cardiac failure, and therefore the intensity of the findings is related to the severity of those conditions. The presence of **placental hydrops** parallels that of fetal hydrops. Thus, the most striking feature of the placenta in erythroblastosis fetalis is the *pallor and marked uniform enlargement*. The villous tissue is diffusely *pale, boggy, and friable* (Fig. 20.1). Rarely, one observes gross icteric staining of placental surface vessels and umbilical cord.

Microscopically, the most striking feature is *villous enlargements and edema* (Fig. 20.2). *Bone marrow elements and hematopoiesis* are present in the fetal circulation (Fig. 20.3). Fetal NRBCs are particularly prominent. Additional histologic features in the placenta are *villous immaturity* (Fig. 20.4), *a marked decrease in the number of fetal vessels, and an increased number and size of Hofbauer cells* (Fig. 20.5). On occasion, one may find

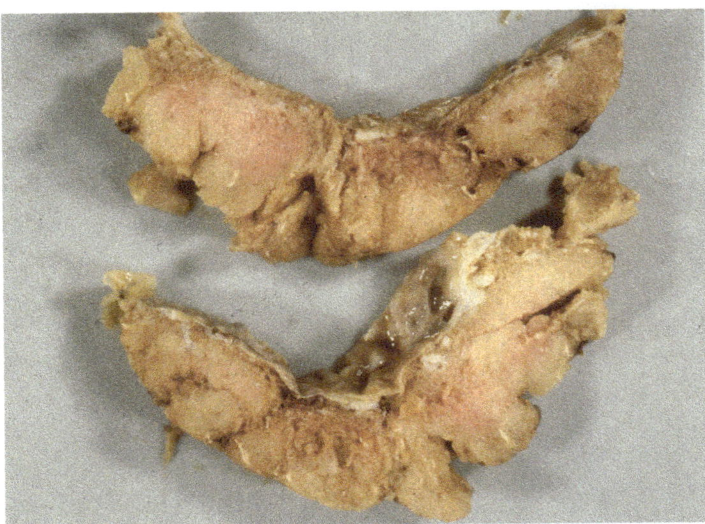

Figure 20.1. Cut sections of a placenta with hydrops in an infant with erythroblastosis fetalis. Note the extreme pallor of the villous tissue.

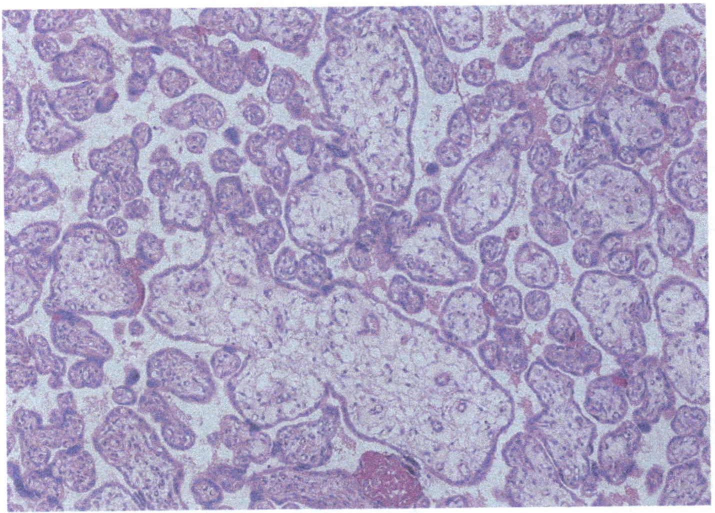

Figure 20.2. Placenta with hydrops demonstrating enlarged villi with edema. H&E ×160.

small amounts of hemosiderin deposited in chorionic *macrophages* betraying the long-standing hemolysis, but this is usually not a prominent finding. *Intervillous thrombi* are also common in erythroblastosis fetalis (see Fig. 19.3 in Chap. 19). It is likely that the villous edema so alters the intervillous blood flow as to cause local eddying and stasis, with thrombosis the end result. Nevertheless, since NRBCs are often found in the thrombi, *fetal bleeding must occur at times* and is likely due to local villous hypoxic injury.

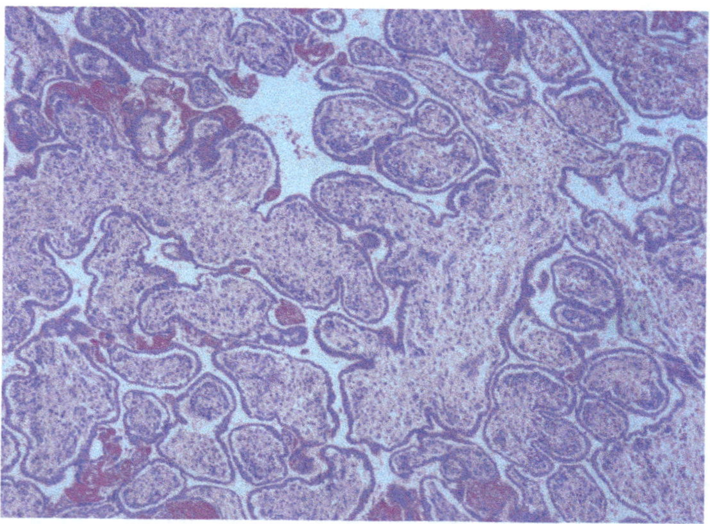

Figure 20.3. Placenta in fetal hydrops. Note the abundant NRBCs in the fetal capillaries. H&E ×640.

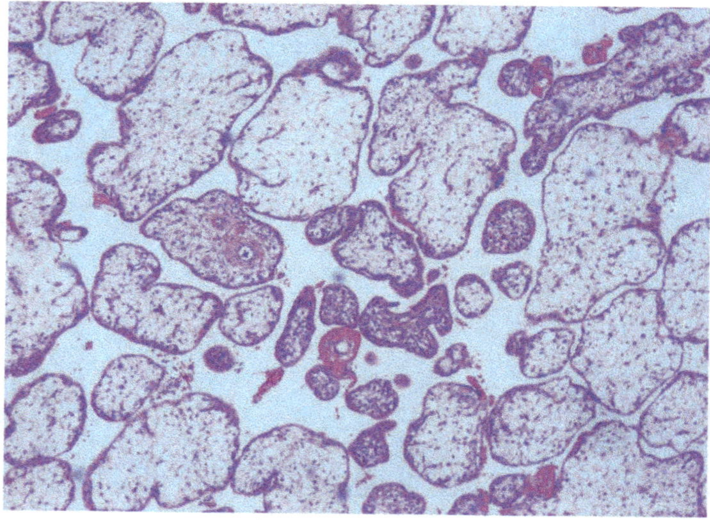

Figure 20.4. Immature appearing, edematous villi in the setting of fetal hydrops. H&E ×100.

Clinical Features and Implications

Fetal hydrops is now readily diagnosed sonographically. If the hydrops is due to hemolysis, it may be quickly reversed through prenatal transfusion (transabdominally or by cordocentesis), thus restoring oxygenation. Although intrauterine transfusions are not without significant risk, the morbidity and mortality of untreated infants is very high. *Hepatosplenomegaly* is prominent, and usually infants have

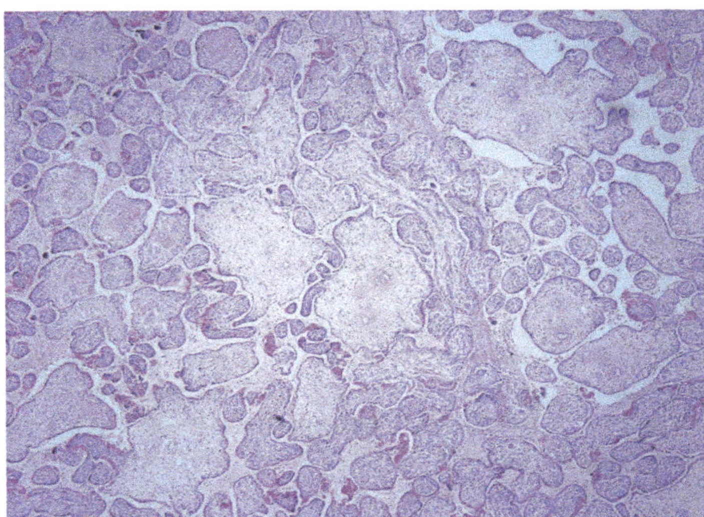

Figure 20.5. Stillborn with typical erythroblastosis fetalis showing edema, abundance of Hofbauer cells and persistent cytotrophoblast. Because of fetal demise, the fetal vessels are obliterated. H&E ×250.

some degree of *hypoproteinemia, thrombocytopenia, and increased beta-cell activity of the islets of Langerhans* (due to insulin binding by the circulating hemoglobin). Elevated serum levels of human chorionic gonadotropin (hCG), human placental lactogen (hPL), and placental protein 5 (PP5) may be present, which are presumably due to the increased placental mass. Occasionally one sees large *maternal ovarian lutein cysts* and *fetal ovarian cysts* due to the elevated hCG.

Hematologic Disorders

Clinical Features and Implications

Normal adult hemoglobin molecules contain two pairs of polypeptide (globin) chains, the **α-chains** and **β-chains**. In embryonic and fetal life, special forms of hemoglobin are prevalent at carefully scheduled times. *Abnormal construction of the globin chains results in altered hemoglobins that may be deficient in oxygen-carrying capacity.* This, in turn, can lead to abnormal red blood cell shapes, as in sickle cell disease. In **α- and β-thalassemias**, *anemia results from a decreased* **production** *of normal hemoglobin.*

Homozygous **α-thalassemia** is inherited as an autosomal *recessive*, and therefore has a recurrence rate of 1 in 4. The pathology in the newborn is essentially identical to that of Rh-disease and it is lethal unless intrauterine blood transfusions are performed. The abnormal gene for α-thalassemia (α-thal$_1$) is common in Indonesians, Filipinos, Thais, Chinese, Germans, African-American, and Canadian Asians. It is also common in Kurdish and Ashkenazi Jews, but in those populations it has not been associated with hydrops. The frequency of this deletion of α-chain genes is greatest in Indonesians and Chinese.

Bart's hemoglobin disease occurs when the *α-chains are replaced by gamma chains (γ-chains)*. The γ-chains are often heterogeneous, and different chain compositions cause different severities of the disease. *Hydrops occurs when the γ-chain gene is homozygous and the four α-chains are replaced by four tau chains (τ-chains)*. The defective hemoglobin is unable to release its oxygen effectively, causing tissue hypoxia, fetal cardiac failure, and hydrops. It is lethal at birth or very shortly thereafter. The fetal red blood cells are frequently *misshapen* and may even be *sickled*. *Cardiac hypertrophy* is often striking, as is the extensive, widespread *extramedullary hematopoiesis*.

In **hemoglobin-H disease**, the hemoglobin molecule consists of *four β-chains*. This particular hemoglobinopathy is prevalent in Asians, and although it causes neonatal anemia, hydrops has not been described. The same is true of **sickle cell anemia** and **sickle cell β-thalassemia**. Both are associated with poor reproductive outcome, but do not feature hydrops as a complication.

Hemoglobin electrophoresis is perhaps the simplest and most widely available tool for the differential diagnosis of the various types of hemoglobin. Chorionic villus sampling (CVS) has made possible the accurate diagnosis of sickle cell disease and thalassemia by direct globin gene analysis. *Appropriate samples of blood should be saved for such studies at autopsy when the etiology of hydrops is uncertain.* The aforementioned methods also much facilitate the diagnosis of heterozygotes.

Pathologic Features

The placentas in these disorders do not differ very much from those with classical erythroblastosis. *Histology alone cannot make the correct differential diagnosis.* The placental enlargement may be massive and is usually *even more enlarged than in classic erythroblastosis*. Placentas weighing up to 3,500 g have been described. The placenta is also *pale, friable, and edematous*. Microscopically, the *cytotrophoblast is prominent* and, in the much-enlarged fetal circulation, large numbers of *red-cell precursors* are found. Pigment is occasionally seen within *chorionic macrophages* either representing hemosiderin or bilirubin from bilirubinuria and liver damage. Preeclampsia is a frequent corollary of this condition, presumably because of the massive placental enlargement.

Trauma

Fetal hemorrhage with resultant hydrops may occur due to various traumatic events. An example is **cordocentesis**, which is usually a benign procedure, but rarely hemorrhage has led to exsanguination. If the infant survives and if severe bleeding has occurred, the resultant anemia can lead to hydrops. Thrombosis of umbilical vessels due to cordocentesis has also been described. In addition, it carries a risk of *transplacental hemorrhage* and, thus, the possibility of *maternal alloimmunization*. **Retroplacental hematoma** (abruptio), although usually associated with maternal bleeding, may sometimes be associated with fetal hemorrhage. Blunt abdominal trauma to the mother without abruption may also be associated with fetal hemorrhage. It is thought that trauma from fetal movement, such as "kicking" the placenta, may cause hemorrhage; however, that has not been proved. Many cases of totally unexplained acute exsanguinations have also occurred.

Miscellaneous Causes of Fetal Hydrops

Occasionally, *tumors or tumor-like lesions may lead to significant fetomaternal hemorrhage, fetal hemorrhage, or hydrops*. For example, placental **choriocarcinomas** (see Chap. 24) may invade villous tissue and cause fetal vascular discontinuity. Discovery of placental choriocarcinomas is usually fortuitous, and perhaps other "unexplained" transplacental hemorrhages would yield similar lesions, if the placenta were examined in more detail. **Chorangiomas** may also be the source of transplacental hemorrhage (see Chap. 22), and hydrops may develop secondary to sequestration of fetal blood cells and due to obstructed venous return from the placenta. **Hemangiomas** of the umbilical cord have also led to hydrops. Other fetal tumors associated with hydrops are listed in Table 20.1.

Fetal hydrops may be associated with various congenital syndromes, in particular, the **Beckwith–Wiedemann syndrome**. *Placentomegaly* is quite common in this disorder, and *hydrops* has been described. The placenta often shows *villi with lacunar, hydropic expansion, and focal chorangiomatosis* (Fig. 20.6). Venous thrombi have been described, as have edematous and excessively *long umbilical cords*. The placental and cord enlargement may be secondary to the dysregulation of normal growth control seen in this syndrome. It is not completely clear what is the etiology of the hydrops in these cases. Hydrops may also be associated with a number of metabolic storage disorders (see below).

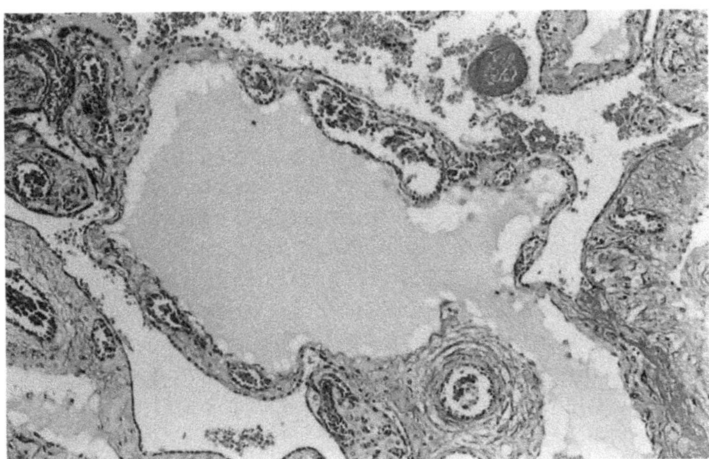

Figure 20.6. Villous alteration in the placenta of a case of Beckwith-Wiedemann syndrome shows a massive cistern, chorangiosis, and congestion. Placentomegaly was also present, and the cord was 69 cm in length with a true knot. Masson trichrome ×160.

Hydrops is associated with various infections (Table 20.2; see Chap. 16). Finally, hydrops may be **idiopathic**. However, as more cases are being investigated, the number of cases that cannot be explained is diminishing. The indications are that, with careful prenatal sonographic surveillance and with the help of more sophisticated autopsy and molecular techniques, this entity may vanish in future. Some of the rarer entities that cause fetal hydrops should be considered before evoking this diagnosis.

Suggestions for Examination and Report
(Fetal or Placental Hydrops)

Gross Examination: A description should be made of the pale, hydropic nature of the placenta. If a fetal demise has occurred, and the etiology is unknown, blood should be submitted for hemoglobin analysis. Furthermore, the presence of a pale placenta or placental hydrops is an indication of fetal anemia even without clinical history. In these cases, and particularly if there has been a fetal demise, it is recommended that the clinicians be contacted to ensure that a Kleihauer–Betke has been done to rule out fetomaternal hemorrhage (see below). It is also prudent to fix a small amount of tissue for electron microscopy in the event the hydrops is due to a metabolic disorder (see below).

Comment: The histologic features are consistent with hydrops. Hydrops has a varied etiology and clinical correlation is necessary for diagnosis.

Fetomaternal Hemorrhage

Pathogenesis

Despite the anatomic separation of the fetal and maternal circulations, transplacental transfer of blood occurs. Transfer of blood from mother to fetus is rare, but the fetus often bleeds into the maternal circulation. The reason for this fetal bleeding is usually obscure. Etiologic factors that have been implicated include *cesarean section delivery, external fetal version, traumatic amniocentesis, maternal trauma, placental abruption, placental tumors (chorangioma, choriocarcinoma), subchorionic hematomas, tight nuchal cord, and tumultuous labor* but most are idiopathic. In the majority of cases, hemorrhage is of a minor degree, but rarely is it a cause of fetal death (approximately 1:2,000 deliveries). The prenatal diagnosis of a **fetomaternal hemorrhage** may be suggested by certain fetal heart tracing abnormalities, such as a sinusoidal rhythm.

Pathologic Features

One should suspect transplacental bleeding when placenta and villous tissue is *unusually pale*. This observation presupposes that the examiner is familiar with the "normal" color of the placental tissue at different stages of gestation. The presence of *intervillous thrombi* may be another clue signaling that hemorrhage has occurred through the placenta and may even signify the point of origin of hemorrhage. In some cases, large intervillous thrombi or many intervillous thrombi may be present, while in other cases they may be absent. Intervillous thrombi may occur for other reasons. The villous tissue is also unusually *thick as well as pale*, but not so overtly hydropic as in thalassemia or erythroblastosis. A marked increased in the NRBCs in the fetal circulation of the placenta are also an important pathologic finding (Fig. 20.7).

Clinical Features and Implications

Significant **fetomaternal hemorrhage** may cause *severe fetal anemia, hemorrhagic shock, hydrops fetalis, maternal isoimmunization, fetal cardiac arrhythmias, and fetal or neonatal death. Cerebral palsy, cerebral infarcts, and microcephaly* have also resulted, presumably due to acute hypotension. In a massive, chronic fetomaternal hemorrhage, hydrops may result from cardiac failure, and brain injury is common. In an acute, massive fetomaternal hemorrhage, fetal death is often the result. Loss of 20% of blood volume is sufficient to produce signs of shock and loss of greater amounts will result in death.

In the event of an *unexplained stillbirth, marked placental pallor, or significant neonatal anemia, the maternal blood should be examined for fetal cells*. This may be done using the **Kleihauer-Betke test**. This technique depends on the fact that fetal hemoglobin is less soluble than maternal (adult) hemoglobin in an acid milieu. Air-dried maternal blood films are fixed, eluted in buffer, and stained. Fetal red blood cells maintain their color but, because the maternal hemoglobin is largely eluted, the maternal cells appear as mere shadows (Fig. 20.8). Ten fields at 250× magnification are reviewed and fetal and maternal cells are counted. The results are reported as a percentage of fetal red blood cells in the

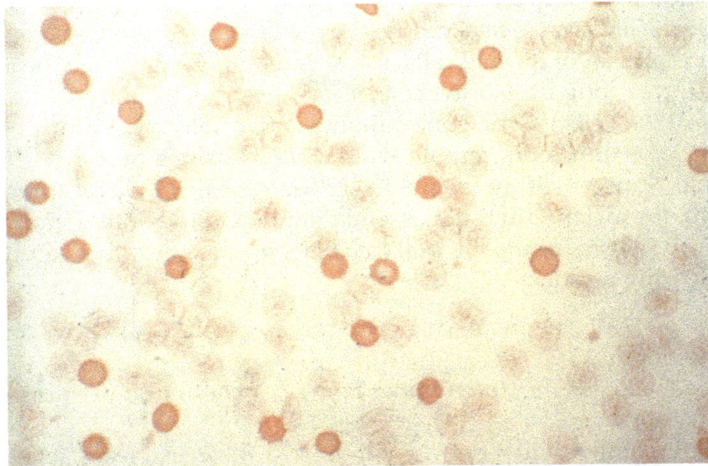

Figure 20.7. Kleihauer-Betke stain of maternal blood. The darkly stained cells are fetal erythrocytes and there are approximately 5% of cells staining. Eosin; Kleihauer. ×1,000.

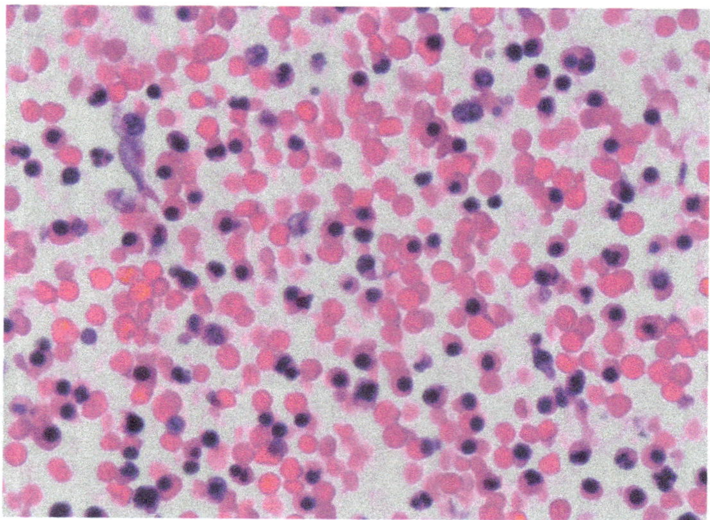

Figure 20.8. Numerous nucleated red blood cells within fetal capillaries. H&E ×200.

maternal circulation and based on a maternal blood volume of approximately 5,000–6,000 mL. One can thus calculate:

$$\_\% \text{ fetal cells} \times 5{,}000 \text{ mL} = \_ \text{ mL of fetal blood in maternal circulation}$$

The blood volume of the infant can be estimated to be approximately 80 mL/kg body weight, with perhaps half again as much present in the placenta. Therefore, the volume of hemorrhage relative to the total fetal blood volume can also be determined. It is important to realize that if a *large quantity of fetal blood* is present in the mother, particularly if it is *equal to or greater than the blood volume of the infant*, a chronic hemorrhage should be suspected.

While the life span of fetal cells in the maternal circulation is somewhat shorter than that of normal cells, transplacental bleeding may be ascertained for as long as *4–6 weeks after delivery* by Kleihauer-Betke tests alone. All the cells will be gone 3 months after delivery. Unfortunately, the test is, at times, inaccurate. Falsely high values may result from maternal sources of hemoglobin F (present in 25% of pregnant women), for instance in β-thalassemia minor. On the other hand, there will be an *underestimation of fetal blood loss* or false-negative results for the following reasons:

- Only 90% of the fetal cells will stain, as 10% already contain hemoglobin A.
- Some fetal cells die, the number being dependent on the time since the hemorrhage.
- ABO incompatibility between mother and fetus clears fetal cells rapidly.
  - For example, if the mother is blood group O and the fetus is A, the fetal cells will be rapidly cleared by maternal anti-A antibody.

Other tests used in the determination of the presence and/or quantification of fetomaternal hemorrhage are **α-fetoprotein** and **flow cytometry**. These tests have also been used after Rh-negative women give birth to an Rh-positive infant to determine the amount of Rhogam prophylaxis necessary.

Suggestions for Examination and Report
(Suspected fetomaternal hemorrhage)

Gross Examination: If the placenta is markedly pale, fetal anemia should be suspected.

Comment: If there is placental hydrops and the presence of numerous NRBCs, a fetomaternal hemorrhage should be suspected and there should be a recommendation for a Kleihauer-Betke test.

Fetal Nucleated Red Blood Cells

It is known that **nucleated red blood cells (NRBCs)** appear in the circulation of *anemic fetuses*, and this is best exemplified in erythroblastosis fetalis (Fig. 20.7). Similarly, there is an increase in NRBCs with *acute blood loss* and in fetuses experiencing *hypoxia*. This feature plays an important role in current medicolegal decisions. One of the most important aspects to the presence of elevated NRBCs in the fetal circulation is how rapid the response is to the loss of red cells and hypoxia, and whether this response is quantitatively reflected in the number of the NRBCs in the circulation.

Studies have shown that NRBCs disappear by the end of the third month of pregnancy. In the histologic evaluation of placentas *only rare NRBCs should be observed in the term placenta*. When NRBCs are present in the fetal blood, and thus in the fetal vessels in the placenta, it is a distinctly abnormal finding. The pathologist should then try to find the reason for their presence. An absolute value *greater than 1×10^9/L should be considered as a potential index of intrauterine hypoxia*. Normally there are about 200–600 NRBCs/mm^3 and 10,000–30,000 white blood cells (WBC). However, *infants of diabetic mothers have increased numbers, as do growth-restricted infants*. NRBCs that already formed may be released initially, but because of the complex sequence of signals to initiate erythropoiesis and release of NRBCs, many hours must pass from the initiation of a hypoxic stimulus to the appearance of *significant* numbers of NRBCs in the circulation.

Suggestions and Examples for Report
(Nucleated Red Blood Cells)

Gross Examination: NRBCs are not evident on gross examination.

Comment: The presence of increased NRBCs may be indicative of fetal anemia and if this can be ruled out, is indicative of intrauterine hypoxia.

Transplacental Passage of Cellular Elements

While transplacental red blood cell passage has the most serious consequences due to anemia and immunization, **transplacental white blood cell transfer** is also of interest. Fetal lymphocytes pass to the mother in most normal pregnancies and may be found years postpartum in the maternal blood or bone marrow. Of course **deported syncytiotrophoblast** traveling from the placenta to the maternal lung has long been known. **Transplacental passage of tumor cells** or metastasis from mother to fetus has also been described many times (see Chap. 22). Chimerism, induced by prenatal **maternal lymphocyte transfer**, has also been reported. A few additional reports of 46 XX cells in the circulation of male fetuses have been forthcoming. Such passage is clearly exceptional. There have also been occasional reports of fetal plethora that were apparently due to **mother-to-fetus blood transfer**; however, numerous studies have affirmed the transfer of small numbers of maternal red blood cells to the fetus without fetal plethora or abnormal placentas.

Fetal Metabolic Storage Disorders

Many of the **metabolic storage disorders** produce inclusions or vacuoles in the tissues of affected individuals. In some, involvement of placental tissues enables prenatal diagnosis via chorionic villus biopsy or from material obtained at amniocentesis. Many of these diseases may cause fetal *hydrops*, the etiology of which remains obscure. Nevertheless, because of the association with storage disorders, *cases of nonimmune hydrops fetalis warrant special attention*. Many of the inclusions are highly water and/or lipid-solvent soluble and can only be identified with proper fixation. *Electron microscopy* and *special enzyme studies* are often necessary to make the definitive diagnosis. Therefore, consideration should be given to fixation of tissue for electron microscopy when one of these disorders is suspected. Importantly, there are numerous cases in which a *storage disorder was suspected only after placental examination* revealed characteristic features. Even without clinical suspicion or evidence of disease, the presence of **foam cells, trophoblastic vacuolization**, and **irregular calcification** *is indicative of an unidentified fetal storage disorder*. Further workup is then warranted.

Pathologic Features

Macroscopically, the placenta will be *enlarged, pale, and/or soft*, particularly in cases associated with hydrops. On microscopic examination, intracellular accumulation of material is revealed as *vacuolization of the cytoplasm* of certain cells, the distribution of which is particular to that storage disorder. Because the cellular glycolipids are highly water-soluble, the empty appearance of the vacuoles is the usual finding in many fetal storage disorders. In the majority of the disorders with placental manifestations, it is primarily the *syncytiotrophoblast* that shows the typical vacuolated cytoplasm (Fig. 20.9). Other trophoblastic cells may show vacuolation as well, including *cytotrophoblast and extravil-*

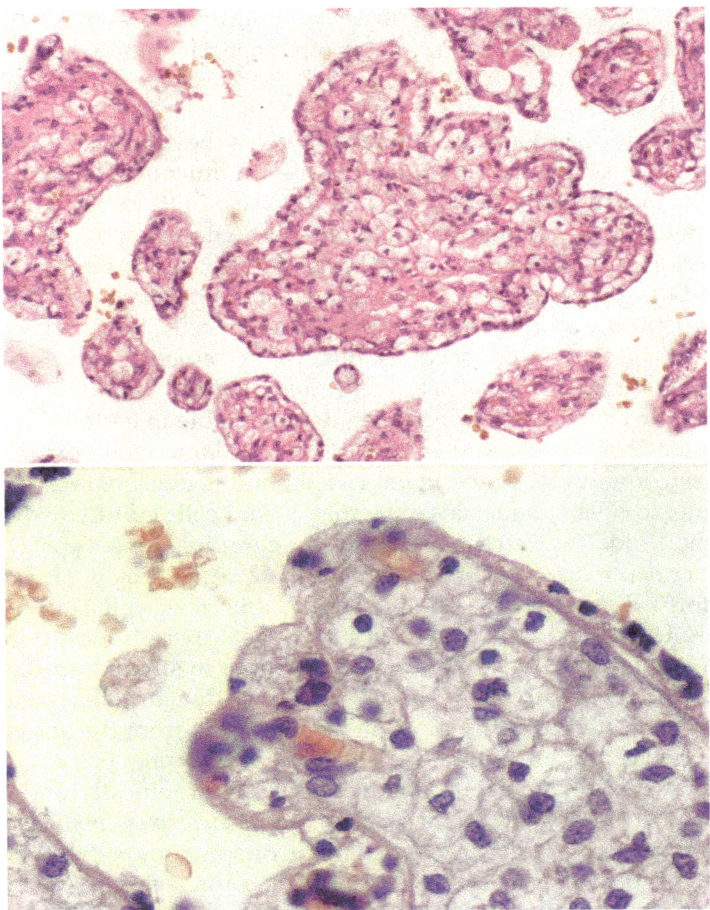

Figure 20.9. (a) Chorionic villi affected by Hurler's Disease (mucopolysaccharidioses I) with vacuolization of syncytiotrophoblast as well as Hofbauer and stromal cells. H&E ×240. (b) Villus affected by mucolipidosis II (I-cell disease). Note the abundance of vacuoles in the syncytium and Hofbauer cells. H&E ×360.

lous trophoblast. Furthermore, *villous fibroblasts, Hofbauer cells, villous capillary endothelial cells, and, rarely, the amnion* may show vacuolization. Endothelial damage, perhaps secondary to lipid accumulation, is seen in a number of storage diseases leading to *thrombosis* of chorionic or fetal stem vessels.

If vacuolization of cells in the placenta is identified, a metabolic storage disorder may be tentatively diagnosed. Based on which cells contain the vacuolization, whether the infant or fetus has hydrops and other clinical information, a differential diagnosis may be compiled. Table 20.2 lists selected storage disorders and the particular placental cells in which vacuolization can be identified. Histochemical stains can be helpful in differentiating some of these disorders, but this has not been studied on placental tissue in every disorder. After making the tentative diagnosis of storage disorder, diagnosis and confirmation of the specific disease must be made via enzyme or other special studies.

Specific Disorders

A few specific disorders are mentioned here, as they show some unique features. For instance, **Morquio disease** or **mucopolysaccharidosis type IV**, unlike many of the storage diseases, only rarely has histologic evidence of storage products in trophoblast, but rather shows *granularity in Hofbauer cells*. The absence of β-galactosidase defines **type 1 G_{M1} gangliosidosis**. Typical inclusions or *zebra bodies* may be ultrastructurally identified in the fetal ganglion cells. Fetal cells will be unremarkable in paraffin sections, but *"empty vacuoles" in the syncytial cytoplasm, the amnionic epithelial cells, and Hofbauer cells* are present. Occasionally, vacuolization has been demonstrable in endothelial cells in villous stem vessels, and *calcified thrombi* in large fetal vessels have also been identified. Since membrane-bound inclusions are present in amnionic cells, diagnosis can be made from cells cultured from the amniotic fluid. **Tay–Sachs' disease (G_{M2}-gangliosidosis type I)** produces *vacuolization of syncytiotrophoblast*. In **G_{M2}-gangliosidosis type II, Sandhoff's disease**, vacuolation is seen in *stromal* as well as the *syncytial* cells. Ultrastructurally, the most striking feature is the occurrence of *parallel membranous arrays in occasional lysosomes* in stromal cells.

Niemann–Pick disease Type A, which is due to sphingomyelin diphosphodiesterase deficiency, can be diagnosed from the absence of the enzyme in amniotic fluid. Unusual *echogenic densities in the placentas* of several cases have been demonstrated sonographically and these placentas have had *thick chorionic plates. Vacuolated syncytium, Hofbauer cells,* and *fibrocytes* contain accumulations of sphingomyelin, which is also present in the umbilical cord and the chorion laeve.

Gaucher's disease is a heterogeneous disease that may cause *fetal hydrops*. The placenta is *large* and *edematous* with macroscopic features similar to that of erythroblastosis fetalis. In the absence of hydrops, there are generally no placental findings. However, some cases may show *Hofbauer cells with minimal vacuolization*. Uncommonly, characteristic histiocytes, or *Gaucher cells*, may be found in fetal vessels in the placenta. Absence of α-galactosidase A results in **Fabry's disease**, a disorder of glycosphingolipid metabolism. The tissues accumulate ceramide trihexose. Although the syncytiotrophoblast does not show vacuolization, the *decidual cells* and *decidual vessels* contain *argyrophilic granules*, which, by electron microscopy, have the appearance similar to zebra bodies. The fetal portions of the placenta are normal.

Mucolipidosis type II or **I-cell disease** is a rare and fatal disorder whose genetic transmission is autosomal recessive. *Periodic acid-Schiff (PAS)-positive lysosomal inclusions* are present in the cells of affected children, including kidney cells, leukocytes, and fibroblasts. The typical "inclusions" cannot be seen in paraffin-embedded sections, but are obvious in epoxy-embedded material. Placental involvement with inclusion-bearing cells in the *villous fibroblast* has also been demonstrated. In paraffin sections of the placenta, the *vacuoles of formerly mucolipid-containing lysosomes* are readily apparent in the *syncytium* and in *Hofbauer cells* (Fig. 20.9). The features are much enhanced by processing the tissues in epoxy resin. In some cases vascular lesions have been present in the *villous stem arteries ranging from fibrinoid necrosis to complete obliteration*. Focal *villous calcification* is also a common finding. As with many of these disorders, diagnosis may be made with electron microscopy.

Unusual placental findings in **Pompe's disease** or **glycogen storage disease type II** consist of *cytoplasmic vacuolation of syncytium, cytotrophoblast, fibroblast, and amnionic connective tissue cells*. By electron microscopy, typical *membrane-bounded, glycogen-filled inclusions in capillary endothelial cells and villous fibroblasts* are found. These inclusions may be found in cells obtained via CVS as early as 10 weeks. In **type IV glycogen storage disease**, vacuoles are only present in the *amnionic epithelium*.

Suggestions for Examination and Report
(Storage disorders with vacuolization of trophoblast or other cells)

Gross Examination: Generally, the placentas in these disorders are grossly unremarkable, but may be pale, enlarged and soft, particularly if hydrops is present. If a disorder is suspected, tissue should be fixed for electron microscopy.

Comment: Vacuolization of trophoblast or other placental cells is highly suggestive of a fetal metabolic disorder and further testing should be suggested.

Placental Changes in Intrauterine Fetal Demise

After death in utero, the fetal tissue begins to undergo autolysis. Certain placental changes also occur that are attributable to fetal death, which are different from the pathologic changes that are the cause of death. Macroscopically, the *fetal surface and fetal membranes may be discolored red-brown* due to hemolysis. Microscopically, the pathologic changes in the placenta that are directly caused by the fetal demise mostly relate to the *cessation of fetal circulation*. This causes *progressive sclerosis of the fetal vessels* and ultimately their *obliteration*. This is particularly true of the villous capillaries and thus leads to widespread *avascular villi*. Studies have shown that these and other changes occur after fetal death in a relatively predictable manner such that the time of fetal death may be roughly estimated by the presence of absence of particular features.

One of the first changes that occur is **intravascular karyorrhexis** in villous capillaries. This consists of particles of nuclear debris, predominantly derived from leukocytes, stained deeply with hematoxylin, present within villous capillaries and small villous vessels (Fig. 20.10). This change is not present if fetal death has occurred less than 6 h prior to delivery. Another early change is **degeneration of the umbilical vascular smooth muscle cells**. This finding may be present within a few hours but is present in virtually all cases by 12 h. It consists of some *loss of nuclear basophilia* and *nuclear pyknosis*. In addition, the *smooth muscle cells become thin and spindled*, also taking on a *"wavy"*

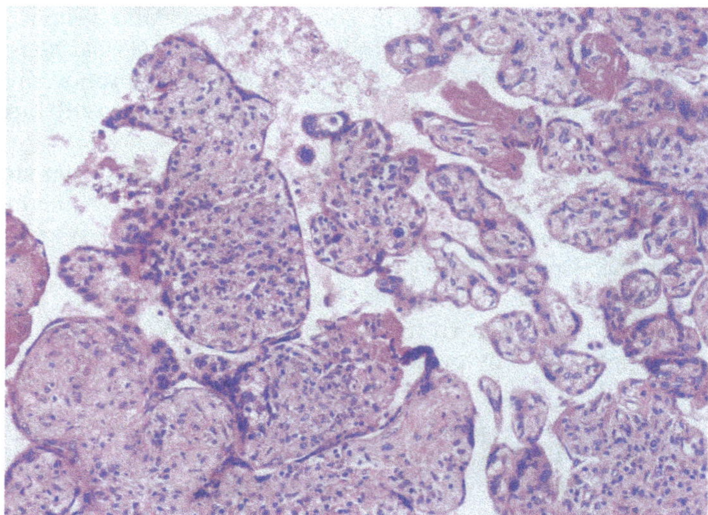

Figure 20.10 Intravascular karyorrhexis with nuclear debris in fetal capillaries. H&E ×140.

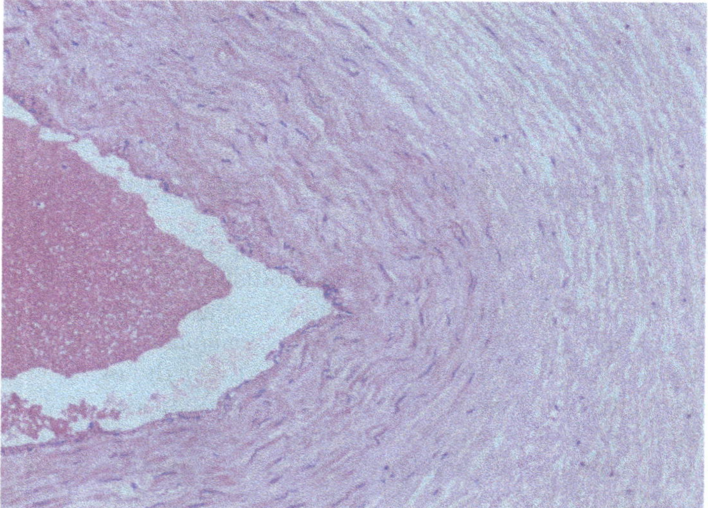

Figure 20.11. Degeneration of vascular smooth muscle of umbilical cord after demise. H&E ×200.

appearance (Fig. 20.11). The loss of fetal circulation also causes **luminal abnormalities of the fetal stem vessels** consisting of *septation of the lumen and obliteration* (Fig. 20.12). The septation commonly appears as the presence of *multiple irregular lumens connected by thin fibrous tissue* containing degenerated blood and occasionally thrombi. If these changes are multifocal and present in 10–25% of stem villi, then the time from fetal death is at least 48 h. The changes do not become exten-

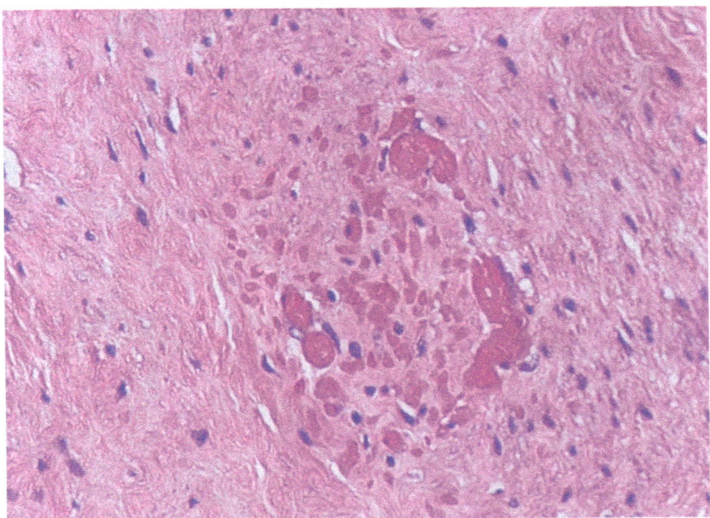

Figure 20.12. Stem vessel luminal abnormalities, septation, and fibromuscular sclerosis with partial obliteration. H&E ×400.

sive, involving more than 25% of the stem villi, until approximately 2 weeks after fetal death. *Sclerosis of the villous stroma or avascular villi* often accompanies obliteration of the fetal vessels. Extensive avascular villi, involving at least 25% of the terminal villi, also occur roughly 2 weeks after fetal demise. The luminal abnormalities described above can also be seen in live-born fetuses when there is cessation of fetal blood flow secondary to fetal vascular thrombosis (see Chap. 21). Therefore, in stillborn fetuses caution should be used in attributed these changes to thrombosis, as they can be due solely to fetal death. Correlation with autopsy findings and known time of death may be helpful in these cases.

Other changes also occur but in a less predictable manner. Some authors have suggested that **increased syncytial knots** are associated with fetal death, while others do not find this association. It is our experience that this change may occur, but when it does it is usually in cases with long-term intrauterine retention of the placenta after fetal death, on the order of weeks to months. It is, however, important to note that although there is some decrease in maternal blood flow after fetal death, flow does not completely stop nor does it impair the viability of the trophoblast. Thus, weeks and even months after fetal death when the villous stroma is completely avascular and hyalinized, the trophoblastic cover can continue to be viable. After fetal death, **villous stromal microcalcification** may be present consisting of fine, *granular calcification of the trophoblastic basement membrane* or fine, punctate granules within the stroma (Fig. 20.13). It is likely that calcium is not the sole mineral that deposits within the villi in this situation. Normally, the fetal vessels transport these minerals away from the placenta,

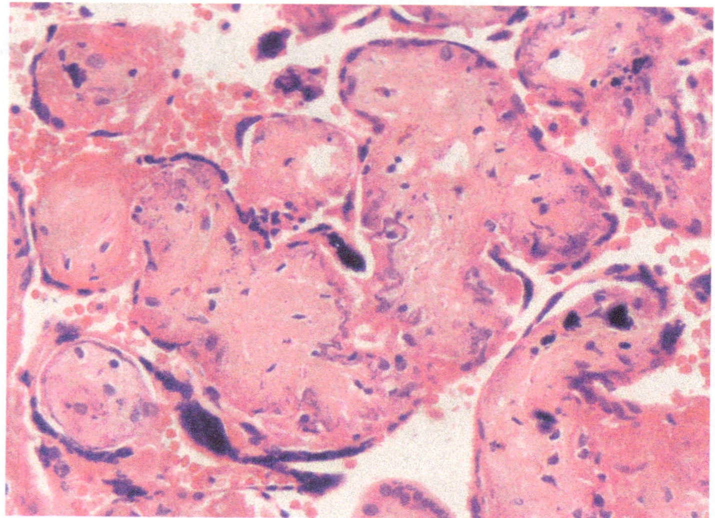

Figure 20.13. Microcalcification of trophoblastic basement membrane. H&E ×200.

but with the loss of fetal circulation, there is accumulation and deposition within the villous stroma and the trophoblastic basement membrane. Other changes that may occur with fetal death include **thickening of the trophoblastic basement membrane** and **degeneration of Wharton's jelly**.

Suggestions for Examination and Report
(Fetal demise)

Gross Examination: The cord and fetal surface may be hemolyzed and discolored red. No additional gross examination or sections need to be submitted if the cause of demise is known. If it is not, 4–5 additional random sections of villous tissue should be submitted to identify possible causes of demise.

Comment: The changes seen should be described and it should be indicated that they are consistent with fetal demise. The approximate timing of fetal death can be included. Certainly a comment on possible placental causes of death should be made based on pathology found on examination.

Table 20.1. Causes of nonimmune hydrops fetalis.

Cardiovascular: congenital heart disease
    Coarctation of the aorta
    Hypoplastic left heart
    Cardiac arrhythmias particularly supraventricular tachycardia
    Premature closure of the foramen ovale
    Endocardial fibroelastosis
    Ebstein's anomaly of the tricuspid valve
Chromosomal (see Chap. 11)
    Turner's syndrome, 45 XO
    Trisomy 13, 15, 16, 18, and 21
    Duplications of the long arms of chromosomes 15 or 17
    Triploidy
Anemia
    Twin to twin transfusion syndrome (see Chap. 10)
    Thalassemia
    Fetomaternal hemorrhage
    Hemolytic anemia
    Fetal hemorrhage
        Disrupted velamentous or other fetal vessels (see Chap. 15)
        Injury to the fetus
Thoracic: space-occupying lesions
    Cystic adenomatoid malformation and pulmonary sequestration
    Diaphragmatic hernia
    Cystic hygroma
    Chylothorax
    Lymphangiectasias
Infection (see Chap. 16)
    Parvovirus
    Cytomegalovirus
    Toxoplasmosis
    Herpes simplex virus
    Syphilis
    Rubella
Congenital tumors (see Chap. 22)
    Congenital neuroblastoma
    Hepatoblastoma
    Sacrococcygeal teratoma
    Leukemia
    Mesoblastic nephroma
    Hemangioma
    Chorangioma
    Choriocarcinoma

Table 20.1. (continued)

Miscellaneous

    Malformations of the genitourinary tract

    Fetal storage disorders

    Thyrotoxicosis

    Small bowel volvulus

    Intussusception

    Trauma

    Beckwith-Wiedemann syndrome

    Chorangiomatosis

    Idiopathic

Table 20.2. Summary of placental findings in metabolic storage diseases.

Disorder	Deficiency	Hydrops	Intracellular vacuolization						Histochemistry			
			ST	ET	HC	FB	EN	AE	PAS	Alcian blue	Colloidal Fe	ORO
Mucopolysaccharidoses									+/−		+	
MPS I (Hurler disease)	α-1-Iduronidase	+	+		+	+						
MPS III (San Filippo disease)	Various		+									
MPS IV (Morquio disease)	Various	+			a							
MPS VII (Sly disease)	β-Glucuronidase	+			+							
Sphingolipidoses												
GM1 gangliosidosis	β-Galactosidase		+	+	+	+		+	+	+	+	+
GM2 gangliosidosis												
Type I (Tay–Sachs disease)	β-Hexosaminidase, α subunit		+		+			+				
Type II (Sandhoff disease)	β-Hexosaminidase, β subunit		+			+						
Niemann–Pick disease, type A	Sphingomyelinase	+	+	+	+	+			+/−			+
Niemann–Pick disease, type B	Sphingomyelinase											
Gaucher's disease	β-Glucosidase	+			M				+			
Fabry disease	α-Galactosidase								+			+

Table 20.2. (continued)

Disorder	Deficiency	Hydrops	ST	ET	HC	FB	EN	AE	PAS	Alcian blue	Colloidal Fe	ORO
Other lipidoses												
Wolman disease	Acid lipase	+	+									+
Cholesterol ester storage disease	Acid lipase	+	+			+						
Niemann–Pick disease, type C	Unknown											
Neuronal ceroid lipofuscinosis	Unknown		+				+	+				
Mucolipidoses												
Type I, sialidosis	Sialidase		+		+	+						
Type II, I-cell disease	N-acetylglucosamine-1-phosphotransferase	+	+	+	+			M	+/−	+/−	+/−	+/−
Type IV	Unknown					+						
Oligosaccharidoses												
Galactosialidosis	β-Galactosialidase	+	+			+						
Sialic acid storage disease (Salla disease)	Sialic acid transporter	+	+	+	+		+	+		+	+	
Glycogen storage disease												
Type II, Pompe disease	α-1,4-Glucosidase		+			+	+		+/−			
Type IV	Amylopectinase						+					

ST syncytiotrophoblast, *ET* extravillous trophoblast or X-cell, *FB* villous stromal fibroblast, *HC* Hofbauer cell, *EN* endothelium, *AE* amnionic epithelium, *PAS* periodic acid-Schiff, *ORO* oil red O, *M* minimal vacuolization[a]Granularity and *not* vacuolization can be seen in Hofbauer cells

Selected References

PHP5, pages 519–551 (Hydrops), pages 552–576 (Transplacental Hemorrhage, Trauma), pages 577–583 (Fetal Storage Disorders).

Bouvier R, Maire I. Fetal presentation of 23 cases of lysosomal storage disease. A collaborative study of the French Society of Fetal Pathology. Pediatr Pathol Lab Med 1997;17:675.

Bowman JM, Lewis M, de Sa DJ. Hydrops fetalis caused by massive maternofetal transplacental hemorrhage. J Pediatr 1984;104:769–772.

Fox H. The incidence and significance of nucleated erythrocytes in the foetal vessels of the mature human placenta. J Obstet Gynaecol Br Commonw 1967;74:40–43.

Genest DR. Estimating the time of death in stillborn fetuses: II. Histologic evaluation of the placenta; a study of 71 stillborns. Obstet Gynecol 1992;80:585–592.

Hellman LM, Hertig AT. Pathological changes in the placenta associated with erythroblastosis of the fetus. Am J Pathol 1937;14:111–120.

Higgins SD. Trauma in pregnancy. J Perinatol 1988;8:288–292.

Isaacs H. Fetal hydrops associated with tumors. Am J Perinatol 2008;25:43–68.

Jones CJP, Lendon M, Chawner LE, et al. Ultrastructure of the human placenta in metabolic storage disease. Placenta 1990;11:395–411.

Lage JM. Placentomegaly with massive hydrops of placental stem villi, diploid DNA content, and omphaloceles: Possible association with Beckwith-Wiedemann syndrome. Human Pathol 1991;22:591–597.

Machin GA. Hydrops revisited: literature review of 1,414 cases published in the 1980s. Am J Med Genet 1989;34:366–390.

Mostoufi-Zadeh M, Weiss LM, Driscoll SG. Nonimmune hydrops fetalis: a challenge in perinatal pathology. Human Pathol 1985;16:785–789.

Potter EL. Intervillous thrombi in the placenta and their possible relation to erythroblastosis fetalis. Am J Obstet Gynecol 1948;56:959–961.

Roberts DJ, Ampola MG, Lage JM. Diagnosis of unsuspected fetal metabolic storage disease by routine placental examination. Pediatr Pathol 1991;11:647–656.

Santamaria M, Benirschke K, Carpenter PM, et al. Transplacental hemorrhage associated with placental neoplasms. Pediatr Pathol 1987;7:601–615.

Schröder J. Review article: transplacental passage of blood cells. J Med Genet 1975;12:230–242.

Stonehill LL, LaFerla JJ. Assessment of fetomaternal hemorrhage with Kleihauer–Betke test. Am J Obstet Gynecol 1986;155:1146.

Chapter 21

Fetal Thrombotic Vasculopathy

General Considerations

The umbilical vessels insert onto the placental surface, branch, run within the chorionic plate, and then, at the periphery, turn abruptly toward the maternal surface, branching repeatedly to finally become villous capillaries. Blood is returned from the villous capillary loops to the umbilical cord by veins that merge into the umbilical vein. In the overwhelming majority of cotyledons, there is *a 1:1 relation between artery and vein* at the periphery, and each artery "supplies" a single cotyledon (placentone). It is remarkable that at least *the larger arteries always cross over the veins on the placental surface*. They can thus be readily identified by macroscopic examination, while histologically it is nearly impossible to make this distinction. It is interesting to note that the circumferential architecture of the placental surface vessels is asymmetrical. This is due to hemodynamic thinning where pressure in the vessels buckle and thin the superficial portions of the vessels, whereas the "fixed" portions resist this pressure. This phenomenon of thinning of the superficial aspect of chorionic vessels is also shared with cord vessels.

R.N. Baergen, *Manual of Pathology of the Human Placenta,*
DOI 10.1007/978-1-4419-7494-5_21, © Springer Science+Business Media, LLC 2011

Thrombosis in the Fetal Circulation

Pathologic Features

Thrombosis

Mural and occlusive thrombi occur frequently in the superficial placental vessels and their villous ramifications. They are more commonly present in the veins and are variably located across the fetal surface and within the placenta. They are only occasionally accompanied by thrombi in the umbilical cord. *Surface thrombi can be recognized by careful gross examination.* When the vessel is hugely distended (Fig. 21.1), the identification of thrombi is easy. Much more frequently overlooked are thrombi identified only by the presence of thickening of the vessel or a white streak within the lumen. When thrombi are fresh, their *gross appearance is that of a slightly enlarged vessel that may have an unusual color, usually tan or white* (Figs. 21.2 and 21.3). It is not as shiny and blue as normal vessels. One is also unable to move the blood mechanically in thrombosed vessels.

Mural thrombosis is much more frequent than complete obliteration of the vessel (Figs. 21.4 and 21.5). Older thrombi may even *calcify* (Fig. 21.6), but variations are frequent, and when thrombosis has occurred a *long time before examination, the vessels may be completely obliterated. They then appear as a rounded fibromuscular structure without a lumen* (Fig. 21.7). True organization of dead tissues, as the pathologist knows from renal or splenic infarcts, does not really occur in placental degenerative lesions. That is, removal of debris by phagocytes and ingrowth of granulation tissue and fibrous tissue are phenomena not seen in true placental infarcts, nor do they occur in thrombosed placental vessels. Rather, these lesions shrink, and some phagocytes may appear, but eventually they become calcified or the vessel atrophies. It may eventually disappear completely, becoming unrecognizable as a former vessel.

Avascular Villi

If the thrombi have been *occlusive for a prolonged time, particularly if the thrombi are present in the arterial circulation,* the villous tree may become avascular as the vessels atrophy (Fig. 21.8). These villi then become **avascular villi**. Avascular villi are considered direct evidence of thrombosis in the fetal circulation, even without the presence of frank thrombi within vessels. Larger foci of avascular villi may be visible *grossly as a triangular area of pallor with the consistency of villous tissue.* The base is usually at the basal plate, and may be easier to visualize in a fixed specimen. Microscopically, the area is sharply demarcated from the surrounding normal villous tissue. Avascular villi differ from true infarction in that the trophoblast is viable as it continues to be perfused by the maternal blood in the intervillous space. There may, however, be increased syncytial knotting in some cases. The villous vessels and stroma atrophy over time due to loss of the fetal circulation. *The stroma is usually pink and hyalinized without vessels. Occasional deposits of hemosiderin may be present.* At the apex of the lesion, one may occasionally find the supplying

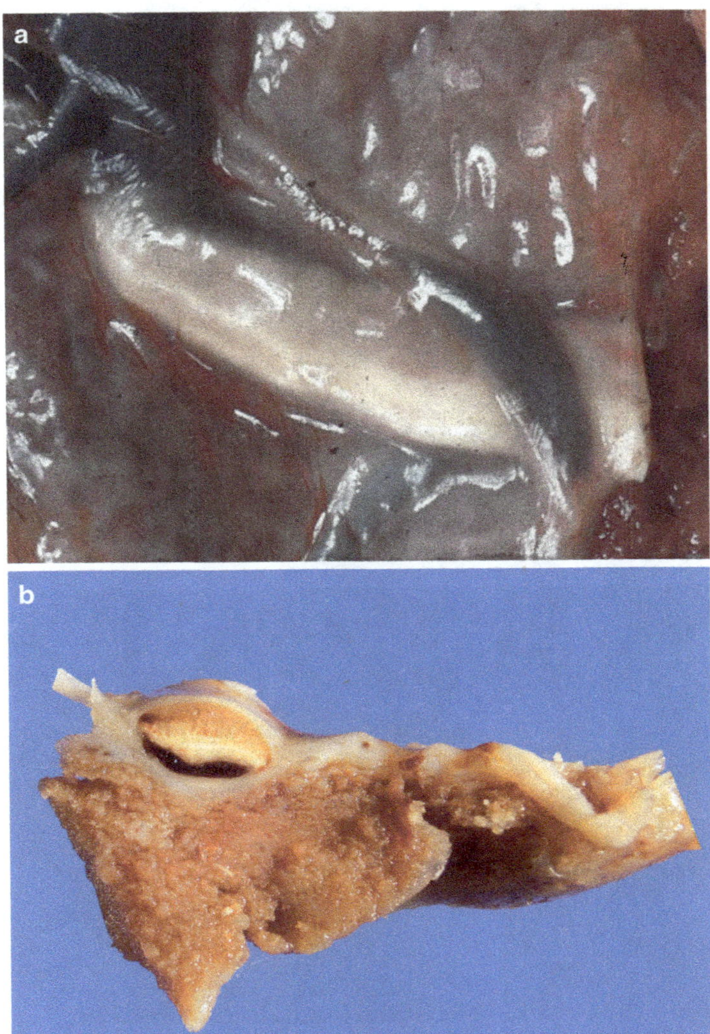

Figure 21.1. (a) Distended surface chorionic vessel with obvious thrombus seen as a white streak. (b) Layered thrombus present apparent on cut section of placental surface.

artery with thrombosis. In older lesions, the distal stem vessels may show thickening of the vascular walls, ultimately with obliteration of the lumen. Caution must be used in cases of stillbirth, as loss of the entire fetal circulation will cause a similar but diffuse change.

Intimal Fibrin Cushions
Intimal fibrin cushions or intimal vascular cushions are microscopically similar to those that pathologists find in the pulmonary vessels of patients with pulmonary hypertension. *Laminated fibrin is deposited in the intima of the vessel and bulges out into the lumen like a "cushion"*

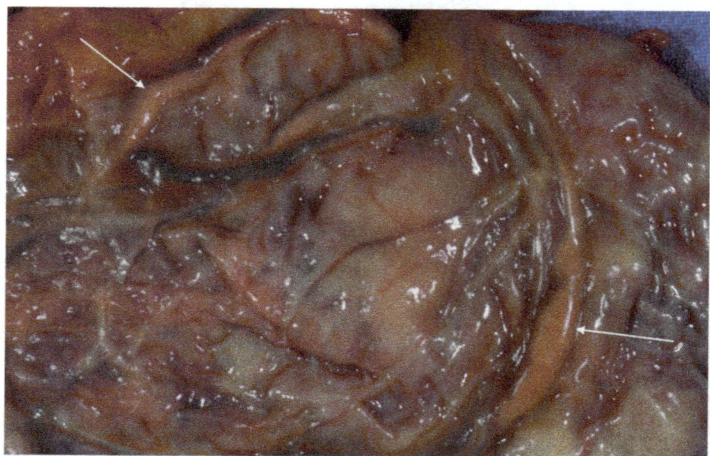

Figure 21.2. Thrombi in fetal surface vessels (*arrows*). The infant developed cerebral palsy.

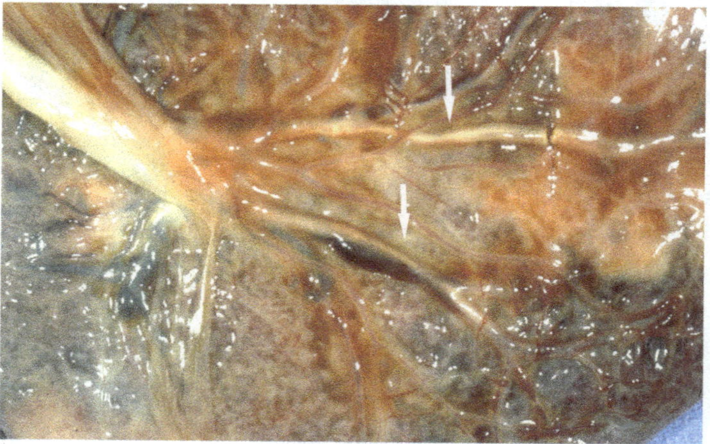

Figure 21.3. Thrombi in chorionic vessels are visible as tan-white streaks (*arrows*).

(Fig. 21.9). These are sometimes just referred to as "mural thrombi." The lumen is usually not obstructed to a significant degree. At times, one may see *accumulation of what appears to be mucopolysaccharide or ground substance within the intima as well*. This appears as pale, blue material separating the vascular smooth muscle from the endothelium. Calcifications may occur in older lesions (Fig. 21.10).

Fibromuscular Sclerosis
A vascular lesion of small vessels called **fibromuscular sclerosis** has been found to be associated with abnormal Doppler flow and growth restriction. It is often seen in conjunction with terminal villus deficiency (see Chap. 18). In this lesion, there is *an increase in the smooth muscle and fibrous tissue of the stem arteries leading to narrowed lumens,*

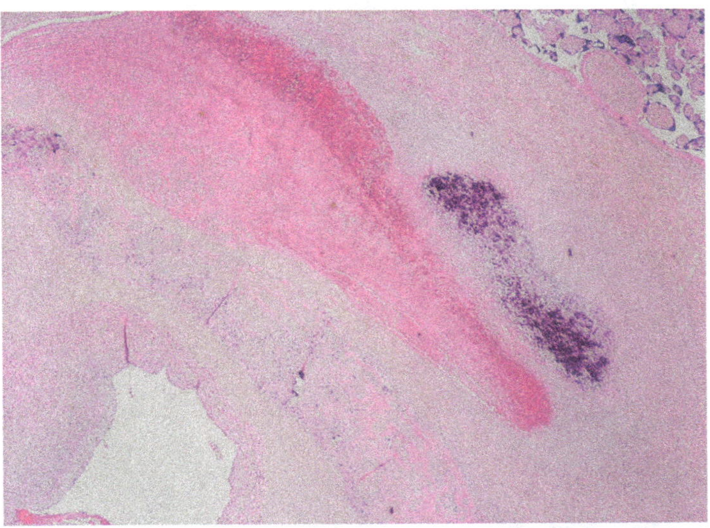

Figure 21.4. Mural thrombi in surface vein with associated calcification. H&E ×20.

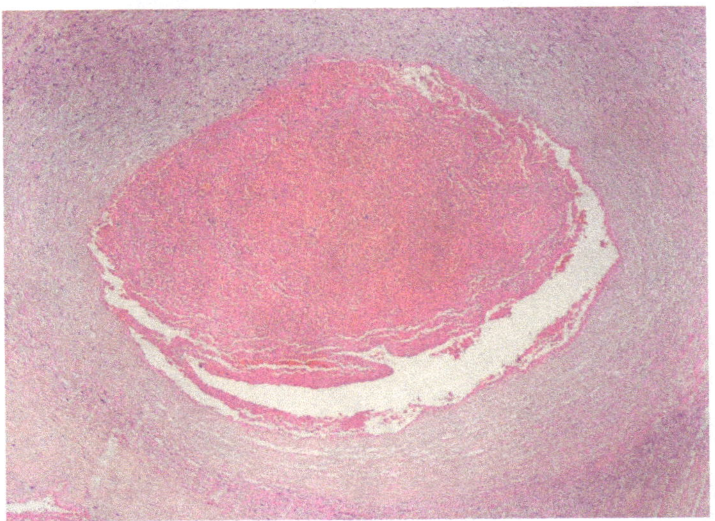

Figure 21.5. Nearly occlusive thrombus in a dilated chorionic vein associated with long cord and stillborn. H&E ×20.

and it is generally a focal phenomenon. Occasionally, complete occlusion may occur.

Hemorrhagic Endovasculopathy: Villous Stromal Karyorrhexis
Finally, there is a pathologic change referred to as **hemorrhagic endovasculitis, hemorrhagic endovasculosis,** or **hemorrhagic endovasculopathy (HEV)**, which includes a variety of different lesions. The most common lesion consists of *extravasated red blood cells (RBCs) in the stroma, karyorrhexis of the nuclei of endothelial and blood cells, and septation* (Fig. 21.11). The integrity of the vascular walls is lost and they

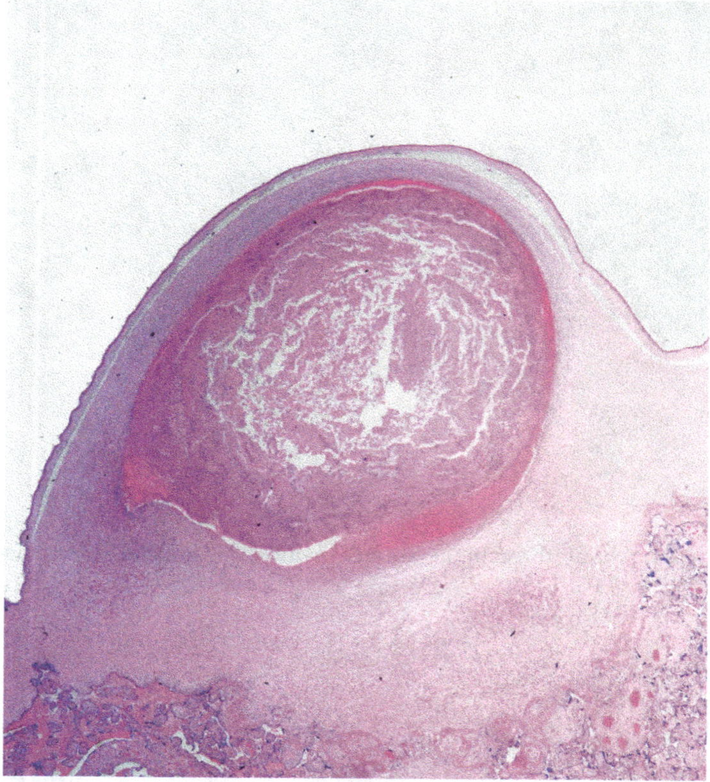

Figure 21.6. Occlusive thrombus in chorionic plate vein. H&E ×26.

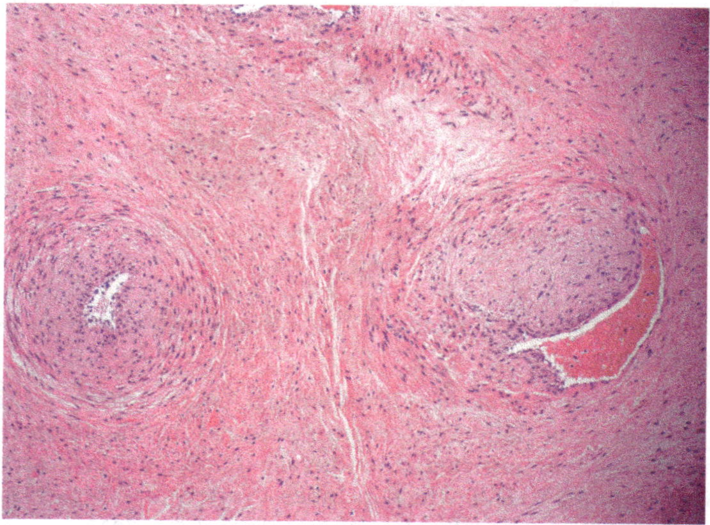

Figure 21.7. Muscular hypertrophy with near occlusions of stem vessels. H&E ×260.

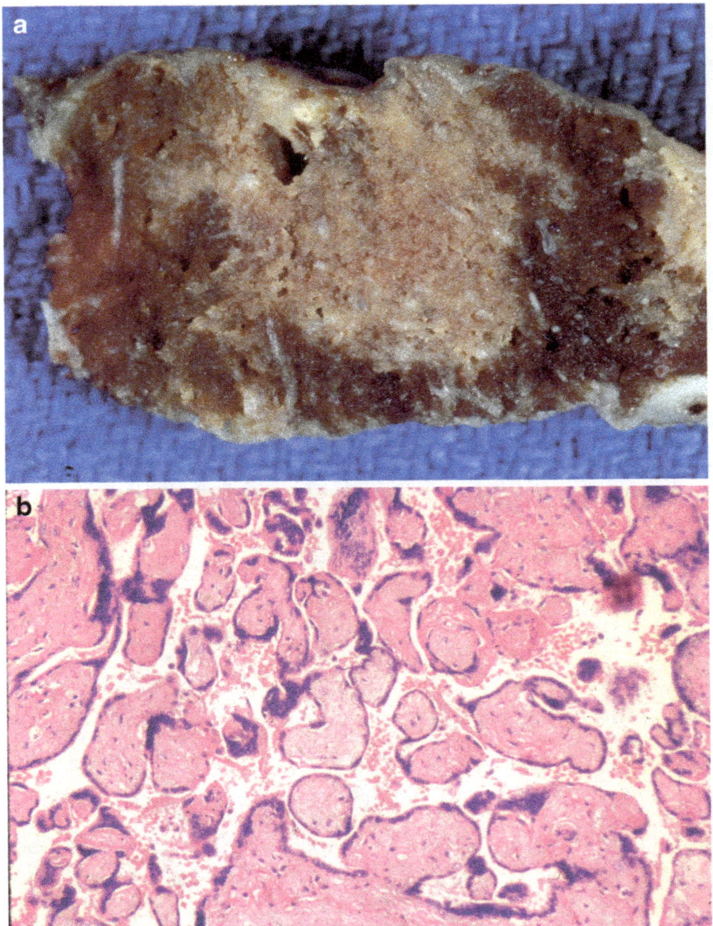

Figure 21.8. (a) Cross section of placenta with large focus of avascular villi. Note the pallor of the lesion, the irregular border, and consistency, which are similar to the adjacent normal villous tissue. (b) Microscopic section of a focus of avascular villi demonstrating hyaline quality of villous stroma, which is devoid of vessels. H&E ×200.

may be hard to identify on histologic section. Like avascular villi, these changes may be present in the setting of fetal demise. In the latter case, they will tend to be more diffuse, but the differences are often subtle. There may be *inflammatory infiltrates in the villi, a lesion sometimes referred to as hemorrhagic **villitis**, in which there is necrosis and/or destruction of the vascular walls* (Fig. 21.12). These lesions may involve all types of vessels, from the large stem vessels down to the villous capillaries. Associations with poor neonatal outcome including neurologic injury have been associated with these lesions. HEV also has a recurrence rate of 28% in subsequent pregnancies.

This lesion has a close association with another lesion, **villous stromal karyorrhexis.** In the latter lesion, there is nuclear degeneration and karyorrhexis within the villous stroma and capillaries (Fig. 21.13).

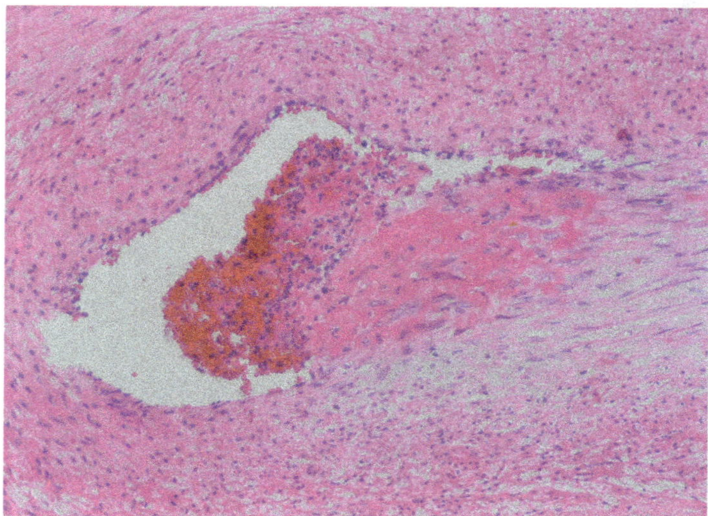

Figure 21.9. Intimal fibrin cushion. H&E ×200.

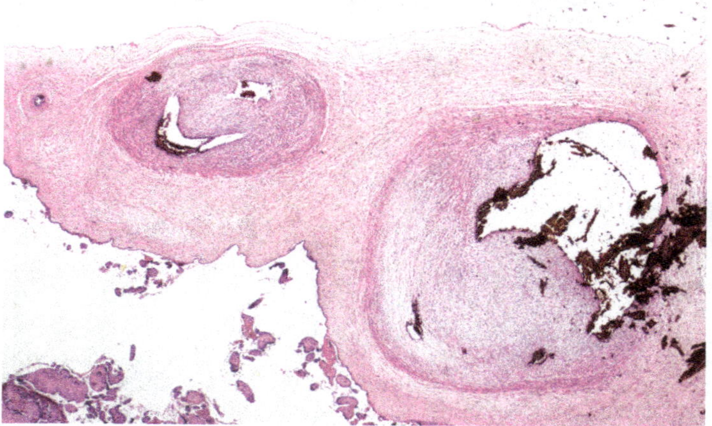

Figure 21.10. Intimal fibrin cushion with calcification in the vessel wall. H&E ×20.

It is thought to be an interim lesion or earlier version of avascular villi before the vessels become completely obliterated. Since villous stromal karyorrhexis and HEV have similar pathologic features and are both associated with thrombosis and sequelae of thrombosis, they are considered by some authors to be similar or even the same lesion.

Pathogenesis

Thrombosis clearly bespeaks a pathologic prenatal environment. Thrombotic lesions may form in the venous or arterial circulation and may involve umbilical vessels (see Fig. 15.24), chorionic vessels, large and small stem vessels, and villous capillaries. Arterial thrombosis is much less common than thrombosis in the venous circulation. *Significant obstruction in the arterial circulation* will rob the "downstream"

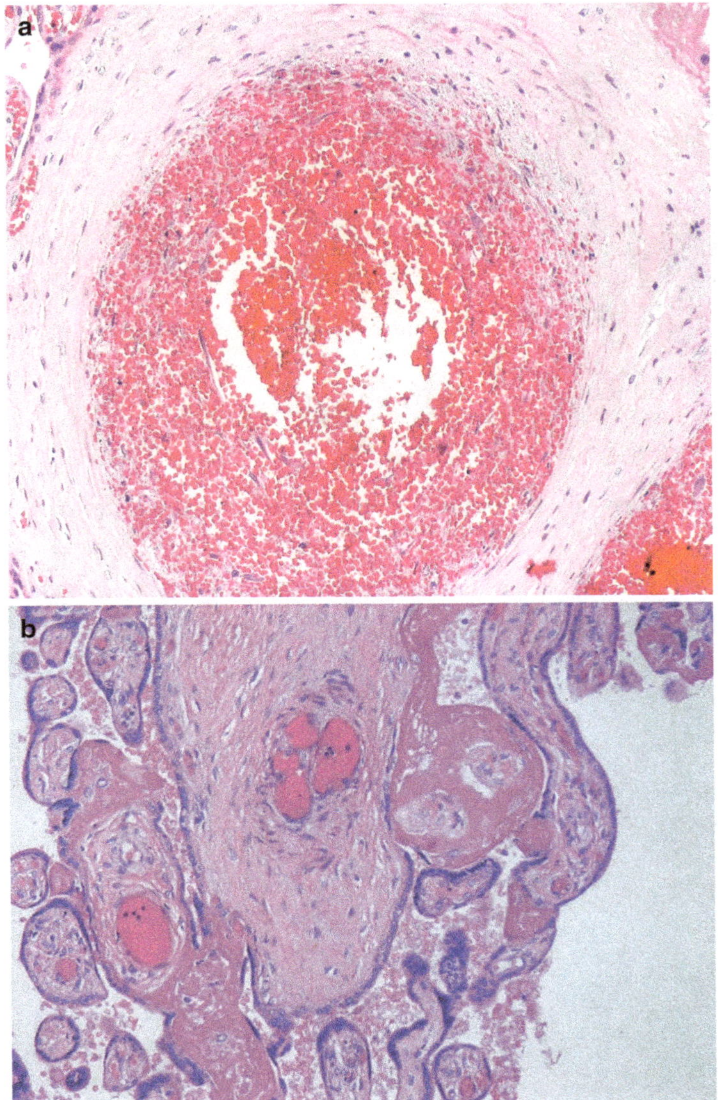

Figure 21.11. HEV. (**a**) Extravasated blood cells are present around this vessel in a stem villus. H&E ×100. (**b**) Septation of the lumen is present in this vessel. H&E ×200.

villi of their vascular supply. Any time the fetal circulation is lost but the maternal circulation is maintained, there will be loss of the fetal vasculature, but the trophoblastic cells will be left intact. The villi then become sclerotic or **avascular** (Fig. 21.8). The presence of avascular villi can be considered direct evidence of the presence of thrombosis.

Thrombi may develop when blood flow through the umbilical cord is compromised, and here the problem is *primarily in the venous circulation*. Cord accidents such as *excessively long cords, excessive spiraling, true umbilical cord knots, cord entanglement, and velamentous cord insertion* are common antecedents. Mechanical obstruction of the cord will initially lead to compression of the umbilical vein, as it is more pliable than the

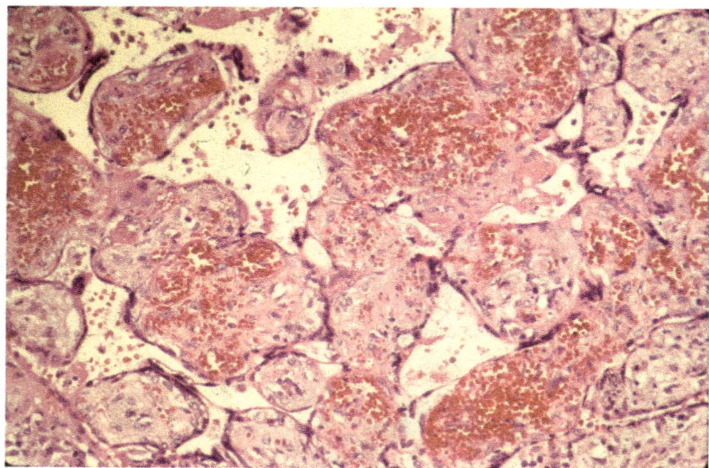

Figure 21.12. So-called hemorrhagic villitis in which there is destruction and necrosis of the vessel wall and karyorrhexis. H&E ×200.

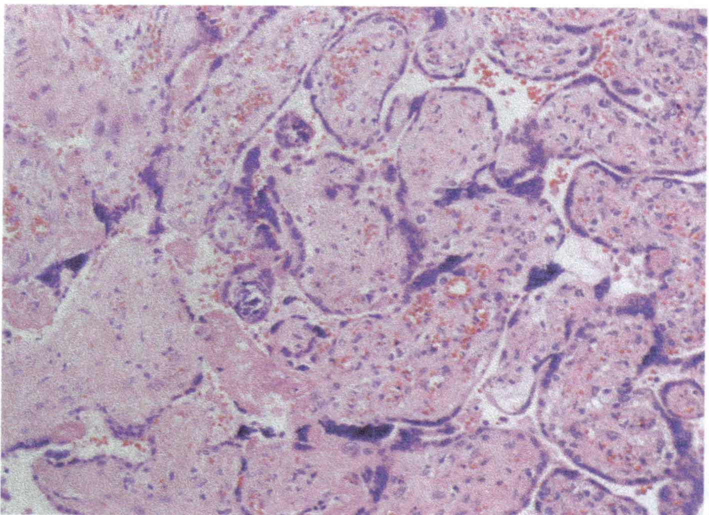

Figure 21.13. Villous stromal karyorrhexis – there is nuclear degeneration and nuclear debris present within the villous stroma and capillaries. The villi are becoming hyalinized and eventually will become completely avascular. H&E ×300.

umbilical arteries. *Occlusion of blood flow in the venous circulation leads to congestion, venous stasis,* and increased intraluminal pressure, which in turn results in endothelial injury and subsequent thrombosis. Venous stasis also may lead to vasospasm, further compromising the circulation. Thrombosis may also be seen in the arterial circulation, and in this case it is more likely to be associated with abnormal coagulative states in the mother or the fetus.

The origin of **intimal fibrin cushions** is not completely clear but it is thought that they either are *"organized" mural thrombi or are an early stage of thrombosis.* The fact that they may be associated with calcifications suggests an older lesion at least in those cases. They are also often associated with venous hypertension. Thrombi and cushions are most common in placental surface veins and in major villous stem vessels (Fig. 21.9). They often have mural thrombi overlying them. It may be that the cushions form first and then, after much distention and elevated pressure, their endothelial surface degenerates and mural thrombosis develops.

Veno-occlusive disease has also been implicated in the development of **HEV**. This entity has aroused much controversy. It was initially identified in the study of many placentas from perinatal deaths and infants with perinatal problems and it was hypothesized that HEV played an important role in the etiology of these tragedies. HEV is, in effect, a *microangiopathy that etiologically and pathologically resembles the glomerulopathy of the hemolytic uremic syndrome* and is often referred to as a *vasodisruptive process*. It is postulated that, as in frank thrombosis, there is *endothelial injury and vessel necrosis, which leads to fragmentation of RBCs and extravasation of these fragments into the villous stroma.* It is strongly associated with thrombosis as well. The etiology of HEV has been hotly debated, in part because the histologic picture is often seen in placentas of stillborns and some of the features can be directly related to loss of fetal circulation to the villous tissue. As indicated above, there is much overlap with villous stromal karyorrhexis both in histology and etiology.

Clinical Features and Implications

Venous thrombosis is associated with *compromise of blood flow through the umbilical cord* secondary to cord entanglement, abnormal insertion, and abnormal length or coiling. Thrombosis may also be seen associated with *maternal or fetal thrombophilias* such as the factor V Leiden mutation, activated protein-C resistance, protein S deficiency, protein C deficiency, lupus anticoagulant, and antiphospholipid antibodies (see Chap. 18). *Maternal diabetes* is occasionally associated with thrombosis in the placenta or neonate, but there are no other morphologic or clinical features to explain the cause of this fetal vascular coagulation. *Severe chorioamnionitis*, particularly when there is a fetal response, may be associated with thrombosis in fetal vessels. This occurs secondary to damage to the endothelium and vessel wall from the inflammatory changes. Finally, thrombosis has also been associated with *vascular anomalies and various forms of trauma.*

Fetal thrombotic vasculopathy (FTV) is a term often used to encompass all thrombotic lesions seen in the placenta. FTV as a whole has been strongly associated with *preeclampsia, intrauterine growth restrictions (IUGR), intrauterine fetal demise (IUFD), seizures, and amputation necrosis.* Prenatal and neonatal thrombosis has been described in the central nervous system (CNS), pulmonary circulation, and renal vessels. The etiology of this thrombosis, at least in some cases, is thromboembolism, which has been documented with placental thrombi embolizing to the fetal circulation. Other etiologies of neonatal thrombosis may be underlying thrombophilias. *Neonatal stroke, cerebral degenerative changes, abnormalities in brain imaging, cerebral palsy, and poor long-term neurologic outcome* are also strongly associated with FTV.

> **Suggestions for Examination and Report**
> (Fetal thrombotic vasculopathy)
>
> **Gross Examination:** When gross thrombi are noted or there is a clinical history of cord problem or thrombosis, additional sections of fetal surface vessels should be submitted. It is suggested that multiple sections of the fetal surface with large caliber fetal vessels (near the umbilical cord insertion) be submitted in these cases.
>
> **Comment:** All the specific lesions identified should be listed. Thrombosis may explain poor perinatal outcome and findings should be correlated with clinical history of coagulopathy, diabetes or cord problems. Particular correlation can be done with cord abnormalities such as true knots, velamentous insertion, excessive coiling or long cords.

Selected References

PHP5, pages 426–434.

Baergen RN, Malicki D, Behling CA, et al. Morbidity, mortality and placental pathology in excessively long umbilical cords. Pediatr Dev Pathol 2001;4:144–153.

Boué DR, Stanley C, Baergen RN. Placental pathology casebook. J Perinatol 1995;15:429–431.

De Sa DJ. Intimal cushions in foetal placental veins. J Pathol 1973;110:347–352.

Gogia N, Machine GA. Maternal thrombophilias are associated with specific placental lesions. Pediatr Dev Pathol 2008;11:424–429.

Heifetz SA. Thrombosis of the umbilical cord: analysis of 52 cases and literature review. Pediatr Pathol 1988;8:37–54.

Kaplan CG. Fetal and maternal vascular lesions. Semin Diagn Pathol 2007;24:14–22.

Kraus FT, Achen VI. Fetal thrombotic vasculopathy in the placenta. Cerebral thrombi, infarct, coagulopathy and cerebral palsy. Hum Pathol 1999;30:759–769.

Rayne SC, Kraus FT. Placental thrombi and other vascular lesions: classification, morphology, and clinical correlations. Pathol Res Pract 1993;189:2–17.

Redline RW. Severe fetal placental vascular lesions in term infants with neurologic impairment. Am J Obstet Gynecol 2005;192:452–457.

Redline RW, Ariel I, Baergen RN, DeSa DJ, Kraus FT, Roberts DJ, Sander CM. Fetal vascular obstructive lesions: nosology and reproducibility of placental reaction patterns. Pediatr Dev Pathol 2004;7:443–452.

Redline RW, Pappin A. Fetal thrombotic vasculopathy: the clinical significance of extensive avascular villi. Hum Pathol 1995;26:80.

Sander CM. Hemorrhagic endovasculitis and hemorrhagic villitis of the placenta. Arch Pathol Lab Med 1980;104:371–373.

Sander CM, Gilliland D, Flynn MA, et al. Risk factors for recurrence of hemorrhagic endovasculitis of the placenta. Obstet Gynecol 1997;89:569–576.

Section VI

Neoplasms and Gestational Trophoblast Disease

This section covers primary and metastatic tumors of the placenta and trophoblastic disease. Chapter 22 discusses the primary tumors seen in the placenta as well as tumors that may metastasize from the mother or the fetus. Gestational trophoblastic disease is discussed in the following chapters. Hydatidiform moles are covered in Chap. 23, choriocarcinoma in Chap. 24, and lesions of extravillous trophoblast in Chap. 25.

Chapter 22

Neoplasms

General Considerations

There are only a few primary neoplasms of the placenta, but there is a wide variety of maternal malignancies that metastasize to the placenta. This reflects the diversity of neoplasms seen in the maternal population. Fetal tumors may also metastasize to the placenta, but these tumors are derived from a smaller group of congenital neoplasms.

Primary Placental Neoplasms

Chorangioma (Angioma)

Pathogenesis
Chorangiomas are basically angiomas that develop within a chorionic villus, most likely a stem villus. They are the most common benign tumor of the placenta. Tumors that have been designated **chorioangiomas, chorangiomas, angiomyxomas, fibroangiomyxomas,** and **fibromas** are essentially the same lesion, usually designated simply, **chorangioma.** The incidence of these tumors is reported to be one in 9,000 to one in 50,000 placentas. When careful study and sectioning of

R.N. Baergen, *Manual of Pathology of the Human Placenta,*
DOI 10.1007/978-1-4419-7494-5_22, © Springer Science+Business Media, LLC 2011

placentas are undertaken, the prevalence may be as high as 1 in 100, as many lesions are small and not grossly identifiable but rather are discovered incidentally on microscopic examination. Chorangiomas occur more frequently in Caucasian mothers than in those of other races. They are seen more often with *multiple gestations* and more often with *neonates who have congenital anomalies*, particularly infants with hemangiomas. This suggests that this tumor may be a congenital malformation or hamartoma, rather than a true neoplasm. Indeed, clonal studies, which would differentiate these lesions, have not been done at this point in time. Interestingly, the incidence of chorangiomas in high-altitude populations such as in Nepal is reported to be from 2.5% to 7.6%, which is much higher than the incidence at lower elevations. This suggests that chorangiomas may have a similar etiology to chorangiosis, which occurs with increased frequency at higher altitudes and in association with chronic hypoxia (see Chap. 19). Furthermore, like chorangiosis, chorangiomas may be associated with *elevated nucleated red blood cells (NRBCs)* in the fetal circulation, suggesting that a hypoxic stimulus leads to the excessive villous capillary proliferation. While still speculative, such angiogenesis may well be regulated by vascular growth factors.

Pathologic Features

Grossly, chorangiomas are sharply circumscribed from the surrounding parenchyma and often *bulge from the fetal surface of the placenta* (Fig. 22.1). When they are embedded deeper in the villous tissue, they are almost always located closer to the fetal surface. They are also more common in a peripheral rather than a central location within the placenta. The color and consistency of the cut surface is variable, from a *dark red, soft appearance similar to a blood clot to a firm, white lesion similar*

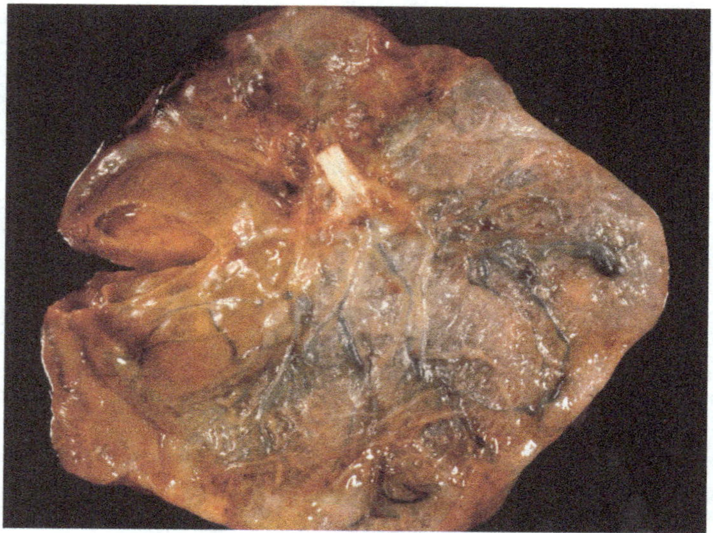

Figure 22.1. Typical chorangioma (*left*) bulging from the fetal surface. The cut surface is hemorrhagic.

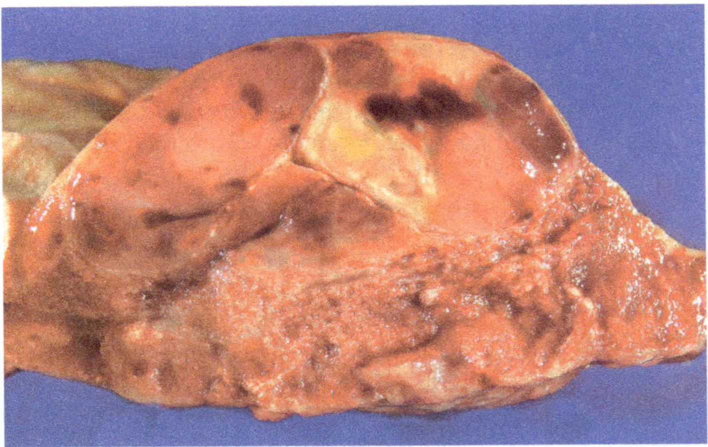

Figure 22.2. Chorangioma. The cut surface is heterogeneous with some areas having the appearance of blood clot, while others appear more fibrous. Normal placental tissue is seen underlying the tumor.

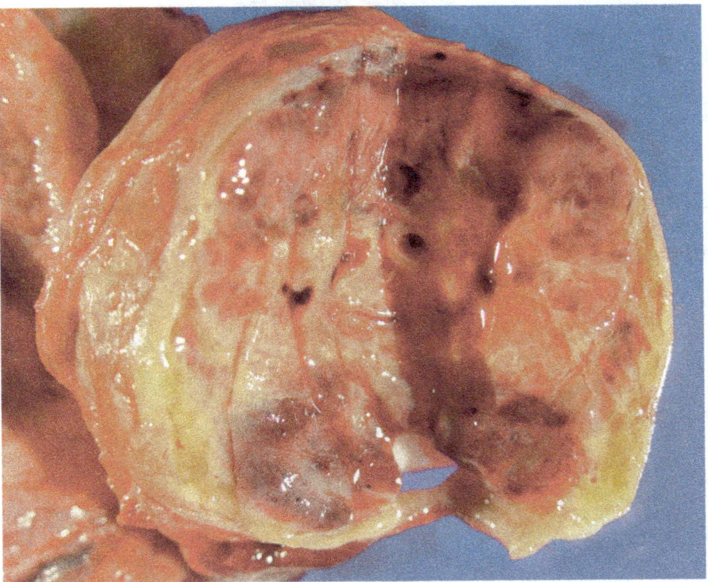

Figure 22.3. A chorangioma with some myxoid change. The lesion was large (10 cm) and was associated with mild neonatal cardiac failure.

to an infarct (Figs. 22.2 and 22.3). If there is associated fetal hydrops (see below), the entire placenta may be enlarged and edematous. Extremely large tumors may occur (Fig. 22.4). The record is probably held by a 1,500-g tumor measuring 30 by 20 by 5 cm, which was associated with placenta previa, hydramnios, preeclampsia, and abruptio placentae. The 32-week gestation fetus weighed 1,000 g and died from anemia and asphyxia.

Microscopically, the typical chorangioma is *composed of a proliferation of fetal blood vessels, usually supported by scant connective tissue* (Figs. 22.5 and 22.6). The vessels comprising the tumor may be capillary or sinusoidal. The *stromal component is variable but is frequently abundant*, and the lesion may then resemble a fibroma (Fig. 22.7). When

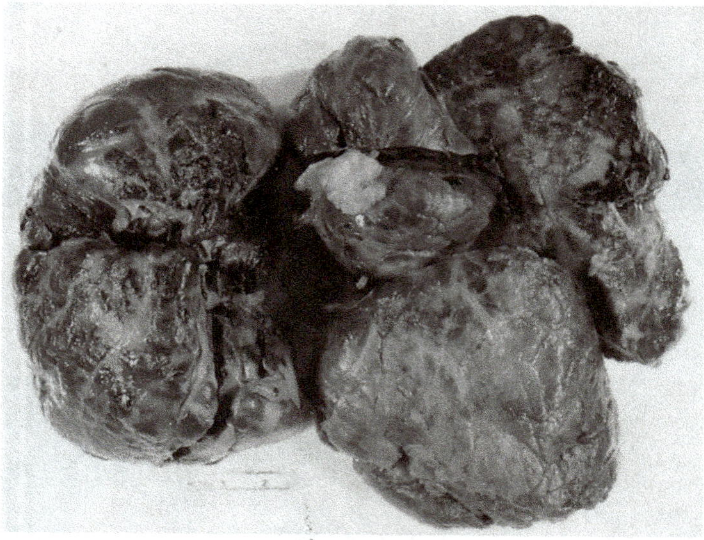

Figure 22.4. Exceptionally large (400 g) chorangioma shelled out from its placenta. The infant was stillborn and had cardiomegaly. The surface in this case had a fibromyxoid appearance.

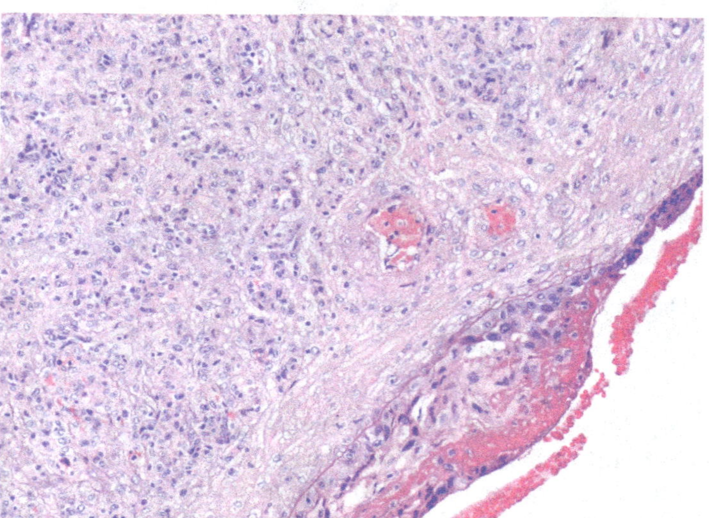

Figure 22.5. Typical microscopic appearance of a chorangioma with numerous small capillaries. The convexity of the tumor is covered by syncytiotrophoblast. H&E ×160.

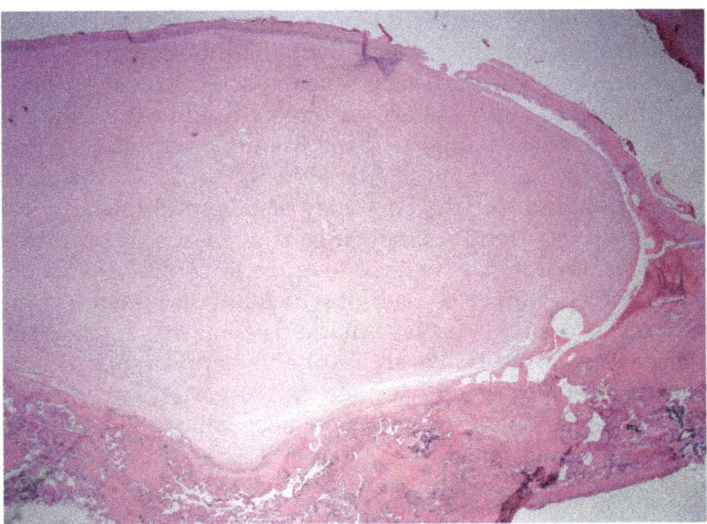

Figure 22.6. This chorangioma is completely infarcted and appears as a well-circumscribed nodule under the chorionic plate. H&E ×40.

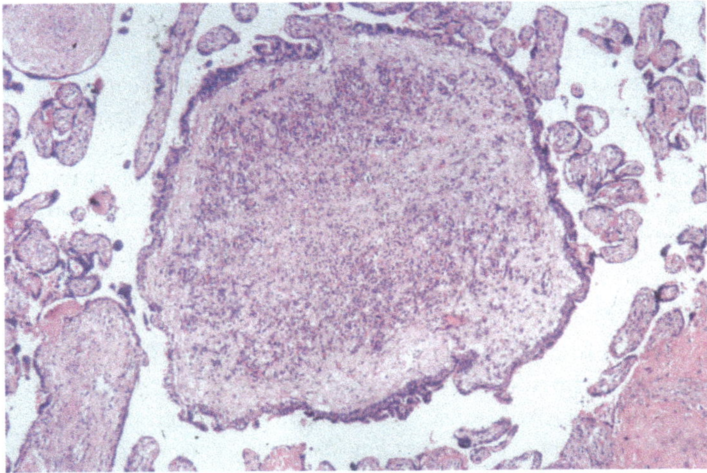

Figure 22.7. Small, incidental chorangioma identified only on microscopic examination. It has a primarily fibromatous appearance. Cellularity of these lesions may sometimes suggest a sarcoma. H&E ×170.

Wharton's jelly-like material participates in formation of the tumor, the appearance is that of a *myxomatous neoplasm*. The latter is particularly frequent when a chorangioma arises near the base of the umbilical cord. In such cases, a mucicarmine stain reveals the presence of mucin. *Capillary, cavernous, endotheliomatous, fibrosing,* and *fibromatous* tumors have been differentiated, but such precision is unwarranted as the clinical outcome depends more on the size of the mass than on its composition. The variable components of the lesions give rise to the difference in appearance grossly. Chorangiomas are invariably *covered by trophoblast*, and one may envisage them to be the proliferation of vessels within a villus whose surface thus expands. Recent studies have suggested that chorangiomas arise from stem villi rather than terminal villi, as previously thought. These tumors often have *degenerative changes, calcification, infarction, and thrombosis* (Fig. 22.7). This may lead to problems in identification. They may also be multiple and in some cases have been recurrent. As they are characterized by an increase in villous vessels, chorangiomas have features in common with chorangiomatosis and chorangiosis, both of which are discussed in Chap. 19. Uncommonly, chorangiomas have marked cellularity, cytologic atypia, and prominent mitoses; however, despite this appearance, the tumors are invariably benign. Metastases and true invasion have never been described. At times, these variants have been called cellular chorangioma or atypical chorangioma.

Clinical Features and Implications

The relation of chorangioma to *hydramnios* and *fetal hydrops*, particularly in large tumors, is well known. Other complications include *stillbirth, fetal growth restriction, anemia, cardiomegaly, heart failure, disseminated intravascular coagulation, transplacental hemorrhage, premature delivery, abruptio, and preeclampsia.* Many complications are secondary to transplacental hemorrhage or sequestration of blood. Most tumors are not associated with sequelae, and the large tumors are more likely to be associated with severe complications. *Thrombocytopenia*, which is often observed in these newborns, is secondary to sequestration of platelets within the tumor. Repetitive multiple chorangiomas have been described in several families, sometimes associated with recurrent fetal demise. Whether isolated chorangiomas can occur repetitively is unknown.

Chorangiocarcinoma

Chorangiocarcinoma is a lesion with features similar to both chorangioma and choriocarcinoma and has been variably reported in the literature. Reported cases have depicted a *solitary lesion typical of a chorangioma whose surface, however, was covered by proliferating trophoblastic cells.* No untoward sequelae have been noted, and there is no chemical or cytochemical evidence of choriocarcinoma. Certainly, in most cases the tumors are truly variants of a benign chorangioma. However, a recent report describes a case of chorangioma associated with areas of marked syncytiotrophoblastic and cytotrophoblastic proliferation histologically consistent with choriocarcinoma. The authors opined that this was a true case of chorangiocarcinoma; however, again no malignant sequelae were noted. It appears that there may be cases in which a chorangioma was in close proximity to choriocarcinoma, representing a type of "collision" tumor. Therefore, the issue is not completely resolved and caution should be taken when presented with a chorangioma with trophoblastic proliferation.

> **Suggestions for Examination and Report**
> (Chorangioma)
>
> **Gross Examination:** Note size, location and gross appearance of the tumor or tumors. Representative sections of the tumor should be submitted.
>
> **Comment:** Large chorangiomas may be associated with anemia, thrombocytopenia, hydrops, growth restriction and stillbirth. In the case of "chorangiocarcinoma", it is preferable to refer to the lesion as "chorangioma with trophoblastic proliferation" with a description and notation that no malignant sequelae have been reported but that the lesion is not well studied. In some cases it may be prudent to suggest that the clinicians check and/or follow maternal serum beta-hCG levels.

Leiomyoma

There have been several reported cases of tumors morphologically and immunohistochemically compatible with **leiomyomas**, located within the placental tissue and covered by decidua at the maternal surface. Easy separation of the tumors from the uterus suggests these may not be uterine primaries. However, molecular studies on one reported case confirmed its maternal origin. Furthermore, no intrinsic structures in the placenta contain smooth muscle. For these reasons, it is likely these are *primary uterine leiomyomas that have become parasitic*, losing their vascular connection to the uterus and stealing a new blood supply from the placenta. These tumors have not been associated with adverse outcome.

Endometrial Stromal Lesions

Rarely, **endometrial stromal sarcomas** and **endometrial stromal nodules** have been identified. They are found either within the membranes or within the basal plate of the placenta. Like leiomyomas, their derivation from uterus, specifically endometrial stroma, has been documented by immunohistochemistry. They likely arise by the same mechanism that leiomyomas do, becoming parasitic and stealing the blood supply from the placenta. Metastasis has been reported in cases associated with endometrial stromal sarcoma.

Teratomas Versus Acardiac Twinning

Masses of tissue composed of *ectodermal, mesodermal, and endodermal elements* have been noted in the fetal membranes, umbilical cord, and chorionic plate of the placenta (see also Chap. 14). In cases where either umbilical cord structures or axial skeleton is present, they are usually considered a component of an acardiac twin. There is, however, disagreement over those cases that do not contain either of these elements. Since proof of neoplastic origin has not been presented, we believe that true teratomas of the placenta likely do not exist and that all these cases represent variants of acardiac twining.

Hepatocellular Adenoma

Several cases of **hepatocellular adenoma** in the placenta have been reported. Grossly they have been *tan-white, sharply delimited* lesions present in intervillous or subchorionic locations. Microscopically, they *are composed of polyhedral cells with the appearance of hepatocytes*. The cells contain glycogen, and some show reactivity with antibodies to α-fetoprotein, $α_1$-antitrypsin, and carcinoembryonic antigen; convincing evidence of hepatic differentiation. No portal areas or central veins are seen, but study by electron microscopy has shown structures that resemble bile canaliculi. These lesions likely originate from displaced yolk sac structures. The clinical course for both fetus and mother is benign.

Heterotopia

Heterotopic tissues, such as **adrenal gland**, and **liver** occasionally occur in the placenta. Suggested mechanisms for the origin of these tissues have included embolic spread via the fetal vasculature, monodermal teratoma, and abnormal mesodermal differentiation. No sequelae have been reported.

Suggestions for Examination and Report
(Miscellaneous neoplasms and heterotopia)

Gross Examination: Grossly, neoplasms usually present as a mass, which should be described and liberally sampled for microscopic examination.

Comment: The diagnosis of the lesion should be given and a comment may be included indicating the lack of clinical sequelae (if it is known).

Maternal Neoplasms Metastatic to the Placenta

Clinical Features and Implications

Maternal malignancy occurs in approximately one in 1,000 pregnancies. Metastasis to the placenta, however, is rare, with less than 100 reported cases in the literature. The most common tumor to metastasize to the placenta is *melanoma*. Carcinomas of the *breast, cervix, gastrointestinal tract, and lung* occur less frequently, and there are rare reports of metastases from the *pancreas, ovary, endometrium, rectum, eye,* and *skin,* as well metastases from *medulloblastoma* and *rhabdomyosarcoma*. *Hematopoietic neoplasms* of various types have also been described. It is interesting to note that melanoma metastasizes so commonly, since it is not frequent in the pregnant population. This phenomenon is probably due to the hematogenous dissemination in melanoma and to the fact that melanoma patients are more likely to have advanced disease. Many placental metastases occur in patients with end-stage disease who presumably had a significant tumor burden, facilitating vascular spread to the placenta.

Transplacental metastasis to the fetus is much rarer than placental metastasis. Here again, *melanoma is most common,* but cases of *lymphoma, leukemia, and pulmonary adenocarcinoma* have been reported. Many cases have resulted in neonatal death, but there are also reports of spontaneous regression. The immunologic ramifications of these cases remain to be studied. *Due to the occurrence of fetal metastasis, although rare, it is recommended that all placentas from patients with a diagnosis of malignancy be examined histologically.*

Pathologic Features

Placental metastases often go unnoticed. In many cases, the lesions are not visible grossly, while in other cases they are overlooked, as they may appear *similar to infarcts.* Microscopically, metastases usually consist of clusters of *malignant cells in the intervillous space* (Fig. 22.8). In some cases, *invasion of the villous structures and even the fetal vasculature may occur.* However, the latter feature does not correlate well with the presence of metastasis to the infant. Often these intervillous collections do not show vascularization, leading some authors to call them "pseudometastases." In the case of maternal **leukemia**, metastasis cannot be documented merely by the presence of leukemic cells in the intervillous space, but must be made by the presence of leukemic cells in the villous tissue and/or fetal vessels.

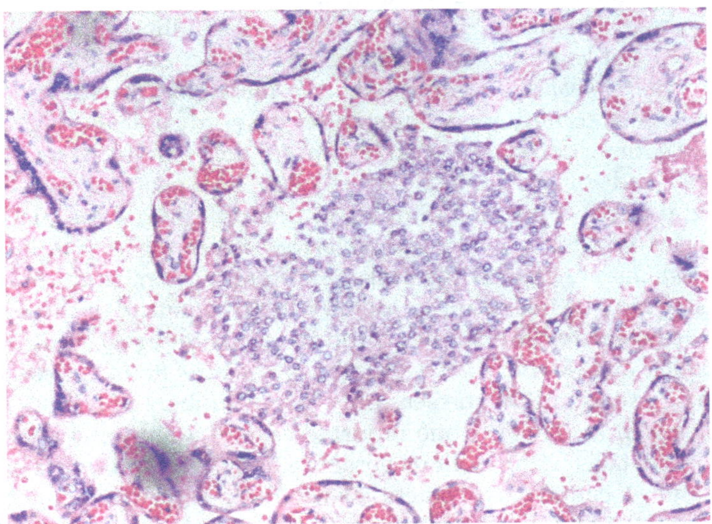

Figure 22.8. Metastatic melanoma to the placenta. Note the large, atypical cells present in the intervillous space. The mother had widespread metastases at the time of delivery and died 1 month later. H&E ×200.

> **Suggestions for Examination and Report**
> (Maternal metastasis to the placenta)
>
> **Gross Examination:** Metastatic lesions are usually not grossly visible, but, if large, may appear similar to an infarct. In the context of a maternal malignancy, any parenchymal lesion should be sampled. If no gross lesions are present, additional random sections should be submitted.
>
> **Comment:** If metastases are present, characterization of the type of metastasis and comparison with the maternal primary is optimal. Immunohistochemistry may be necessary to fully evaluate the malignant cells. In addition, involvement of the villous stroma or fetal vessels should also be noted. The fact that fetal metastasis is a possible, although rare complication, may also be stated. Follow up in the infant may be suggested if placental lesions are present.

Fetal Neoplasms Metastatic to the Placenta

Malignant Fetal Tumors

Congenital malignancies include **neuroblastoma, lymphoma, leukemia, sarcomas, brain tumors, hepatoblastoma,** and **teratomas.** Metastases from these neoplasms to the placenta are rare but do occur. Congenital **neuroblastoma** has repeatedly been shown to cause fetal heart failure, hydrops and death, but the pathogenesis of hydrops remains to be identified. Grossly, the *placenta is markedly enlarged.* On histologic examination, the villi are *enlarged and edematous, and have increased numbers of Hofbauer cells with persistent villous cytotrophoblast. Cords of neuroblastoma cells may be found in fetal capillaries* sometimes accompanied by erythroblasts (Fig. 22.9). Neuroblastoma cells may also infiltrate the villous tissue. Fetal hydrops and placentomegaly may also be seen in association with fetal **hepatoblastoma.** Similar to neuroblastoma, the placental metastases consist of *malignant, immature-appearing cells filling the villous capillaries.* Due to the lack of differentiation, immunohistochemistry may be necessary to identify the true nature of these cells. **Sacrococcygeal teratomas** may produce *placentomegaly, fetal edema, hydramnios, and elevated human chorionic gonadotropin (hCG) levels.* On histologic examination, one sees only large numbers of *NRBCs in the villous capillaries.* There is one reported case of a teratoma with placental metastasis within villous vessels. Lastly, fetal **leukemia** occurs rarely and placental involvement is even rarer. When it does occur, it is also associated with placentomegaly. On microscopic examination, villous capillaries are packed with leukemic cells, which may extend into the villous stroma (Fig. 22.10). Diagnosis can be quite difficult on placental tissue alone.

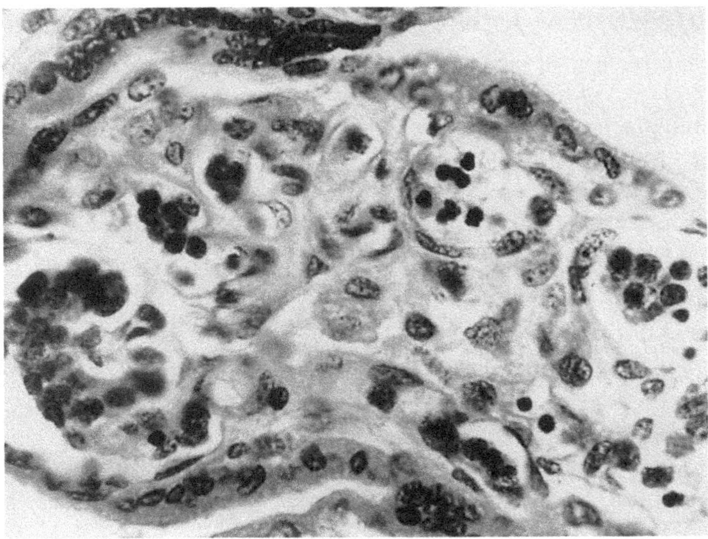

Figure 22.9. Villus from a case of congenital neuroblastoma. The enlarged villus has numerous neuroblastoma cells within the villous capillaries, some of which show rosetting. H&E ×400.

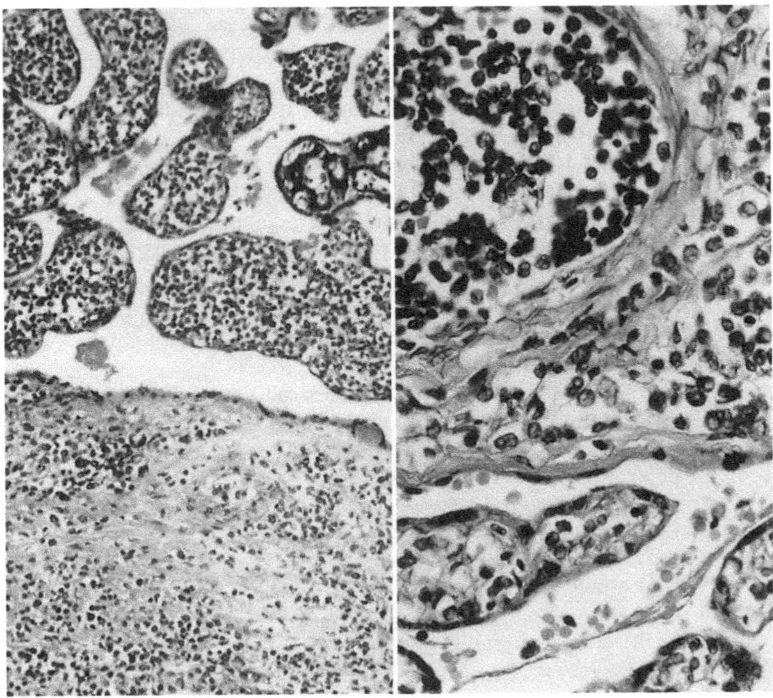

Figure 22.10 Placenta from a macerated stillborn with presumed leukemia. The villous capillaries are packed with leukemic cells, and some stromal infiltration is seen. H&E: *left* ×60, *right* ×160.

Benign "Metastatic" Lesions

Fetal giant pigmented nevi have been described in the placenta, usually as *multiple foci of pigmented nevus cells in the villi.* Occasionally, there is extensive placental involvement, but the lesions are considered benign. The cells may derive from early neural crest cell migration.

Suggestions for Examination and Report
(Fetal neoplasms metastatic to the placenta)

Gross Examination: When a fetal malignancy is known, additional sections of placenta should be submitted for identification of metastases.

Comment: Diagnosis of the neoplasm is essential and may require immunohistochemistry. As with maternal malignancy, the location and extent of involvement should also be mentioned.

Selected References

PHP5, pages 863–870 (Chorangiomas), pages 870–871 (Other Benign Tumors), pages 600–604 (Maternal Neoplasms), pages 530–532 (Fetal Tumors).

Baergen RN, Johnson D, Moore T, et al. Maternal melanoma metastatic to the placenta. Arch Pathol Lab Med 1997;121:508–511.

Benirschke K. Recent trends in chorangiomas, especially those of multiple and recurrent chorangiomas. Pediatr Dev Pathol 1999;2:264–269.

Doss BJ, Vicari J, Jacques SM, et al. Placental involvement in congenital hepatoblastoma. Pediatr Dev Pathol 1998;1:538–542.

Ernst LM, Hui P, Parkash V. Intraplacental smooth muscle tumor: a case report. Int J Gynecol Pathol 2001;29:284–288.

Guschman M, Vogel M, Urban M. Adrenal tissue in the placenta. A heterotopia caused by migration and embolism? Placenta 2000;21:427–431.

Khalifa MA, Gersell DJ, Hansen CH, et al. Hepatic (hepatocellular) adenoma of the placenta: a study of four cases. Int J Gynecol Pathol 1998;17:241–244.

Lentz SE, Coulson CC, Gocke CD, et al. Placental pathology in maternal and neonatal myeloproliferative disorders. Obstet Gynecol 1998;91:863–864.

Leung JC, Mann S, Salafia CM, et al. Sacrococcygeal teratoma with vascular placental dissemination. Obstet Gynecol 1999;93:856.

Lynn AA, Parry SI, Morgan M, et al. Disseminated congenital neuroblastoma involving the placenta. Arch Pathol Lab Med 1997;121:741–744.

Majlessi HF, Wagner KM, Brooks JJ. Atypical cellular chorangioma of the placenta. Int J Gynecol Pathol 1983;1:403–408.

Qureshi F, Jacques SM. Adrenocortical heterotopia in the placenta. Pediatr Pathol Lab Med 1995;15:51–56.

Chapter 23

Hydatidiform Moles

General Considerations

Understanding early trophoblastic development is essential to the discussion and categorization of trophoblastic lesions. Therefore, a brief review is presented here (see also Chap. 8). After fertilization, the blastocyst differentiates into embryonic and extraembryonic cells, the latter becoming **trophoblast**, and the forerunner of the placenta.

R.N. Baergen, *Manual of Pathology of the Human Placenta*,
DOI 10.1007/978-1-4419-7494-5_23, © Springer Science+Business Media, LLC 2011

The trophoblastic cells further differentiate into villous and nonvillous or extravillous trophoblast. **Villous trophoblast** consists of *villous cytotrophoblast and syncytiotrophoblast.* **Cytotrophoblast** is a term also used for the trophoblastic stem cells of the cell columns, the so-called stem trophoblast, but it is thought that once the cells form the inner layer of the chorionic villi they are then differentiated toward villous trophoblast. **Extravillous trophoblast** is composed of the trophoblast of the *chorionic plate, chorion laeve, cell islands, septa, implantation site,* and *basal plate.* Currently, the term "intermediate" trophoblast is commonly used to represent all types of extravillous trophoblast. Unfortunately, however, it has also been used to refer to a type of *villous* trophoblast that is transitional between cytotrophoblast and syncytiotrophoblast or between cytotrophoblast and villous cytotrophoblast. This is incorrect because nonvillous or extravillous trophoblast, or "intermediate trophoblast," by definition **cannot** be villous trophoblast. Therefore, the use of the term "intermediate trophoblast" should be abandoned. Simply stated, *villous and extravillous trophoblast are derived from different pathways of trophoblastic differentiation, and lesions arising from these cells have different morphological features, clinical attributes, and biologic behavior.*

Trophoblastic lesions comprise a complex and challenging group of lesions that are unique in pathology for the following reasons:

- They are composed, partly or exclusively, of genetic maternal derived from another individual (paternally derived genes).
- They are **gestational** and have **nongestational** counterparts that arise from gonadal germ cells rather than a conceptus.
- The nonneoplastic cells have features usually only associated with malignancy:
  - Destructive **stromal invasion** (in the implantation site)
  - Distant **deportation** of cells into the maternal circulation during pregnancy
  - **Cytologic features of malignancy**

Trophoblastic lesions are classified into several groups (Table 23.1). **Hydatidiform moles** are *nonneoplastic lesions derived from villous trophoblast.* They are divided into complete, partial, and invasive types. **Choriocarcinoma**, a malignant tumor of gestational trophoblastic origin, also *derives from villous trophoblast.* The remaining lesions, placental site trophoblastic tumor, exaggerated placental site, and placental site nodule derive from extravillous trophoblast.

Hydatidiform Moles

Pathogenesis

Hydatidiform moles are not neoplasms. They are, however, *associated with an increased risk for the development of* **persistent gestational trophoblastic disease**, specifically **choriocarcinoma**, a highly malignant tumor of trophoblastic origin (see Chap. 24). Traditionally, moles have been subdivided into complete and partial hydatidiform moles. **Complete hydatidiform moles** have a genetic complement that is *androgenetic, i.e., all the genetic material is paternally derived.* In most instances, they result from *an ovum that has lost its nucleus, an "empty egg," which is then fertilized by a single sperm. Subsequent duplication of the haploid spermatozoal complement* leads to a diploid genotype (Fig. 23.1a). Thus, the majority of complete moles have a 46XX karyotype. A small number of complete moles have a 46XY karyotype. These, along with a minority of 46XX moles, arise from *dispermy, i.e., fertilization of an empty egg by two sperm with fusion of the two male pronuclei* (Fig. 23.1b). These

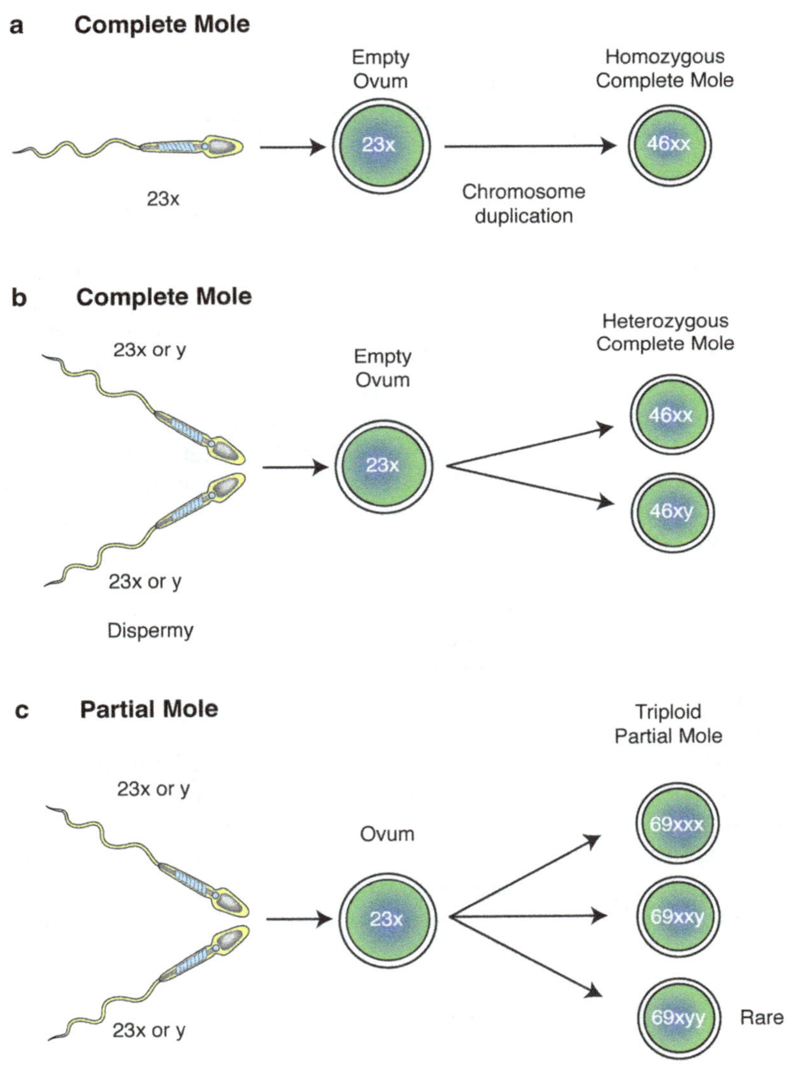

Figure 23.1. Origin of complete and partial hydatidiform moles. (**a**) Complete moles most commonly arise from fertilization of an empty ovum by a single sperm that then undergoes chromosomal duplication. (**b**) Less commonly complete moles arise from dispermy in which two sperm fertilize an empty ovum. (**c**) Partial moles arise from two sperm that fertilize a single ovum.

are sometime referred to as "heterozygous" complete moles. Moles with a 46YY karyotype are not found, and it is assumed that these conceptuses do not further develop. Dispermy represents about 15% of all complete moles. Triploid and tetraploid complete moles occur rarely; these are also derived solely from paternal DNA.

In comparison, **partial hydatidiform moles** are *usually triploid*. They develop from *fertilization of an ovum by two sperm, leading to a paternal to maternal chromosome ratio of 2:1* (Fig. 23.1c). Thus, partial moles generally have a 69XXX or 69 XXY karyotype. Rarely a 69XYY partial mole is identified. Tetraploid partial moles have also been described and have a paternal to maternal chromosome ratio of 3:1. The important differentiating feature between partial and complete moles is that complete moles are "completely" paternal DNA and partial moles have an altered maternal to paternal ratio, always with more paternal than maternal DNA.

Imprinting plays a pivotal role in the development of hydatidiform moles. Studies in mice have shown *that paternally derived genes are important for placental development, while maternal genes have more influence over fetal development.* Therefore, excess paternal genetic material leads to excessive growth of trophoblastic (placental) over fetal tissues, which is the sine qua non for the diagnosis of molar pregnancies. The fetus, if it can even be identified, is usually small, with stunted growth. Complete moles, having *only* paternal DNA, have more extreme trophoblastic proliferation than partial moles, which maintain some maternal DNA, albeit in the minority. On the other hand, *nonmolar triploid abortuses have a 2:1 maternal to paternal chromosome ratio* and derive from nondisjunction of maternal chromosomes. Since there is a maternal excess of genetic material, they do not show the trophoblastic proliferation seen in moles. Furthermore, in contrast to partial moles, the placenta is often quite small and stunted while the fetus is relatively normal in size, even though congenital anomalies are the rule. Maternal triploidy represents only about 10–15% of triploid conceptuses overall.

Since identification of an excess paternal contribution is *essential* in the diagnosis of molar pregnancies, various techniques have been developed to confirm paternal origin. These include **polymerase chain reaction, DNA fingerprinting, restriction fragment length polymorphism (RFLP) assessment,** and use of **short tandem repeat-derived DNA polymorphisms.** In addition, **flow cytometry** readily allows the diagnosis of triploidy although it cannot differentiate between paternal and maternal contributions.

Incidence and Epidemiologic Factors

The incidence of molar pregnancies in the United States is approximately 1 in 1,000 to 1 in 2,000 pregnancies. There are clear ethnic and geographic differences, with complete moles being particularly common in Hawaii, the Philippines, India, and Japan. The frequency is higher toward the beginning and the end of childbearing age, with the highest incidence in women over 45, but moles have been described in women as young as 12 and as old as 60 years of age. Many other epidemiologic factors have been associated with an increased risk of molar pregnancy. These include race, ethnicity, ABO blood groups, diet, and previous treatment with certain drugs. However, no single, specific etiologic factor has been confirmed. There *is* an increased incidence of moles with a history of a previous molar pregnancy, which may be explained by a *genetic propensity for loss of chromosomal material from ova.* This is supported by reports of women with multiple recurrent moles from different fathers.

Complete Hydatidiform Moles

Pathologic Features

Macroscopically, complete moles have abundant tissue with *grossly identifiable translucent vesicles* that represent enlarged, hydropic villi. The vesicles are classically described as "grape-like" and may measure 2 cm in diameter or more (Figs. 23.2 and 23.3). Most or all of the villi show hydropic swelling, and often the uterine cavity is filled with molar tissue (Fig. 23.3). Procedural manipulation may, at times, result in collapse of some or all of the vesicles. These macroscopically identifiable villi are virtually never seen in hydropic abortuses.

On microscopic examination, the villi are *diffusely hydropic* due to massive fluid accumulation. This occurs primarily in the terminal villi. *Cisterns are present are consist of central acellular spaces within the hydropic villi* which form when the connective tissue of the villi dissociates (Fig. 23.4). *Trophoblastic hyperplasia is universally present and is*

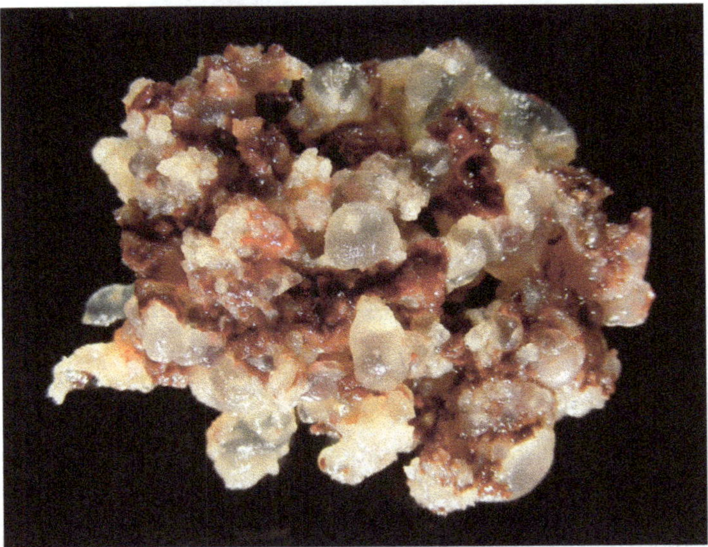

Figure 23.2. Complete hydatidiform mole. Note bulbous swelling of terminal villi.

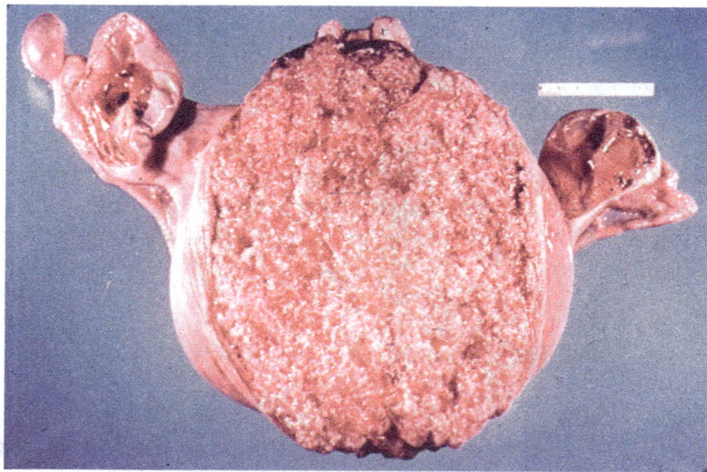

Figure 23.3. Hydatidiform mole in situ. Note the distention of the uterus and the bilateral theca lutein cysts of the ovaries. The vesicular nature of the molar villi is apparent grossly.

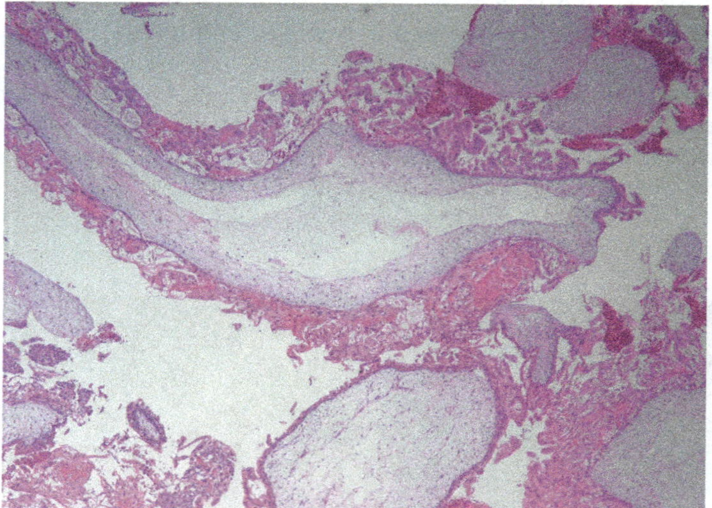

Figure 23.4. Complete mole demonstrating a large hydropic villus with cistern formation, an acellular region surrounded by loose stroma that is usually devoid of blood vessels. There is marked circumferential trophoblastic proliferation as well. H&E ×120.

a requirement for diagnosis. Proliferation varies from villus to villus, but is usually *circumferential around the entire villous perimeter and involves both cytotrophoblast and syncytiotrophoblast* (Fig. 23.5). This feature is key in the differential diagnosis with hydropic abortus (see below). *Trophoblastic atypia* is present, manifesting as nuclear pleomorphism and cytoplasmic vacuolization in syncytiotrophoblast. Mitotic figures

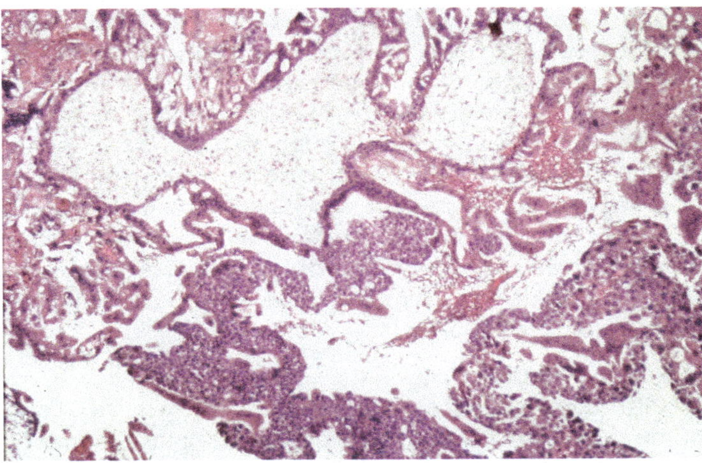

Figure 23.5. Marked circumferential trophoblastic proliferation in a complete mole. H&E ×100.

may be present, even in syncytiotrophoblast. Focally, degenerative change of the trophoblast may be present, the villous surface becoming enmeshed in fibrinoid. Many Hofbauer cells may be identified in the villous stroma. *Intervillous thrombi* are also common due to the aberrant intervillous circulation. The implantation site frequently shows an exuberant proliferation of implantation trophoblast. This exaggerated physiologic response, called an **exaggerated placental site** (see Chap. 25), is seen commonly enough in complete moles for its presence to be helpful in the differential diagnosis.

There have been many attempts at grading molar pregnancies in an effort to determine which moles are most likely to develop choriocarcinoma. Classifications based on trophoblastic atypia, proliferation, and so on have been proposed. However, grading has not been found to be of use so far in predicting behavior. The most important criterion in predicting prognosis is differentiation between partial and complete moles.

Embryonic and Fetal Tissue in Complete Hydatidiform Moles

Traditional teaching has been that complete moles are never associated with an embryo. Even though in the majority of cases embryos are absent, fetal blood vessels and fetal nucleated red blood cells may be encountered in many complete moles, and in rare cases an embryo may be present. This is logical since the stroma of the villi in complete moles, as with other conceptuses, is derived from **embryonic** mesenchyme. Thus, an embryo must have been present, at least initially. There are several reasons that embryos are rarely seen in complete moles. First, early embryonic death is common in complete moles. Since most moles are homozygous for all their genes, and most individuals carry several recessive lethal genes, it makes sense that some of these lethal genes would lead to early death. Second, small, stunted embryos may not be identified the massive villous tissue and so they may be missed. Third, it is clear from studies of early abortion that the incidence of complete moles is much lower than would be expected. This is probably due to the subtlety of diagnostic features seen in early moles (see below). Therefore, early on when an embryo might still be visible, the diagnosis of a mole is less likely to be made. A documented case is shown in Fig. 23.6 in which a complete mole was identified with a tiny embryo, and the patient later developed disseminated choriocarcinoma. The conclusion is that although embryonic or fetal tissue is rare in complete moles, it is does occur. Therefore, the presence of these elements **does not rule out a complete mole**.

Clinical Features and Implications

Patients with complete moles usually present between the 11 and 25th week of pregnancy with a markedly elevated serum β-human chorionic gonadotropin (β-hCG). The levels are much higher than expected for the gestational age, in some cases reaching over 1,000,000 mI/mL. There may be associated *vaginal bleeding or an enlarged and distended uterus* ("size greater than dates"). Sonographically, there is *usually* no embryo or demonstrable heart activity and the presence of multiple echogenic signals described as a *speckled or snowstorm*. Sonographic examination used in conjunction with serum β-hCG levels gives a diagnostic accuracy reaching 90%. Complete moles, in comparison to partial moles, have higher levels of serum β-hCG, present more often in the first trimester and more often have increased uterine size for gestational age, and occur more commonly in women over the age of 40.

Complete moles have been associated with various clinical conditions in the mother, some of which are attributable to the elevated

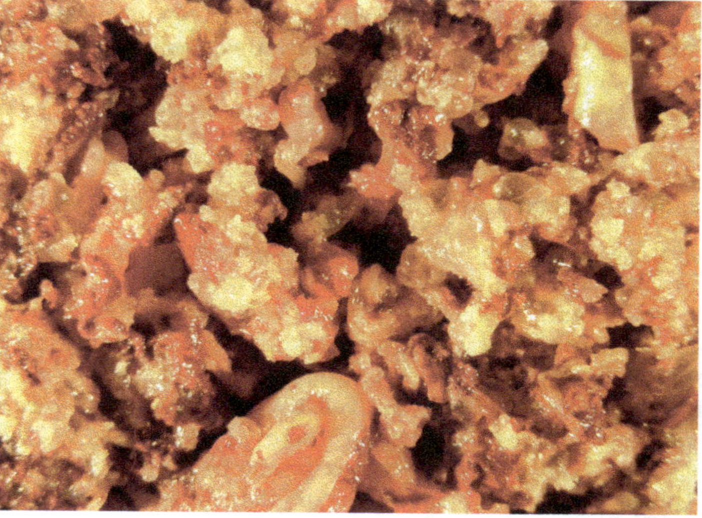

Figure 23.6. Photograph of a partial hydatidiform mole. Note the admixture of swollen, cystic villi with more normal appearing villous tissue.

hCG levels. **Multiple theca lutein cysts** or **hyperreactio luteinalis** in the ovary are present in 25–60% of patients with complete moles. These "functional" ovarian cysts may grow up to 35 cm in diameter, causing significant ovarian enlargement (Fig. 23.3). The cysts are usually multiple, with thin walls and filled with clear or hemorrhagic fluid. Microscopically, *multiple follicle cysts are lined by luteinized theca cells*. Granulosa cells may also show luteinization. The *ovarian stroma is usually edematous and contains scattered luteinized cells as well* (Fig. 23.7). The cysts regress spontaneously after termination of the pregnancy. Moles are also associated with *preeclampsia, eclampsia, pregnancy-induced hypertension, hyperemesis gravidarum, hyperthyroidism, and pulmonary edema* – conditions that spontaneously resolve after evacuation. At least some of these conditions are attributable to the elevated β-hCG levels.

Development of **persistent gestational trophoblastic disease** occurs in approximately 15–20% of women with a diagnosis of complete mole. Most develop persistent or invasive moles (see below), and 1–2% develop **choriocarcinoma**. Early and complete evacuation of the mole is the first line of therapy. Patients with a complete mole are usually followed with serial serum β-hCG levels and concurrent contraception for 6 months to a year or until they fall within the normal range. The reason for contraception is that rises in the titers caused by pregnancy may be confused with the development of persistent disease. If the β-hCG titers do not normalize of if they rise, persistent trophoblastic disease is usually diagnosed without the benefit of a tissue diagnosis and chemotherapy is given without pathologic confirmation.

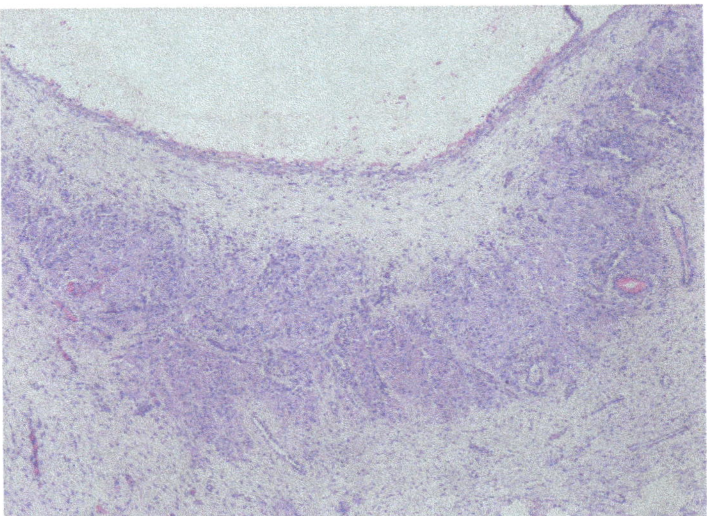

Figure 23.7. Hyperreactio luteinalis of the ovary in a patient with a complete mole. The ovaries were markedly enlarged by numerous luteinized follicle cysts and many luteinized cells in the stroma. A portion of a follicle cyst wall is seen here. H&E ×40.

Early Complete Hydatidiform Moles

With the advent of sonography and the early diagnosis and evacuation of moles, specimens at younger gestational ages are being sent for pathologic evaluation with increasing frequency. **Early complete hydatidiform moles** represent a greater challenge in diagnosis, as *the pathologic features are more subtle and less well developed.* They are thus more difficult to differentiate from partial moles and hydropic abortuses. It is likely that many of these have gone unrecognized in the past. Younger moles tend to *have smaller, less edematous villi, which are more bulbous, club shaped, or cauliflower shaped* than older moles (Fig. 23.8). The *villous stroma often shows a light blue discoloration or myxoid like change. Increased stromal debris and apoptosis has also been described. Cisterns are poorly formed, and trophoblastic proliferation is not as pronounced* as in the more "mature" mole. Capillary remnants and fetal blood vessels are also more easily found.

Biparental Complete Hydatidiform Moles

Recently, families have been described in which recurrent moles are common. Further study revealed that unlike the usual complete moles, which are completely androgenic, these were **biparental.** This phenomenon is due to an abnormal autosomal recessive gene affecting imprinting. Although the underlying mutation has not been fully described, linkage studies have shown that the gene, which lies on the long arm of chromosome 19, allows greater expression of paternal genes leading to, morphologically, a complete mole. Further study is ongoing.

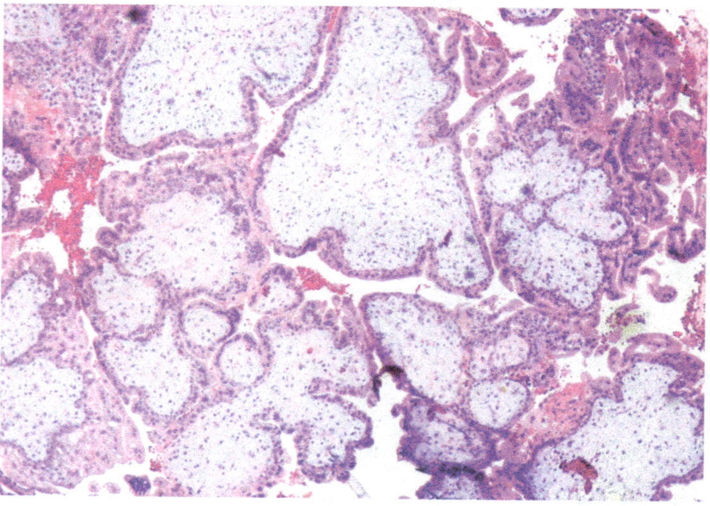

Figure 23.8. Early complete mole with club-like villi, moderate edema, and moderate trophoblastic proliferation. The stroma has a myxoid appearance. H&E ×100.

Ectopic Molar Pregnancy

Partial and complete moles may arise in the fallopian tube, ovary, or other ectopic sites. Moles arising in the fallopian tube are likely to result in *tubal rupture* if not treated promptly. The practice of administering methotrexate to patients with early ectopic pregnancies has interesting implications in the development and behavior of ectopic moles that have yet to be studied. *Overall, moles arising in ectopic locations have similar recurrence rates and risk of development of persistent gestational trophoblastic disease as their intrauterine counterparts.*

Partial Hydatidiform Mole

Pathologic Features

Partial hydatidiform moles are *most commonly triploid with two sets of paternal genes and one set of maternal genes.* The gross and microscopic features are *similar to those of the complete mole but the features are less striking.* The partial mole is less voluminous and is composed of *normal-appearing villous tissue intermixed with larger, distended villi or vesicles.* An associated embryo or fetal tissue is identified more commonly than in complete moles. Microscopically, partial moles have an *admixture of relatively normal immature villi and distended hydropic villi.* The villous outlines are scalloped and the villi are irregularly edematous. *Although cisterns are present, they tend to be scarce. Trophoblastic pseudoinclusions,* which are due to tangential sectioning of the irregular villous outlines, are easily identified (Fig. 23.9). *Focal villous fibrosis may be present.* As with complete moles, trophoblastic proliferation is required for diagnosis, but *the degree of trophoblastic proliferation and atypia is less* in partial moles (Fig. 23.10). The trophoblastic proliferation has been described as being more lace-like than that seen in complete

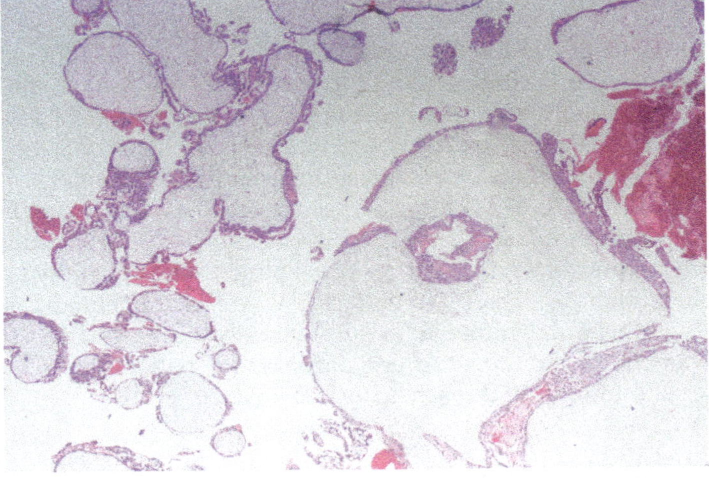

Figure 23.9. Partial hydatidiform mole showing trophoblastic "pseudoinclusions" and irregular invaginations of this villus. H&E ×200.

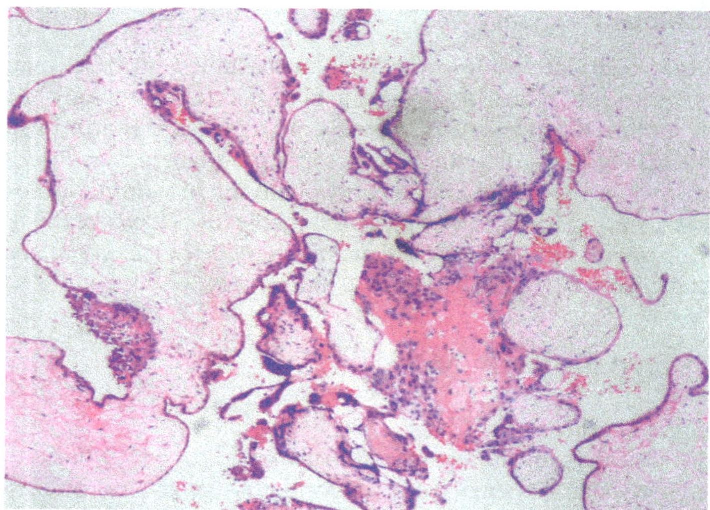

Figure 23.10. Partial mole demonstrating only modest trophoblastic proliferation. Two populations of villi, typical of partial moles, are seen here. H&E ×40.

moles. *Villous capillaries can usually be found*. Many features, such as trophoblastic pseudoinclusions, are occasionally seen in the chromosomally abnormal abortus.

Four major features have been suggested for partial moles, and if the following diagnostic criteria are not met, consideration should be given to ancillary studies:

- An admixture of two populations of villi (normal and hydropic)
- Enlarged villi with "cavitation" or cisterns
- Irregular villi with scalloped borders and trophoblastic pseudoinclusions
- Focal, mild trophoblastic hyperplasia

Clinical Features and Implications
Patients with partial moles usually present between the 18 and 20th week of gestation *with vaginal bleeding suggestive of a missed abortion*, "size less than dates," and *moderate elevations in serum β-hCG*. They also may show findings on sonographic examination similar to those seen for complete moles. Partial moles are associated with **persistent gestational trophoblastic disease** in less than 5% of cases, usually in the form of persistent molar tissue. These patients are generally treated with chemotherapy. There are only a few well-documented cases of patients with partial moles who subsequently developed malignant disease or choriocarcinoma. After a partial mole, patients are followed with serial β-hCG until it reaches normal levels.

Differential Diagnosis

There is much overlap in the histologic appearance of partial and complete moles, and even experienced pathologists may have difficulty in differentiating between them. Problems usually occur between complete and partial moles, between partial moles and hydropic abortuses, and in diagnosing early moles. These differential diagnoses are discussed below and summarized in Table 23.2.

Hydropic Abortus Versus Partial Mole

Hydropic abortuses tend to have *less tissue than partial moles and do not show grossly identifiable vesicles.* The latter are not present in all partial moles, but are usually present admixed with more normal-appearing tissue. Microscopically, hydropic abortuses and partial moles both show moderate *hydropic change in a portion of chorionic villi.* The swollen villi of the abortus will be covered by thinned and *attenuated trophoblast* (Fig. 23.11) and this occurs when the villi swell after embryonic death and the trophoblast is literally stretched over the circumference of the villus. Proliferation of trophoblast may be seen in early abortuses but is clearly *polar*, growing from one aspect of the villus (Fig. 23.11). These are usually anchoring villi and represent an area of growth in the early placenta (see Chap. 8). In partial moles, there is *proliferation of trophoblast, which although focal, is circumferential* around the villous perimeter (Fig. 23.10). The abortus will show a spectrum of villi, from small normal villi all the way to large hydropic villi, while the *partial mole shows two distinct populations of villi.*

Partial Mole Versus Complete Mole

Complete moles tend to have more *voluminous tissue* than partial moles, with *easily identifiable vesicles* on gross examination (Fig. 23.2). Microscopically, the complete mole shows significantly *more trophoblastic proliferation that involves all the villous tissue* rather than *the focal proliferation* in partial moles. Complete moles have more *nuclear pleomorphism and anaplasia as well.* The proliferation in partial moles

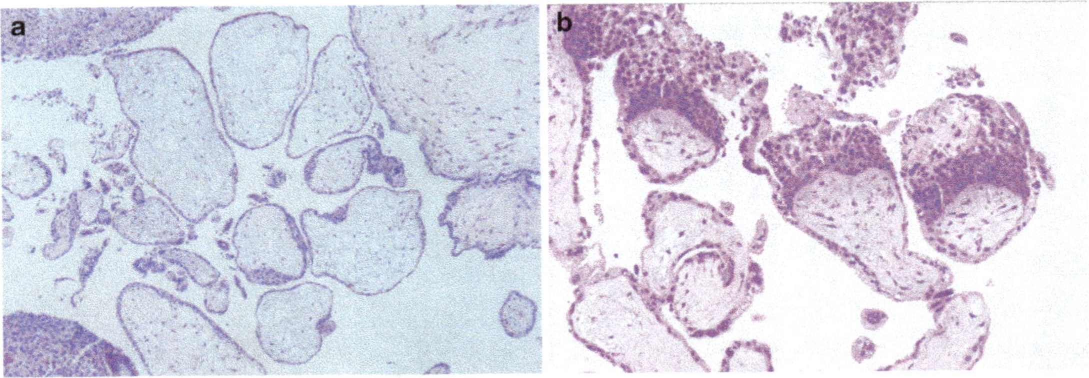

Figure 23.11. (**a**) Hydropic abortus with marked swelling of the villi. In contrast to a molar pregnancy, the trophoblastic cover is thin and attenuated. H&E ×40. (**b**) "Polar" proliferation of trophoblast, rather than circumferential proliferation may be present and is a feature that distinguishes hydropic abortuses from partial moles. H&E ×100.

is *clubbed or lacy* (Fig. 23.12) rather than the more solid proliferations seen in complete moles. Partial moles also have *two distinct populations of villi*: (1) a population of normal villi; and (2) villi with *edema, irregular villous contours, invaginations, and trophoblastic pseudoinclusions* (Fig. 23.9). The latter are not generally seen in complete moles. Finally, although embryonic or fetal tissue, blood vessels, and nucleated red blood cells may be seen in both complete and partial moles, they are much more common in partial moles.

Early Mole Versus Hydropic Abortus Versus Partial Mole

In early moles (particularly those less than 10 weeks), the histologic features are more subtle and therefore may be confused with hydropic abortuses or a partial mole. Hydropic abortuses have a complete range of villi, from large hydropic villi to small, normal villi. The hydropic villi may have *cisterns*, but these are covered by *thin, attenuated trophoblast*. On the other hand, early moles have a uniform population of villi with *bulbous, cauliflower-like or clubbed villi, myxoid-like stroma, and poorly formed cisterns*. They may often be smaller than those seen in partial moles. Blood vessels are more common, and the villous stroma is more cellular than in older moles and the villi have an appearance reminiscent of mesenchymal villi (see Chap. 7). The most important feature in differentiating an abortus from an early mole is that the latter shows *trophoblastic proliferation*, albeit less than an older mole.

Partial Mole Versus Twin Pregnancy with Complete Mole

Rarely, in twin pregnancy, one of the twins is a mole and the other normal. The distinction from a partial mole may be quite difficult, particularly if the tissue is disrupted. Both will have two populations of villi, some hydropic and some normal (Fig. 23.13), and both may

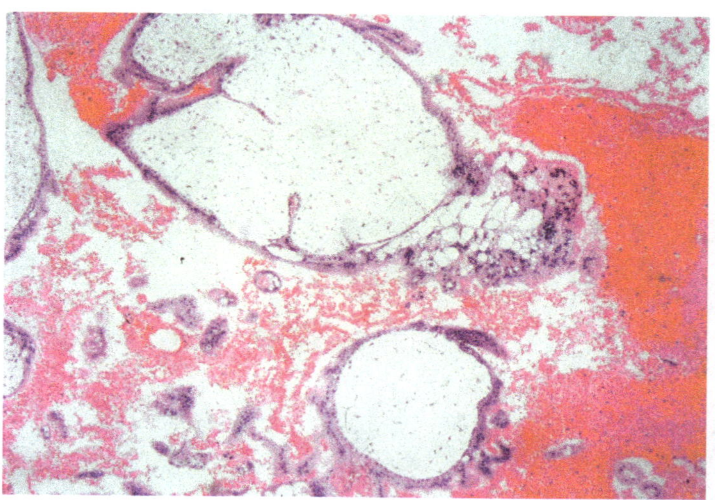

Figure 23.12. Partial mole showing irregular proliferation of trophoblast with lacy extensions. H&E ×40.

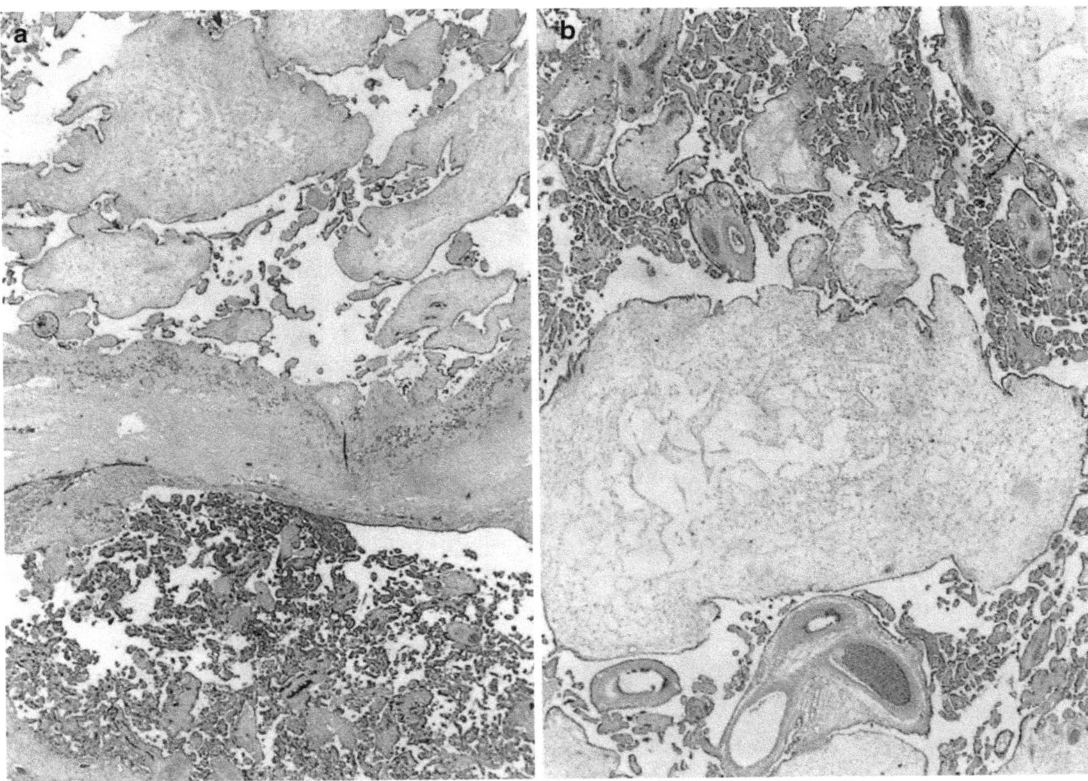

Figure 23.13. (a) Sharp division of molar villi (*top*) and normal villi (*bottom*) in twin gestation. H&E ×16. (b) Focal admixture of molar and normal villi. H&E ×16.

have fetal tissue. *The most important feature in differentiation is the presence of marked trophoblastic proliferation and atypia* in the complete mole. Of course, twin pregnancies occur in which a partial mole is combined with a normal pregnancy. Accurate diagnosis may be impossible unless the placentas may be grossly differentiated from each other.

Ancillary Testing

Since the histologic features are not completely reliable, in certain cases accurate categorization may be improved by performing ploidy analysis. Ploidy may be helpful in the following situations:

- Partial versus complete mole
  - Diploid → complete mole
  - Triploid → most likely a partial mole
- Partial mole versus hydropic abortus
  - Diploid → hydropic abortus
  - Triploid → most likely a partial mole

Caution is advised, as these rules are not strict. Particularly, *rare* complete moles are triploid or tetraploid. In addition, nonmolar triploidy may occur with a maternal excess of DNA, or **maternal triploidy.** These do not show the trophoblastic proliferation typical of moles and so are not usually confused histologically with moles.

Recently, *a maternally transcribed but paternally imprinted gene* has been described that is a cyclin-dependent kinase (CDK) inhibitor $p57^{KIP2}$ protein, referred to as **p57KIP2** or **p57.** This protein is strongly expressed in maternal tissues such as decidua and is expressed in cytotrophoblast and villous stromal cells if a maternal component is present, such as in partial moles and hydropic abortuses. However, it is **not** expressed in androgenetic complete moles, or in the rare biparental complete moles. Therefore, since this antibody is commercially available, immunohistochemistry for p57 may be helpful in the differential diagnosis of difficult cases. One must be careful, however, as rarely a biparental complete mole may occur. In addition, recently a case of a complete mole with retained maternal chromosomes resulting in positivity for p57 has been reported. A summary of the findings of flow cytometry and p57 is shown in Table 23.3. If flow cytometry or other methods are not available or the diagnosis is still unclear, a report reflecting uncertainty may be prudent and the patient may then be followed with β-hCG monitoring.

Suggestions for Examination and Report
(Hydatidiform moles)

Gross Examination: The presence of enlarged villi or vesicles should be noted and is most consistent with a molar pregnancy. If the clinical history suggests molar pregnancy (elevated hCG or typical sonography), and vesicles are not visible grossly, additional sections should be submitted. It is recommended that additional sections of moles be submitted in any cases so that there is sufficient tissue for histologic diagnosis. Identification of fetal or embryonic tissue should also be documented.

Comment: If the diagnosis is equivocal, additional sections can be submitted initially. If the issue is not then clarified, additional testing such as flow cytometry or p57 immunostaining should be employed. If the diagnosis is still in question or if ancillary testing is not available, and the differential is between complete and partial mole, the diagnosis of a **"hydatidiform mole"** can be made with a comment that differentiation between partial and complete is not possible. A suggestion should also be made for serial β-hCG testing, at least until the levels normalize. If the differential is between a hydropic abortus and a partial mole and cannot be resolved, a descriptive diagnosis should be rendered such as **"chorionic villi with hydropic change and trophoblastic proliferation, see comment."** The comment should then address the differential, again with the suggestion for serial β-hCG measurements.

Invasive Hydatidiform Mole

Pathogenesis

Invasive mole is a rare entity composed of *trophoblastic cells and molar villi, which invade the uterus and have the potential for invasion of adjacent structures.* Invasive moles usually develop subsequent to a molar pregnancy and are most often diagnosed by ultrasonography or other imaging technique. The patients may present with elevated serum β-hCG during follow-up after a molar pregnancy and often have vaginal bleeding. Since invasive moles are characterized by molar villi invading through the myometrium, they may be viewed as a *placenta accreta/increta of a molar pregnancy* (see Chap. 12). Their biologic behavior is very similar to choriocarcinoma.

Pathologic Features

Microscopically, *molar villi are admixed with proliferating cytotrophoblast and syncytiotrophoblast.* The villi invade the myometrium without intervening decidual tissue (Figs. 23.14 and 23.15). *Deep myometrial invasion is typical and uterine perforation is relatively common.* Invasive moles are often associated with abundant hemorrhage and necrosis, similar to that seen in choriocarcinoma. Differentiation between an invasive mole and choriocarcinoma is straightforward as, by definition, molar villi are present in invasive moles and not in choriocarcinoma.

Clinical Features and Implications

Invasive moles usually occur after a previously diagnosed molar pregnancy, and most commonly a rise in the serum β-hCG heralds the onset. Their behavior is similar to choriocarcinoma and usually requires similar therapy with chemotherapeutic agents, but hysterectomies are more commonly done with invasive moles. They may develop metastases, usually to the lungs, and late metastases have been reported. Prognosis is based on the nature of the mole and the efficacy of its initial removal. Rare cases of spontaneous regression have been described.

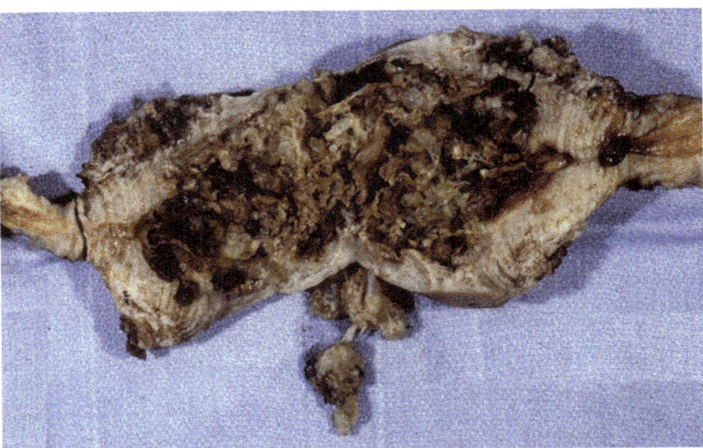

Figure 23.14. Hysterectomy specimen with a large, invasive, hemorrhagic lesion containing molar tissue.

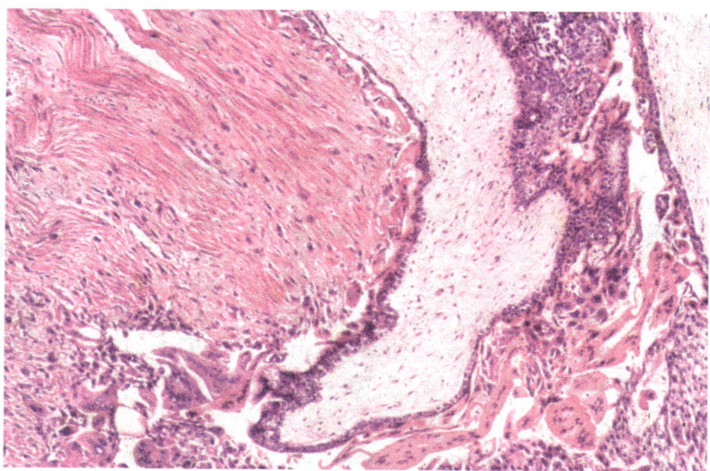

Figure 23.15. Invasive mole showing a molar villus invading the myometrium. Note the trophoblastic proliferation at the right. H&E ×200.

Suggestions for Examination and Report
(Invasive hydatidiform mole)

Gross Examination: When an invasive mole is suspected, generous sampling of the endomyometrium is advised as well as any grossly identifiable molar villi.

Comment: If an invasive mole is diagnosed, a comment on the extent of involvement is suggested.

Table 23.1. World Health Organization classification of gestational trophoblastic disease.

Hydatidiform mole

    Complete mole

    Partial mole

    Invasive mole

    Metastatic mole

Trophoblastic neoplasms

    Choriocarcinoma

    Placental site trophoblastic tumor

    Epithelioid trophoblastic tumor

Nonneoplastic, nonmolar trophoblastic lesions

    Placental site nodule and plaque

    Exaggerated placental site

From Tavassoli FA, Devilee P. World Health Organization classification of tumours: Pathology and Genetics. Tumours of the Breast and Female Genital Organs. Lyon, France: IARC Press, 2003

Table 23.2. Differential diagnosis of complete and partial hydatidiform moles.

Characteristic	Hydropic abortus	Complete mole	Early complete mole	Partial mole
Ploidy[a]	Diploid	Diploid	Diploid	Triploid
Paternal/maternal chromosome ratio[a]	1:1	2:0	2:0	2:1
Embryo/fetus	May be present	Rarely present	Rarely present	May be present
Clinical presentation	Missed abortion	Size > dates	± Missed abortion	Size < dates
Serum β-hCG	Normal or low	Markedly elevated	Moderately to markedly elevated	Moderately elevated
Histology				
Villous enlargement	Moderate	Marked	Mild to moderate	Moderate with admixture of normal villi
Villous population	Range of villi from small to hydropic	Relatively uniform population of large hydropic villi	Relatively uniform population of mildly enlarged villi	Two populations of villi, one normal and one moderately hydropic
Villous shape	Round	Round	Clubbed or bulbous	Scalloped with trophoblastic pseudoinclusions
Cisterns	Usually absent	Common	Rare	Rare
Trophoblastic proliferation	None	Marked circumferential	Moderate circumferential	Mild to moderate and focal
Trophoblastic atypia	None	Common	Common	Minimal
Fetal blood vessels/ nucleated red blood cells	Usually absent	Rare	May be present	Common
Persistent gestational trophoblastic disease	No	Up to 20% May develop choriocarcinoma	Up to 20% May develop choriocarcinoma	Less than 5%, usually not requiring chemotherapy

[a]Most common presentation, but variations may occur. See text for more information

Table 23.3. Differential diagnosis: ancillary testing.

	Ploidy[a]	p57
Hydropic abortus	Diploid	+
Partial mole	Triploid	+
Complete mole	Diploid	−

[a]Ploidy is indicated for the majority of cases as occasionally maternal triploidy or triploid complete moles may occur

Selected References

PHP5, Chapter 22, pages 797–836.

Ambrani LM, Vaidya RA, Rao CS, et al. Familial occurrence of trophoblastic disease – report of recurrent molar pregnancies in sisters in three families. Clin Genet 1980;18:27–29.

Baergen RN, Kelly T, McGinnis MJ, et al. Complete hydatidiform mole with a coexisting embryo. Hum Pathol 1996;27:731–734.

Fukunaga M. Immunohistochemical characterization of p57^{KIP2} expression in early hydatidiform moles. Hum Pathol 2002;33:1188–1192.

Genest DR. Partial hydatidiform mole: clinicopathologic features, differential diagnosis, ploidy and molecular studies, and gold standards for diagnosis. Int J Gynecol Pathol 2001;20:315–322.

Hui P, Martel M, Parkash V. Gestational trophoblastic diseases: recent advances in histological diagnosis and related genetic aspects. Adv Anat Pathol 2005;12:116–125.

Kajii T, Kurashige H, Ohama K, et al. XY and XX complete moles: clinical and morphological correlations. Am J Obstet Gynecol 1984;150:57–64.

Kajii T, Ohama K. Androgenetic origin of hydatidiform mole. Nature 1977;268:633–634.

Keep D, Zaragoza MV, Hassold T, et al. Very early complete hydatidiform mole. Hum Pathol 1996;27:708–713.

Lage JM, Driscoll SG, Yavner DL, et al. Hydatidiform moles: application of flow cytometry in diagnosis. Am J Clin Pathol 1988;89:596–600.

Lawler SD, Fisher RA, Dent JA. Prospective genetic study of complete and partial hydatidiform moles. Am J Obstet Gynecol 1991;164:1270–1277.

Li HW, Tsao SW, Cheung ANY. Current understandings of the molecular genetics of gestational trophoblastic diseases. Placenta 2002;23:20–31.

Sebire NJ. Histopathological diagnosis of hydatidiform mole: contemporary features and clinical implications. Fetal Pediatr Pathol 2010;29:1–16.

Szulman AE, Surti U. The syndromes of hydatidiform mole. I. Cytogenetic and morphologic correlations. Am J Obstet Gynecol 1978;131:665–671.

Szulman AE, Surti U. The syndromes of hydatidiform mole. II. Morphologic evolution of the complete and partial mole. Am J Obstet Gynecol 1978;132:20–27.

Zaragoza MV, Keep D, Genest DR, et al. Early complete hydatidiform moles contain inner cell mass derivatives. Am J Med Genet 1997;70:273–277.

Chapter 24

Choriocarcinoma

General Considerations

Choriocarcinoma is a rare tumor with an incidence of one in 25,000–40,000 pregnancies. It may develop after an abortion, a term or preterm pregnancy, an ectopic pregnancy, or a hydatidiform mole. In their oft-depicted diagram (Fig. 24.1), Hertig and Mansell estimated that the lesion was preceded by a *complete hydatidiform mole in 50%, an abortion in 25%, a normal pregnancy in 22.5%, and an ectopic pregnancy in 2.5%*. Choriocarcinoma is more common in young women and in those 40 years of age or older. There is as wide a geographic variation in its incidence as there is for hydatidiform moles.

Clinical Features and Implications

The most common presenting symptom is *abnormal vaginal bleeding*, usually developing several months following a pregnancy. Long latency periods of up to 14 years or more have been reported. Some patients present with *elevated serum β-human chorionic gonadotropin (β-hCG), a radiographically detectable lesion or metastatic disease* with symptoms reflecting the site of the metastasis.

Before the advent of chemotherapy, the prognosis of choriocarcinoma was dismal, with a 5-year survival of 32%, which dropped to 19% if metastatic disease was present. Survival has improved dramatically since the introduction of efficacious chemotherapeutic agents, and the *overall survival for all gestational trophoblastic disease (GTD) is greater than 90%*. Some women successfully treated for choriocarcinoma have gone on to have normal pregnancies. Prognosis is primarily

R.N. Baergen, *Manual of Pathology of the Human Placenta,*
DOI 10.1007/978-1-4419-7494-5_24, © Springer Science+Business Media, LLC 2011

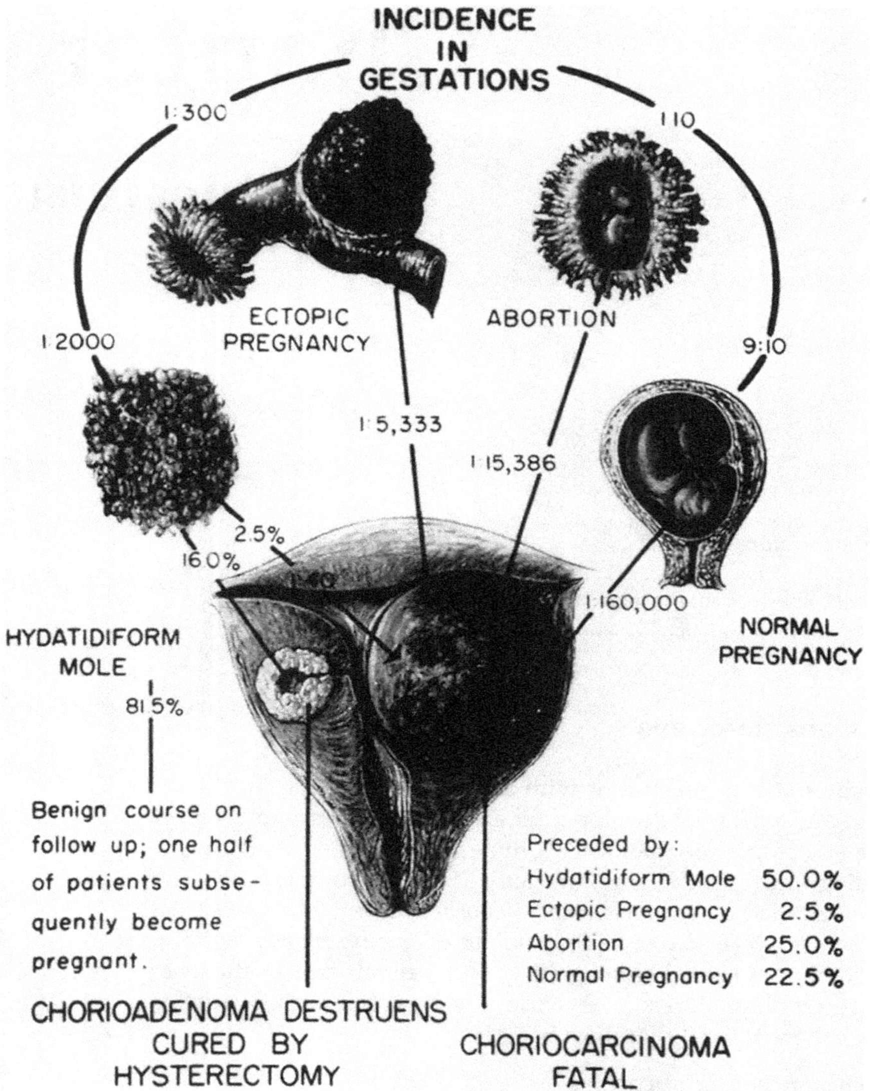

Figure 24.1. Frequency of choriocarcinoma relative to its various precursors (from Hertig and Mansell 1956, with permission).

based on the stage (Table 24.1). A staging system for GTD devised by the International Federation of Gynecology and Obstetrics has been recently revised to include the modified World Health Organization risk factor scoring system (Table 24.2). *Older age, longer interval from preceding pregnancy, antecedent term pregnancy, high serum β-hCG levels, location and number of metastases, and history of failed treatment are all poor prognostic indicators.* This scoring system along with staging forms the basis for treatment. In general, patients with a score of 7 or more are considered high risk and treated with more aggressive multiagent chemotherapy.

Pathologic Features

Grossly, choriocarcinoma may vary from an inconspicuous tumor only a few millimeters in diameter to large, bulky tumors. It presents as a *friable, hemorrhagic, and often necrotic mass* with an infiltrating border (Fig. 24.2). The tumors may be so large as to completely fill the uterine cavity (Fig. 24.3). On microscopic examination, choriocarcinoma consists of *solid sheets of cytotrophoblast and multinucleated syncytium without stroma* (Fig. 24.4). As the tumor has no intrinsic vascular stroma, it takes its blood supply from invasion of host vessels. This great propensity for *vascular invasion* leads to the prominent *hemorrhage and necrosis* characteristic of choriocarcinoma (Fig. 24.5). So much blood may be present in some tumors that one may have to search long for the tumor cells, which are often at the periphery of the lesion. Classically, *broad sheets or smaller nests of cytotrophoblast form the central portions of the tumor, the periphery being syncytium*, recapitulating the normal relationship of trophoblast in the early embryo (Fig. 24.6). Commonly, there is a completely haphazard mixture of trophoblastic cells that irregularly infiltrate the surrounding tissue. The **syncytiotrophoblast** contains *multiple irregular, hyperchromatic nuclei with dense, eosinophilic cytoplasm*. Nuclear pleomorphism is common. Because of its dilated cytoplasmic cisternae, the *syncytium is frequently vacuolated*

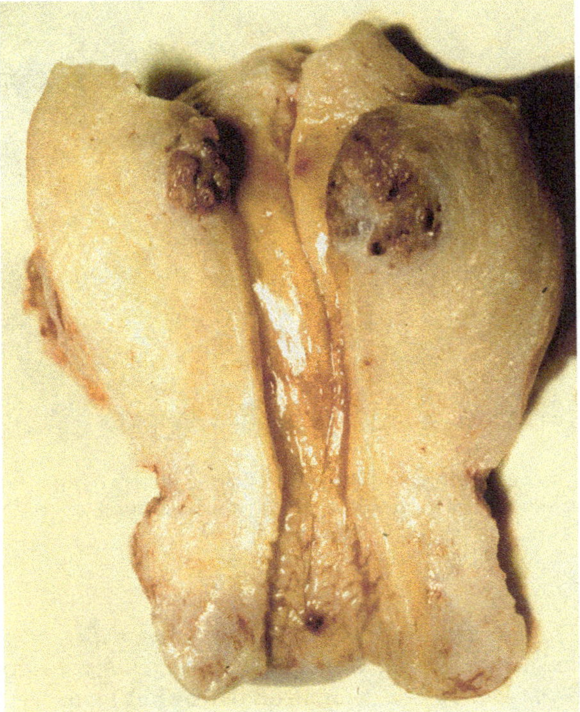

Figure 24.2. Opened uterus showing an irregular, necrotic and hemorrhagic tumor involving the endomyometrium (Baergen and Rutgers 1997, with permission).

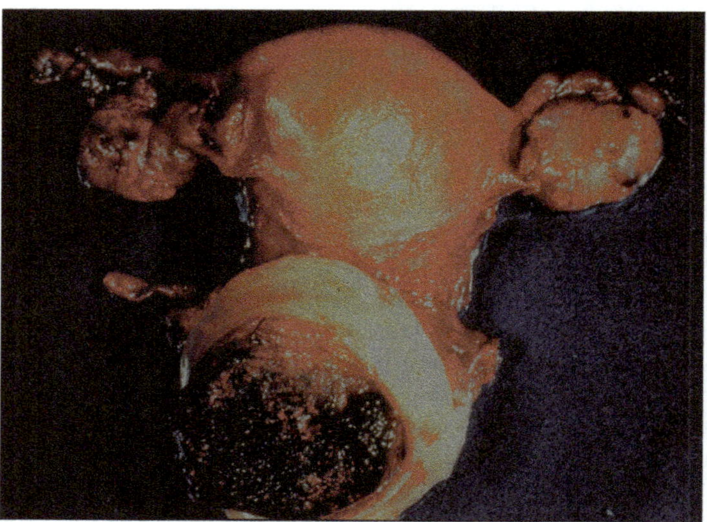

Figure 24.3. Hemorrhagic choriocarcinoma completely filling the uterine cavity.

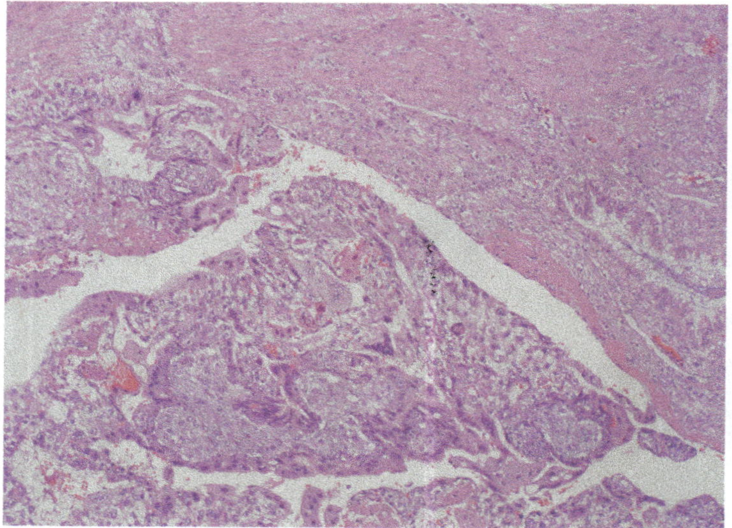

Figure 24.4. Choriocarcinoma of the uterus. Solid sheets of neoplastic cytotrophoblast and syncytiotrophoblast with marked nuclear pleomorphism. H&E ×160.

(Fig. 24.7). The **cytotrophoblastic cells** are *large, with moderate clear to lightly eosinophilic cytoplasm, large round nuclei, clumped chromatin, and one or more nucleoli.* A few **transitional trophoblastic cells** may be present in choriocarcinoma, even though they are not the hallmark of the lesion. Those cells are truly intermediate between cytotrophoblast and syncytium but are **not** the "intermediate trophoblast" of the implantation site (extravillous trophoblast). Differentiation of

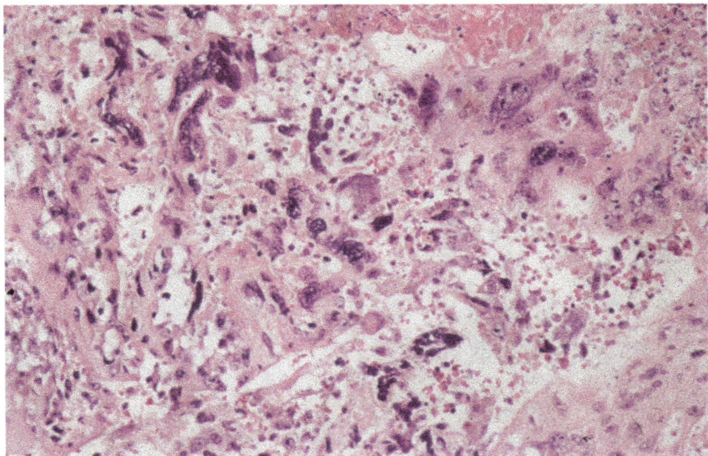

Figure 24.5. Choriocarcinoma demonstrating marked nuclear atypia. Characteristic associated necrosis is present in the upper portion of the figure. H&E ×200.

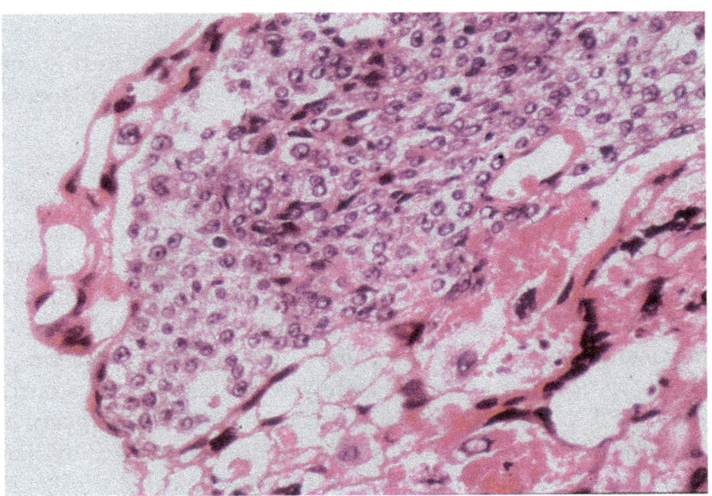

Figure 24.6. Choriocarcinoma, recapitulating the normal arrangement seen in chorionic villi, with syncytial cells surrounding groups of cytotrophoblast. H&E ×200.

choriocarcinoma from lesions of extravillous trophoblast is discussed in Chapter 25 and summarized in Tables 25.1–25.3.

Occasionally confusion with early abortion specimens may occur as the latter will contain sheets of proliferating trophoblastic cells with mitotic activity. Choriocarcinoma has no villous stroma or blood vessels, and these can easily be found in the early abortus. One does not usually make the diagnosis of a choriocarcinoma in the presence

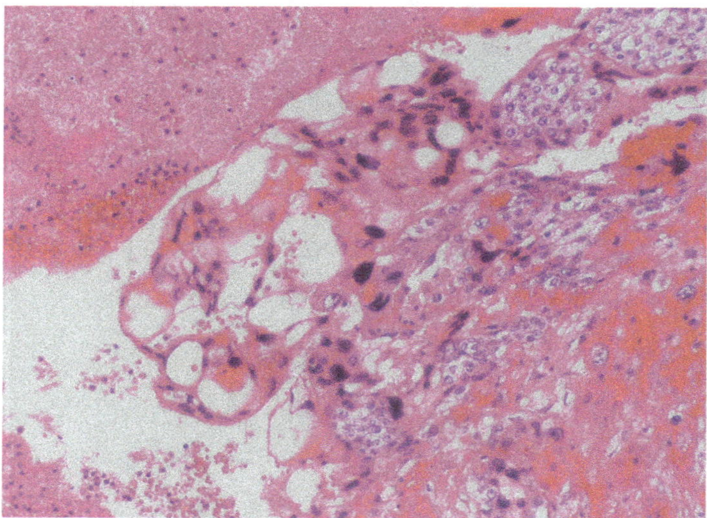

Figure 24.7. Vacuolated syncytiotrophoblast with marked atypia, characteristic for choriocarcinoma. Hemorrhage and necrosis is also present. H&E ×200.

of chorionic villi, although clearly they must develop in this context. The exception is choriocarcinoma in a term or near term placenta (see below).

Metastasis

Metastases occur largely from *hematogenous dissemination through the venous system to the lungs*, and in some cases into the systemic circulation. Therefore, metastatic lung lesions are present in 94% of patients with metastases. The *vagina* is also often involved. Other, less common, metastatic sites include *brain, liver, kidney, spleen, intestines, broad ligament, ovary, pelvis, and cervix*. Rarely metastases have occurred in the *oral gingival, subungual region, gastrocnemius muscle, coronary artery, aorta, and choroid of the eye*. Histologically, metastatic lesions tend to be *better circumscribed* but are otherwise histologically similar to the primary (Figs. 24.8 and 24.9). Occasionally, a metastasis is identified without an identifiable primary. Spontaneous resolution of the primary lesion can occur as well as spontaneous remission of metastasis, although these have been reported only infrequently.

Choriocarcinoma-In Situ: Placental Choriocarcinoma

Pathogenesis

When choriocarcinoma develops during a term or near-term pregnancy, an intraplacental lesion is likely present and may be identified in some cases. This lesion has been referred to as a **choriocarcinoma-in situ**. The lesion clearly arises in the placenta (Fig. 24.10), but these intraplacental lesions are usually invasive within the placenta and often metastatic at the time they are discovered. Therefore, the

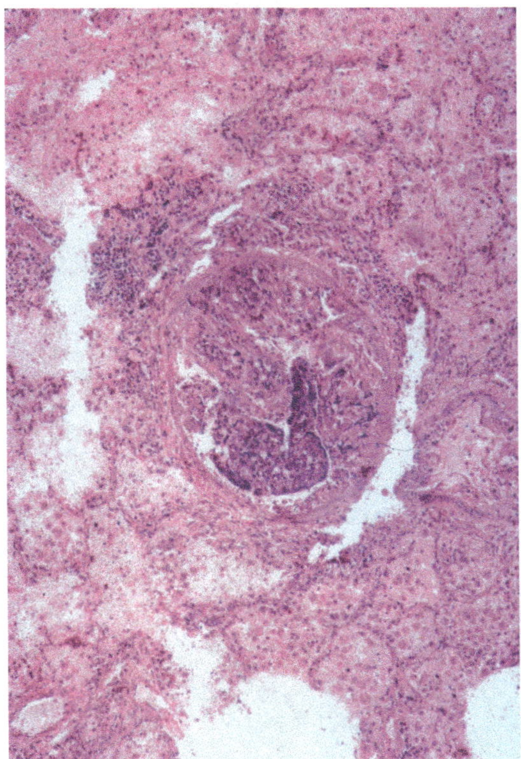

Figure 24.8. Choriocarcinoma metastatic to the lungs. This vessel is filled with solid nodules of choriocarcinoma. Some inflammatory reaction is also present in the vascular wall. H&E ×40.

term **choriocarcinoma-in situ** is not appropriate and the preferred designation is **placental choriocarcinoma**. These lesions are the probable origin of many of the choriocarcinomas that develop after a term pregnancy. However, one must keep in mind that some choriocarcinomas that develop after a term pregnancy may actually have arisen from a prior pregnancy. Since routine placental examination is not performed on every placenta, it is quite likely that many of these lesions are missed. Furthermore, the subtlety of the gross appearance of these lesions may result in them being overlooked when the placenta is examined.

Pathologic Features
Placental choriocarcinomas are usually *inconspicuous grossly and are often mistaken for an infarct as they will have a similar appearance.* Some are quite small and thus only identified by microscopic examination. Microscopically, they show proliferation of both cytotrophoblast and syncytiotrophoblast in the intervillous space (Figs. 24.11 and 24.12), which is typical for this lesion. Usually there is focal involvement of the adjacent chorionic villi. Invasion of the villous stroma or fetal vessels may also be present.

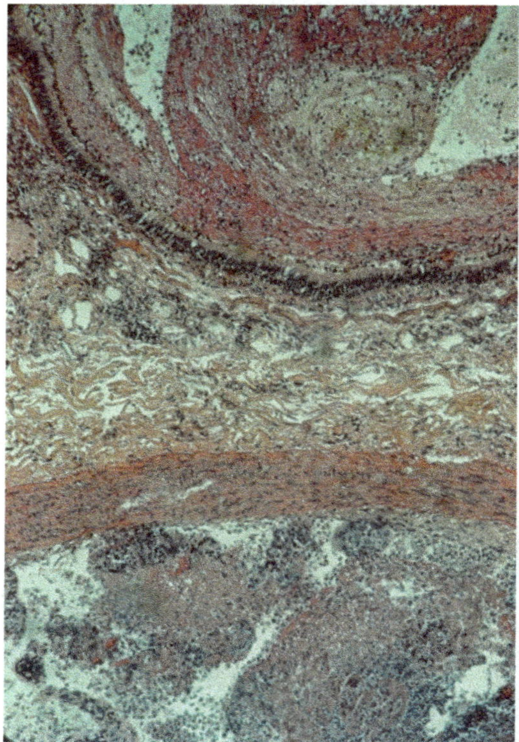

Figure 24.9. Metastatic choriocarcinoma to the lungs. Tumor is present within the lumen of a large vessel (*bottom*) and exudate is present with a bronchus (*top*) Trichrome ×40.

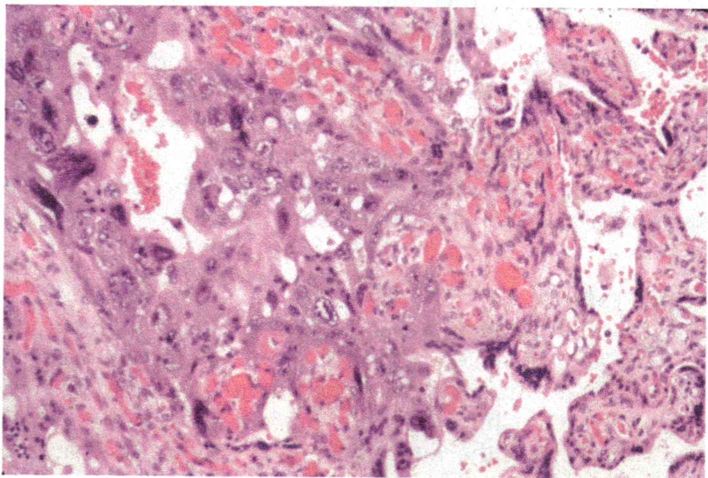

Figure 24.10. Term placenta with proliferation of trophoblast, consistent with intraplacental choriocarcinoma. H&E ×200.

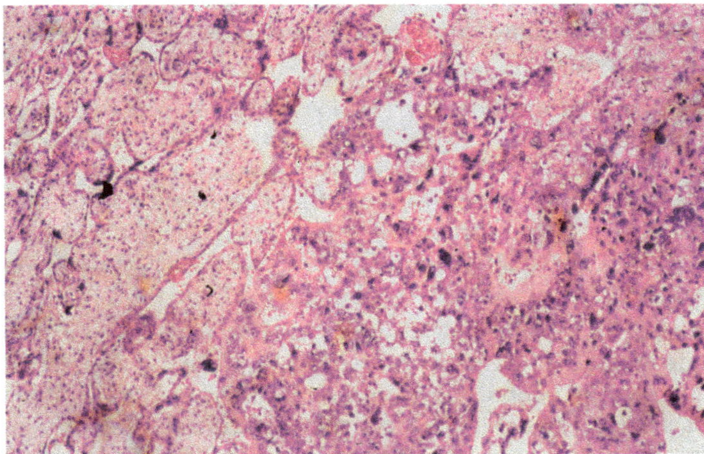

Figure 24.11. Mature placenta with placental choriocarcinoma ("choriocarcinoma-in situ"). Sheets of atypical trophoblast proliferate between the chorionic villi within the intervillous space. H&E ×80.

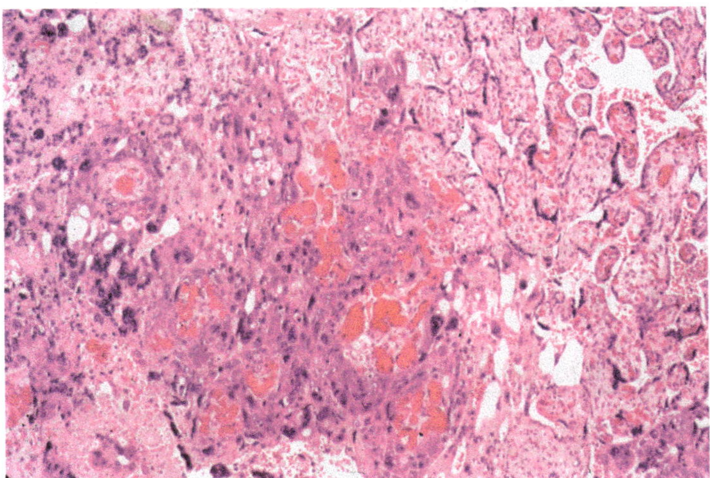

Figure 24.12. Placental choriocarcinoma demonstrating the cytologic atypia pleomorphism. H&E ×200.

Clinical Features and Implications

The reported cases of placental choriocarcinoma have had a varied outcome. In some cases, mother and infant showed no ill effect, while in other cases metastatic lesions, particularly to the lungs, required treatment. Placental choriocarcinoma can *metastasize to both the mother and the fetus*, and may be fatal to both. *Massive transplacental fetal hemorrhage* has also been reported. Occasionally, tumor in the placenta is not identified despite metastasis in the neonate. In some of these cases, this was certainly due to lack of placental examination. Due to the subtle nature of the gross appearance of these lesions, it is likely that many cases go undiagnosed.

> **Suggestions for Examination and Report**
> (Choriocarcinoma)
>
> **Gross Examination:** Uterine choriocarcinomas are hemorrhagic and necrotic and may require many sections for identification of viable tumor cells. Often, the primary lesion is not resected or even noted and it is the metastatic lesions that find its way to the pathology laboratory. Generous sampling is advised. Placental choriocarcinomas are not usually visible grossly or have an inconspicuous appearance.
>
> **Comment:** If placental choriocarcinoma is present, a comment may be made about the possibility of maternal or fetal metastases. In the rare case of a resection of a primary uterine choriocarcinoma or a metastasis, information about the extent of disease spread is necessary in order that proper staging be performed (see Table 24.1).

Table 24.1. Staging of gestational trophoblastic disease.

Stage	Definition
I	Disease confined to the uterus
II	Disease outside the uterus but limited to the genital structures (i.e., pelvis, vagina)
III	Metastatic disease to the lungs
IV	Metastatic disease to sites other than the lungs

Modified from Kohorn EI. The new FIGO 2000 staging and risk factor scoring system for gestational trophoblastic disease: description and critical assessment. Int J Gynecol Cancer 2001;11:73–77

Table 24.2. FIGO 2000 scoring system for gestational trophoblastic disease.

FIGO score	0	1	2	3
Age at diagnosis	≤39 years	>39 years		
Type of antecedent pregnancy	Hydatidiform mole	Abortion	Term pregnancy	
Interval from antecedent pregnancy	<4 months	4–6 months	7 to 12 months	>12 months
Serum β-hCG mIU/mL	<1,000	1,000–10,000	10,000–100,000	>100,000
Tumor size	≤4 cm	>4 cm		
Sites of metastases	None	Spleen or kidney	Gastrointestinal tract	Brain or liver
Number of metastases	0	1–3	4–8	>8
Response to chemotherapy	Full response	Full response	Failure with single drug chemotherapy	Failure with multiagent chemotherapy

Risk is assessed by adding factors according to the above system. Scores of seven or greater constitute a high-risk group that is treated more aggressively

Modified from Kohorn EI. The new FIGO 2000 staging and risk factor scoring system for gestational trophoblastic disease: description and critical assessment. Int J Gynecol Cancer 2001;11:73–77

Selected References

PHP5, Chapter 23, pages 837–846, 852–862.

Baergen RN. Gestational choriocarcinoma. Gen Diagn Pathol 1997;143:127–142.

Baergen RN, Rutgers JL. Trophoblastic lesions of the placental site. Gen Diagn Pathol 1997; 143:143–158.

Driscoll SG. Choriocarcinoma: an "incidental finding" within a term placenta. Obstet Gynecol 1963;21:96–101.

Gardiner HAR, Lage JM. Choriocarcinoma following a partial hydatidiform mole: a case report. Hum Pathol 1992;23:468–471.

Hertiz AT, Mansell H. Tumors of the female sex orangs Part I. Hydatidiform mole and choriocarcinoma. In, Atlas of Tumor Pathology. Sect IX. Fasc. 33. Armed Forces of Pathology, Washington, D.C., 1956.

Jacques SM, Qureshi F, Doss BJ, et al. Intraplacental choriocarcinoma associated with viable pregnancy: pathologic features and implications for the mother and infant. Pediatr Dev Pathol 1998;1:380–387.

Kendall A, Gillmore R, Newlands E. Chemotherapy for trophoblastic disease: current standards. Curr Opin Obstet Gynecol 2002;14:33–38.

Kohorn EI. The new FIGO 2000 staging and risk factor scoring system for gestational trophoblastic disease: description and critical assessment. Int J Gynecol Cancer 2001;11:73–77.

Lage JM, Roberts DJ. Choriocarcinoma in a term placenta: pathologic diagnosis of tumor in an asymptomatic patient with metastatic disease. Int J Gynecol Pathol 1993;12:80–85.

Scully RE, Bonfiglio TA, Kurman RJ, et al. Histologic typing of female genital tract tumours, 2nd ed. New York: Springer-Verlag, 1994.

Seckl MJ, Newlands ES. Treatment of gestational trophoblastic disease. Gen Diagn Pathol 1997;143:159–171.

Silverberg SG, Kurman RJ. Tumors of the uterine corpus and gestational trophoblastic disease. Atlas of tumor pathology, Third Series, Fascicle 3. Washington, DC: AFIP, 1992.

Wells M. The pathology of gestational trophoblastic disease: recent advances. Pathology 2007;39:88–96.

Chapter 25

Lesions of Extravillous Trophoblast

General Considerations

Lesions of extravillous trophoblast (EVT) have been known for over 100 years. The first lesion that was described, "syncytial endometritis," is a nonneoplastic lesion that is merely an exuberant proliferation of the EVT in the implantation site. It was later renamed **exaggerated placental site**. Another lesion of EVT was described shortly thereafter, the "syncytioma." Other designations, such as chorioma, atypical chorionepithelioma, chorionepitheliosis, and trophoblastic pseudotumor, have also been used. It was first thought that it was also a benign, nonneoplastic proliferation of EVT, hence the designation of pseudotumor. Reports of lesions with aggressive behavior and metastasis, however, have led to its reclassification as a potentially malignant neoplasm. It is since been renamed **placental site trophoblastic tumor**. Much more recently, two additional lesions of EVT have been described: a benign nonneoplastic lesion called the **placental**

R.N. Baergen, *Manual of Pathology of the Human Placenta,*
DOI 10.1007/978-1-4419-7494-5_25, © Springer Science+Business Media, LLC 2011

site nodule, and a variant of placental site trophoblastic tumor, the **epithelioid trophoblastic tumor.**

Placental-Site Nodule

Clinical Features and Implications

The **placental-site nodule** (PSN) is a benign, nonneoplastic lesion thought to represent EVT retained in the uterus after pregnancy. PSNs occur primarily in reproductive-age patients, but may be seen in postmenopausal patients. They may follow a normal pregnancy, abortion, or mole, and may be diagnosed several weeks to many years after the preceding pregnancy. Many patients have a history previous gynecologic surgery such as cesarean section, therapeutic abortion, or curettage. In one study, a significant number of patients had a history of bilateral tubal ligation. One half of the patients present with *abnormal bleeding,* and in the remainder, the lesions are *incidental findings in curettage or hysterectomy specimens.* The lesions are often found in the lower uterine segment and cervix. Serum β-human chorionic gonadotropin (β-hCG) levels are not elevated. *Follow-up on patients with PSNs has been benign,* and progression to gynecologic malignancy or trophoblastic disease is generally thought not to occur. However, one recent report describes a lesion with features of both PSN and epithelioid trophoblastic tumor (see below) and the authors suggested that this indicated malignant transformation of a PSN. This has yet to be confirmed by other reports.

Pathologic Features and Pathogenesis

Placental-site nodules are usually *too small to be visible by gross inspection.* When they are visible, they consist of single or multiple, small, focally *hemorrhagic pale-tan nodules or plaques in the endometrium or the superficial myometrium measuring from 1 to 4 mm in diameter.* They are commonly located in the lower uterine segment or the cervix. Microscopically, PSNs consist of *well-circumscribed, rounded nodules or plaques with prominent hyalinization and fibrinoid deposition* (Fig. 25.1). They may have *central hyalinization with a more cellular peripheral zone of EVT* (Fig. 25.2). The cells are arranged singly or in clusters, and contain *eosinophilic or amphophilic cytoplasm that is often vacuolated and appears degenerative.* The cell borders are often indistinct, merging with the extracellular material. The *nuclei may be degenerative or smudgy* in appearance as well (Fig. 25.3). Occasionally they are pale and vesicular, lobulated, or infrequently, bizarre. *Mitotic activity is minimal or absent* and nodules stained immunohistochemically for Ki-67, show positivity in less than 5% of cells (Ki-67 labeling index). The nodule also may contain scattered chronic inflammatory cells and fibroblasts. In over one-half of the cases, small extensions or *"pseudopods" consisting of EVT admixed with eosinophilic, fibrinoid material extend into the surrounding tissue.* The fibrinoid material in particular is similar to keratinization and may mimic invasive squamous carcinoma. The frequent location of PSNs in the cervix may thus be problematic. The adjacent endometrium is usually proliferative or secretory. PSNs are not associated with chorionic villi or elevation in serum β-hCG levels.

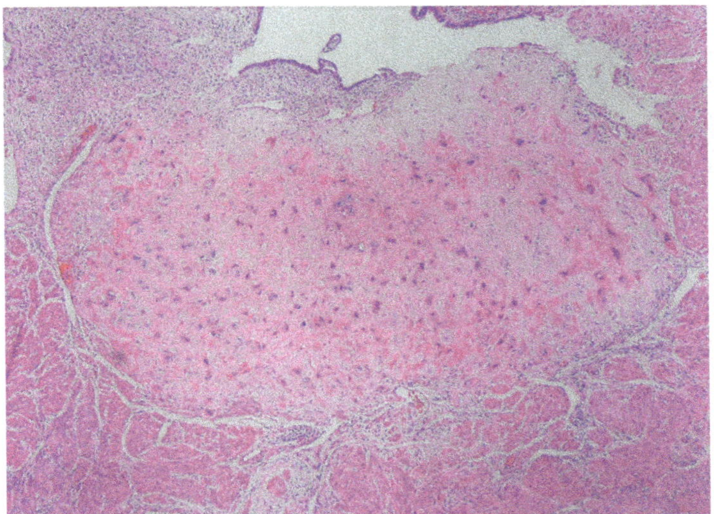

Figure 25.1. Incidental placental site nodule/plaque in a hysterectomy specimen. H&E ×40.

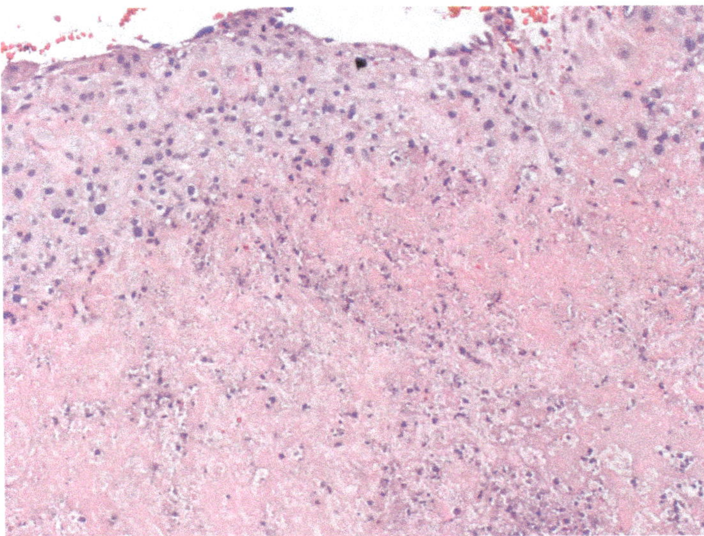

Figure 25.2. Placental site nodule showing hyalinization and degenerative change. Extravillous trophoblast is present in the *upper portion* of the figure. H&E ×200.

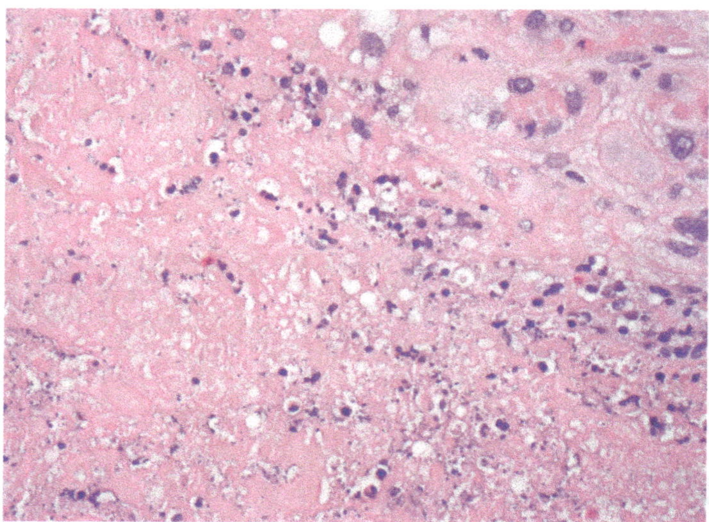

Figure 25.3. Placental site nodule with degenerated and vacuolated nuclei. H&E ×360.

Exaggerated Placental Site

Clinical Features and Implications
Exaggerated placental site (EPS) is a *nonneoplastic, albeit exuberant, proliferation of EVT in the implantation site, associated with pregnancy.* It occurs in 1.6% of first trimester abortion specimens and represents an *"excessive" physiologic response* of EVT. The original name of syncytial endometritis for lesion reflects the presence of many placental site giant cells in the implantation site.

Pathologic Features
Exaggerated placental site is *not identifiable on gross examination.* On microscopic examination, the architecture of the endometrial and myometrial tissue in the placental site is maintained. The trophoblastic cells *proliferate in and around the endometrial glands and smooth muscle fibers without destructive invasion* (Fig. 25.4). The extravillous trophoblastic cells have moderately abundant *eosinophilic or amphophilic cytoplasm and nuclei, which are sometimes irregular or hyperchromatic.* Occasional multinucleated cells are also present. *Mitotic activity is minimal or absent,* and the Ki-67 labeling index is low. Intermixed with the trophoblastic cells are variable numbers of smooth muscle cells, decidual cells, and inflammatory cells, and the *fibrinoid material* that is so characteristic of EVT. These lesions occur concomitant with pregnancy, and therefore *chorionic villi are almost always present.* Their presence is an important clue in diagnosis. The significance of this lesion lies primarily in its common association with complete hydatidiform moles and in its differentiation from other trophoblastic lesions. *Differentiation of EPS from a normal implantation site is rather arbitrary, as there are no specific criteria.* This is in part because "normal" placental sites are rarely sampled or

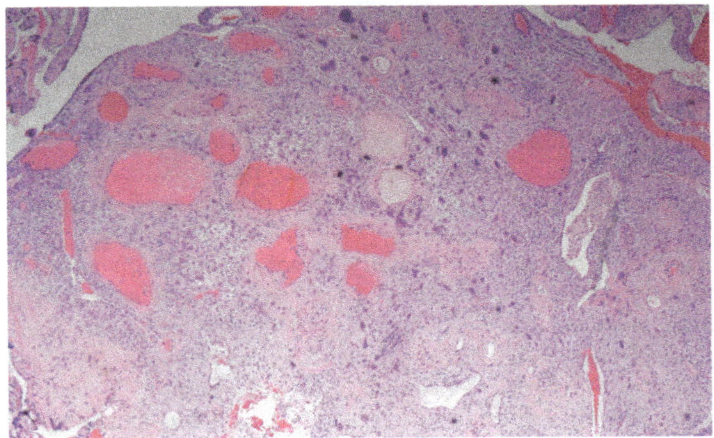

Figure 25.4. Exaggerated placental site. Note preservation of glandular architecture and the exuberant trophoblastic proliferation. Multinucleated trophoblast are also present. H&E ×20.

observed by pathologists. Diagnosis may be made when the proliferation of EVT is significantly more prominent than usual.

Placental-Site Trophoblastic Tumor

Clinical Features
Placental-site trophoblastic tumor (PSTT) is a rare gestational tumor deriving from EVT. Like other trophoblastic lesions, PSTTs occur predominantly in reproductive-age women and have been reported in patients as young as 18 and as old as 62 years of age. PSTTs may occur after abortions, term pregnancies, or moles. In contrast to choriocarcinoma in which 50% develop after a hydatidiform mole, only 5–8% of PSTTs develop after a molar pregnancy. The interval from the previous known pregnancy has been reported to be as little a several months to as long as 18 years.

Patients most commonly present with *abnormal uterine bleeding or amenorrhea*. In comparison to choriocarcinoma, in which virtually all patients have marked elevations in serum β-hCG levels, in PSTT, *β-hCG levels are only moderately elevated and only in 80% of patients*. The presence of *uterine enlargement, abnormal bleeding, and a positive pregnancy test* often leads to the presumptive diagnosis of pregnancy, missed abortion, or ectopic pregnancy. In rare cases, patients may present with abdominal pain, virilization, spider angiomata of the skin, infertility, galactorrhea, or renal failure.

Pathologic Features
Lesions arise primarily in the *myometrium and endomyometrium* but occasionally may involve, or extend to, the cervix. They vary in size from a *few millimeters to large, bulky masses measuring up to 10 cm in diameter*. Most commonly, they have ill-defined borders (Fig. 25.5), but

occasionally they may be grossly well circumscribed. On cut section, the tumor is generally *soft, tan-white to yellow. Focal hemorrhage and necrosis are sometimes identified;* however, the hemorrhage and necrosis are much less conspicuous than in choriocarcinoma. PSTTs are deeply invasive into the uterine wall in 60% of patients, and extension to the serosa may result in *uterine perforation* at presentation or curettage. Some tumors have extended through the uterine wall to involve the fallopian tube or broad ligament.

Microscopic examination typically reveals an *infiltrative mass* within the endomyometrium composed of *infiltrating sheets and cords of predominantly mononuclear EVT, which separate and split apart individual smooth muscle fibers* (Fig. 25.6). *The histologic appearance is quite variable,* both from tumor to tumor and within the same tumor. The tumor cells are predominantly *polygonal with moderately abundant dense amphophilic, eosinophilic, or clear cytoplasm* (Fig. 25.7). Tumor cells may also be *spindled,* and in some tumors, the majority of cells are spindled. A minority of the EVT may be binucleated or trinucleated, and contain nuclei similar to those within the mononuclear cells. Often scattered throughout

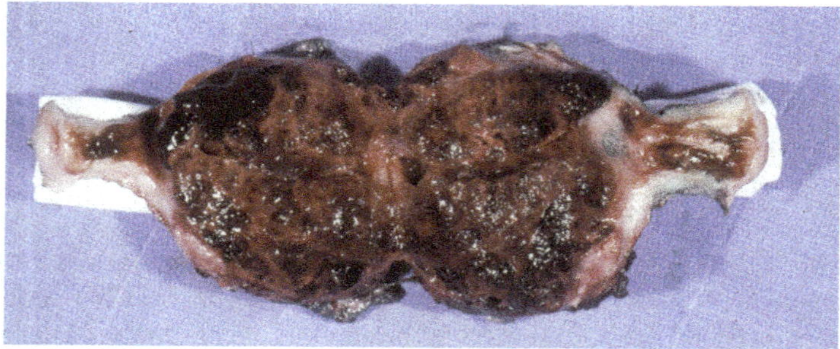

Figure 25.5. PSTT. An ill-defined, hemorrhagic, and necrotic tumor fills the endometrial cavity.

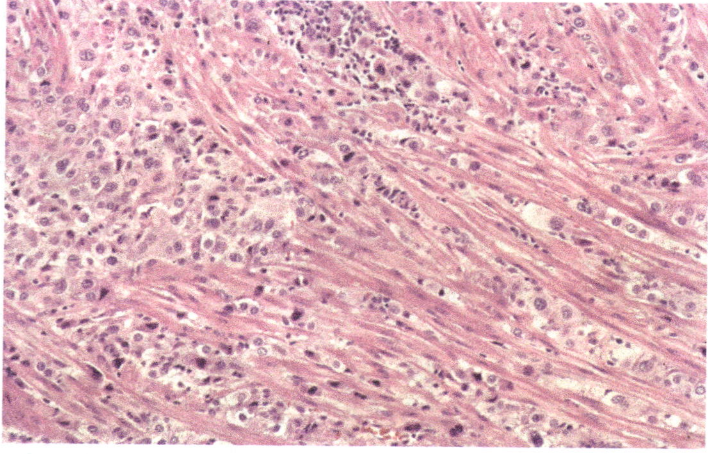

Figure 25.6. PSTT. Sheets of EVT proliferate between and split apart smooth muscle fibers. H&E ×200.

the tumor are multinucleated cells with irregular, hyperchromatic, or smudgy nuclei similar to syncytiotrophoblast; however, these are generally scarce. The cells may be relatively monomorphic (Fig. 25.8) or show marked nuclear pleomorphism and atypia (Fig. 25.9). Nuclear folding and intranuclear pseudoinclusions may also be seen. *Nucleoli, though, are usually small and indistinct,* but focally may be quite large and prominent. The mitotic rate ranges from less than 1 to more than 30 mitoses per 10 high-power field (hpf). Atypical mitotic figures are seen in up in 90% of cases.

Coagulative tumor cell necrosis, hemorrhage, and focal inflammation are seen in over two thirds of these tumors. One of the *most characteristic features is the presence of extracellular fibrinoid material* similar to that present in the normal implantation site. This feature is also present in over 90% of cases (Fig. 25.10). In approximately two thirds of cases,

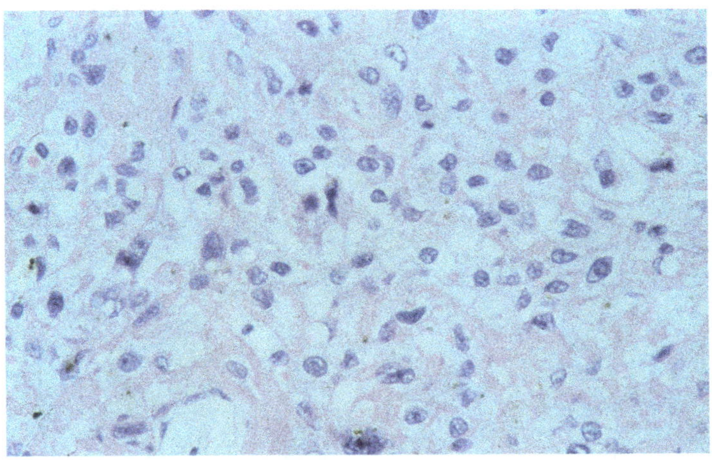

Figure 25.7. Variant of PSTT with clear cytoplasm. H&E ×300.

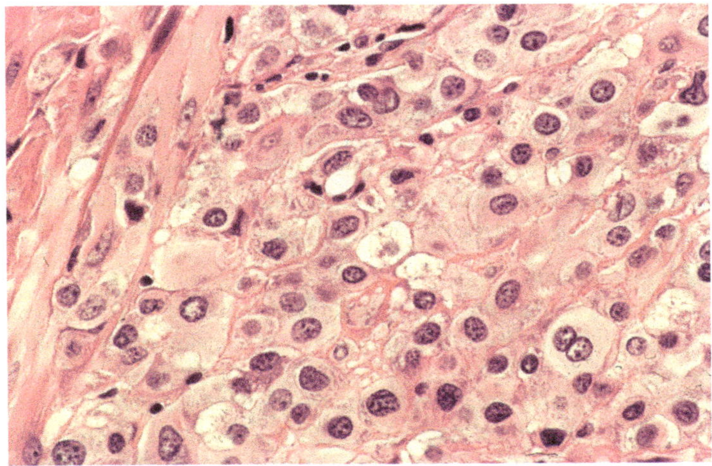

Figure 25.8. Relatively monomorphic population of EVT with minimal atypia in PSTT. H&E ×160.

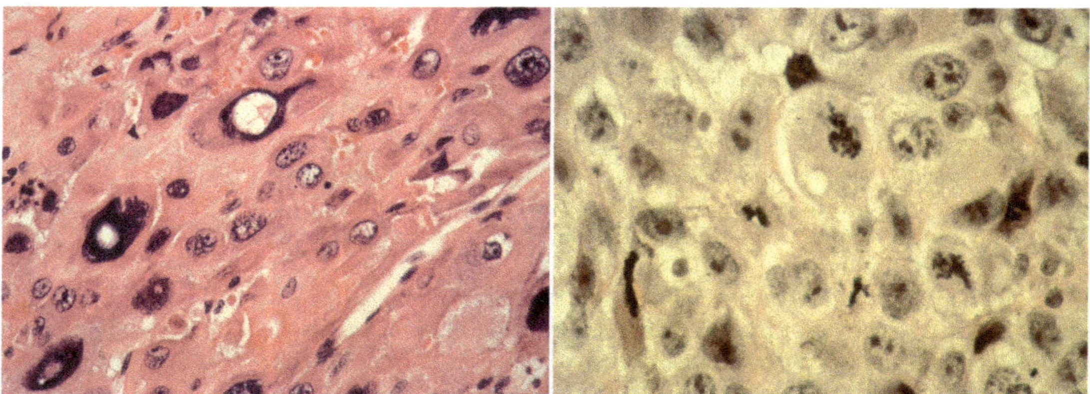

Figure 25.9. PSTT. Marked nuclear pleomorphism (*left*) is present in this tumor, which also shows with easily identifiable mitotic figures (*right*). H&E ×400.

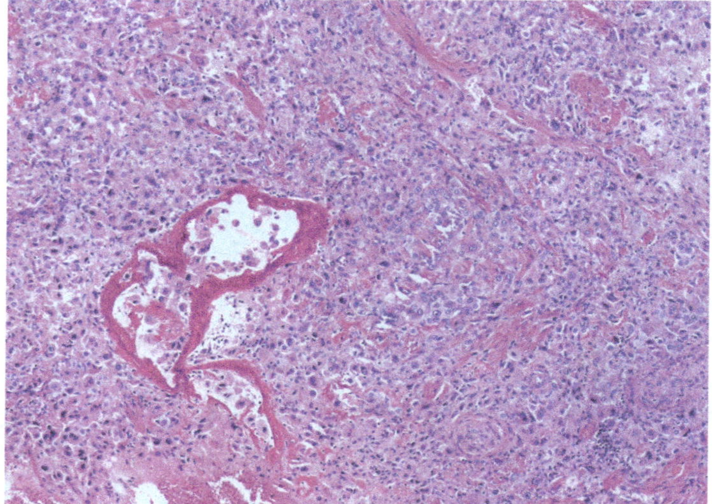

Figure 25.10   PSTT. Prominent fibrinoid deposition is present. H&E ×100.

there is a peculiar form of *vascular invasion* that recapitulates the normal implantation site in that there is replacement of the vascular wall by trophoblast and the presence of intraluminal trophoblast (Fig. 25.11). The uninvolved endometrium is usually decidualized or secretory, but occasionally is proliferative or inactive.

Clinical Implications
Most PSTTs behave in a benign manner. The remaining 10–15% of patients shows aggressive disease with metastasis and even death. Metastases have been reported in the *lungs, liver, vagina, gastrointestinal tract, pelvis, bladder, brain, ovary, omentum, diaphragm, spleen, pancreas, pelvic lymph nodes, and bone marrow.* Lung metastases are the most common. Metastasis to the brain is usually fatal due to intracranial hemorrhage. Late metastasis or recurrence has been reported 5 years after initial diagnosis. Prognosis is heavily dependent on Stage. Survival at 10 years is 90% in stage 1 tumors, 52% in stage II tumors, and 49% in stage III and IV tumors.

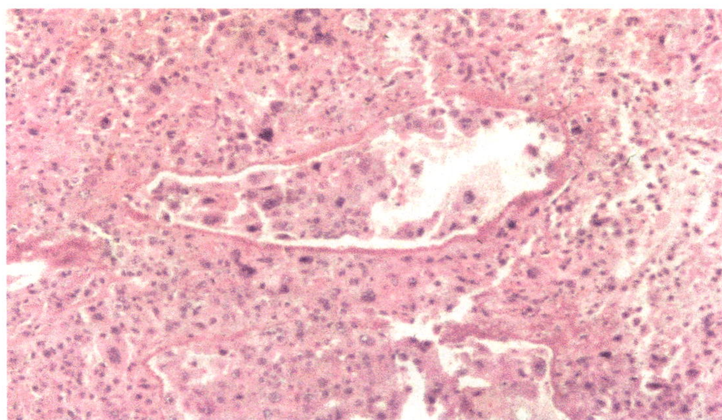

Figure 25.11. PSTT. Typical "vascular invasion." H&E ×200.

Unfortunately, at present there is no way of accurately predicting which tumors will behave in a malignant manner. Recent attempts to find clinical and histologic features that could serve as prognostic factors have generally been disappointing. This having been said, some features are more common in patients that develop distant metastases. The most important prognostic factor is the International Federation of Gynecology and Obstetrics (FIGO) trophoblastic staging. Histologic factors that have been associated with poor prognosis are *deep myometrial invasion, cervical involvement, increased mitotic activity, and clear cytoplasm.* Clinical factors associated with a poorer prognosis are *more advanced age at diagnosis, increased interval from preceding pregnancy, preceding term pregnancy, and high maximum serum levels of β-hCG.* Recently, occurrence of the tumor more than 48 months after preceding pregnancy was the most important prognostic factor other than stage. Caution must be used when predicting the behavior of individual tumors, as some tumors with low mitotic rates have metastasized and some with pelvic extension or metastasis have ultimately had an indolent or even benign course without treatment.

In most patients with disease confined to the uterus, e.g., stage I, the treatment of choice is *hysterectomy.* Conservative local excision has been advocated for some patients with limited disease. Unfortunately, patients with metastatic PSTT have not experienced the success seen in patients with choriocarcinoma who have been treated with chemotherapy. Some patients with advanced disease have been cured, but outcome is variable. Generally speaking, patients at higher stages are usually treated with combined surgery and multiagent chemotherapy. Patients may be followed for treatment response or to monitor the disease with serial serum β-hCG determinations because the levels fall to normal in remission and rise with disease recurrence or metastasis. This is not useful in all patients, as 20% of patients do not have an elevation in serum β-hCG.

Differential Diagnosis

Placental-site trophoblastic tumor must be distinguished from other lesions of EVT, from choriocarcinoma, and from nontrophoblastic lesions, particularly poorly differentiated carcinomas. Clinical features that may be used in differentiating extravillous trophoblastic lesions are summarized in Table 25.1, pathologic features in Table 25.2, and immunohistochemical findings in Table 25.3.

Differential Diagnosis: PSTT Versus Lesions of EVT

Since PSN, EPS, and PSTT derive from EVT, differentiation between lesions may sometimes be difficult. PSTTs are infiltrative tumors with mitotic activity, hemorrhage, necrosis, and vascular invasion, and are quite cellular. PSNs, on the other hand, are well-circumscribed nodules with hyalinization and a degenerative appearance that can usually be recognized as benign lesions, despite the presence of irregular extensions into the adjacent tissue or pseudopods. Neither EPSs nor PSNs produce a mass lesion or grow in an infiltrative pattern. Neither PSTTs nor PSNs contain chorionic villi, a feature that usually distinguishes both from an EPS.

Immunohistochemical studies of PSN, EPS, and PSTT confirm origin from EVT, with positivity for epithelial markers such as cytokeratin and EMA, positivity for trophoblastic markers such as human placental lactogen (hPL), human chorionic gonadotropin (hCG), placental alkaline phosphatase (PLAP), Mel-CAM (CD146), and α-inhibin. PSNs show diffuse positivity for PLAP and P63 and only focal positivity for hPL and Mel-CAM, while PSTTs show the opposite pattern with diffuse positivity for hPL and Mel-CAM and only focal positivity for PLAP and hCG, and negativity for P63. This is similar to the staining pattern of *EVT in the chorion laeve, and it has been suggested that PSNs derive from those cells.* The difference in immunohistochemical profiles is summarized in Table 25.3. Ki-67 is also useful as PSN has a labeling index of <5%, while PSTT may have a labeling index of up to 14%.

Clinical information may be essential in the differentiation of these lesions. PSTT usually presents clinically as a mass, so information gained from physical examination or various types of imaging studies may be very helpful in adjudicating difficult cases. Patients with PSN do not have elevations in serum β-hCG, while those with EPS will have elevations consistent with an intrauterine pregnancy. Since 80% of patients with PSTT have elevations, this may help distinguish these lesions. *When it is difficult to distinguish PSTT from a PSN, serum β-hCG levels should be requested.*

Differential Diagnosis: PSTT Versus Choriocarcinoma

The main difference between *choriocarcinoma and PSTT is that the former consists almost exclusively of villous trophoblast while the latter consists almost exclusively of extravillous trophoblast.* Although rare "monophasic" variants of choriocarcinoma have been described, choriocarcinoma typically consists of cytotrophoblast and syncytiotrophoblast with a typical biphasic pattern, as opposed to the monophasic proliferation of the EVT seen in PSTT.

Immunohistochemistry is helpful in differentiating EVT from villous trophoblast, as PSTTs will be positive for markers of EVT, while mononuclear cytotrophoblast is generally negative for those markers and hCG. Syncytiotrophoblast is not difficult to distinguish from EVT due to its multinucleation, the presence of atypical hyperchromatic nuclei, and strong immunoreactivity for hCG. However, occasional multinucleated syncytial cells may be seen in PSTT that stain positive for hCG. In addition, rare trophoblastic tumors have been described that have features of both PSTT and choriocarcinoma. These may represent tumors of stem cell trophoblast that have divergent differentiation.

Differentiation of PSTT from Other Tumors

Often, the infiltrative and malignant nature of PSTT is obvious, but its origin remains obscure. It may be misinterpreted as a type of poorly differentiated carcinoma or even a sarcoma. *The fibrinoid produced by EVT often suggests keratin, and as a result PSTT may be confused with squamous cell carcinoma.* This is particularly problematic when the tumor is present in the cervix. Although both tumors are cytokeratin positive, markers for EVT will be negative in squamous carcinomas. Occasionally, *PSTT may be confused with a sarcoma, in particular epithelioid leiomyosarcoma, or with a mesothelioma showing deciduoid morphology.* Immunohistochemistry will also easily differentiate between these tumors.

Epithelioid Trophoblastic Tumor

Clinical Features and Implications

The **epithelioid trophoblastic tumor** (ETT) is a recently described tumor believed to *arise from EVT of the chorion laeve.* It has immunohistochemical similarities to PSN and thus may represent its neoplastic equivalent. Clinical features are indistinguishable from PSTT. Patients generally are in the reproductive age group and present with vaginal bleeding. Most patients have an elevated β-hCG. The interval from preceding pregnancy is up to 18 years. *Approximately 25% of the reported cases have been malignant,* similar to that reported for PSTT. *Treatment and follow-up have also been similar to PSTT.*

Pathologic Features

On gross examination, ETTs are *tan to yellow, fleshy, infiltrative nodules in the endomyometrium* measuring up to 5 cm in diameter. Like PSNs, they are *commonly seen in the lower uterine segment.* They tend to show more necrosis than typical PSTTs. On histologic section, ETTs have a distinctive appearance with nests of *small, relatively uniform trophoblastic cells clustered around small vessels with surrounding geographic necrosis* (Fig. 25.12). The tumor cells are smaller and more monomorphic compared to those in a typical PSTT. The cells usually have *clear or vacuolated cytoplasm, and the nuclei contain finely dispersed chromatin with identifiable nucleoli.* The mitotic rate is variable. Many ETTs focally show a pattern reminiscent of typical PSTT.

Extrauterine Lesions of Extravillous Trophoblast

As with hydatidiform moles and choriocarcinoma, *lesions of EVT may occur in ectopic locations, such as the fallopian tube, ovary, mesosalpinx, and broad ligament.* Reported cases have included both PSNs and PSTTs. They are similar in appearance and behavior to their uterine counterparts and are *presumed to arise from previous ectopic pregnancies.* They are frequently associated with chronic salpingitis and endometriosis.

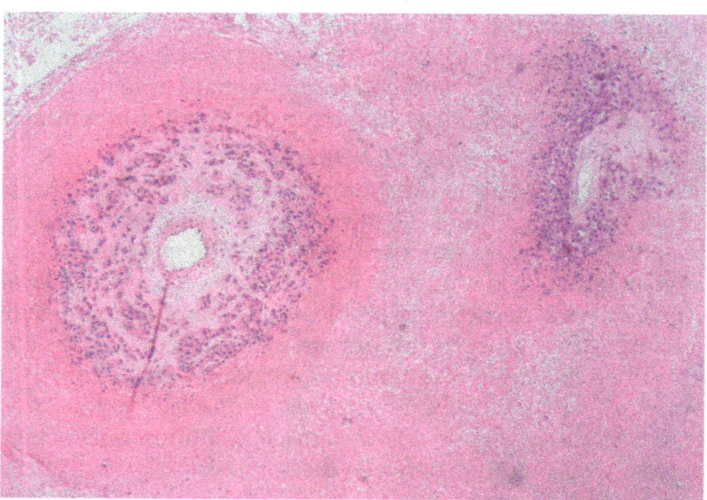

Figure 25.12. Epithelioid trophoblastic tumor consisting of a relatively mono-morphic population of extravillous trophoblast surrounded by geographic necrosis. H&E ×20.

Another lesion, called **"trophoblastic implants,"** "residual tro-phoblastic tissue," or "persistent ectopic pregnancy," has also been described. Trophoblastic implants occur in up to 29% of patients with ectopic pregnancies treated conservatively with laparoscopic salpingostomy. They may be found in the adnexa, pelvic peritoneum, or even the omentum, and are *thought to represent residual extrauter-ine implantation sites that have not undergone full involution or excision.* Grossly, they appear as *hemorrhagic nodules* and may be confused with endometriosis by the surgeon. Microscopically, they consist of *degenerative nodules composed of EVT admixed with chorionic villi.* They do not show the hyalinization of PSNs, nor the infiltrative features, cytologic atypia, and proliferative activity of PSTTs. Serum β-hCG levels are often elevated. Patients may require additional surgery for excision of the lesions, but clinical follow-up has been benign.

Suggestions for Examination and Report
(Extravillous trophoblastic lesions)

Gross Examination: PSN and EPS are not grossly identifiable. PSTTs and ETTs are generally evident as infiltrative masses in the endomyometrium. Sufficient sections should be taken to adequately sample the tumor given its variable histologic pattern and to pro-vide sufficient information for staging.

Comment: Immunohistochemistry is particularly useful in the diagnosis of these lesions. If diagnosis of a PSTT or ETT cannot defi-nitely be made, serum β-hCG levels may be requested. If positive, it is helpful in making the diagnosis as well as for follow up. If nega-tive, a neoplastic process cannot be ruled out. With PSN and EPS, a comment may be made about the benign nature of the lesion.

Table 25.1. Clinical features of trophoblastic lesions.

	PSN	EPS	PSTT/ETT	CCA
H/O previous mole	–	–	5–8%	50%
Serum β-hCG	Normal	Appropriate for pregnancy	Moderately elevated in 80%	Markedly elevated
Symptoms	50% have abnormal uterine bleeding	Related to pregnancy	Bleeding, uterine enlargement, or mass	Bleeding, uterine enlargement
Location	Often in lower uterine segment or cervix	Endometrium	Endomyometrium	Endomyometrium
Treatment	None	None	Hysterectomy; chemotherapy if malignant	Chemotherapy
Metastasis	None	None	Occurs in 10–15% of cases	Potential for metastasis
Prognosis	No sequelae	No sequelae	Guarded if malignant	>90% responsive to chemotherapy

PSN placental site nodule, *EPS* exaggerated placental site, *PSTT* placental-site trophoblastic tumor, *ETT* epithelioid trophoblastic tumors, *CCA* choriocarcinoma

Table 25.2. Histopathologic features of trophoblastic lesions.

	PSN	EPS	PSTT	ETT	CCA
Forms a mass	–	–	+	+	+/–
Chorionic villi present	–	+	Very rare	Very rare	–[a]
Fibrinoid	+	+	+	–	–
Hemorrhage	–	+/–	+	+	++
Necrosis	–	+/–	+	++	++
Vascular invasion	–	–	+	+	+
Degenerative changes	+	–	–	–	+
Extravillous trophoblast	+	+	+	+	–
Syncytiotrophoblast	–	+	–[b]	–	++
Nuclear pleomorphism	–	–	++	–	++
Mitotic activity	Minimal or absent	Minimal or absent	+	+	+

[a]Villi are present only in placental or in-situ choriocarcinoma (see Chap. 24)
[b]Multinucleated cells similar to syncytiotrophoblast may be present

Table 25.3. Immunohistochemistry of trophoblastic lesions.

	PSN	EPS	PSTT	ETT	CCA
Cytokeratin	+	+	+	+	+
EMA	+	+	+	+	+
hCG	Weak focal	+	Weak focal	Weak focal	+++
hPL	Focal	Diffuse	Diffuse	Focal	Focal
PLAP	Diffuse	Focal	Focal	Diffuse	
Mel-CAM	Focal	Diffuse	Diffuse	Focal	
Major basic protein	+/−	+	+	+	−
P63	+	−	−	+	+/−
α-inhibin	+	+	+	+	−
Ki-67	<5%		5–15%	5–15%	

Selected References

PHP5, Chapter 23, pages 846–853.

Allison KH, Love JE, Garcia RL. Epithelioid trophoblastic tumor: review of a rare neoplasm of the chorionic-type intermediate trophoblast. Arch Pathol Lab Med 2006;130:1875–1877.

Baergen RN, Rutgers JL. Trophoblastic lesions of the placental site. Gen Diagn Pathol 1997;143:143–158.

Baergen RN, Rutgers JL, Young RH. Extrauterine lesions of intermediate trophoblast. Int J Gynecol Pathol 2003;22:362–367.

Finkler NJ, Berkowitz RS, Driscoll SG, et al. Clinical experience with placental site trophoblastic tumors at the New England Trophoblastic Disease Center. Obstet Gynecol 1988;71:854–857.

Huetter PC, Gersell DJ. Placental site nodule: an analysis of 40 cases. Mod Pathol 1993;4:74A;abstract 422.

Kurman RJ, Main CS, Chen H-C. Intermediate trophoblast: a distinctive form of trophoblast with specific morphological, biochemical and functional features. Placenta 1984;5:349–370.

Roberts JP, Lurain JR. Treatment of low-risk metastatic gestational trophoblastic tumors with single-agent chemotherapy. Am J Obstet Gynecol 1996;174:1917–1924.

Rutgers JL, Baergen RN, Young RH, et al. Placental site trophoblastic tumor: clinicopathologic study of 64 cases. Mod Pathol 1995;8:96A.

Schmid P, Nagai Y, Agarwal R, et al. Prognostic markers and long-term outcome of placental-site trophoblastic tumours: a retrospective observational study. Lancet 2009;374:48–55.

Scully RE, Young RH. Trophoblastic pseudotumor: a reappraisal. Am J Surg Pathol 1981;5:75–76.

Shih I-M, Kurman RJ. Epithelioid trophoblastic tumor. A neoplasm distinct from choriocarcinoma and placental site trophoblastic tumor simulating carcinoma. Am J Surg Pathol 1998;22:1393–1403.

Shitabata PK, Rutgers JL. The placental site nodule: an immunohistochemical study. Hum Pathol 1993;25:1295–1301.

Young RH, Kurman RJ, Scully RE. Placental site nodules and plaques. A clinicopathologic analysis of 20 cases. Am J Surg Pathol 1990;14:1001–1009.

Section VII

Legal Considerations and New Directions

This final section differs from the previous sections in that it discusses the application of placental pathology rather than pathology itself. Chapter 26 discusses legal aspects to placental examination. It is not intended as advice on how to perform expert review in legal cases, but rather as a guide for the practicing pathologist. It is hoped that it will give the reader a sense of the importance of placental pathology in understanding perinatal outcome, and provide guidance on maximizing the benefit to the patient as well as the potential expert who might examine the case in the future. The subject of Chap. 27 is future directions and is written by Kurt Benirschke. This chapter covers new and fascinating discoveries and advances in the field of placental pathology.

Chapter 26
Legal Considerations

General Considerations

Numerous litigations against hospitals and obstetricians take place in which the placental findings become an important issue for lawyers when advising the disputing parties on perinatal circumstances. These litigations are initiated most often on behalf of children with cerebral palsy, children with some level of neurologic impairment, children with malformations, stillborns, or children with other less than optimal

R.N. Baergen, *Manual of Pathology of the Human Placenta,*
DOI 10.1007/978-1-4419-7494-5_26, © Springer Science+Business Media, LLC 2011

or expected outcomes. A number of lawsuits are filed merely because there is an unexpected or poor outcome and not because there is the perception that medical negligence has occurred. There is ongoing controversy over the etiology and timing of neurologic injury in infants. This is due, at least in part, to poorly defined antenatal "risk factors" and limitations in the ability to identify fetal distress during labor and delivery.

There is no doubt that there has been an increase in the overall incidence of cerebral palsy because of the increasing prematurity of babies for whom care is provided. Moreover, with increased usage of assisted reproductive technology, there are more multiple births, which are often preterm and have increased morbidity and mortality. They are also delivered by much older mothers, and these are all factors of importance in cerebral palsy. Our understanding of how cerebral palsy develops is still imperfect. The study of the causes of cerebral palsy is a difficult aspect of medicine, as no single etiology can possibly be assigned. Conclusions made from the 56,000 pregnancies in the Collaborative Perinatal Study were that chronic, rather than acute, hypoxia has a greater influence in causing abnormal brain development. Cerebral palsy obviously has great social importance; the disease often represents a major tragedy to the families involved, let alone to the child.

The Placenta in Litigation

The placenta is a reflection of intrauterine life, providing a wealth of information on prenatal events. It may be helpful in understanding adverse outcome in several ways. First, the *placenta itself may be abnormal and thus the cause of the adverse outcome*. This is the case in primary lesions of the placenta, such as maternal floor infarction, as well as maternal diseases, such as preeclampsia. At times, the placenta itself is functionally normal, but *reflects an adverse intrauterine environment*. Such is the case with severe fetomaternal hemorrhage, in which the placenta is markedly pale and hydropic due to the severe fetal anemia. Finally, the placenta may *show no abnormality* and thus may not be helpful in determining causation. In the latter case, certain pathologic processes may be ruled out and the specific etiology must be sought elsewhere.

It is now apparent to many health care providers that, when caring for problematic neonates or when difficulties in labor and delivery are encountered, the placenta should be examined professionally. The legal profession has also recognized that placental examination is helpful in adjudicating litigations relating to neurologic injury. Although experts in perinatal pathology may be asked to review these cases, the general pathologist usually receives the placenta and examines it first. All too often, when placental consultation is requested, the placental material available is insufficient for an expert opinion. Recommendations have been made (see Chap. 3) on how to collect and examine placentas. It is regrettable that, occasionally, erroneous testimony is given in good faith because the consultant did not have the benefit of a complete gross examination and was not made aware of the perinatal circumstances. Of course, a pathologist should not be put into the position of making judgments on monitor strips and the like, but must have a general idea of the entirety of these complex cases before the placental examination can be meaningfully interpreted.

It is most important that placentas be *adequately sampled for histology*. When selecting the villous tissue, it is important that more than the obviously infarcted or pathologic areas be sampled; most infarcts look alike microscopically. For an appreciation of the placental status, *the more normal-appearing villous tissue is usually most informative*. It is often beneficial to have *photographs of the placenta* available, particularly when confronted with the record of a poorly described or inadequately studied placenta. If photography is impractical, a drawing of salient findings, e.g., to indicate the insertion of the umbilical cord or the presence of twin vascular anastomoses, is often more helpful than a poor description of the gross features. Another important aspect to gross examination is the evaluation of the *extent or involvement of any macroscopic lesions*. The percentage of villous tissue involved as well as the location (peripheral versus central) of the lesions should always be noted. If adequate initial examination is performed, proper interpretation can be made, even if it occurs at a later date.

Twinning Problems

Multiple births have not only a much higher incidence of prematurity and demise, but also suffer an increased frequency of cerebral palsy compared with singletons. It should be understood that the umbilical cords of twins must be labeled at delivery, so that it becomes possible to assign specific placental lesions to individual infants. Central nervous system (CNS) damage of prenatal onset appears to be more common in **monozygotic–monochorionic** twins than in dizygotic twins, and this is primarily *due to the vascular anastomoses* between the placentas. If one wants to understand the origin of the lesions, *it is imperative that the membrane relation and vascular anastomoses of all twins be firmly established during placental study*. The anastomoses are best recorded by making a drawing of these connections; they cannot otherwise be easily reconstructed. This point is particularly important when one twin has died prenatally. Coagulative, destructive events in the survivor are then especially common due to **acute twin-to-twin transfusion** (see Chap. 10) commencing soon after the death of the co-twin. The notion that "thromboplastic" substances are released from the circulation of the dead twin and cause strokes and other adverse events in the survivor has been shown to be incorrect.

Twins also suffer from **chronic twin-to-twin transfusion syndrome**, an important aspect of monozygotic twinning (Chap. 10). Firm diagnosis requires the demonstration of dominant arteriovenous shunts in the placenta as well as correlative clinical information. Chronic twin-to-twin transfusion usually leads to polyhydramnios in the recipient twin and oligohydramnios in the donor as well as discordant growth. It is associated with premature delivery and often results in fetal demise, usually of the donor twin. When this occurs, the chronic transfusion is reversed and the plethoric recipient twin becomes the anemic donor twin as it acutely exsanguinates into the stillborn twin. This is often referred to as **"acute-on-chronic" twin-to-twin transfusion.** Brain damage or death is often the fate of the surviving twin.

The highest mortality in twins attends **monoamnionic–monochorionic** twins due to *frequent entanglement of their cords.* This complication often kills one or both fetuses; in others, venous return problems are evident by the presence of fetal vascular thrombosis. Monoamnionic twins also have vascular anastomoses and thus may suffer from rapid shifts of blood from one twin to the other, which may lead to acute anemia and hypotension in utero.

Inflammatory Processes

Acute Chorioamnionitis

Ascending infections, as evidenced by the presence of **acute chorioamnionitis** and **acute funisitis,** *are much overrepresented in children who develop cerebral palsy and neurologic impairment.* These pathologic findings have also been correlated with prenatal cystic lesions in the brain. Studies have suggested that the mechanism may be the result of vasoconstriction, engendered by the release of prostaglandins, tumor necrosis factor, or other vasoactive agents and cytokines that come either from the inflammatory exudate or from bacterial products in the amniotic cavity. Moreover, various inflammatory mediators have been shown to cause direct neuronal injury, astrogliosis, and inhibition of oligodendrocyte maturation. Since ascending infection often leads to premature delivery, the infants are also susceptible to the risk factors associated with prematurity. Chorioamnionitis is an occasional cause of thrombosis in fetal surface vessels (see Chap. 16). The correlation with cerebral palsy is stronger is cases in which there is a fetal inflammatory response, specifically a severe fetal inflammatory response, i.e., when there is inflammation in the chorionic vessels, inflammation in the umbilical vessels, and particularly when there is thrombosis of these vessels. Adequate sampling of the membranes, fetal surface, and fetal surface vessels is essential to determining the extent of the infection and its possible impact on fetal morbidity and mortality.

Chronic Villitis

Chronic villitis may be of infectious or of unknown etiology. In suspected viral infections, it is difficult to identify the specific infection by histopathological study alone. Immunohistochemistry, polymerase chain reaction (PCR), DNA hybridization, or other methods may then be used to identify specific organisms. Unfortunately, some viruses, such as human immunodeficiency virus, leave no characteristic alterations in the placenta. **Cytomegalovirus** infection is perhaps the most common prenatal virus infection of relevance to cerebral palsy-type lesions. Significant damage to the fetal brain and other organs occurs frequently from this infection, and the placenta often shows characteristic chronic villitis with plasma cells (see Chap. 16). Nevertheless, these changes are frequently widely scattered in the placenta, sometimes affecting only a few villi, and thus may be difficult to find. Infection with **herpes virus** before birth may lead to destructive encephalopathy, porencephaly, and neonatal death. However, when these infants come to autopsy, neither culture nor electron microscopy will identify the now vanished agent.

Villitis of unknown etiology (VUE) is an alteration of villi in which there is an infiltrate of lymphocytes, macrophages, and rare plasma cells, and it is associated with villous destruction (see Chap. 16). As the name suggests, the underlying pathophysiologic process is unknown. It is often indistinguishable from infectious villitis. VUE reduces the area of placental exchange and, if severe, may be associated with *fetal death and growth restriction*. If there is associated obliterative vasculopathy, there is significant association with cerebral palsy. The dire significance of VUE is not in doubt, and it has a tendency to recur in future pregnancies. It may be difficult at times to differentiate VUE from infectious villitis.

Vascular Abnormalities

Fetal Thrombotic Vasculopathy

Abnormalities of the umbilical cord and placental surface vessels are important findings in placental examinations. It is particularly important to look for thromboses in the fetal surface vessels of every placenta. Many surface **vascular thrombi** are evident macroscopically by the yellow-white streak that is present in a chorionic vessel. Thrombi are more difficult to spot in the umbilical cord. Thrombi may be associated with *cord entanglements, velamentous cords, excessively long cords, or markedly twisted cords* (see Chap. 15). They are also associated with *maternal lupus anticoagulant, maternal diabetes, and thrombophilias*. Vascular thrombosis may be a feature of certain infections such as *acute chorioamnionitis, cytomegalovirus infection, and toxoplasmosis*. There are many other placentas with extensive thrombosis, in which the etiology of the thrombi remains obscure. Thrombosis may be associated with CNS damage, and the thrombi may embolize to the fetus, causing tissue infarcts and strokes. However, unless such an infant comes to autopsy, embolic sequelae are usually not evident. Complete vascular obliteration leads to "atrophy" of the villous district subserved by the vessel. It is the frequent cause of **avascular hyalinized villi** (see Chap. 21) which may thus reduce the quantity of available "exchange membrane"; for this reason, chronic thrombosis correlates *with growth restriction and hypoxia*. **Hemorrhagic endovasculopathy** or **villous-stromal karyorrhexis** (see Chap. 21) has also been specifically associated with adverse neurologic outcome. These lesions have been given the name *fetal thrombotic vasculopathy*. Fetal thrombotic vasculopathy and extensive avascular villi have also been shown to be significantly associated with neurologic impairment. For the purpose of legal adjudication, it is important to recognize this point and to acknowledge that fetal thrombotic vasculopathy is usually a long-standing event and that it can usually not be anticipated before birth.

Umbilical Cord

The cord displays many lesions that have a significant impact on fetal well-being (see Chap. 15). It may also be discolored from hemolysis, especially when thrombi are present or when prenatal bleeding has occurred. True cord **hematomas**, often caused by other lesions in the cord such as **hemangiomas** and **aneurysms**, may lead to hypoxia and subsequent neurologic injury primarily to *compression of the umbilical vessels* and embarrassment of blood flow through the cord. These are uncommonly seen. Compression from **true knots** or **prolapsed cords** may cause significant obstruction and may be accompanied by *marked distention of blood vessels on one side but not the other*, betraying the prenatal compromise of the circulation. The cord may also show **excessive twisting** or **excessive length**. That such excessive spiraling *can lead to fetal death* is not in doubt. More problematic is the chronic effect that may ensue from cord obstruction such as reduced venous return and subsequent fetal *surface vessel (venous) thrombi. Associations with neurologic injury are seen with excessively short cords, excessively long cords, excessively twisted cords, minimally twisted cords, cord entanglements, cord prolapse, and true knots*. **Velamentous insertion** of the umbilical cord and marginal insertions with membranous vessels may also cause significant anemia and hypoxia if the membranes vessels rupture or *thrombose*. Dire fetal sequelae may occur including death or neurologic injury. The abnormalities of the umbilical cord that are associated with adverse outcome are often macroscopic lesions, and so adequate documentation of these findings in the gross description is essential. Photographs are especially helpful.

Meconium – the "Green" Placenta

Prenatal meconium discharge is common and occurs in about 17% of all births. Its presence at birth is a frequent reason for allegations that birth was delayed or inappropriately handled, the suggestion being that it is evidence of fetal distress. In fact, **meconium** discharge, in most cases, is **not** associated with fetal distress or cerebral palsy. *In a mature placenta, meconium discharge occurs primarily because the fetus is mature enough to discharge meconium and thus is physiologic, and not pathologic because of intrauterine stress.* Meconium is extremely rare in immature placentas, and when present **may** be an indication of intrauterine hypoxia. However, when a damaged or stillborn infant is under consideration and its birth is not accompanied by meconium discharge, the question of why the baby did not release meconium is never asked. Interestingly, most stillbirths have no meconium staining, even though, ultimately, anoxia was presumably the cause of their death. The evaluation of the timing of meconium discharge is often discussed and several studies have been performed to investigate this. Unfortunately, the results have not been consistent. Furthermore, the timing of meconium discharge is complicated by the fact that at least in some cases, repeated discharges occur. The legal profession often overemphasizes the importance of meconium discharge, without appreciating the complexity of this process and of cerebral palsy.

Rather than meconium discharge occurring because of fetal distress, it is likely that the *meconium may damage the fetus by acting as a vasoconstrictive agent on the umbilical and superficial placental vessels.* In so doing, it may reduce the venous return of oxygenated blood from the placenta. These avenues are now being explored experimentally. Therefore, when the umbilical cord is meconium stained, *additional sections of the discolored cord should be submitted to identify meconium-induced myonecrosis of the umbilical vessels* (see Chap. 14). Meconium-associated myonecrosis of chorionic plate vessels and umbilical vessels is strongly associated with neurologic impairment. Furthermore, there is some speculation that the real damage of the meconium aspiration syndrome in neonates is a chemical injury to the alveolar epithelium, similar to its effect on amnion and cord vessels leading to a chemical pneumonitis. It is noteworthy that not all meconium-stained placentas are accompanied by fetal meconium aspiration. It must be emphasized that meconium may have been discharged many hours before delivery, and most of it may already have been transported away from the fetal surface when the placenta becomes available for study.

When the membranes or fetal surface of a placenta from a premature infant is discolored green, one must consider the possibility that this discoloration is due to **hemosiderin** and related precursor pigments. Hemosiderin deposits frequently accompany the *peripheral hemorrhages of circumvallate placentas, retromembranous hematomas, marginal hemorrhage, and fetal hemolysis* (see Chap. 14). An iron stain of the placenta quickly reveals the nature of the pigment when doubt exists.

Uteroplacental Malperfusion

Abruptio Placentae

Abruption is a clinical term for premature separation of the placenta from the uterus. The most common underlying etiology is maternal hypertensive disease and thus it is often seen in the context of other lesions of uteroplacental malperfusion. Many cases of placental separation are clinically silent and can be observed only when the maternal surface is carefully scrutinized. The pathologic correlation of abruption is a retroplacental hematoma. A fresh **retroplacental hematoma** will show *indentation of the villous tissue.* In an older lesion, the clot will be drier, stringy, and compacted. When placental separation is focal and has occurred long before delivery, the clot may have largely disappeared, or is replaced by a brown, filmy material. The clot will become adherent to the placental surface within a few hours of separation and then will begin to compress the placental surface. The underlying villous tissue becomes ischemic immediately on separation of the placenta; however, the effects are not visible under the microscope many hours later with collapse of the intervillous space and villous agglutination. Therefore, in abruptios less than 6–12 h old, identification of the retroplacental clot is much easier on gross examination. With increasing time, infarction develops with smudging of the trophoblast nuclei and loss of nuclear basophilia, and eventually the villous tissue becomes pale and ghost-like (see Chap. 18). Sudden separation of more than 50% of the placenta usually results in fetal death. If an abruptio develops over time, the fetus can adjust somewhat, and so larger, but more slowly developing, abruptios may not result in stillbirth. Neurologic injury may still occur. Chronic abruption with hemorrhage and hemosiderin deposition at the periphery of the placenta has also been shown to be associated with neurologic injury.

Infarcts

Small infarcts at the edge of the placenta at term are common and are of little significance. **Multiple infarcts** scattered throughout the placenta, however, signify maternal disease of some sort. This finding assumes particular importance in prematurely delivered infants in whom infarcts are rare. Most commonly, the cause of such infarcts is *preeclampsia or maternal hypertensive disease,* but the lesions due to *lupus anticoagulant* and *thrombophilia* may have a similar appearance (see Chap. 18). When infarcts are found in the absence of maternal disease, their cause requires further study. To understand the fetal impact of infarcts, it is necessary that a *percentage estimate of the amount of infarcted villous tissue* be recorded. If sufficient placental tissue is infarcted, fetal hypoxia develops with the potential for brain injury and even death.

Miscellaneous

Maternal Floor Infarction – Massive Perivillous Fibrin Deposition

Maternal floor infarction is strongly correlated with fetal growth restriction, fetal demise, and neurologic injury in the neonate (see Chap. 19). Gross examination reveals a firm, stiff placenta with abundant deposition of fibrinoid visible on cut section. Appropriate histologic study verifies the existence of excessive fibrinoid deposits. It is clear from histologic examination that the surface exchange area in these placentas is severely limited, and so it is easy to understand how this condition could lead to growth restriction or other sequelae.

The disorder is of unknown etiology and has a tendency to recur in subsequent pregnancies.

Chorangiosis

Chorangiosis is an abnormal condition correlated with *prolonged fetal oxygen deprivation*. It has been associated with *many perinatal problems*. Although minor forms of chorangiosis are reasonably common, its value for our understanding of the fetal/placental/maternal relations has so far been underestimated. That it is associated with hypoxia is supported by the finding of chorangiosis in women gestating at very high altitude, in patients with heart disease, and in other situations in which there is hypoxia, as well as in animal studies. Other correlations exist with *fetal death, diabetes, umbilical cord problems, and other perinatal problems*. It is important to realize that because chorangiosis involves proliferation and formation of new capillaries, it must take weeks to develop.

Nucleated Red Blood Cells

After approximately 28 weeks, the fetal circulation of the placenta contains very few **nucleated red blood cells** (NRBCs). When they are found in sections of the mature placenta, the pathologist must seek an explanation for their presence. It may be obvious that there is evidence of *hemolytic disease or that transplacental bleeding or chronic infection* existed, but often the cause of an excessive number of NRBCs is not immediately evident. Presumably, the human fetus reacts to oxygen deficiency, as it does to anemia, by first releasing and then increasing production of NRBCs from the hepatic or bone marrow stores. There is no consensus as to exactly how acutely this reaction occurs, and to what degree. Probably there is an initial release of already formed, slightly immature NRBCs within a relatively short period. If hypoxia is sustained, the production of red cells is increased and the immature forms are produced and released in increasing numbers. In the case of fetal hemorrhage, some degree of an initial NRBC response may be detectable already *within an hour*. It is thought that the rise of the NRBC count is much slower when due to hypoxia. When the initial NRBC count is very high, it indicates a more severe and prolonged hypoxia. This finding, like chorangiosis, is an indicator of significantly decreased placental reserves.

Placental Pallor

The color of the villous tissue reflects the fetal hemoglobin content. Placentas of diabetic mothers are dark and congested because of fetal plethora, and those of immature infants are lighter. **Pale placentas** occur primarily from infants with hydrops or severe anemia. The latter may be due to *fetomaternal hemorrhage or to fetal bleeding from ruptured velamentous vessels, from a ruptured umbilical cord, or from the fetus itself*. If fetomaternal hemorrhage is suspected, an immediate Kleihauer-Betke stain on maternal blood is strongly suggested (see Chap. 20) to assess the amount of fetal blood loss, and in fact this test should be routinely done in any case of severe placental or fetal pallor or anemia that is unexplained. Significant hypotension and hypoxia may transpire, and this is an important cause of brain injury. But, unfortunately, the diagnosis cannot be made until after delivery. If the amount of fetal blood present in the maternal circulation exceeds 50% of the fetal blood volume, the hemorrhage is likely chronic in nature, as an acute hemorrhage of this magnitude would lead to fetal death. Shock can develop when as little as 20% of the blood volume is suddenly lost. The adjustment of the fetal hematocrit may take some time after fetal blood loss, but we have only the most superficial knowledge of how quickly the hematocrits adjust after fetal bleeding. Occasionally infants become hydropic due to high-output cardiac failure from large **placental chorangiomas**, and these are readily apparent when the placenta is examined and sectioned. Other causes may be maternal trauma, external version, amniocentesis, or rarely abruption.

Villous Changes

Another relevant feature is **villous immaturity or dysmaturity**, the discrepancy of apparent villous maturation with chronological age. In this situation there is delayed maturation and *an increase in villous size, an increase in stromal cells, decreased syncytial knots, and, frequently, increased vascularity*. Irregularly matured villi are frequent in the placentas of a variety of chromosomal abnormalities (see Chap. 11) and maternal diabetes. Alternatively, accelerated villous maturity, as evidenced by **increased syncytial knotting** or **terminal villus deficiency**, signify deficient uteroplacental blood flow of some duration and thus reduced oxygen to the fetus (see Section "Uteroplacental Malperfusion", above). The implication to the fetus must be made in light of other pathologic findings and clinical history. Focal **severe villous edema** has been associated with *premature delivery, neonatal hypoxia, neonatal death, and neurologic injury*. However, further studies are needed to clarify the etiology and development of both villous edema and villous immaturity.

Timing of Fetal Death

In cases of fetal death, the timing of intrauterine death may be important to determine. Genest (1992) has depicted the changes seen after fetal death can provide information on the timing of intrauterine retention after death. The evaluation is based on the fact that autolysis of fetal organs occurs at differing rates. By evaluating the loss of nuclear basophilia in various organs, one can estimate the time of fetal death. Evaluation of the extent of maceration of the fetus as well as stromal karyorrhexis and avascular villi in the placenta is also helpful in determining the timing of death and intrauterine retention.

Conclusion

During legal proceedings, pathologists are frequently asked to determine causation as well as place a time frame for the lesion under discussion. They may be required to specify how quickly villi can become infarcted, what is the exact temporal evolution of thrombi, how long has acute chorioamnionitis been present, and so on. These and other probing questions are often difficult to adjudicate, and the answers may present problems for a conscientious witness. It requires experience, general knowledge, and expertise, and in some cases it may be best to state the lack of our knowledge than to express unwarranted opinions that are contradicted in the courtroom or by other experts. This uncertainty is also an indication for the pathologist to seek new information from appropriate cases in which clinical data corroborate a particular finding.

Selected References

PHP5, Chapter 28, pages 1001–1026.

Altshuler GA. Conceptual approach to placental pathology and pregnancy outcome. Semin Diagn Pathol 1993;10:204–221.

Baergen RN. The placenta as witness. Clin Perinatol 2007;34:393–407.

Bejar R, Vigliocco G, Gramajo H, et al. Antenatal origin of neurologic damage in newborn infants. Part II. Multiple gestations. Am J Obstet Gynecol 1990;162:1230–1236.

Benirschke K. The placenta in the litigation process. Am J Obstet Gynecol 1990;162:1445–1450.

Benirschke K. The use of the placenta in the understanding of perinatal injury. In: Fisher DSM, ed. Risk management techniques and neonatal practice. Futura Publishing, Armonk, NY, 1996:325–345.

Genest DR. Estimating the time of death in stillborn fetuses: II. Histologic evaluation of the placenta; a study of 71 stillborns. Obstet Gynecol 1992;80:585–592.

Grafe MR. The correlation of prenatal brain damage with placental pathology. J Neuropathol Exp Neurol 1994;53:407–415.

Kaplan CG. Forensic aspects of the placenta. In: Dimmick JE, Singer DB, eds. Forensic aspects in pediatric pathology. Perspectives of pediatric pathology, Vol. 19. Basel: Karger, 1995:20–42.

Kraus FT. Cerebral palsy and thrombi in placental vessels of the fetus: insights from litigation. Hum Pathol 1997;28:246–248.

Marin-Padilla M. Developmental neuropathology and impact of perinatal brain damage. II: White matter lesions of the neocortex. J Neuropathol Exp Neurol 1997;56:219–235.

Naeye RL, Localio AR. Determining the time before birth when ischemia and hypoxemia initiated cerebral palsy. Obstet Gynecol 1995;86:713–719.

Naeye RL, Peters EC, Bartholomew M, et al. Origins of cerebral palsy. Am J Dis Child 1989;143:1154–1161.

Redline RW. Cerebral palsy in term infants: a clinicopathologic analysis of 158 medicolegal case reviews. Pediatr Dev Pathol 2008;11:456–464.

Redline RW. Placental pathology: a systematic approach with clinical correlations. Placenta 2008;22:S86–S91.

Redline RW. Severe fetal placental vascular lesions in term infants with neurologic impairment. Am J Obstet Gynecol 2005;192:452–457.

Chapter 27

New Directions: What is New in Placental Studies?

by Kurt Benirschke, MD

The answer to the question in the chapter subtitle depends very much on the knowledge of the examiner of placentas. From my perspective, perhaps the most interesting aspects have been the placental changes that are now being observed in multiple gestations and that result from the different practices of assisted reproductive technology (ART), in-vitro fertilization (IVF), and, especially, intracytoplasmic sperm injection (ICSI). The increased frequency with which excessive numbers of multiples are produced has been widely commented upon, and in recent publications it has been recommended that only single ovum transfers be practiced in ART, rather than the more frequent method of multiple blastocyst transfer. The attending prematurity rate and the frequently serious sequelae of marked prematurity have been the principal reasons for this recommendation. Additionally, because of uterine space limitations when multiple blastocysts compete for implantation sites, some placentas may become "squeezed" by the other placenta(s) and thus acquire less room for their expansion. This may then lead to fetal growth restriction and the more frequent and abnormal (velamentous) cord insertion seen in the placentas of multiples. We recently studied 127 sets of triplet placentas that had more single umbilical arteries (SUAs), more circumvallation, more chorangiomas, and, interestingly, more placentas with increased syncytial knots. More recently we saw a normal-appearing newborn with SUA who had a major contribution of cells that were mosaic for an 18q deletion. Thus one may ask, How normal are children with SUA?

Even more interesting, however, is the increased frequency of monochorionic twin placentas developing with these ART practices. Thus, when three blastocysts were transferred, four embryos may develop. Apparently, one of the embryos had split, to result in a set of monozygotic twins. We also found that when three embryos were implanted, sometimes we ended up with two of the triplets being monochorionic,

R.N. Baergen, *Manual of Pathology of the Human Placenta*,
DOI 10.1007/978-1-4419-7494-5_27, © Springer Science+Business Media, LLC 2011

probably due to the death of one embryo with splitting of another and a former quadruplet gestation. The reason for this apparent induced "splitting" has been difficult to explain, but Steinman (2003) has suggested a model that needs future investigation. He proposed that adhesion molecules that normally keep the blastomeres together are weakened in their effectiveness. He believes that this is dependent on the calcium concentration in the culture media that are being used and that contain the blastocysts before their transfer; he incriminates the anticoagulant ethylene diamine tetraacetic acid (EDTA) used for the prevention of coagulation as a possible culprit. Since we still do not have any reliable cause for the process of monozygotic twinning in general, this suggestion needs serious consideration by the community of physicians employing ART. Other suggestions are that there may be a discrepancy of the timing of the embryonic development and the uterine readiness, or even that the handling and potential disruption of the zona pellucida are at fault. It has also been suggested that the splitting of embryonic cells into equal numbers of cells during the MZ twinning event may not be as equal as is usually assumed. This may explain the cause of discordant MZ twin fetal anomalies, and specifically it may be the reason for the development of the twin–twin transfusion syndrome (TTTS) and acardiac twins (Benirschke 2009).

Another development recently discovered in several placental studies is dizygotic twins (DZ) with monochorionic placentation (DiMo) that also may then possess vascular anastomoses (Souter et al. 2003). The finding of DiMo placentas has, in the past, been held to be diagnostic of MZ twinning. That notion now needs revision. Moreover, the cases of blood chimerism, starting with Mrs. McKay many years ago, need reexamination and new special care needs to be exercised by the placental pathologist. Mrs. McKay was found to be a blood chimera while she was pregnant, and when asked about possibly having had a twin, she recalled that her male co-twin had died while very young (Dunsford et al. 1953). His blood group could then still be ascertained and, presumably, she would also still have had a chimeric XY lymphocyte cell line. Similar cases have since come to light, and indicate that this can also happen spontaneously. Thus, truly competent placental studies to demonstrate possible anastomoses are needed; on the other hand, these may also lead to the twin-twin transfusion syndrome (Assaf et al, 2010).

In the recent past, much progress has also been made in the therapy of TTTS. It has emerged that serial amniocentesis for the relief of hydramnios is not truly efficacious in the treatment of the "disease," and more centers now have gone over to the more effective laser coagulation of the causative arteriovenous (A-V) shunts in the placenta. The anastomoses are not always easy to identify through the small optics used during fetoscopy, and to select the right ones is a challenge (Chmait et al. 2010). It is therefore strongly recommended that future fetoscopic surgeons familiarize themselves with the vascular anatomy of the placental surface before attempting this challenging procedure. It has also emerged that artery-to-artery anastomoses are largely protective against the development of TTTS. What is less well appreciated, however, is that the neonatal diagnosis of TTTS may be difficult, as blood may shift rapidly during delivery between the twins' circulations.

Thus, false hematologic values can emerge that may not betray the prenatal, in utero, circumstances. This has legal ramifications in particular, and we have repeatedly suggested that it is imperative to adjudicate the cases through an examination of the twins' heart sizes (Benirschke and Masliah 2001). In the true TTTS, there is a major discrepancy of the heart sizes beginning already prior to the emerging hydramnios or other symptoms of TTTS, especially when they are adjusted for gestational age. Thus cardiac size discrepancy, rather than hematologic values, is a more reliable measure of the existence of the TTTS, and this relates to the lower blood pressure of the donor twin. Also, it has now become well established that the prenatal central nervous system (CNS) damage that may occur in TTTS, especially when one twin dies in utero, is the result of a transient severe hypotension because transplacental "hemorrhage" into the dead twin occurs from the living twin; that twin may recover, albeit with CNS damage. This CNS damage is not the result of a coagulation syndrome, as was formerly suspected. It has even been witnessed sonographically as a reversal of flow in such cases. Indeed, prenatal sonography has become an essential tool also in the assessment of the "dividing membranes" of twins, with the twin delta peak sign in DiDi twins (T-sign in DiMo twins) and the ascertainment of possible disruption of the amnionic membranes. Attempts at defining heart sizes of twins should be the future goal.

While speaking of chimerism, the other notable development is the recognition of several maternal autoimmune diseases as being the result of maternal blood chimerism by fetal cells that was initiated during the woman's prior pregnancy. It is envisaged that some fetal lymphocytes (perhaps even stem cells) transfer to the mother; this occurs most likely regularly during all gestations, in small numbers. When significant human leukocyte antigen (HLA) diversity is present, perhaps these transferred white blood cells later direct their attention against the maternal antigens in her future life and "reject" the carrier. Indeed, an important case reported by Srivatsa et al. (2001) indicates that, in a case of postpartum thyroiditis, even the maternal thyroid epithelium may be replaced by fetal cells. The magnitude of this process is under active investigation, but a correlation with the type and possible complications of prior gestations has rarely been possible. Thus, in view of the occasionally massive fetal hemorrhage (into maternal blood with Kleihauer-positive maternal blood that results) that we occasionally witness in the perinatal period, it might be asked whether the resultant induced chimerism is perhaps more often responsible for maternal autoimmune diseases in the future of those particular mothers (Johnson et al. 2001). Therefore, attention might be paid more specifically to the future diseases that might affect the mothers with major fetal blood transfer. It has since also been found that during pregnancy the maternal serum carries a substantial amount of cell-free DNA (Lo et al. 1997). It presumably arises from deported syncytial emboli that occur regularly during gestation and then undergo apoptosis in the lung. It is also the reason why that DNA disappears within 2 days after placental delivery. Cell-free DNA may also be useful for prenatal diagnosis, and is often used for genotyping the fetus in Rh-negative women.

There has been a remarkable reduction of perinatal mortality since the development of surfactant therapy for prematurely born infants. The old "hyaline membrane disease" has virtually disappeared from our perinatal autopsies as a consequence. Neonatal autopsies are now largely limited to significant structural abnormalities, chromosomal errors, and severely premature infants, those weighing less than 1,000 g. The placental pathologist notices that the latter infants are almost always associated with chorioamnionitis, or the placental sections show at least significant deciduitis. Remarkable progress has been made clinically in identifying the presence of this ascending infection (e.g., sonographic assessment of the cervix, interferon measurements, and identification of the many interleukins present in the cervical os), but few advances have been made in the precise identification of the responsible organisms, let alone in the therapy for these frequently recurrent infections. It has been my contention that the process is initiated by the existence of chronic endocervicitis and that this is then followed by deciduitis of the "forelying" membranes. Subsequently, local phospholipid production leads to cervical dilatation, to foreshortening of the cervix, and to premature labor. Cerclage, occasionally practiced in this clientele, has been only minimally effective, nor has the initiation of antibiotic therapy at the time of cervical "incompetence" been helpful. This disease process has not diminished in frequency and is now the most important cause of significant prematurity. It needs additional attention by the reproductive specialists. Because of the frequent recurrence of this cause of significant prematurity, these patients may benefit from antibiotic therapy in between pregnancies, and this probably should include the husbands, since inapparent nongonorrheal urethritis may accompany these gestations. At least it is worthy of a major clinical trial. We also need to make much greater efforts in identifying the organisms that cause the inflammation.

Much progress is being made in the identification of genes that regulate placental development – in the mouse, that is (Cross et al. 2003). Despite all the publications on putative causes of pregnancy-induced hypertension (PIH; preeclampsia), we are not truly closer to understanding its etiology. It is often speculated that PIH relates to the immunologic disparity of placental and maternal genotypes, but this has not been borne out with sufficient clarity, despite the occasional mutations occurring in the HLA-G complex. Hope exists that, once genetic regulation of murine placentation is better understood, we can decipher human placental development also. But we are not there yet. Microarrays are beginning to be employed without yet defining genes for specific diseases. This regulation is of more than casual interest, as it also involves the determinants of paternal placental "imprinting" and may be of concern to those readers with an interest in cloning and interspecific embryo transfers and in hopes of understanding the complex mechanisms that must underlie the evolution of the many different types of placentas. Aspects of comparative placentation and their evolution have long been hotly debated without clear resolution, and they are currently mostly descriptive (http://medicine.ucsd.edu/cpa). Greater attention might profitably be paid to the often deeply invasive trophoblast in some of the South American rodents and their possible immunologic consequences. The genetic disparity of these litters from the dams should be more fully investigated because they have claimed little attention to date.

We have made remarkably little progress concerning the etiology of chromosomal errors and their correlation with placental phenotype. For one thing, the high frequency of spontaneous abortions due to aneuploidies in the human population is not mirrored in other species that have been studied. In fact, it seems to be low in primate research centers where breeding is supervised and conceptions are known (Small and Smith 1983), and this is also true from my observations with wild animals at the San Diego Zoo. Abortions occur extremely rarely, and chromosomal errors as their cause are practically unknown or they can be enumerated easily. The reasons for these discrepancies are of potential importance to human reproductive performance and need better explanations than they now receive. But it is also true that we lack an understanding of why major trisomies cause often specific congenital anomalies in the embryo, while they appear to cause few if any characteristic placental changes. To be sure, the "partial mole" due to triploidy can be cited as an exception; but other major chromosomal errors are not known to be reflected in specific placental phenotypes. Perhaps we need to make a greater effort in their recognition and must more carefully compare cytogenetic findings with placental characteristics. Other than sporadic villous changes (edema, abnormal shape, vascular prominence) or the presence of a single umbilical artery, not much is known, not even a correlation with placental weights exists, and the same applies to "confined placental mosaicism," for which no good histology supports the abnormal placental regions.

When unusual moles have been characterized cytogenetically, a number of mosaic or chimeric genotypes have been identified. A beginning is made by the methods of differentiating partial moles from complete moles through the employment of chromosomal in situ hybridization (Lai et al. 2004). And while it is easy to state that complete hydatidiform moles have an exclusively paternal genome, the reasons for this feature (other than speculations about imprinting) are unresolved. It has become clear now that all complete moles must have had an embryo, at least at one time in early development. Not only have some been demonstrated, but this must also be deduced from the connective tissue these moles contain. But what are the precise reasons (e.g., structural anomalies, imprinting) for the death of these embryos? And why are moles so much more common in Asian populations, and why have they never been seen in any other species? These are questions to which placental pathologists should address some of their thoughts and research efforts.

Another important "black box" at present is the etiology of maternal floor infarction (MFI), a condition that can occasionally now be recognized sonographically. In this condition, excessive amounts of fibrinoid are deposited, and frequently MFI is associated with excessive proliferation of extravillous trophoblast. The precise nature of the fibrinoid has not been sufficiently explored, and the reasons for the frequent recurrences are similarly unknown. It is here where more definitive knowledge of trophoblast regulation that we hope to obtain from the mouse model might be applied. Perhaps the same can be said of villitis of unknown etiology. As with MFI, the condition is occasionally recurrent and leads to growth restriction and may lead to fetal death. Search for an infectious etiology has been negative, and the only detailed study that has identified the population of inflammatory cells within the villi was incomplete (Redline and Patterson 1993) but has more recently been clarified as representing maternal T-lymphocytes (Myerson et al. 2006). These studies suggested that in male births, there was no Y-signal in the affected villous inflammatory cell population. But that was done on histologic sections, not on fresh material. Thus, the exact nature of the infiltrating cell population remained unknown. Clearly, immunologists need to participate in identifying these cells more precisely than we have been able to do so far. A much more intensive study of this problem is now in order.

Placenta accreta was rare many years ago, and placenta percreta was virtually unheard of. Now, both play an important role in gynecologic pathology. We see many cases of placenta percreta annually, and most are identified sonographically long before labor commences. Usually, the uterus is removed in placenta percreta; the placenta is found to lie anteriorly and has dehisced (prolapsed) through a former cesarean section scar. It has not "invaded"; it just sticks out of the uterus because the thin scar tissue has become even thinner as the uterus expands in all directions during the next pregnancy. Most of this is the result of the greater frequency with which cesarean section delivery is done, and the frequently practiced avoidance of a trial of labor after one cesarean section (vaginal birth after cesarean [VBAC]). Are there other causes? Certainly there is no evidence that the trophoblast is truly invasive and destructive at its implantation site; abdominal pregnancies alone support that notion. But perhaps the uteri are less adequately repaired after cesarean section? At least that is what I believe; the rapidity of closure, the single stitch approach, and the nature of the suture material may be responsible for the higher frequency of percretas. One fact is clear, however, the progress made in sonography techniques, the recognition of placental "lakes," apparent hemangiomas, or abnormal-appearing implantation sites by ultrasound has much enhanced early recognition of this potentially serious complication of pregnancy.

Other advances in sonography might be highlighted as they also affect placental pathology studies and give insight into prenatal life. The coiling and entanglement of the umbilical cord (especially in MoMo twins) are now recognized earlier; blood flow can be adjudicated (and reversal can be documented – end-diastolic flow), we will learn to identify more precisely the sites of anastomoses in twin gestations and perhaps, with color power angiography, we will even better assess the development and abnormalities of the villous tree (Konje et al. 2003). The prospects are excellent, and placental pathologists should stay abreast of these developments so as to enable them to make more meaningful studies and diagnoses.

Finally, we have had an interest in understanding the causes that determine the length of the umbilical cord (normal is 55 cm) and its helical twists. Both aspects warrant more attention than is generally appreciated. Excessively long cords may lead to knots and to encircling around the fetus, and they may cause fetal demise. More often they are also associated with excessive spiraling of the cord; 2.5 twists per 10 cm are the normal, but we have seen many cords with excessively marked twisting associated with intrauterine growth restrictions (IUGR) and fetal demise. What determines the cord's length? We know that immobile fetuses (muscular diseases, osteogenesis imperfecta, etc.) have short umbilical cords, and thus we assume that the length of the umbilical cord may be determined by fetal mobility. But why is the cord occasionally much longer than 55 cm? A gestation that we have observed recently with a long and excessively twisted cord and an IUGR neonate was in a mother who was an avid runner during pregnancy, and we wonder whether the length of the cord may not reflect excessive fetal mobility. Future studies are needed.

References

Assaf SA, Randolph LM, Benirschke K, Wu S, Samadi R, Chmait RH. Discordant blood chimerism in dizygotic monochorionic laser-treated twin-twin transfusion syndrome. Obstet Gynecol. 2010 Aug;116 Suppl 2:475–6.

Benirschke K. The monozygotic twinning process, the twin-twin transfusion syndrome and acardiac twins. Placenta 2009;30:923–928.

Benirschke K, Masliah E. The placenta in multiple pregnancy: outstanding issues. Reprod Fertil Dev 2001;13:615–622.

Chmait RH, Khan A, Benirschke K, Miller D, Korst L, Goodwin TM. Perinatal survival following preferential sequential selective laser surgery for twin-twin transfusion syndrome. J Matern Fetal Neonatal Med 2010;23:10–16.

Cross JC, Baczyk D, Dobric N, Hemberger M, Hughes M, Simmons DG, Yamamoto H, Kingdom JCP. Genes, development and evolution of the placenta. Placenta 2003;24:123–130.

Dunsford I, Bowley CC, Hutchison AM, Thompson JS, Sanger R, Race RR. A human blood group chimera. Br Med J 1953;2:81.

Johnson KL, Nelson JL, Furst DE, McSweeney PA, Roberts DJ, Zhen DK, Bianchi DW. Fetal cell microchimerism in tissue from multiple sites in women with systemic sclerosis. Arthritis Rheum 2001;44:1848–1854.

Konje JC, Huppertz B, Bell SC, Taylor DJ, Kaufmann P. 3-dimensional colour power angiography for staging human placental development. Lancet 2003;362:1199–1201.

Lai CYL, Chan KYK, Khoo U-S, Ngan HYS, Xue W-C, Chiu PM, Tsao S-W, Cheung ANY. Analysis of gestational trophoblastic disease by genotyping and chromosome *in situ* hybridization. Mod Pathol 2004;17:40–48.

Lo YM, Corbetta N, Chamberlain PF, Rai V, Sargent IL, Redman CW, Wainscoat JS. Presence of fetal DNA in maternal plasma and serum. Lancet 1997;350:485–487.

Myerson D, Parkin RK, Benirschke K, Tschetter CN, Hyde SR. The pathogenesis of villitis of unknown etiology: analysis with a new conjoint immuno-histochemistry-in situ hybridization procedure to identify specific maternal and fetal cells. Pediatr Dev Pathol 2006;9:257–265.

Redline RW, Patterson P. Villitis of unknown etiology is associated with major infiltration of fetal tissue by maternal inflammatory cells. Am J Pathol 1993;143:473–479.

Small MF, Smith DG. Chromosomal analysis of perinatal death in *Macaca mulatta* and *Macaca radiata*. Am J Primatol 1983;5:381–384.

Souter VL, Kapur RP, Nyholt DR, Skogerboe K, Myerson D, Ton DR, Opheim KE, Easterling TR, Shields LE, Montgomery GW, Glass IA. A report of dizygous monochorionic twins. NEJM 2003;349:154–158.

Srivatsa B, Srivatsa S, Johnson KL, Samura O, Lee SL, Bianchi DW. Microchimerism of presumed fetal origin in thyroid specimens from women: a case-control study. Lancet 2001;358:2034–2038.

Steinman G. Mechanism of twinning VI. Genetics and the etiology of monozygotic twinning in in vitro fertilization. J Reprod Med 2003;48:583–589.

Appendix A
Abbreviations and Definitions

Abbreviations

ACLA	Anticardiolipin antibody
AEDF	Absent end-diastolic flow
AFI	Amniotic fluid index
AFLP	Acute fatty liver of pregnancy
AGA	Appropriate for gestational age
APLA	Antiphospholipid antibody
AROM	Artificial rupture of membranes
ART	Assisted reproductive technology
BPD	Biparietal diameter
BPP	Biophysical profile
BTBV	Beat-to-beat variability
CPD	Cephalopelvic disproportion
CPM	Confined placental mosaicism
CS	Cesarean section
CVS	Chorionic villus sampling
EDC	Estimated date of "confinement"
EDD	Estimated date of delivery
EFW	Estimated fetal weight
EGA	Estimated gestational age
FGR	Fetal growth restriction
FHR	Fetal heart rate
FLM	Fetal lung maturity
FM	Fetal movement
FMH	Fetomaternal hemorrhage
FW	Fetal weight
GBBS	Group B beta *Streptococcus*
GBS	Group B *Streptococcus*
GDM	Gestational diabetes mellitus
GDMA1	Gestational diabetes mellitus, not requiring insulin or oral agents
GDMA2	Gestational diabetes mellitus, requiring insulin or oral agents

R.N. Baergen, *Manual of Pathology of the Human Placenta,*
DOI 10.1007/978-1-4419-7494-5 © Springer Science+Business Media, LLC 2011

GTD	Gestational trophoblastic disease
GxPxxxx	Gravity, parity; numbers indicate: term, preterm, abortion, living
hCG	Human chorionic gonadotropin
HELLP	Hemolysis, elevated liver enzymes, low platelets
hPL	Human placental lactogen
ICSI	Intracytoplasmic sperm injection
IDM	Infant of diabetic mother
IUFD	Intrauterine fetal demise
IUGR	Intrauterine growth restriction (formerly "retardation")
IUP	Intrauterine pregnancy
IVDA	Intravenous drug abuse
IVF	In vitro fertilization
LAC	Lupus anticoagulant
LFCS	Low flap cesarean section
LGA	Large for gestational age
LOF	Low outlet forceps
LTCS	Low transverse cesarean section
MFI	Maternal floor infarction
MSAFP	Maternal serum alpha-fetoprotein
MSF	Meconium-stained fluid
NIHF	Nonimmune hydrops fetalis
NRNST	Nonreactive nonstress test
NST	Nonstress test; antenatal test of fetal well-being
NSVD	Normal spontaneous vaginal delivery
OA	Occiput anterior (presenting part)
OCT	Oxytocin challenge test
OP	Occiput posterior (presenting part)
PEC	Preeclampsia
PET	Preeclampsia, toxemia
PIH	Pregnancy-induced hypertension
PLAP	Placental alkaline phosphatase
PNC	Prenatal care
PPROM	Preterm premature rupture of membranes; may be prolonged (>24 h) as well
PROM	Preterm (prior to term) or premature (prior to labor) rupture of membranes
PTL	Preterm labor
PUBS	Percutaneous umbilical blood sampling
PUPPP	Pruritic urticarial papules and plaques of pregnancy
REDF	Reversed end-diastolic flow
SGA	Small for gestational age
SROM	Spontaneous rupture of membranes
SVD	Spontaneous vaginal delivery
TTTS	Twin-to-twin transfusion syndrome
UC	Uterine contractions
UC	Umbilical cord
UPD	Uniparental disomy
US	Ultrasound
VAVD	Vacuum-assisted vaginal delivery

VBAC   Vaginal birth after cesarean delivery
Vtx   Vertex presentation of the fetus during delivery.
VUE   Villitis of unknown etiology

Glossary

Amnioinfusion	Usually saline injected intraamniotically in situations with thick meconium in an attempt to dilute the meconium.
Apgar scores	Evaluation of infant after delivery and used as a predictor of fetal well-being. Commonly done at 1 and 5 min. Zero, one, or two points given for color, tone, cry, respiratory effort, and reflex irritability.
Beat-to-beat variability	In fetal heart monitoring. Normally strip should show a certain amount of variability in rate from beat to beat. Lack of this variability is an indication of "nonreassuring fetal status."
Biophysical profile	Test of fetal well-being. Includes nonstress test (NST, see below) and assessment of amniotic fluid volume. Highest is 10; 7 and above is considered reassuring.
Cord prolapse	When the cord is the presenting part and precedes the fetus during delivery. Results in cord occlusion if the head is allowed to compress the cord against the cervix.
Deceleration	Fetal heart monitoring abnormality. May be early, variable, or late. Variable usually considered due to cord compression. Late decelerations commonly thought to be "uteroplacental insufficiency" and are ominous findings.
Doppler velocimetry	Studies of blood flow, usually through the umbilical artery, to measure systolic and diastolic flow (see "End-diastolic flow").
End-diastolic flow	End-diastolic blood flow through the umbilical artery may be absent or reversed with significant placental malperfusion. Absent or reversed EDF has been associated with IUGR and poor outcome.
Incompetent cervix	Defined as painless cervical dilation in the second trimester or early third trimester, with prolapse and ballooning of the membranes into the vagina, followed by ruptured membranes and delivery. Often recurs and is usually due to an anatomical defect.
L/S ratio	Lecithin/sphingomyelin ratio, used to evaluate fetal lung maturity, measured on samples of amniotic fluid.
Nonstress test	Evaluation of fetal well-being by assessment of fetal heart rate acceleration detected by Doppler coordinated with fetal movements as perceived by the mother. It is a test of fetal well-being.

Percutaneous umbilical cord sampling	Sampling of fetal blood by introduction of a needle through the abdomen into the umbilical cord.
Placenta previa	Placental implantation over the cervical os, may be partial.
Quadruple screen	Prenatal screen for anomalies performed on maternal serum; includes beta-human chorionic gonadotropin (hCG), estriol, alpha-fetoprotein, and dimeric alpha-inhibin; reported as multiples of the median.
Stress test	Also called contraction stress test, is a test of utero-placental function. Contractions are enhanced by IV oxytocin and fetal heart rate is monitored. A positive or abnormal test is when fetal heart rate decelerations are noted.
Tocolysis	Use of various drugs to inhibit preterm labor.
Triple screen	Prenatal screen for anomalies performed on maternal serum. Includes beta-hCG, estriol, and alpha-fetoprotein. Reported as multiples of the median.
Twin peak sign	Peak seen on the fetal surface of twin placentas that represents the fibrin ridge seen between fused diamnionic–dichorionic twin placentas.
Vasa previa	Velamentous vessels over cervical os

Appendix B

Table 3.1. Indications for placental examination.

Maternal indications

History of reproductive failure – ≥1 spontaneous abortions (Abs), stillbirths, neonatal deaths, or premature births

Maternal diseases

Coagulopathy
Hypertension (preeclampsia, pregnancy induced or chronic)
Diabetes mellitus
Prematurity (<2 weeks)
Postmaturity (>42 weeks)
Oligohydramnios
Polyhydramnios
Fever or infection
Repetitive bleeding
Abruptio placentae

Fetal and neonatal indications

Stillbirth or perinatal death
Fetal growth restrictions (intrauterine growth restrictions, IUGR)
Hydrops
Severe neonatal central nervous system (CNS) depression or neurologic problems such as seizures
Apgar score of 3 or less at 5 min
Suspected infection
Congenital anomalies
Thick meconium

Placental indications

Any gross abnormality of the placenta, membranes or umbilical cord, such as masses, thrombi, excessively long, short or twisted umbilical cord, etc.

Optional recommendations

Prematurity between 32 and 36 weeks
Low 1-min Apgar score
Fetal distress or non-reassuring fetal status
Multiple birth

Adapted from the College of American Pathologists (Altshuler and Deppisch 1991)

Table 3.2. Macroscopic lesions of the fetal membranes (see Chap. 14).

Type of lesion	Diagnosis		Comment	Figure number
Discoloration				
Green, green-yellow	Meconium		Check for staining of umbilical cord (see Table 3.4)	14.15a
Opaque, white to yellow	Acute inflammation (chorioamnionitis)		Check for odor Consider culture	16.2
Brown to yellow	Hemosiderin		Old bleeding – retromembranous or retroplacental hematoma	14.19a
Red-brown, red-pink	Hemolysis		Most often due to fetal demise or freezing	–
Focal lesions	*Description*	*Diagnosis*		
Plaques	Red to brown, shaggy	Retro-membranous hematoma	May be secondary to ruptured membranes, decidual bleeding or iatrogenic due to amniocentesis	14.12
	Yellow to white, ragged	Decidual necrosis	May be due to decidual vascular lesions but most commonly nonspecific	–
	Tan, roundish, plaque-like	Fetus papyraceous	Ascertain placentation if possible	10.1–10.3
	Pasty, hydrophobic material	Vernix caseosa	Usually secondary to membrane rupture and is of little consequence	14.8
Strings or bands of membrane	Usually tethered to base of umbilical cord	Amnionic bands	Chorionic plate will be devoid of amnion May be associated with isolated amputations, various fetal anomalies or cord entanglement Take photograph	14.24–14.29

Table 3.3. Macroscopic lesions of the fetal surface and chorionic plate (see Chaps. 14, 21 and 22).

Description	Diagnosis	Comment	Figure number
Plaques or nodules			
White, hydrophobic plaques	Squamous metaplasia	Adherent to surface DDx: amnion nodosum	14.21a
Translucent, white or yellow nodules	Amnion nodosum	Can be scraped off Due to oligohydramnios DDx: squamous metaplasia	14.22
Oval, chalky disk, under amnion	Yolk sac remnant	Normal embryonic remnant	14.7a
Firm, white subchorionic nodules or plaques	Subchorionic fibrin/fibrinoid	Usually of no consequence	3.4 3.8
Well-circumscribed, hemor-rhagic, fibrous or myxoid nodule	Chorangioma	Note size, consistency Villous tissue may be pale due to associated hemorrhage	3.8 22.1–22.4
Cyst	Subchorionic cyst	Usually of no consequence	14.4, 14.5

(continued)

Table 3.3. (continued)

Description	Diagnosis	Comment	Figure number
Plaques or nodules			
Hemorrhage or hematoma	Amnionic cyst	Usually of no consequence	14.2
	Subchorionic hematoma	Note size and % surface	3.8, 14.13
		If large, may be associated with demise	14.14
	Subamnionic hematoma	Usually iatrogenic	3.8, 14.11
		Look for source of bleeding – disrupted fetal vessels in chorionic plate (rare)	
Chorionic vessels			
White streak or firmness in vessel	Thrombosis	Extra sections of fetal surface vessels	21.1–21.3
		May be associated umbilical cord problems	
Dilated and tortuous vessels	Acute cord compression	May be associated with cord problems, e.g., hypercoiling, long cords, knots, entanglements, etc.	–
	Mesenchymal dysplasia	May be associated with cystically dilated villi	19.18a

DDx differential diagnosis

Table 3.4. Macroscopic lesions of the umbilical cord (see Chap. 15).

Description	Diagnosis	Gross examination	Figure number
Insertion			
Insertion at placental margin	Marginal	Usually of no consequence unless there are associated velamentous vessels (velamentous insertion)	15.17
Insertion into/within membranes	Velamentous	Measure from insertion to placental margin	15.17
		Note disruption, hemorrhage or thrombosis of vessels	15.18
		Submit separate membrane roll of velamentous vessels	15.21
			15.22
Cord divides before insertion	Furcate	Check that all vessels are intact	15.17
			15.19
Cord inserts and runs in membranes without branching	Interpositional	Usually of no consequence	15.17
			15.20
***Length*: Normal 55 cm**			
<40 cm	Short cord	Difficult to diagnose without measurement of total cord length at delivery	–
>70–80 cm	Long cord	Check for associated chorionic plate vascular thrombosis	15.9
***Diameter*: Normal 1–1.5 cm**			
Increased	Thick cord	If focal, may represent a cyst	15.10
		May be associated with diabetes, macrosomia or hydrops	

(continued)

Table 3.4. (continued)

Description	Diagnosis	Gross examination	Figure number
Diameter: Normal 1–1.5 cm			
Decreased	Thin cord	May be associated with growth restriction	15.8
Focal constriction	Stricture	Measure diameter and take sections through stricture	15.8
		Check for associated chorionic plate vascular thrombosis	
Knot	True knot	Document	15.12
		Loose or tight	15.13
		Congestion on one side of the knot	15.16
		If, after untying, cord stays coiled	
		Take sections through untied knot	
	False knot	Redundant vessels of no consequence	15.15
Twisting or coiling			
Excessive twist		Check for associated thrombosis or stricture	15.6
		May be associated with adverse outcome	15.7
Minimal or no twist		May be associated with adverse outcome	15.6
Vessels: Normally three			
Two vessels	Single umbilical artery	Avoid sections near insertion site due to arterial anastomosis	15.23
Four vessels	Persistent vein	Avoid sections with false knots	–
Thrombosis	Thrombosis	Ensure it is not in an area of cord clamping or due to false knotsSerially section and submit	15.24
		Take photograph	
Discoloration: Normal – white			
Pink, red, or red-brown	Hemolysis	Usually due to fetal demise or freezing of the placenta	–
Brown, yellow-brown	Hemosiderin	Due to old bleeding	14.19a
Green or yellow-green	Meconium	Note if focal or diffuse	14.15a
		Take extra sections of stained cord	
Yellow	Bile	Note in report	14.18
		May be due to maternal hyperbilirubinemia	
Chalky deposits	Calcification	Usually due to infection – necrotizing funisitis	16.21
Mass			
Cyst	Embryonic remnants	Measure and take extra sections	15.2
White, tan, or yellow surface nodules	*Candida* infection	Take additional sections of lesions	16.16
Hemorrhage	Hemorrhage, hematoma, or hemangioma	Ensure it is not in an area of cord clamping	15.26
			15.27
Miscellaneous			
Edema	Edema	If localized, may represent a cyst	15.10
		May be associated with macrosomia or hydrops	
Rupture	Rupture	Look for associated lesions that could explain rupture, such as hematoma, meconium, masses, etc.	15.26

Table 3.5. Macroscopic lesions of the maternal surface (see Chaps. 16, 18, and 19).

Description	Diagnosis	Comment	Figure number
White, chalky, stippled, gritty lesions	Calcifications	Normal finding	3.7
Shaggy, tan loosely adherent plaques	Decidual necrosis	Usually a nonspecific finding but may be associated with decidual vascular disease	–
Adherent blood clot	Retroplacental hematoma (abruptio placentae)	Note size and % of maternal surface involved	3.8 18.13
		Note compression of villous tissue	18.14
		Note if old or recent	19.5
		Note if there is an underlying infarct	19.6
	Marginal hematoma	Often due to ascending infection (acute chorioamnionitis)	3.8 16.3
		Note size and % of maternal surface involved	
		Note compression of villous tissue	
Yellow discoloration; firm, corrugated surface	Maternal floor infarction (massive perivillous fibrinoid)	Note % involvement of placental parenchyma	19.13 19.14
		Note if diffuse or multifocal	
Firm, white or reddish lesions	Infarct, intervillous thrombus or fibrin deposition	Note size and % involvement	3.8
		Take extra sections of lesions	18.7–18.9 19.6

Table 3.6. Abnormalities of placental shape and macroscopic lesions of the villous tissue (see Chaps. 13, 18–23).

Description	Diagnosis	Comment	Figure number
Shape alterations			
Two equal lobes	Bilobed	Check membranous vessels to ensure they are intact and without thrombosis	13.1 13.2
Two or more unequal lobes	Succenturiate lobe	Check membranous vessels to ensure they are intact and without thrombosis	13.1 13.3
Extremely large, thin placenta	Membranacea	May be associated with bleeding and/or placenta accreta	13.1 13.12
Membranes do not insert into placental margin	Circumvallate or circummarginate	Note if partial or complete	13.4–13.6
		Measure distance from insertion to placental margin	13.8
	Extrachorial or extramembranous pregnancy	Measure distance from insertion to placental margin	13.9 13.10
Full thickness defect in placenta	Fenestra	Usually of no consequence	13.1 13.13
Ring shaped placenta	Zonary placenta	Usually of no consequence	13.1 13.14

(continued)

Table 3.6. (continued)

Description	Diagnosis	Comment	Figure number
Diffuse lesions of villous tissue			
Firm, net-like, white deposits throughout villous tissue	Maternal floor infarction/massive perivillous fibrin deposition	Note extent – % of villous tissue involved	19.15–19.17
		Note if multifocal or diffuse	
		Note involvement of maternal floor	
Mottling of villous tissue	Chronic villitis	Usually very subtle	3.8
		Note the extent – % of villous tissue involved	16.29
Focal lesions			
Well-circumscribed, round lesion with granular surface	Recent infarct (pink to red discoloration)	Note if single or multiple	3.8
		Note % of placenta involved	18.8
	Old infarct (white discoloration)	Note if single or multiple	3.8
		Note % of placenta involved	18.7–18.9
			19.6
Well-circumscribed, angular lesion with shiny surface	Intervillous thrombus	Usually of no consequence	3.8
		If large or multiple may be associated with fetomaternal hemorrhage	19.1
			19.2
Well-circumscribed nodular lesion with consistency of blood clot, myxoid or "fibrous" tissue	Chorangioma	Benign hemangioma Usually of no consequence unless large	3.8
			22.1–22.4
Poorly demarcated white, granular lesion	Intervillous abscess	Associated with bacterial infection, most commonly *Listeria*	16.12
Cystically dilated villi	Mesenchymal dysplasia	Dilated, tortuous vessels on fetal surface may also be present	19.18a
	Hydatidiform moles	Additional sections should be taken	23.2
			23.3
		Consider cytogenetics, flow cytometry, etc.	23.6
Nodular lesion with consistency of blood clot, myxoid or "fibrous" tissue	Chorangioma	Benign hemangioma	3.8
			22.1–22.4
	Chorangiomatosis	Multiple lesions – various clinical associations	19.10
***Color of villous tissue* – reflective of fetal hematocrit**			
Pale	Fetal anemia	May be associated intervillous thrombi	20.1
		May be associated with fetomaternal hemorrhage or hydrops	
	Twin-to-twin transfusion	Note type and size of vascular anastomoses	9.7
			10.13
Congestion	Villous congestion	May be associated with maternal diabetes or obstruction of venous return (possible umbilical cord problems)	17.3

Table 3.7. Normative values.

Pregnancy week postmenstrual	Crown–rump length (mm)	Foot length (cm)	Embryonic/fetal weight (g)	Placental weight (g)	Fetal/placental weight ratio	Placental thickness (cm)	Placental diameter (cm)	Umbilical cord length (cm)
3								
4								0.2
5	2.5							0.4
6	5							0.7
7	9							1.2
8	14		1.1	6	0.18			2.0
9	20		2	8	0.25			3.3
10	26		5	13	0.38			5.5
11	33		11	19	0.58			9.2
12	40		17	26	0.65			12.6
13	48	1.2	23	32	0.72		5.0	15.8
14	56	1.7	30	41	0.73	1.0	5.6	18.8
15	65	1.9	40	50	0.80	1.1	6.2	21.5
16	75	2.2	60	60	1.00	1.2	6.9	24.0
17	88	2.5	90	70	1.29	1.2	7.5	26.4
18	99	2.8	130	80	1.63	1.3	8.1	28.7
19	112	2.9	180	101	1.78	1.4	8.7	30.9
20	125	3.3	250	112	2.23	1.5	9.4	33.0
21	137	3.6	320	126	2.54	1.5	10.0	35.0
22	150	3.9	400	144	2.78	1.6	10.6	36.9
23	163	4.2	480	162	2.96	1.7	11.2	38.7
24	176	4.5	560	180	3.11	1.8	11.9	40.4
25	188	4.7	650	198	3.28	1.8	12.5	42.0
26	200	5.0	750	216	3.47	1.9	13.1	43.5
27	213	5.3	870	234	3.72	1.9	13.7	45.0
28	226	5.5	1,000	252	3.97	2.0	14.4	46.4
29	236	5.8	1,130	270	4.19	2.0	15.0	47.7
30	250	6.0	1,260	288	4.38	2.1	15.6	49.0
31	263	6.2	1,400	306	4.58	2.1	16.2	50.2
32	276	6.5	1,550	324	4.78	2.2	16.9	52.0
33	289	6.7	1,700	342	4.97	2.2	17.5	53.0
34	302	6.9	1,900	360	5.28	2.3	18.1	54.0
35	315	7.1	2,100	378	5.56	2.3	18.7	54.9
36	328	7.4	2,300	396	5.81	2.4	19.4	55.7
37	341	7.6	2,500	414	6.04	2.4	20.0	56.5
38	354	7.8	2,750	432	6.37	2.4	20.6	57.2
39	367	8.0	3,000	451	6.65	2.5	21.3	57.9
40	380	8.1	3,400	470	7.23	2.5	22.0	58.5

Portions of this table were modified from Kalousek et al. (1992)

Table 4.1. Lesions of the Fetal Membranes (Chapter 14).

Description	Diagnosis	Comment	Figure number
Pigment in macrophages			
Yellow-brown	Meconium	Often associated with degenerative change of the amnion	4.1
			14.15b
			14.16
Brown, particulate, refringent	Hemosiderin	Look for source of bleeding – often from decidua	14.19b
		Iron stain may be needed to confirm	
Inflammation – see also Table 16.1			
	Acute inflammatory cells	Acute chorioamnionitis	16.4
		Gram stain done rarely – usually negative	16.5
	Chronic inflammatory cells	Chronic chorioamnionitis	16.20
		May be associated with chronic villitis	16.32
		Often only present in decidua	
	Acute inflammatory cells with necrosis	Subacute chorioamnionitis – acute chorioamnionitis of longer duration	16.10
Hemorrhage	Retromembranous hematoma	May be associated with rupture of membranes, but usually nonspecific finding	14.12
Cyst			
Epithelial	Amnionic cyst	No clinical significance	14.1
Squamous	Epidermoid cyst	No clinical significance	14.2
Extravillous trophoblast	Subchorionic cyst	No clinical significance	14.3
Epithelial change			
Squamous change	Squamous metaplasia	Normal finding near term	4.1
			14.21b
Anucleate squames and debris forming nodules	Amnion nodosum	Usually secondary to severe oligohydramnios and associated with fetal renal anomalies	4.1
			14.23
Vacuolization	Gastroschisis	Specific finding associated with gastroschisis	4.1
			14.20
Degenerative change of epithelium	Meconium	Degenerative change may indicate that meconium discharge is more remote	4.1
			14.16
Miscellaneous			
Cartilage, bone, skin	Teratoma	May represent acardiac twin	–
	Embryonic remnants	No clinical significance	–
	Fetus papyraceous	Document and identify membranes relationships if possible	10.4
Anucleate squames and debris	Vernix caseosa	No clinical significance	14.9
		Often occurs with membrane rupture	14.10
Necrotic tissue	Decidual necrosis	May be associated with decidual vasculopathy or hemorrhage but often non-specific	–
Inflammation in decidua	Acute deciduitis	May be associated with acute chorioamnionitis, otherwise is nonspecific	16.6
	Chronic deciduitis	May be associated with chronic villitis	16.20
		Diagnosis usually made only with intense infiltrate and/or presence of plasma cells	
Abnormal vessels	Decidual vasculopathy	May be associated with other changes of placental malperfusion	18.1–18.5

Table 4.2. Umbilical cord (see Chap. 15).

Description	Diagnosis	Comment	Figure number
Skin, cartilage, bone	Teratoma	May represent an acardiac twin	–
Vessels	Hemangioma	May be associated with hematoma or rupture	15.25
Epithelial elements	Embryonic remnants	Allantoic duct remnant	15.1
		Omphalomesenteric duct remnant	15.3–15.5
		Vitelline vessel remnant	
Edema	Focal – embryonic cyst	Usually develops from embryonic remnants	15.2
	Diffuse – edema	May be associated with fetal hydrops	15.10
Acute inflammation	Acute funisitis	Fetal inflammatory response	16.7
See also Table 16.1	*Candida* infection	Focal lesions of umbilical cord surface	16.17
		Usually not associated with acute chorioamnionitis	
		PAS or Gomori methenamine silver (GMS) to confirm	
	Necrotizing funisitis	May be associated with calcification	16.8
		Classically seen in syphilis but may be seen in other infections	16.22
Pigmented macrophages	Meconium	Meconium filled macrophages rarely identified in cord despite gross staining	–
		May be associated with myonecrosis of umbilical vascular smooth muscle	
Single umbilical artery	Single umbilical artery	May be associated with other fetal anomalies	15.23
Four umbilical vessels	Supernumerary vessel	Rare, may be associated with fetal anomalies	–
Thrombosis	Thrombosis	Often associated with thrombosis in chorionic or stem vessels	15.24b
Hemorrhage	Hematoma	May be associated with other cord lesions	15.27
		May compress umbilical vessels (particularly the umbilical vein) leading to vascular embarrassment	
Thinned vessels	Varix or aneurysm	May lead to hemorrhage or rupture	15.30
Vascular necrosis	Meconium induced vascular necrosis	Usually due to prolonged meconium exposure in utero	14.17

Table 4.3. Chorionic plate (see Chaps. 14, 21, and 22).

Description	Diagnosis	Comment	Figure number
Oval, lacy structure	Yolk sac remnant	Embryonic remnant of no clinical significance	1.8 14.7b
Fetal skeleton	Fetus papyraceous	Note membrane relationship if possible	10.4
Fibrinoid	Subchorionic fibrinoid	If excessive, may be associated with placental malperfusion or maternal floor infarction	3.4
Cyst	Subchorionic cyst	Usually of no clinical significance	14.6
Hematoma	Subchorionic hematoma	If large, may be associated with stillbirth	–
	Subamnionic hematoma	Fresh blood under amnion, most commonly an artifact secondary to excessive traction on cord during delivery	–
		Rarely due to disruption of fetal chorionic vessels	
Vascular mass	Chorangioma	Benign vascular neoplasm – similar to hemangioma	22.5–22.7
Chorionic vessels			
Thrombosis	Thrombosis	Look for other associated thrombotic lesions in villous tissue: avascular villi, villous stromal karyorrhexis	21.4–21.7 21.10
Inflammation See also Table 16.1	Acute chorioamnionitis	Ascending infection May be associated with thrombosis	16.4 16.5 16.9
	Chronic chorioamnionitis	Often associated with chronic villitis	16.32
	Subacute chorioamnionitis	Due to long standing ascending i nfection	16.10
Degeneration of muscle	Meconium induced damage	Usually due to long standing meconium	14.17

Table 4.4. Intervillous space.

Description	Diagnosis	Comment	Figure number
Blood clot	Intervillous thrombus	If large or multiple, may be associated with fetomaternal hemorrhage	3.8 19.3
Fibrin/fibrinoid	Increased perivillous fibrin	If excessive, may represent maternal floor infarction	19.12 19.15 19.16 19.17
Inflammation – see also Tables 16.1 and 16.2	Intervillous abscess	Most commonly due to *Listeria* infectionRarely due to maternal sepsis	3.8 16.13
	Chronic intervillositis	Idiopathic disorder with infiltrate of histiocytes and lymphocytes	16.33

(continued)

Table 4.4. (continued)

Description	Diagnosis	Comment	Figure number
Abnormal or atypical cells	Malignancy – fetal or maternal metastatic	Cells may present as clusters in inter-villous space or invade villi	3.8 22.8–22.10
		Immunohistochemistry may be necessary for specific diagnosis	
	Intraplacental choriocarcinoma	Markedly atypical syncytiotrophoblast and cytotrophoblast	24.10–24.12
Collapse of inter-villous space	Early villous ischemic change	Often associated with infarction	18.10
Expansion of intervillous space	Villous hypoplasia – terminal villus deficiency	Often associated with other changes of placental malperfusion	18.16

Table 4.5. Chorionic villi.

Description	Diagnosis	Comment	Figure number
Villous morphology			
Increased syncytial knots	Increased syncytial knots	Associated with placental malperfusion	18.15 18.17
Delayed maturation	Villous immaturity	Associated with maternal diabetes	17.4
		May be associated with IUGR, IUFD	
Straight, unbranched villi	Villous hypoplasia/ terminal villus deficiency	Indicative of profound decrease in perfusion	18.15 18.16
		Usually associated with abnormal Doppler (absent or reversed end diastolic flow)	
Invagination, irregular contour	Trophoblastic inclusions	Suggestive of chromosomal defect	11.7
		Also seen in hydatidiform moles	23.9
Clear space inside villi	Cisterns	Hydatidiform moles	23.4
		Beckwith–Wiedemann syndrome	20.6
		Mesenchymal dysplasia	19.19
Degeneration, smudging of nuclei	Ischemia	Evidence of early infarction	18.11
		Associated with placental malperfusion	
Ghost villi	Infarction	Old infarction	18.12
Vacuolization of trophoblast or other cells	Storage disorder	Various cells may show vacuolization	20.9
		See Table 20.1	
Trophoblastic proliferation	Hydatidiform mole	Associated with hydropic villous changeSee Tables 23.2 and 23.3	23.4 23.5 23.8 23.9 23.10 23.12
Edema	Villous edema	Focal villous edema (if diffuse, may be seen in hydrops – see below)	19.21 20.5

(continued)

Table 4.5. (continued)

Description	Diagnosis	Comment	Figure number
Villous stroma			
Inflammation	Acute villitis	Generally due to *Listeria* infection	16.13
See also		May be due to maternal sepsis	
Tables 16.1 and 16.2	Chronic villitis	Differential diagnosis is chronic villitis of unknown etiology versus infectious etiology	16.18 16.19 16.23 16.25 16.30 16.31
Fine stippled calcification of stroma or basement membrane	Microcalcification	Seen in fetal death, twin–twin transfusion and hydrops	20.13
Hyalinization of stroma	Avascular villi	Associated with thrombosis in fetal circulation	21.8
Hemorrhage	Intravillous hemorrhage	May be secondary to acute injury, ischemia, abruption	19.4
Red blood cells in stroma	Villous stromal karyorrhexis/hemorrhagic endovasculopathy	Generally associated with other thrombotic lesions	19.4 21.12 21.13
Edema or hydropic change	Mesenchymal dysplasia	Developmental abnormality of villous tissue	19.19
		Also associated with tortuous chorionic vessels	
	Molar pregnancy	Marked hydropic change	23.4
		Trophoblastic hyperplasia is necessary for the diagnosis – see Tables 23.2 and 23.3	23.5 23.8 23.9 23.10 23.12
	Villous edema	May be secondary to acute injury or ischemia	19.21 20.5
	Villous immaturity	Diffuse villous immaturity for gestational age	19.20
	Hydropic abortus	Seen in early pregnancy and may be confused with a hydatidiform mole	11.8 11.9 23.11
	Hydrops	Placental and/or fetal hydrops (diffuse edema)	20.2 20.3
		May be secondary to fetomaternal hemorrhage	
	Immature intermediate villi	Residual immature villi in term placenta may be confused with villous edema	7.4

(continued)

Table 4.5. (continued)

Description	Diagnosis	Comment	Figure number
Villous capillaries			
Increased vessels	Diffuse – chorangiosis	Placental response to hypoxia	19.8
	Multifocal – chorangiomatosis	Focal, segmental, or multinodular diffuse	19.11
	Single lesion–chorangioma	Localized lesion – increased capillaries representing a benign neoplasm	22.5–22.7
	Diffuse – congestion	Not true increase in vessels but may be confused with chorangiosis	19.9
		Associated with decreased venous return and maternal diabetes	
Disruption of vessels	Villous stromal karyorrhexis/hemorrhagic endovasculopathy	Associated with disruption of vessels and extravasated red blood cells and thrombosis	21.11–21.13
Thrombosis	Thrombosis	May be associated with other thrombotic lesions	21.12 21.13
Nucleated red blood cells	Nucleated red blood cells	Fetal response to hypoxia or anemia	20.7

Table 4.6. Basal plate.

Description	Diagnosis	Comment	Figure number
Increased fibrinoid	Maternal floor infarction – massive perivillous fibrin deposition	Some fibrinoid is normal	19.12
		If excessive may represent a "maternal floor infarction"	19.15
		May be associated with proliferation of extravillous trophoblast	19.16 19.17
Necrosis	Decidual necrosis	Look for associated lesions such as hemorrhage or decidual vasculopathy	–
Inflammation	Acute deciduitis	May be associated with acute chorioamnionitis	16.6
	Chronic deciduitis	May be associated with chronic villitis	16.20
Hemorrhage	Retroplacental hematoma	Underlying tissue may be ischemic or infarcted	3.8
		May be associated with other changes of placental malperfusion	18.14 19.7
Abnormal vessels	Decidual vasculopathy	Usually associated with other changes of placental malperfusion	18.1–18.5
Adherent myometrium	Placenta accreta	Diagnosis based on lack of decidua between chorionic villi and myometrium	12.6

Table 4.7. Placental lesions in specific clinical situations.

Clinical situation	Placental conditions	Maternal conditions	Fetal conditions
Preterm delivery	Placental malperfusion Infarction Decreased weight Retroplacental hematoma Circumvallate membrane insertion Maternal floor infarction Acute chorioamnionitis	Poor nutrition Uterine anomalies	Fetal anomalies

(continued)

Table 4.7. (continued)

Clinical situation	Placental conditions	Maternal conditions	Fetal conditions
Intrauterine growth restriction	Maternal floor infarction Villitis of unknown etiology Fetal thrombotic vasculopathy Shape abnormalities Umbilical cord Excessively long cord Velamentous insertion	Drug use Tobacco Alcohol Poor nutrition Uterine anomalies Systemic disease Diabetes mellitus with vascular disease Preeclampsia Gestational hypertension Renovascular disease Autoimmune disease Thrombophilias	Genetic conditions Confined placental mosaicism Chromosomal disorders Genetic disorders
Intrauterine fetal demise	Maternal floor infarction Villitis of unknown etiology Fetal thrombotic vasculopathy Abruptio placentae Umbilical cord Entanglement True knots Torsion Constriction Rupture Excessive length or twisting Velamentous insertion and rupture	Systemic disease Diabetes mellitus with vascular disease Preeclampsia Gestational hypertension Renovascular disease Autoimmune disease Thrombophilias	Infection TORCH Ascending infection Fetomaternal hemorrhage

Table 6.1. Villous characteristics.

Villous type	When present	When maximum	% Volume at term	Size	Characteristic features
Mesenchymal villi	5 weeks-term	0–8 weeks	<1%	120–250 μm (<8 weeks) 60–100 μm (>8 weeks)	Primitive stroma, thick trophoblastic cover, few vessels
Immature intermediate villi	8 weeks-term	14–20 weeks	5–10%	100–200 μm May be up to 400 μm	Reticular stroma with fluid-filled stromal channels
Stem villi	12 weeks-term	Term	20–25%	150–300 μm	Fibrotic stroma, myofibroblastic perivascular sheath, large vessels
Mature intermediate villi	Third trimester	Third trimester	25%	80–150 μm	Cellular stroma with <50% capillaries
Terminal villi	Third trimester	Term	40–50%	60 μm	>50% capillaries

Table 8.1. Differences between the proliferative and invasive phenotype of extravillous trophoblast.

	Proliferative phenotype	Invasive phenotype
Invasion	−	+
Proliferation	+	−
Contact on or near fetal stromal basal lamina	+	−
Expression of proliferation markers	MIB-1, EGFR (c-erbB-1)	c-erbB-2
Integrin expression	Epithelial types ($\alpha6\beta4$, $\alpha3\beta1$)	Interstitial types ($\alpha5\beta1$, $\alpha1\beta1$, $\alpha v\beta3$, $\alpha v\beta5$)
Secretion of extracellular matrix	Polar	Apolar

Table 11.1. Maternal serum markers and risk of anomalies.

Abnormality	AFP	hCG	UE3	DIA
NTD	↑	−	−	−
Trisomy 21	↓	↑	↓	
Trisomy 18	↓	↓	↓	−

Note: *Arrows* indicate increase or decrease compared to normal results at that gestational age, results are reported as multiples of the median.

AFP alphafetoprotein, *hCG* human chorionic gonadotropin, *UE3* unconjugated estriol, *DIA* dimeric alpha inhibin, *NTD* neural tube defect

Table 12.1. Histologic changes of normal placental site involution.

Time post-partum	Gross size (cm)	"Slough"	Glands	Decidua	Veins	Arteries
<1 day	From 18 to 9	Hemorrhage	Few, inactive	Viable	Hyalinized	Fibrinoid necrosis, minimal inflammation
1–3 days	7–8	Early necrosis	Mild reactive change	Necrosis and inflammation	Thrombosed	Obliterative endarteritis, hyalinization
3–5 days	6	Necrosis with inflammation	Regenerating glands, moderate reactive change	Increased necrosis and inflammation	Organizing	Hyalinization, intimal proliferation
5–8 days	4.5	Well demarcated	Marked reactive change, increased numbers of glands, placental site giant cells	Necrosis and inflammation	Organizing thrombi	Hyalinization
4–20 weeks	2.0	None	Inactive glands, hemosiderophages	None	Recanalized, hyalinized	Remnants of hyalinized vessels

Table 16.1. Miscellaneous bacteria in ascending infection.

Bacteria	Morphology	Pathologic features	Potential clinical sequelae	Comment
Actinomyces	GP filamentous anaerobe	Foul smelling placenta Severe ACA may be necrotizing Identifiable organisms	Preterm labor	May show massive invasion by organism
Bacteroides fragilis	GN anaerobe	ACA	Meningitis	Other neonatal infections described
Brucella		No characteristic lesion	Abortion Fetal infection may be fatal or self-limited	Acquired from animal and animal products
Campylobacter	GN aerobe	ACA Villous necrosis Acute villitis	Recurrent abortions Fetal death	Common enteric pathogen
Corynebacteria	GP diphtheroids	ACA Gray-brown plaques on placental surface with invading organisms	Sepsis not described	Normal vaginal flora Occasional infection
Coxiella burnetii (Q fever)	GN obligate intracellular	Severe necrotizing villitis	Congenital infection Fetal death	Rare zoonosis Organisms may be identified in placenta
Ehrlichiosis	GN obligate intracellular	No lesions	Neonatal infection (of granulocytes)	Probable transplacental infection
Francisella tularensis		Granulomatous lesions	Granulomatous lesions	
Gardnerella	G variable	Occasionally mild ACA	Preterm delivery Fetal demise (rare)	Common vaginal organism
Group A *Streptococcus* (*S. pneumoniae*, *Enterococcus*)	GPC	ACA	Pneumonia	Common
Haemophilus influenzae	GNR	ACA	Preterm delivery Pneumonia Sepsis	Uncommon May mimic group B *Streptococcus* infection
Neisseria gonorrhoeae	GN diplococcus	ACA associated with cervical infection	Sepsis Ophthalmia neonatorum	Uncommon
Rickettsia	GN obligate intracellular	No lesions	Full recovery	Very rare
Salmonella	GNR	ACA	Meningitis Pneumonia Fetal demise	Mothers are symptomatic or carriers
Shigella	GNR	ACA	Sepsis Enterocolitis	Uncommon
Staphylococcus	GPC	ACA	Neonatal sepsis	Common pathogen
Streptobacillus	GNR	ACA	Rare	Causes "rat bite fever" or Haverhill fever

G Gram, *P* positive, *N* negative, *C* cocci, *R* rods, *ACA* acute chorioamnionitis, *AF* acute funisitis

Table 16.2. Miscellaneous organisms causing villitis.

Organism	Category	Pathologic features	Potential clinical sequelae	Comment
Borrelia (relapsing fever)	Spirochete	No lesions	Found in neonatal and placental blood	Follows bite of infected tick Geographically widespread
Borrelia burgdorferi Lyme disease (erythema migrans)	Spirochete	Rare plasma cells Increased nucleated red blood cells	Stillbirth Congenital anomalies	
Leptospira	Spirochete	No lesions	Abortion	Rare
Blastomyces	Fungus	Granulomas Chronic villitis	No neonatal infection reported	
Coccidioides immitis	Fungus	Fungal spherules Acute inflammatory response Fibrinoid deposition and necrosis Infarction and necrosis	Fetal death reported Disseminated infection	
Cryptococcus	Fungus	Colonies of organisms in intervillous space Scant inflammation No villous invasion	Cryptococcosis or meningitis in mother Infants not affected	Associated with lupus and immunodeficiency
Coxsackie B	Virus	Villous necrosis Severe intervillositis	Fetal hydrops Myocarditis Meningitis	Rare fetal infection May not show placental lesions
ECHO	Virus	Chronic villitis Chronic intervillositis Mural thrombosis	Congenital infection	Rare
Epstein–Barr virus	Virus	Deciduitis Lymphoplasmacytic villitis Trophoblastic necrosis Endothelial damage	Early abortion Congenital anomalies (rare)	Uncommon
Hepatitis	Virus	Yellow green discoloration of placenta Bilirubin in Hofbauer cells and chorionic macrophages Relative villous immaturity Focal syncytial necrosis	Abortion Fetal ascites Meconium peritonitis	Usually hepatitis B
Human immunodeficiency virus	Virus	No lesions	Prematurity Endometritis	Transmission rate to fetus 24%
Influenza	Virus	No lesions		Transplacental infection occurs
Mumps	Virus	Severe villous necrosis Small cytoplasmic inclusion bodies in decidua	Possible congenital anomalies	Virus isolated from placenta

(continued)

Table 16.2. (continued)

Organism	Category	Pathologic features	Potential clinical sequelae	Comment
Poliomyelitis	Virus	No lesions		Virus isolated from the placenta
Rubella	Virus	Endothelial damage in villi Obliteration of stem vessels Focal trophoblastic necrosis Villous inflammation and sclerosis Swollen Hofbauer cells (in early infection)	Congenital anomalies in early infection	
Rubeola	Virus	Not described	Not teratogenic	Rare
Smallpox	Virus	Villous, membrane and trophoblastic necrosis Intervillous fibrinoid deposits Calcification	Fetal mortality Fetal demise Early abortion	May occur with primary vaccination
Varicella	Virus	Chronic villitis Occasional multinucleated giant cells Rare granulomas Remote infection: occluded stem vessels	Cutaneous scars Limb hypoplasia Chorioretinitis Cataracts Hydrops Visceral calcifications	
Babesia microti	Protozoa	No lesions	Infection of neonatal red blood cells	Very rare
Leishmania major (Kala-Azar)	Protozoa	Thrombosis of villous vessels Amastigotes within and outside macrophages Trophoblastic degeneration No inflammation		Occasional congenital infection
Trichomonas vaginalis	Protozoa	No specific lesions	Preterm delivery Low birth weight Neonatal infection Pneumonia	Rare
Trypanosoma cruzi (Chagas disease)	Protozoa	Enlarged, pale placenta Chronic destructive villitis Chronic intervillositis Amnionic epithelium, Hofbauer cells, or syncytium may contain amastigotes	Stillbirth Maternal myocarditis, esophagitis, and encephalitis	Transmitted by triatomid the "kissing" bug
Enterobius vermicularis	Nematode	Embryo with worm in abdomen and no inflammation	One case reported	
Schistosomes	Trematode	Eggs with granulomas Occasional worms		

Table 17.1. Reported features of maternal disorders.

Disorder	Clinical prenatal features	Pathology
Connective tissue disorders		
Dermatomyositis	–	Subamnionic necrosis, infarcts, ↑fibrinoid
Ehlers–Danlos	PM, PROM	?Fragile membranes
Myositis ossificans	PROM	–
Periarteritis nodosa	–	NL
Rheumatoid arthritis	IUGR	Small infarcts, calcification
Scleroderma	IUFD, Ab, PM, abruptio, maternal death	Infarcts, DV, ↑fibrinoid
Takayasu's arteritis	–	–
Renal and liver disease		
Chronic renal disease	–	Small, abnormal decidual vessels
Acute fatty liver of pregnancy	PEC, coagulation abnormalities	Gross bilirubin staining
Cholestasis of pregnancy	IUFD, PM	Meconium macrophages
Hyperlipidemia	IUGR	Rare foam cells in intervillous space
Miscellaneous inherited disorders		
Cystic fibrosis	–	–
Cystinosis	–	Vacuolization of decidual cells
Cystinuria	IUGR	–
Gaucher's disease	Thrombocytopenia	NL
Gordon's syndrome	–	NL
Impetigo herpetiformis	IUFD	"Placental insufficiency"
Niemann–Pick disease	–	NL
Phenylketonuria	–	NL
Pruritus gravidarum	Cholestasis, PM, IUFD	Meconium macrophages
Sarcoidosis	–	Granulomas
Smith–Lemli–Opitz	–	NL
Wilson's disease	–	NL
Hematologic disorders		
Heart disease	fetal/placental weight ratio, IUGR	Infarcts, intervillous thrombi
β-Thalassemia	Ab, IUFD	Occasional infarcts
Factor VII deficiency	–	–
Folate deficiency	Ab, abruption	Retroplacental hematoma
Hemorrhagic hereditary telangiectasia	–	–
High altitude	–	Placentomegaly, increased syncytial knots, chorangiosis
ITP	Postpartum hemorrhage	Intervillous thrombus, infarcts, decidual vasculopathy
Leukoagglutinins	–	–
Maternal anemia	–	Placentomegaly or small placenta with increased syncytial knots
SC disease (sickle thalassemia)	Ab, IUFD	Infarcts
Sickle cell disease	PEC, sepsis, perinatal mortality, IUGR, abruptio	Small placenta, sickle cells in intervillous space, increased syncytial knots, infarcts, increased fibrin, villous edema, retroplacental hematoma
Sickle cell trait	Similar to disease but less severe	Similar to sickle cell disease but less severe
TTP	IUFD, high mortality	Hyaline thrombi in decidual vessels
Von Willebrand's disease	–	–

(continued)

Table 17.1. (continued)

Disorder	Clinical prenatal features	Pathology
Endocrine disorders		
Cushing's disease	Ab, IUFD, PM	NL
Diabetes insipidus	Severe oligohydramnios	–
Diabetes mellitus	Macrosomia, PM, Ab, IUGR, congenital anomalies, fetal vascular thrombopathy	Placentomegaly, dysmature villi, hypervascular villi, NRBCs, thrombosis
Thyroid disease (general)	PEC, abruptio, IUGR, IUFD	Infarcts
Thyroid-hyperthyroidism	Polyhydramnios, fetal distress	Meconium macrophages
Thyroid-hypothyroidism	Ab, congenital anomalies, postpartum hemorrhage	–
Zollinger–Ellison	–	NL
Maternal drug use		
Alcohol	IUGR, fetal alcohol syndrome, abruptio	Acute chorioamnionitis, meconium macrophages, chorangioma, umbilical cord remnants
Cocaine	Abruptio, IUGR, maternal hypertension, PM, PEC	Retroplacental hematoma
Heroin	IUGR	Acute chorioamnionitis, meconium macrophages
LSD	Ab, chromosome breakage	NL
Tobacco	IUGR, Ab, PROM, IUFD, abruptio	Single umbilical artery, abnormal cord insertions, calcifications
Marijuana	–	–

"–" Not been reported, *Ab* abortion, *IUFD* intrauterine fetal demise, *IUGR* intrauterine growth restriction, *NL* normal, *PEC* preeclampsia, *PM* prematurity, *PROM* premature rupture of membranes

Table 20.1. Causes of non-immune hydrops fetalis.

Cardiovascular: congenital heart disease
    Coarctation of the aorta
    Hypoplastic left heart
    Cardiac arrhythmias particularly supraventricular tachycardia
    Premature closure of the foramen ovale
    Endocardial fibroelastosis
    Ebstein's anomaly of the tricuspid valve
Chromosomal (see Chap. 11)
    Turner's syndrome, 45 XO
    Trisomy 13, 15, 16, 18, and 21
    Duplications of the long arms of chromosomes 15 or 17
    Triploidy
Anemia
    Twin to twin transfusion syndrome (see Chap. 10)
    Thalassemia
    Fetomaternal hemorrhage
    Hemolytic anemia
    Fetal hemorrhage
        Disrupted velamentous or other fetal vessels (see Chap. 15)
        Injury to the fetus
Thoracic: space-occupying lesions
    Cystic adenomatoid malformation and pulmonary sequestration
    Diaphragmatic hernia
    Cystic hygroma
    Chylothorax
    Lymphangiectasias

(continued)

Table 20.1. (continued)

Infection (see Chap. 16)
   Parvovirus
   Cytomegalovirus
   Toxoplasmosis
   Herpes simplex virus
   Syphilis
   Rubella
Congenital tumors (see Chap. 22)
   Congenital neuroblastoma
   Hepatoblastoma
   Sacrococcygeal teratoma
   Leukemia
   Mesoblastic nephroma
   Hemangioma
   Chorangioma
   Choriocarcinoma
Miscellaneous
   Malformations of the genitourinary tract
   Fetal storage disorders
   Thyrotoxicosis
   Small bowel volvulus
   Intussusception
   Trauma
   Beckwith-Wiedemann syndrome
   Chorangiomatosis
   Idiopathic

Table 20.2. Summary of placental findings in metabolic storage diseases.

Disorder	Deficiency	Hydrops	Intracellular vacuolization Histochemistry									
			ST	ET	HC	FB	EN	AE	PAS	Alcian blue	Colloidal Fe	ORO
Mucopolysaccharidoses									+/−		+	
MPS I (Hurler disease)	α-1-Iduronidase	+	+		+	+						
MPS III (San Filippo disease)	Various		+									
MPS IV (Morquio disease)	Various	+			a							
MPS VII (Sly disease)	β-Glucuronidase	+			+							
Sphingolipidoses												
GM1 gangliosidosis	β-Galactosidase		+	+	+	+		+	+	+	+	+
GM2 gangliosidosis												
Type I (Tay–Sachs disease)	β-Hexosaminidase, α subunit		+		+			+				
Type II (Sandhoff disease)	β-Hexosaminidase, β subunit		+			+						
Niemann–Pick disease, type A	Sphingomyelinase	+	+	+	+	+			+/−			+
Niemann–Pick disease, type B	Sphingomyelinase											

(continued)

Table 20.2. (continued)

Disorder	Deficiency	Hydrops	ST	ET	HC	FB	EN	AE	PAS	Alcian blue	Colloidal Fe	ORO
										Intracellular vacuolization Histochemistry		
Gaucher's disease	β-Glucosidase	+			M				+			
Fabry disease	α-Galactosidase								+			+
Other lipidoses												
Wolman disease	Acid lipase	+	+									+
Cholesterol ester storage disease	Acid lipase	+	+			+						
Niemann–Pick disease, type C	Unknown											
Neuronal ceroid lipofuscinosis	Unknown		+				+	+				
Mucolipidoses												
Type I, sialidosis	Sialidase		+		+	+						
Type II, I-cell disease	*N*-acetylglucosamine-1-phosphotransferase	+	+	+	+			M	+/−	+/−	+/−	+/−
Type IV	Unknown					+						
Oligosaccharidoses												
Galactosialidosis	β-Galactosialidase	+	+			+						
Sialic acid storage disease (Salla disease)	Sialic acid transporter	+	+	+	+		+	+		+	+	
Glycogen storage disease												
Type II, Pompe disease	α-1,4-Glucosidase	+				+	+		+/−			
Type IV	Amylopectinase								+			

ST syncytiotrophoblast, *ET* extravillous trophoblast or X-cell, *FB* villous stromal fibroblast, *HC* Hofbauer cell, *EN* endothelium, *AE* amnionic epithelium, *PAS* periodic acid-Schiff, *ORO* oil red O, *M* minimal vacuolization[a] Granularity and *not* vacuolization can be seen in Hofbauer cells

Table 23.1. WHO classification of gestational trophoblastic disease.

Hydatidiform mole
   Complete mole
   Partial mole
   Invasive mole
   Metastatic mole
Trophoblastic neoplasms
   Choriocarcinoma
   Placental site trophoblastic tumor
   Epithelioid trophoblastic tumor
Nonneoplastic, nonmolar trophoblastic lesions
   Placental site nodule and plaque
   Exaggerated placental site

From Tavassoli FA, Devilee P. World Health Organization classification of tumours: Pathology and Genetics. Tumours of the Breast and Female Genital Organs. Lyon, France: IARC Press, 2003

Table 23.2. Differential diagnosis of complete and partial hydatidiform moles.

Characteristic	Hydropic abortus	Complete mole	Early complete mole	Partial mole
Ploidy[a]	Diploid	Diploid	Diploid	Triploid
Paternal/maternal chromosome ratio[a]	1:1	2:0	2:0	2:1
Embryo/fetus	May be present	Rarely present	Rarely present	May be present
Clinical presentation	Missed abortion	Size > dates	± Missed abortion	Size < dates
Serum β-hCG	Normal or low	Markedly elevated	Moderately to markedly elevated	Moderately elevated
Histology				
Villous enlargement	Moderate	Marked	Mild to moderate	Moderate with admixture of normal villi
Villous population	Range of villi from small to hydropic	Relatively uniform population of large hydropic villi	Relatively uniform population of mildly enlarged villi	Two populations of villi, one normal and one moderately hydropic
Villous shape	Round	Round	Clubbed or bulbous	Scalloped with trophoblastic pseudoinclusions
Cisterns	Usually absent	Common	Rare	Rare
Trophoblastic proliferation	None	Marked circumferential	Moderate circumferential	Mild to moderate and focal
Trophoblastic atypia	None	Common	Common	Minimal
Fetal blood vessels/nucleated red blood cells	Usually absent	Rare	May be present	Common
Persistent GTD	No	Up to 20% May develop choriocarcinoma	Up to 20% May develop choriocarcinoma	Less than 5%, usually not requiring chemotherapy

[a]Most common presentation, but variations may occur. See text for more information
GTD- gestational trophoblastic disease

Table 23.3. Differential diagnosis – ancillary testing.

	Ploidy[a]	p57
Hydropic abortus	Diploid	+
Partial mole	Triploid	+
Complete mole	Diploid	−

[a]Ploidy is indicated for the majority of cases as occasionally maternal triploidy or triploid complete moles may occur

Table 24.1. Staging of gestational trophoblastic disease.

Stage	Definition
I	Disease confined to the uterus
II	Disease outside the uterus but limited to the genital structures (i.e., pelvis, vagina)
III	Metastatic disease to the lungs
IV	Metastatic disease to sites other than the lungs

Modified from Kohorn EI. The new FIGO 2000 staging and risk factor scoring system for gestational trophoblastic disease: description and critical assessment. Int J Gynecol Cancer 2001;11:73–77

Table 24.2. FIGO 2000 scoring system for gestational trophoblastic disease.

FIGO score	0	1	2	3
Age at diagnosis	≤39 years	>39 years		
Type of antecedent pregnancy	Hydatidiform mole	Abortion	Term pregnancy	
Interval from antecedent pregnancy	<4 months	4–6 months	7 to 12 months	>12 months
Serum β-hCG mIU/mL	<1,000	1,000–10,000	10,000–100,000	>100,000
Tumor size	≤4 cm	>4 cm		
Sites of metastases	None	Spleen or kidney	Gastrointestinal tract	Brain or liver
Number of metastases	0	1–3	4–8	>8
Response to chemotherapy	Full response	Full response	Failure with single drug chemotherapy	Failure with multiagent chemotherapy

Risk is assessed by adding factors according to the above system. Scores of seven or greater constitute a high risk group that is treated more aggressively

Modified from Kohorn EI. The new FIGO 2000 staging and risk factor scoring system for gestational trophoblastic disease: description and critical assessment. Int J Gynecol Cancer 2001;11:73–77

Table 25.1. Clinical features of trophoblastic lesions.

	PSN	EPS	PSTT/ETT	CCA
H/O previous mole	–	–	5–8%	50%
Serum β-hCG	Normal	Appropriate for pregnancy	Moderately elevated in 80%	Markedly elevated
Symptoms	50% have abnormal uterine bleeding	Related to pregnancy	Bleeding, uterine enlargement, or mass	Bleeding, uterine enlargement
Location	Often in lower uterine segment or cervix	Endometrium	Endomyometrium	Endomyometrium
Treatment	None	None	Hysterectomy; chemotherapy if malignant	Chemotherapy
Metastasis	None	None	Occurs in 10–15% of cases	Potential for metastasis
Prognosis	No sequelae	No sequelae	Guarded if malignant	>90% responsive to chemotherapy

PSN placental site nodule, EPS exaggerated placental site, PSTT placental site trophoblastic tumor, ETT epithelioid trophoblastic tumors, CA choriocarcinoma

Table 25.2. Histopathologic features of trophoblastic lesions.

	PSN	EPS	PSTT	ETT	CCA
Forms a mass	–	–	+	+	+/–
Chorionic villi present	–	+	Very rare	Very rare	–[a]
Fibrinoid	+	+	+	–	–
Hemorrhage	–	+/–	+	+	++
Necrosis	–	+/–	+	++	++
Vascular invasion	–	–	+	+	+
Degenerative changes	+	–	–	–	+
Extravillous trophoblast	+	+	+	+	–
Syncytiotrophoblast	–	+	–[b]	–	++
Nuclear pleomorphism	–	–	++	–	++
Mitotic activity	Minimal or absent	Minimal or absent	+	+	+

PSN placental site nodules, EPS exaggerated placental site, PSTT placental site trophoblastic tumor, ETT epithelioid trophoblastic tumor, CCA choriocarcinoma

[a]Villi are present only in placental or "in situ" choriocarcinoma (see Chapter 24)

[b]Multinucleated cells similar to syncytiotrophoblast may be present

Table 25.3. Immunohistochemistry of trophoblastic lesions.

	PSN	EPS	PSTT	ETT	CCA
Cytokeratin	+	+	+	+	+
EMA	+	+	+	+	+
hCG	Weak focal	+	Weak focal	Weak focal	+++
hPL	Focal	Diffuse	Diffuse	Focal	Focal
PLAP	Diffuse	Focal	Focal	Diffuse	
Mel-CAM	Focal	Diffuse	Diffuse	Focal	
Major basic protein	+/−	+	+	+	−
P63	+	−	−	+	+/−
α-inhibin	+	+	+	+	−
Ki-67	<5%		5–15%	5–15%	

PSN placental site nodules, *EPS* exaggerated placental site, *PSTT* placental site trophoblastic tumor, *ETT* epithelioid trophoblastic tumor, *CCA* choriocarcinoma

Index

A

Abdominal circumference, fetal, 14
Abdominal wall defect, limb-body wall complex
    associated in, 243
Abnormal primary implantation, 267
ABO incompatibility, 380, 388
Abortion
    hypothyroidism, 326
    induced
        clinical features and implications, 166–167
        criminal, 166
        pathologic features, 167–169
        therapeutic, 166
    infection-associated
        Campylobacter infection, 316
        Ureaplasma infection, 296
    recurrent/habitual, 7, 166, 174
    septic, 167
    spontaneous
        clinical features and implications,
            170–171
        incomplete, 166
        inevitable, 166
        missed, 166
        pathogenesis, 170
        pathologic features, 170–173
        threatened, 166
    and subchorionic hematoma, 229
    and thalassemia, 325
    threatened, definition of, 166
Abortus, hydropic, 439
Abruptio placenta, 344
    alcohol abuse, 329
        cocaine use, 329–330
        hypothyroidism, 326
        pheochromocytoma, 328

scleroderma, 322
    smoking, 330
concealed, 359
definition of, 344
hemosiderin associated with, 482
multiple pregnancy, 127
pathogenesis, 359
pathologic features, 360–362
and retroplacental hematoma, 359–362
Abscesses, intervillous, 293
Acardiac twins
    clinical features and implications, 146
    examination and report, 148
    incidence, 143, 145
    pathogenesis, 145–146
    pathologic features, 146
    vascular anastomoses, 145
Accessory lobe, 204
Accreta, placenta, 217
Actinomyces infection, 316
Acute chorioamnionitis, 283–299, 478
    chlamydia, 296
    clinical, 284
    definition, 285–286
    Escherichia coli, 294–295
    examination and report, 291
    fusobacterium, 295
    mycoplasma, 296
    preterm delivery, 283
    subacute chorioamnionitis, 290–291
Acute endometritis, 191
Acute fatty liver of pregnancy, 331
Acute funisitis, 287, 478
Acute twin-to-twin transfusion syndrome,
    158–159, 477
ADAM complex, 240

R.N. Baergen, *Manual of Pathology of the Human Placenta*,
DOI 10.1007/978-1-4419-7494-5, © Springer Science+Business Media, LLC 2011

GPSR Compliance
The European Union's (EU) General Product Safety Regulation (GPSR) is a set
of rules that requires consumer products to be safe and our obligations to
ensure this.

If you have any concerns about our products, you can contact us on

ProductSafety@springernature.com

In case Publisher is established outside the EU, the EU authorized
representative is:

Springer Nature Customer Service Center GmbH
Europaplatz 3
69115 Heidelberg, Germany

www.ingramcontent.com/pod-product-compliance
Lightning Source LLC
Chambersburg PA
CBHW081101300126
38987CB00041B/196